THE CAMBRIDGE HISTORICAL DICTIONARY OF DISEASE

THE CAMBRIDGE
HISTORICAL DICTIONARY OF
DISEASE

Edited by

KENNETH F. KIPLE

Bowling Green State University

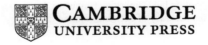

CAMBRIDGE UNIVERSITY PRESS
Cambridge, New York, Melbourne, Madrid, Cape Town, Singapore,
São Paulo, Delhi, Dubai, Tokyo, Mexico City

Cambridge University Press
The Edinburgh Building, Cambridge CB2 8RU, UK

Published in the United States of America by Cambridge University Press, New York

www.cambridge.org
Information on this title: www.cambridge.org/9780521808347

First published 2003

A catalogue record for this publication is available from the British Library

Library of Congress Cataloguing in Publication Data
The Cambridge historical dictionary of disease / edited by Kenneth F. Kiple.

p.   cm.

Includes bibliographical references and index.
ISBN 0-521-80834-0 – ISBN 0-521-53026-1 (pbk.)
1. Disease – History – Dictionaries.   I. Kiple, Kenneth F., 1939–
RC41   .C365   2003
616'.009 – dc21   2002031368

ISBN 978-0-521-80834-7 Hardback
ISBN 978-0-521-53026-2 Paperback

In memory of K. David Patterson

Contents

Contents

Contents

Contents

Contents

Preface

The Cambridge World History of Human Disease (CWHHD) was first published by Cambridge University Press in 1993 and reprinted in 2001. Part VIII, the last section of the work, comprises a history and description of the world's major diseases of yesterday and today in chapters that are organized alphabetically from "Acquired Immune Deficiency Syndrome (AIDS)" to "Yellow Fever." The pages that follow in this *Dictionary* represent an effort to make these essays, along with three chapters from other parts of the CWHHD on "Heart-Related Diseases," "Cancer," and "Genetic Disease," available to a wider audience in paperback form. To achieve this in one manageable volume, the chapters were condensed, and bibliographies and graphics are omitted. As a consequence, readers requiring more than a dictionary treatment of an illness will still need the CWHHD.

A revised edition of that work is still a few years in the future; thus, most of the chapters in the *Dictionary* have not been updated. Indeed, because they are less than a decade old (admittedly still a long time in science), most would not have benefited substantially from what in effect would have been a partial revision of just one part of the larger work, and a revision that would have to be repeated for the upcoming full-scale revision. A few diseases, however, such as AIDS, Alzheimer's disease, Ebola virus disease, and tuberculosis, have been subjects of intense scrutiny, generating much media coverage, even best-selling books. In these instances, postscripts seemed essential to sketch out recent major events in their respective histories.

There were legions of authors and board members to thank whose collective effort brought forth the CWHHD. I thank them all again. Obviously much of that effort undergirds this volume. I also thank Steve Beck, who has worked on our various projects for many years. He did a wonderful job of paring the essays to fit this volume. In addition, I am grateful to Cambridge University Press Publishing Director Frank Smith for his support of this first paperback to emerge from the CWHHD.

Finally, the late K. David Patterson was involved in that project as both enthusiastic board member and prolific author, and this book (containing many of his essays) is dedicated to him.

Kenneth F. Kiple

1. Acquired Immune Deficiency Syndrome (AIDS)

Acquired immune deficiency syndrome (AIDS), first identified in 1981, is an infectious disease characterized by failure of the body's immunologic system. Affected individuals become increasingly vulnerable to many normally harmless microorganisms, eventually leading to severe morbidity and high mortality. The infection, spread sexually and through blood, has a high fatality rate, approaching 100 percent. Caused by a human retrovirus known as HIV-1, AIDS can now be found throughout the world – in both industrialized countries and developing nations. Public-health officials throughout the world have focused attention on this pandemic and its potentially catastrophic impact on health, resources, and social structure. Treatments for the disease have been developed, but no cure or vaccine currently exists.

Characteristics

Beginning in the late 1970s, physicians in New York and California reported increasing incidence of a rare cancer, **Kaposi's sarcoma**, and a variety of infections including **pneumocystis pneumonia** among previously healthy young homosexual men. Because of the unusual character of these diseases, which are typically associated with failure of the immune system, epidemiologists began seeking clues that might link these cases. AIDS was first formally described in 1981, although it now appears that the virus causing the disease was silently spreading in a number of populations during the previous decade. Early epidemiological studies suggested that homosexual men, blood recipients (especially hemophiliacs), and intravenous drug users were at greatest risk. Research focused on searching for an infectious agent transmitted sexually or through blood. In 1983, in French and American laboratories, an unknown human retrovirus was identified and named HIV-1 for "human immunodeficiency virus." Although the biological and geographic origins of the organism remain obscure, the AIDS epidemic appears to mark the first time it has spread widely in human populations. No evidence exists for casual transmission of HIV.

Following identification of HIV-1, tests to detect antibodies against it were devised in 1984. Although these tests do not detect the virus itself, they are generally effective in identifying infection because high levels of antibody are produced in most infected individuals. The enzyme-linked immunosorbent assay (ELISA), followed by Western blot testing, has enabled the screening of donated blood to protect the blood supply from HIV, as well as testing for epidemiological and diagnostic purposes.

As **HIV infection** precedes the development of AIDS, often by several years, the precise parameters of the epidemic have been difficult to define. Although "cofactors" that may determine the onset of symptoms remain unknown, evidence suggests that HIV-infected individuals will eventually develop AIDS.

Researchers have identified three epidemiological patterns of HIV transmission, which roughly follow geographic boundaries. Pattern I includes North America, Western Europe, Australia, New Zealand, and many urban centers in Latin America. In these industrial, highly developed areas, transmission has been predominantly among homosexual and bisexual men. Since the introduction of widespread blood screening, transmission via blood in these areas now occurs principally among intravenous drug users who share injection equipment. Although little evidence exists of widespread infection among heterosexuals in these countries, heterosexual transmission from those infected intravenously has increased, leading to a rise in pediatric cases resulting from perinatal transmission.

Within the United States, distribution of AIDS has been marked by disproportionate representation of minorities and the poor. As the principal mode of transmission has shifted to intravenous drug use, AIDS has increasingly become an affliction of the urban underclass. Surveys reveal that 50 percent or more of intravenous drug users in New York City are infected with HIV. Women are typically infected by intravenous drug use or by sexual contact with a drug user.

In pattern II countries, comprised of sub-Saharan Africa and, increasingly, Latin America, transmission of HIV occurs predominantly through heterosexual contact. In some urban areas in these countries, up to 25 percent of all sexually active adults are reported to be infected, and a majority of female prostitutes are seropositive. Transfusion remains a mode of transmission because universal blood screening is not routine. Unsterile injections and medical procedures may also contribute to the spread of infection. In these areas, perinatal transmission is an important aspect of the epidemic.

Pattern III countries, including North Africa, the Middle East, Eastern Europe, Asia, and the Pacific, initially experienced less morbidity and mortality from the pandemic. Apparently, HIV-1 was not present in these areas until the mid-1980s. The nature of world travel, however, has diminished the significance of geographic isolation as a means of protecting a population from contact with a pathogen.

In 1985, a related virus, HIV-2, was discovered in West Africa. Although early reports suggested that HIV-2 is less pathogenic, the natural history of this agent remains unclear, as does its prevalence.

HIV cripples the body's immunologic system, making an infected individual vulnerable to other disease-causing agents in the environment. The most common of these opportunistic infections in AIDS patients has been pneumocystis pneumonia, previously seen principally in patients receiving immunosuppressive drugs. In addition to pneumocystis, AIDS patients are prone to other infectious agents such as **cytomegalovirus**, *Candida albicans* (a yeastlike fungus), and *Toxoplasma gondii* (a protozoan parasite). Moreover, a resurgence of **tuberculosis** has been reported in nations with high AIDS incidence.

Immunologic damage occurs by depletion of a specific type of white blood cell called a helper T4 lymphocyte. Destruction of these cells accounts for the vulnerability to normally harmless infectious agents. In some cases, infection of the central nervous system with HIV may cause damage to the brain and spinal column, resulting in severe cognitive and motor dysfunction. In its late manifestations, AIDS causes severe wasting. Death may occur from infection, functional failure of the central nervous system, or starvation.

HIV infection has a wide spectrum of clinical manifestations. After infection, an individual may remain free of symptoms for years, even a decade or longer. Some individuals experience fever, rash, and malaise at the time of infection when antibodies are first produced. Patients commonly present with general **lymphadenopathy**, weight loss, diarrhea, or an opportunistic infection. Diagnosis is confirmed by finding antibodies for HIV or by a decline in T4 cells. Most experts now agree that HIV infection itself be considered a disease, regardless of symptoms.

Because the virus becomes encoded within the genetic material of the host cell and is highly mutable, the problem of finding safe and effective therapies has been extremely difficult. Studies have attempted to determine the anti-HIV properties of many drugs, but the ethical and economic obstacles to clinical trials with experimental drugs are formidable. Given the immediacy of the epidemic, it is difficult to structure appropriate randomized clinical trials, which often take considerable time, to assess the safety and efficacy of a drug. Since the beginning of the epidemic, clinical research has refined the treatment of opportunistic infections.

History

In its first decade, AIDS created considerable suffering and generated an ongoing worldwide health crisis. During this brief period, the epidemic was identified and characterized epidemiologically, basic modes of transmission specified, a causal organism isolated, and effective tests for infection developed. In spite of this remarkable progress, which required the application of sophisticated epidemiological, clinical, and scientific research, the barriers to controlling AIDS are imposing and relate to the most complex biomedical and political questions. AIDS has already sorely tested the capabilities of research, clinical, and public-health institutions throughout the world.

Because HIV is related to other recently isolated primate retroviruses, such as simian T lymphotropic virus (STLV)-III in African green monkeys, many have speculated that HIV originated in Africa. Antibodies to HIV were discovered in stored blood dating back to 1959 in Zaire. According to experts, it is likely that HIV has existed for many years in isolated groups in central Africa. Because outside contacts were minimal, the virus rarely spread, and epidemics could not be sustained. Once a sizable reservoir of infection was established, however, HIV became pandemic. As with other sexually transmitted diseases, such as **syphilis**, no country wished the stigma of association with the virus's "origin."

The epidemic began at a moment of relative complacency, especially in the developed world, concerning epidemic infectious disease. Not since the **influenza** of 1918–20 had an epidemic appeared with such devastating potential. The developed world had experienced a health transition from infectious to chronic disease and had focused its resources and attention on systemic, noninfectious ailments. Thus, AIDS appeared at a historical moment comprising little social or political experience in confronting such a public-health crisis. The epidemic fractured a widely held belief in medical security.

Not surprisingly, early sociopolitical responses were characterized by denial. Initial theories, when few cases had been reported, centered on aspects of "fast-track" gay sexual culture that might explain the outbreak of immune-compromised men. Additional cases among blood recipients, however, soon led the U.S. Centers for Disease Control and Prevention to the conclusion that an infectious agent was the likely link. Nevertheless, in the earliest years of the epidemic, few wished to confront openly the possibility of spread beyond the specified "high-risk" groups. During this period, when government interest and funding lagged, grassroots organizations, especially in the homosexual community, were created to meet the growing need for education, counseling, patient services, and – in some instances – clinical research. Such groups worked to overcome the denial, prejudice, and bureaucratic inertia that limited governmental response.

As the nature and extent of the epidemic became clearer, however, hysteria sometimes replaced denial. Because the disease was powerfully associated with behaviors identified as immoral or illegal (or both), the stigma of those infected was heightened. Victims were often divided into categories: those who acquired their infections through transfusions or perinatally, the "innocent victims"; and those who engaged in high-risk, morally condemnable behaviors, the "guilty perpetrators" of disease. Since the early recognition of behavioral risks for infection, there has been a tendency to blame those who became infected through drug use or homosexuality, behaviors viewed as "voluntary." Some religious groups in the United States and elsewhere saw the epidemic as an occasion to reiterate particular moral views about sexual behavior, drug use, sin, and disease. AIDS was viewed as "proof" of a certain moral order.

3

AIDS victims have been subjected to a range of discriminatory behavior, including loss of employment, housing, and insurance. Since the onset of the epidemic, violence against gays in the United States has increased. Despite the well-documented modes of HIV transmission, fears of casual transmission persist. In some communities, parents protested when HIV-infected schoolchildren were permitted to attend school. In one instance, a family with an HIV-infected child was driven from a town by the burning of their home.

By 1983, as potential ramifications of the epidemic became evident, national and international scientific and public-health institutions began to mobilize. In the United States, congressional appropriations for research and education began to rise significantly. The National Academy of Sciences issued a consensus report on the epidemic in 1986. A presidential commission held public hearings and eventually issued a report calling for protection of AIDS sufferers against discrimination and a more extensive federal commitment to drug treatment. The World Health Organization (WHO) established a Global Program on AIDS in 1986 to coordinate international efforts in epidemiological surveillance, education, prevention, and research.

Despite growing recognition of the epidemic's significance, considerable debate continued over the most effective public-health responses. Although some nations – such as Cuba – experimented with programs mandating isolation of HIV-infected individuals, the World Health Organization lobbied against coercive measures. Given the lifelong nature of HIV infection, effective isolation would require lifetime incarceration. With the available variety of less restrictive measures, most nations rejected quarantine as both unduly coercive and unlikely to achieve control. Traditional public-health approaches to communicable disease, including contact tracing and mandatory treatment, have less potential for control because no means exist to render an infected individual noninfectious.

Because biomedical technologies to prevent transmission appear to be some years away, the principal public-health approaches to controlling the pandemic rest on education and behavior modification. Heightened awareness of the dangers of unprotected anal intercourse among gay men, for example, has led to a significant decline in new infections among this population. Nevertheless, as many public-health officials have noted, encouraging the modification of risk behaviors, especially those relating to sexuality and drug abuse, presents no simple task, even in the face of a dread disease.

In the developing world, AIDS threatens to reverse recent advances in infant and child survival. The epidemic is likely to have a substantial impact on demographic patterns. Because the disease principally affects young and middle-aged adults (ages 20–49), it has already had tragic social and cultural repercussions. Transmitted both horizontally (via sexual contact) and vertically (from mother to infant), it has the potential to depress the growth rate of human populations, especially in areas of the developing world. In this respect, the disease could destabilize the work force and depress local economies.

AIDS has clearly demonstrated the complex relationship of biological and behavioral forces in determining patterns of health and disease. Altering the course of the epidemic by human design has already proved to be no easy matter. The lifelong infectiousness of carriers; the private, biopsychosocial nature of sexual behavior and drug abuse; and the stigma already attached to those at greatest risk – all have made effective public policy intervention even more difficult. Finally, the very nature of the virus itself – its complex and mutagenic nature – makes a short-term technological breakthrough unlikely.

The remarkable progress in understanding AIDS is testimony to the sophistication of contemporary bioscience; the epidemic, however, is also a sobering reminder of the limits of that science. Any historical assessment of the AIDS epidemic must be considered provisional.

Nevertheless, it is already clear that AIDS has forced us to confront a new set of biological imperatives.

Allan M. Brandt

Postscript

By way of a caveat, recent estimates of the number of HIV/AIDS infections, the competing theories of origin, conflicting interpretations of new evidence, and announcements of therapeutic and preventive progress are sometimes contradictory and thus constitute especially treacherous terrain.

Beginning with the estimates, in June of 1990 the WHO estimated that there were some 8 million HIV cases worldwide; the following year that estimate was raised to between 10 million and 12 million. Toward the end of the decade the WHO warned that the number of cases would reach between 20 million and 30 million cases by the year 2000. In retrospect, it seems that this estimate was much too conservative; by 1997 the number of cases already exceeded 30 million. By 2001, HIV had infected some 56 million individuals worldwide and killed more than 20 million of them. Left behind were an estimated 36 million living with HIV/AIDS and millions more expected to become infected in the early years of the twenty-first century.

Of the 30 million cases in 1997, almost 21 million were in sub-Saharan Africa alone (where in some places, such as Botswana, upwards of 36 percent of the adult population has become infected with HIV), while South and Southeast Asia and the Pacific accounted for another 6 million cases. In all, the developing world contained 95 percent of the cases, and in 1998 it was estimated that 70 percent of all new infections and 80 percent of all AIDS deaths occurred in sub-Saharan Africa. By 2001, average life expectancy south of the Sahara had declined by 10 years and infant death rates had doubled. Illustrative of the impact of AIDS mortality is the example of Zambia, where a dire shortage of schoolteachers has developed because they are dying of AIDS faster than replacements can be trained.

In the United States – although the millions of cases of HIV infection that had been gloomily predicted by some did not materialize – 774,647 cases were reported between 1981 and 2001, and there were 448,060 deaths. By age and sex, the breakdown of those infected was 79 percent adult males, and by ethnicity 61 percent were black or Hispanic. The major avenues of transmission have been through male homosexual contact (48 percent) and intravenous drug abuse (26 percent), although HIV infection via heterosexual contact – generally between infected males and uninfected females – is on the rise. Today the fastest growing groups of newly infected individuals are reported to be women and their children, and gay black males – the latter group accounting for 42 percent of all new infections. The U.S. cases are almost all HIV-1. Despite fears of HIV-2 also spreading in North America, only 64 cases have been documented, and these were all directly linked with West Africa.

Among HIV/AIDS researchers a consensus gradually emerged that **simian immunodeficiency virus** (SIV) had somehow managed to jump the species barrier from African primates (for whom it seems to be a relatively benign infection) to first infect humans in Central and West Africa and, somewhere along the line, became human immunodeficiency virus or HIV-1 and its subtypes (the most common form worldwide) and HIV-2.

Another question had to do with how the species barrier was hurdled. Again a consensus took shape; SIV had entered the blood of Africans engaged in chimpanzee butchering, after which it became HIV-1 (although the possibility of SIV evolving into HIV in the chimpanzee was not ruled out). Moreover, lineages of HIV transmitted by sooty mangabeys (also called the green monkey) were believed to have reached humans in like fashion to become HIV-2. Some, however, suspected that medicine had something to do with HIV becoming a human infection and, therefore, that AIDS had an iatrogenic or medical cause.

Initially, the WHO **smallpox** vaccination campaign in Africa from 1967 to 1980 came under scrutiny for the possibility that HIV had been propelled through countless bodies with the repeated use of inadequately sterilized needles, or even that the vaccine had been contaminated. These hypotheses, of course, dealt with HIV transmission and did not really confront the question of its origin. Another hypothesis, however, did – this one focusing on the **polio** vaccination campaign conducted in Africa (and elsewhere) during the late 1950s. In the (then Belgian) Congo, chimpanzee kidneys were used to culture the poliovirus, which in turn, it was argued, could have contaminated the oral polio vaccine used in a widespread vaccination effort during 1957–58. Buttressing the case was that this region subsequently became the major epicenter of the burgeoning AIDS epidemic. Also bolstering it was the announcement in 1999 by a group of University of Alabama researchers that they had determined that a kind of chimpanzee once common in West Africa was indeed the source of HIV.

Yet other recent evidence was not so supportive. Most recently, in 2001, it was announced that a vial of the suspected polio vaccine had been found and that analysis had revealed no trace of HIV. Moreover, a study published in 2000 in *Science* had already cast considerable doubt on the contaminated vaccine hypothesis by showing that HIV-1 may well have been present in human African populations since at least the 1930s – almost 30 years before the polio vaccination campaign in the Congo. That date, however, is for the time that the HIV-1 group of viruses began to diversify, and not for when they were transmitted to humans. Thus, vital questions of transmission and origin remain unresolved – that of origin because even if chimpanzees did pass on HIV to humans, they may also have been infected from yet another source.

Great strides have been made recently toward the goals of treatment and prevention. In 1986, the drug azidothymidine (AZT) was shown to extend the period of latency for AIDS. It is one of five drugs called nucleosides licensed by the U.S. Food and Drug Administration, all of which are inhibitors of the viral enzyme reverse transcriptase (RT), which performs reverse transcription – the conversion of RNA into DNA that HIV must undergo to be infective. In the second half of the 1990s, protease inhibitors (which cripple a viral enzyme vital to HIV reproduction) came into use and two nucleoside inhibitors and one protease inhibitor were blended together into what was called the "antiviral cocktail." The results were miraculous. Individuals on the verge of death were going back to jobs and resuming normal lives, the mortality rate from AIDS in the United States fell dramatically, and it seemed that a major battle against the disease had been won.

But it was an incomplete victory, because the "cocktail" can produce unpleasant side effects, and just one missed dose can give the virus the opportunity to quickly mutate into a strain that resists the drugs. In fact, drug-resistant strains of HIV are already complicating AIDS treatment, which has led to different combinations of "cocktail" ingredients, each of which interferes with certain steps in the HIV infection process. Still other drugs have been brought effectively to bear on some of the "killer" opportunistic infections such as pneumocystis pneumonia and tuberculosis, which are the principal cause of AIDS deaths worldwide. But whether the miracle will continue indefinitely remains to be seen. The therapy is new and consequently the long-term success rate is unknown. Moreover, a per-patient annual cost of some 10,000–12,000 U.S. dollars limits this costly drug treatment to a relatively few victims in the developed world. Thus far, pressure on pharmaceutical manufacturers to make low- or no-cost drugs available to the developing world's millions stricken with HIV/AIDS has produced little in the way of results.

Work is also being done to develop a vaccine that could be both protective by preventing infection and therapeutic for those infected, by prolonging survival and decreasing immune system destruction. At the turn of the twenty-first century, vaccines were being tested that had proven effective in protecting monkeys from HIV, and large-scale trials were under way to test them for human safety. In addition, Merck and Company, with its enormous resources, announced in 1999 that it would begin human trials on two vaccines. However, provided that a safe vaccine does become available, the problems of administering it – especially to the millions at high risk in the developing world – are daunting because it appears that one primary injection will be required, followed by three booster shots. The good news, of course, is that the question seems no longer to be whether there will be a vaccine, but rather when a vaccine will be available.

Moreover, gene therapy holds out promise of inhibiting HIV by introducing a gene into cells that interferes with the viral regulatory proteins, or even one that will protect cells from HIV infection. But all of these measures, even when they do bear fruit, will probably be too late to stop AIDS from becoming the biggest killer-disease in human history.

Kenneth F. Kiple

2. African Trypanosomiasis (Sleeping Sickness)

African trypanosomiasis, or "sleeping sickness," is a fatal disease caused by a protozoan hemoflagellate parasite, the trypanosome. It is transmitted through the bite of a tsetse fly, a member of the genus *Glossina*. Sleeping sickness is endemic, sometimes epidemic, across a wide band of sub-Saharan Africa, the so-called tsetse belt that covers some 11 million square kilometers. Although the disease was not scientifically understood until the first decade of the twentieth century, it had been recognized in West Africa as early as the fourteenth century.

Chemotherapy to combat trypanosomiasis has remained archaic, with no significant advances made and, indeed, very little research done between the 1930s and the 1980s. However, in the mid-1980s field trials of a promising new drug demonstrated its efficacy in late-stage disease when there is central nervous system involvement. In addition, there have been exciting recent developments in the field of tsetse eradication with the combined use of fly traps and odor attractants.

Characteristics

An acute form of sleeping sickness caused by *Trypanosoma brucei rhodesiense* with a short incubation period of 5–7 days occurs in eastern and southern Africa. A chronic form (*Trypanosoma brucei gambiense*) of western and central Africa can take from several weeks to months or even years to manifest itself. There are many species of tsetse flies, but only six act as vectors for the human disease. The *Glossina palpalis* group, or riverine tsetse, is responsible for the transmission of *T. b. gambiense* disease. The *Glossina morsitans* group, or savanna tsetse, is the vector for *T. b. rhodesiense*, the cause of the rhodesiense form of sleeping sickness. Although tsetse flies are not easily infected with trypanosomes, once infected they remain vectors of the disease for life.

After being bitten by an infected fly, most victims experience local inflammation, or the trypanosomal chancre; parasites migrate from this site to multiply in blood, lymph, tissue fluids, and eventually the cerebrospinal fluid. The blood trypanosome count oscillates cyclically, with each successive wave, manifesting different surface antigens. In this manner, trypanosomes evade the antibodies raised against them by the host. Eventually, all organs are invaded, with central nervous system involvement, ultimately leading to death.

The epidemiological pattern of sleeping sickness varies considerably from place to place, but two features are well recognized. First, trypanosomiasis is exceptionally focal, occurring at or around specific geographic locations; and second, the number of tsetse flies is apparently not as important for disease incidence as is the nature of the human-fly contact.

The focal nature of sleeping sickness means that the ecological settings in which it occurs are of vital importance for understanding its epidemiology. Seemingly impossible to destroy, many historical foci tend to flare up in spite of concentrated eradication efforts since the 1930s. Very often, villages and regions that were affected decades ago remain problem areas today. The disease involves humans, parasites, tsetse flies, and wild and domesticated animals, and increasing population movements have complicated the epidemiology. Tsetse species have varying food preferences, ranging from the blood of wild and domestic animals to that of humans, but they require a daily blood meal, thereby making a single fly potentially highly infective.

Gambiense sleeping sickness is classically a disease of the frontier of human environments, where human-created habitat meets sylvan biotope. Humans are the principal reservoir of *T. b. gambiense*, and they maintain the typical endemic cycle of the disease. It is now known, however, that some animals, including domestic pigs, cattle, sheep, and even chickens, can act as reservoirs. The key to understanding the gambiense form is its chronicity and the fact that there are usually very low numbers of parasites present in the lymph and other tissue fluids. Gambiense disease can be maintained by a mere handful of peridomestic flies – that is, those that have invaded bush or cultivations near human settlements. This is known as close human-fly contact.

Riverine *G. palpalis* are most commonly found near waterways and pools; during dry seasons, when humans and flies are brought together through their shared need for water, the flies become particularly infective. Other common foci for the disease are sacred groves, which are often small clearings in the forest where the high humidity allows the flies to venture farther from water sources.

The virulent rhodesiense sleeping sickness is a true zoonosis maintained in wild animal reservoirs in the eastern African savannas. In the case of *T. b. rhodesiense*, the usual mammalian hosts are wild ungulates, with humans as adventitious hosts. Transmission of rhodesiense disease is more haphazard and directly relates to occupations such as searching for firewood, hunting, fishing, honey gathering, poaching, cultivation, cattle keeping, and being a game warden or a tourist. Whereas the gambiense form of the disease is site related, the rhodesiense form is occupation related, which helps to explain why the latter characteristically affects many more men and boys than women and girls. However, when a community moves near bush infested with infected flies, the entire population is at risk.

The animal reservoir of trypanosomes is an important factor in the epidemiology and history of sleeping sickness. It is well established that the trypanosomiases are ancient in Africa. Indeed, it is conjectured that the presence of sleeping sickness may explain why the ungulate herds of the African savanna have survived human predators for so long; the wild-animal reservoir of trypanosomes firmly restricted the boundaries of early human settlement. Although the wild ungulate herds became trypotolerant, domestic cattle still succumb to the disease, and the vast majority of research and funding has been aimed at solving the problem of animal – not human – sleeping sickness.

In evolutionary terms, the presence of trypanosomes in Africa may have precluded the development of some ground-dwelling faunas, thus encouraging certain resistant primates, including the early ancestors of humankind, to fill the empty ecological niches. If so, then humans were exposed to trypanosomal infection at the time of their very remote origin. The parasites are on the whole poorly adapted to humans, which accounts for the variety of clinical symptoms and ever-changing epidemiological patterns. A perfectly adapted parasite does not kill its host – at least in the short run.

An estimated 50 million people in 42 countries are at risk for trypanosomal infection, while it is estimated that only about 5 million to 10 million people have access to some form of protection against or treatment for the disease. Sleeping sickness is endemic across the wide band of sub-Saharan Africa known as the "tsetse belt" lying roughly between 20° north and 20° south of the equator, where it also can attain epidemic proportions.

The actual number of cases will never be known, as it is a disease of remote rural areas, and even today people in such places often die undiagnosed and uncounted. Most national statistics are grossly underreported, with the World Health Organization being notified of about only 10 percent of new cases. The current estimate of incidence is 20,000 to 25,000 cases annually. Most of the victims are concentrated in Zaire, Uganda, and southern Sudan. Some villages had infection rates of up to 25 percent. In the late 1970s and 1980s, severe outbreaks occurred in Cameroon, Angola, the Central African Republic, the Ivory Coast, and Tanzania, as well as in Sudan, Zambia, Uganda, and Zaire.

Although trypanosomiasis has been studied for more than 80 years, much is still unknown about the pathology of the disease. Three phases follow the bite of an infected fly: first the chancre itself; then the hemolymphatic or "primary stage"; and finally the meningocephalitic or "secondary stage." On average, people infected with *T. b. gambiense* live 2–3 years before succumbing, although there are recorded cases of infection spanning as much as 2 decades. In contrast, infection with the more virulent *T. b. rhodesiense*, if untreated, usually leads to death within 6–18 weeks.

The disease manifests a bewildering array of clinical symptoms, which can vary from place to place. Progressing through the two stages, there is increasing parasitemia with eventual involvement of the central nervous system. Clinical symptoms can include fever, headache, and psychiatric disorders such as nervousness, irascibility, emotionalism, melancholia, and insomnia, which reflect neuronal degeneration. Other symptoms include loss of appetite, gross emaciation, sleep abnormalities, stupor, and the characteristic coma from which sleeping sickness

derives its name. Some of the initial symptoms of sleeping sickness are also characteristic of early **malaria**, which can make differentiation between the two diseases difficult in the field. A common, easily recognizable symptom is swelling of lymph nodes. Another common symptom is called "moon face," an edema caused by leaking of small blood vessels. A most common complication during trypanosomiasis is **pneumonia**, which is a frequent cause of death. The chronic gambiense form can take as long as 15 years to develop after the victim has left an endemic area.

The prospect of a vaccine for human trypanosomiasis is bleak. The phenomenon of "antigenic variation" greatly reduces the prospect of producing an effective vaccine, and at present very little research is under way on vaccine development.

History

The history of sleeping sickness in Africa is long and complex, and its complicated ecology has dramatically affected demographic patterns in sub-Saharan Africa. The parameters and density of human settlement have been limited in many regions until the present time, while cattle-keeping has been prevented across vast regions of the continent, thereby seriously affecting the nutrition of entire populations.

The "African lethargy," or "sleepy distemper," as trypanosomiasis has been called, was well known to Europeans in West Africa from as early as the fourteenth century, through good descriptions given by Portuguese and Arab writers. For centuries slave traders rejected Africans with the characteristic swollen cervical glands, for it was common knowledge that those with this symptom sooner or later died in the New World or North Africa. As European exploration and trade along the West African coast increased between 1785 and 1840, the disease was reported in Gambia, Sierra Leone, and western Liberia, whereas between 1820 and 1870 it was also commonly noted along the Liberian coast.

2. African Trypanosomiasis (Sleeping Sickness)

Certainly the disease was an important factor in the history of colonial Africa. In the beginning, colonial administrators were concerned mainly with the health of Europeans and those few Africans in their service. But the threat of epidemics of sleeping sickness eventually forced colonial authorities to take much more seriously the health of entire African populations.

In those colonies affected by sleeping sickness, medical services often developed in direct response to this one disease, which resulted in the development of "vertical" health service – programs aimed at controlling a specific disease while neglecting other crucial public health issues. As recently as the 1970s, the World Health Organization urged developing countries to move toward "horizontal" health services that take into account the multifactoral nature of disease and health.

Sleeping sickness, along with malaria and **yellow fever**, played an important role in the development of the new specialties of parasitology and tropical medicine. In 1898, Patrick Manson, the "father of tropical medicine," published the first cogent discussion of the new scientific discipline. He explained that tropical diseases were very often insect-borne parasitical diseases, the chief example being trypanosomiasis.

Trypanosomiasis at the time was very much on the minds of colonial officials. In the decade between 1896 and 1906, devastating epidemics killed more than 250,000 Africans in the new British protectorate of Uganda, as well as an estimated 500,000 residents of the Congo basin. Understandably, the new colonial powers, including Britain, France, Germany, Portugal, and King Léopold's Congo Free State, perceived sleeping sickness to be a grave threat to African laborers and taxpayers, which in turn could dramatically reduce the utility of the new territories. Moreover, the fears were not limited to the continent of Africa; the British also speculated that sleeping sickness might spread to India, the "jewel" of their empire.

Thus ensued one of the most dramatic campaigns in the history of medicine, as scientific research teams were dispatched to study sleeping sickness. They began with the Liverpool School of Tropical Medicine's expedition to Senegambia in 1901 and the Royal Society's expedition to Uganda in 1902; other expeditions followed until World War II.

Many of these were sent by new institutions especially designed to investigate the exotic diseases of warm climates. The British, for example, opened schools of tropical medicine at Liverpool and London in 1899, while other such schools came into being in Germany, Belgium, France, Portugal, and the United States. This new field of scientific endeavor offered the opportunity for bright young men to gain international acclaim and a place in the history of medicine.

It should be noted that sleeping sickness was not the only disease to receive such attention as Europeans sought to establish themselves permanently in regions of the globe where health conditions were difficult and mortality was high. There were major discoveries by Manson, who was the first to demonstrate insects as vectors of human disease (**filariasis**); and by Ronald Ross, who found that the malaria parasite was transmitted by the *Anopheles* mosquito. Yet, despite the fact that endemic malaria was probably the cause of far more morbidity, the trypanosomiases attracted much attention in the new field of tropical medicine for the next 2 or 3 decades.

International meetings were convened to discuss sleeping sickness, beginning with one at the British Foreign Office in 1907. As the number of "tryps" specialists increased, sleeping sickness became a key factor in the international exchange of research findings in tropical medicine. The Sleeping Sickness Bureau was opened in London in 1908 to facilitate communication of research findings on all aspects of the disease. Its work continues to the present time.

After World War I and the formation of the League of Nations' Health Organization (the antecedent of the World Health Organization), two major conferences in 1925 and 1928 were convened to focus on African sleeping sickness. These conferences, following the pattern of the nineteenth-century sanitation and hygiene conferences, sought international collaboration and cooperation in implementing public-health solutions. In Africa, special research centers on tsetse flies and sleeping sickness appeared in many colonies including Uganda, Kenya, Tanganyika (now Tanzania), Belgian Congo (Zaire), Nigeria, Ghana, and French Equatorial Africa (Chad, Central African Republic, Congo-Brazzaville, and Gabon). Sleeping sickness thus became an important catalyst for cooperation among the colonial powers in Africa, which in turn aided the rapid growth of tropical medicine as a field. In fact, sleeping sickness early in the twentieth century attracted international attention to Africa with an urgency that was repeated in the early 1980s with **AIDS**.

Response to the disease occurred within the private sector as well. Concerned at the possible loss of increasingly important African markets, the European business community encouraged and sometimes initiated research into tropical diseases. For example, the principal founder of the Liverpool School of Tropical Medicine in 1899 was the influential and powerful capitalist Alfred Lewis Jones, chairman of a Liverpool-based shipping line that plied a lucrative trade along the West African coast. The businessman shared the imperialist's dismay at the potential devastation that could be caused by sleeping sickness, and together they were keen to support attempts to prevent the decimation of African populations.

The politics of colonialism often reflected contemporaneous perceptions of the epidemiology of sleeping sickness. By 1900, for example, it was widely accepted that the disease had been endemic in West Africa for centuries but had only recently begun spreading into the Congo basin and eastward.

From the earliest days of colonial settlement, it was not uncommon to blame sleeping sickness for the abandoned villages and depopulated regions that Europeans encountered during their push into the interior. It usually did

not occur to the intruders that in many cases Africans were withdrawing from areas because of the brutal nature of colonial conquest. Half a century would pass before researchers began to examine the deeper socioeconomic and political causes of the dramatic changes in the African disease environment that had resulted in the spread and increased incidence of sleeping sickness.

Medical experts at the turn of the nineteenth century tended to favor the theory of circumstantial epidemiology, which held that diseases were spread mainly through human agency within specific sets of circumstances. Because of a lack of effective treatments, the principal methods of control of epidemic disease consisted of segregation or isolation and disinfection with acrid smoke or strong fumes such as sulfur and vinegar. Disease was perceived as an invader to be demolished. This view accounts for much of the imagery and idiom of war used in early public-health campaigns. A major adjunct to this theory was the belief that once the circumstances had been identified, most diseases in Africa could and would be controlled, even eliminated, with techniques and technology developed in Europe. The European colonials assumed they would succeed where Africans had failed and that they would transform the continent by conquering the problems of tsetse and the trypanosome, among others. Most colonists believed that much of the backwardness they saw in African society was attributable, at least in part, to endemic diseases such as sleeping sickness.

Powerful notions of the potential of Western technology for solving health problems in Africa, sleeping sickness among them, have survived until quite recently. Rarely, if ever, did colonial authorities consider the possibility that Africans not only possessed some ideas about the ecology of sleeping sickness but had gained fairly effective control of their environment. An example of one such African strategy was the warnings to early European travelers not to travel through certain regions during daylight hours when tsetse flies were active and might infect their transport animals. Moreover, throughout the tsetse-infested regions, there were instances of African residence patterns that allowed coexistence with the ubiquitous tsetse flies yet avoided population concentrations conducive to epidemic outbreaks. European colonizers, by contrast, often disrupted – or destroyed – indigenous practices and survival strategies with the result that endemic sleeping sickness spread and sometimes became epidemic with disastrous effects.

The colonial powers, however, held their own version of the history of sleeping sickness and its evolution. Prior to their arrival, ancient, intractable foci of the disease had existed in West Africa and in the Congo basin around which, from time to time, the disease would flare into epidemic proportions. Colonials believed that it really began to spread only after the European newcomers had suppressed local wars and slave raiding among African peoples and established law and order. This in turn allowed many Africans, for the first time ever, to move freely and safely away from their home regions. Protected by Pax Brittannica, Pax Belgica, and the like, the increased movements of Africans carried sleeping sickness from old endemic foci to new populations. There was some basis for this hypothesis, especially in West Africa such as in Ghana and Rukuber of Nigeria. This widely accepted notion of the spread of sleeping sickness had an important consequence in the enormous effect expended by the Europeans in trying to regulate African life at every level, and especially to limit strictly any freedom of movement.

John Ford, a British entomologist who spent more than 25 years researching sleeping sickness, was one of the first to challenge this "classical view" of the pacification of Africa and the spread of the disease. He argued that it was not the pacific character of European colonization but, on the contrary, its brutal nature, that greatly disrupted and stressed African populations. In particular, the balanced ecological relationships among humans, tsetse flies, and trypanosomes were disrupted by European activities with the result that endemic sleeping sickness flared into epidemic proportions. Vivid examples of the results of such ecological upheaval were the sleeping sickness epidemics in Uganda and the Congo basin that had killed hundreds of thousands.

Epidemics continued throughout much of the colonial period, especially prior to World War II, when there were serious outbreaks in both West and East Africa. Public-health regulations to control the disease affected other areas of administration. In some colonies, sleeping sickness programs became so extensive and bureaucratic that they came into conflict with other departments, exacerbating competition for scarce staffing and financial resources within colonial administrations. In addition, sleeping sickness regulations were often responsible for confrontations between the private and public sectors as members of the former were increasingly hindered in their attempts to exploit the people and resources of Africa.

Two major patterns emerged in the colonial campaigns against sleeping sickness. In one, the focus was on tsetse eradication, whereas in the other, the focus was on the medicalization of victims. Most campaigns were a combination of features from both approaches. Within this framework, national variations emerged in the colonial campaigns. The British took a more broadly ecological approach to control of the disease, whereas the French and the Belgians took a more "medical" approach to the problem of human infection. British policy was to break the chain of sleeping sickness transmission by separating people from flies. Thus, while British administrators implemented social policies aimed at protecting people from disease, the scientific community, especially the new entomologists, searched for solutions to the "tsetse fly problem" in Africa. The compulsory mass resettlement of Ugandans, which probably helped save lives, from lakeshore communities in Buganda and Busoga in 1908, and the huge Anchau (northern Nigeria) scheme begun in 1936 are good examples of breaking transmission chains. Likewise, in some regions where it was ecologically feasible, Belgians resettled groups of people such as those along the Semliki River in eastern Congo.

Unfortunately, in the context of recently conquered and colonized Africans, who had rural subsistence economies and whose culture and tradition were intricately linked to locale, compulsory relocation sometimes had calamitous effects on those it was meant to protect. In the Belgian Congo an extraordinary amount of legislation and effort was directed at the control of populations in relation to sleeping sickness. It is not surprising that many Africans regarded sleeping sickness as the colonial disease because of the sometimes overwhelming amount of administrative presence it elicited.

French and Belgian efforts were directed chiefly at "sterilizing the human reservoir" of trypanosomes through mass campaigns of medicalization, or injections. To achieve this, they conducted systematic surveys of entire populations, hoping to locate, isolate, and treat all victims. Eugène Jamot, a French parasitologist, developed this method in Ubangui-Chari (French Equatorial Africa) and later introduced it in affected parts of Cameroon and French West Africa. In 1916, he organized an ambitious sleeping sickness campaign based on mobile teams, which systematically scoured the country for victims of the disease to be injected.

A grid system was devised to ensure complete surveys, and the mobile teams worked with true military efficiency. Between July 1917 and August 1919, more than 90,000 individuals had been examined, and 5,347 victims were identified and treated. Jamot's design for a sleeping sickness service was soon adopted by the Belgians in the Congo, and by 1932 there were five such teams operating annually in northern Congo alone. Admirable as it was for its sheer scale of organization, the policy of mass medicalization did not affect the fundamental ecology of the parasites; indeed, this approach had

the effect of removing the store of antibodies from humans that had been built up through long contact with the parasites.

Sterilization of the human reservoir was made possible in 1905 when the first trypanocidal drug became available in the form of an arsenical compound, atoxyl. Discovered by the German chemist Paul Ehrlich and adapted for use with sleeping sickness by Wolferstan Thomas of the Liverpool School of Tropical Medicine, atoxyl, alone or in combination with other compounds, remained the only chemotherapy for 2 decades. Atoxyl was toxic for 38 percent of patients, with dreadful side effects suffered by those whom it did not kill outright, among them the blinding of 30 percent of those injected. Later, new drugs – suramin (1916-20), tryparsamide (1919–25), and pentamidine (early 1940s) – came into use for early-stage rhodesiense and gambiense disease. Another most problematic arsenical with serious side effects, including up to 5 percent mortality, was and is used for second-stage disease. This drug, melarsoprol (along with suramin and pentamidine), has remained the drug of choice since the 1940s.

In the early 1960s, which saw independence for many African territories, colonial rulers concurred that human sleeping sickness was under control in Africa. But political upheavals, accompanied by the breakdown of medical infrastructures and large-scale population displacements, once again seriously affected the epidemiology of the disease. Some countries – Zaire, Uganda, Sudan, and Ivory Coast, for instance – witnessed epidemics of sleeping sickness, and it has been estimated that by 1969 there were up to 1 million victims in the Congo alone.

Tsetse flies and the trypanosomes that cause sleeping sickness will continue actively to shape the future of humankind in Africa. Because the most effective means of control is continual and thorough surveillance, present-day health planners and administrators must be aware of the history of this disease and the ease with which that history can repeat itself.

Maryinez Lyons

3. Ainhum

The word **ainhum** is derived from a term in the Nagos language of East Africa meaning "to saw." It describes the development of constricting bands about digits, almost always the fifth, or smallest, toe, which ultimately undergoes self-amputation. Typically the disease is bilateral (i.e., affecting both small toes).

Ainhum is ordinarily a disease of middle-aged black Africans of both sexes accustomed to going barefoot. The disease is common in Nigeria and East Africa and has been reported less frequently in other tropical areas, including India, Burma, Panama, the Antilles, and Brazil.

Ainhum was noticed frequently among slaves in Brazil and was first described in detail in 1867 by J. da Silva Lima, who also named the disease. Silva Lima's description is outstandingly accurate and has not been bettered. In one case, he wrote that the toe had taken the shape of a small oval potato; the covering skin was coarse and scabrous and tender to touch. As the disease progressed, a strong constriction appeared at the base of the toe, and, as blood flow to the toe was impeded, the bones ceased to exist. In time, spontaneous amputation occurred.

The cause of ainhum is unknown. Chronic trauma, infection, hyperkeratosis, decreased vascular supply, and impaired sensation may alone or in combination produce excessive fibroplasia and lead to ainhum. It is an acquired condition, although a hereditary predisposition has not been ruled out. Surgery is the mainstay of therapy: In most cases, prompt amputation may save the patient pain and infection.

Donald B. Cooper

4. Alzheimer's Disease

In 1906, Alois Alzheimer first described a neurological disorder of the brain associated with global deterioration of cognitive functioning and resulting in severe social impairment. Once thought rare, senile **dementia** of the Alzheimer's type is the most commonly acquired progressive brain syndrome. **Alzheimer's disease** begins with insidious intellectual and memory loss as the brain becomes shrunken from nerve cell loss and advances over 5–15 years to a chronic vegetative state. Progressive cognitive, psychological, and social dysfunction has a profound effect on family and friends. Alzheimer's disease may be the fourth leading cause of death in the United States. D. K. Kay and colleagues showed the average survival for demented men to be 2.6 years after the diagnosis of illness, whereas the survival period for nondemented men of the same age was 8.7 years. However, there is great variability in survival statistics from different studies.

Although Alzheimer's disease is the leading cause of dementia, its etiology remains unknown, and treatment is supportive. The illness is a major problem among the elderly. Approximately 4 percent of the population over the age of 65 is affected, and, by age 80, prevalence reaches 20 percent. As the elderly population of the United States increases, the number of persons with Alzheimer-type dementia will also increase. Even though pathological changes in presenile and senile forms of the illness are similar, there is evidence that early- and late-onset Alzheimer-type dementia differ clinically.

Characteristics

Alzheimer-type senile dementia is associated with behavioral signs and symptoms that divide into corresponding stages. In the early stage, subjective memory deficit may be difficult to differentiate from benign senile forgetfulness. However, elderly persons with benign forgetfulness are unable to recall unimportant details, whereas patients with Alzheimer-type senile dementia forget important and unimportant information randomly.

Typically, patients with Alzheimer's disease forget where things are placed, become lost easily, and have difficulty remembering appointments. Both recent and remote memory are affected. When patients recognize their cognitive and social losses, many develop feelings of hopelessness and despondency. As Alzheimer-type senile dementia progresses, the patient enters a confusional phase with more global impairment of cognitive functioning. Changes in higher cortical functions, such as language, spatial relationships, and problem solving, become more apparent.

During the confusional phase, obvious denial begins to replace anxiety, and cognitive deficits are noticeable to family and friends. In the final phase, the patient becomes aimless and may hallucinate or be restless and agitated. Language disorders can occur in late stages. Abnormal neurological reflexes, indicative of loss of higher neural inhibition, are common. Not all patients with Alzheimer-type senile dementia demonstrate the classic evolution of symptoms. Although almost all patients have some memory impairment, other focal cortical deficits may predominate initially. Spatial relationship impairment is common early. The patient may also complain of word-finding difficulty or demonstrate mild problems in speaking and understanding. In cases where damage to the frontal lobes of the brain predominates, the patient presents with judgment problems.

In the absence of biological markers for the illness, it is not surprising that clinical diagnosis may be less than accurate and, in fact, may be correct in as few as one-half of Alzheimer-type senile dementia cases. Not only do cognitive changes associated with normal aging overlap those found in the early stages of dementia, but also a wide spectrum of conditions may produce dementia. In any given patient, several conditions leading to progressive cognitive decline may occur simultaneously. The clinical diagnosis of Alzheimer-type senile dementia always requires documentation of progression. Reports from family and friends provide the most valid measures of cognitive decline in elderly persons and support the clinician's judgment that global intellectual deterioration has occurred.

Progression is usually gradual but with fluctuation of symptom severity. The patient may react very dramatically to changes in the living situation, to losses of friends or relatives, or even to admission to the hospital for evaluation. These acute changes probably represent withdrawal of orienting stimuli and emotional distress rather than progression of the disease process.

Psychometric tests may be useful in delineating patterns of cognitive deficit at various stages of severity and in identifying the qualitative aspects of performance deficit. Although laboratory tests are sometimes used to support the diagnosis of Alzheimer's disease, the laboratory is actually more useful in excluding other causes of cognitive deterioration. Atrophy of the cerebral cortex is often seen on computed tomography, but it is frequently overinterpreted.

Alzheimer's disease may be difficult to distinguish from the progressive dementias that are caused by many other disease conditions. For example, dementia is common in patients with terminal **cancer** and may result from a variety of causes.

The evaluation of a patient presenting with dementia often reveals untreatable causes, but treatable dementia is discovered in 20–25 percent of such patients. Of the many treatable causes of dementia, **multi-infarct dementia** may be the most difficult to differentiate from Alzheimer's disease. Risk factors for **stroke** should be evaluated and controlled when possible in every patient with early dementia.

Depression is the most common treatable illness that may masquerade as Alzheimer-type senile dementia. Cognitive abilities return to baseline levels when depression is treated. Because some patients with early dementia have secondary depression, dementia and pseudodementia may be difficult to differentiate. The depression that occurs in the early stages of Alzheimer-type senile dementia tends to resolve as the disease progresses. Pseudodemented, depressed patients are apt to have poor attention, inconsistent cognitive changes, absence of cortical signs, weight loss, sleep disturbance, guilt, poor self-esteem, a past personal family psychiatric history, and a more rapid onset.

In contrast, patients with cortical dementia of the Alzheimer type often show insidious onset, slow progression, early loss of insight, **amnesia** for remote and recent events, spatial disorientation, reduction in spontaneous speech, and occasionally aphasia. Agnosia, apraxia, increased muscular tension, and abnormal neurological reflexes may also be present.

A wide variety of gross morphological and microscopic changes occur in the brains of patients with Alzheimer's disease. Unfortunately, many of these changes are difficult to distinguish from alterations that occur in the brains of normal elderly persons, who also show some atrophy of white matter and, to a lesser extent, gray matter.

Although it is generally recognized that genetic influences are important in Alzheimer's disease, the exact nature of these genetic influences also remains unclear. Some families have a large number of members with the clinical or pathological diagnosis of Alzheimer's disease. The most important practical point regarding these kindreds is that most of them meet criteria for autosomal dominant inheritance. Penetrance of the gene exceeds 90 percent in most of these families. As a result, the children of an affected person have a 50 percent risk of developing dementia if they survive to the age at which dementia begins in that family. The exact proportion of familial cases is unknown, but they may account for as many as 10 percent of all cases of Alzheimer-type dementia. There is some familial clustering in families without dominant inheritance. It appears that concordance for dementia is somewhat higher in monozygotic versus dizygotic twins, suggesting genetic factors. On the other hand, concordance is not 100 percent, so environmental factors must have a role. Because age of onset varies within a twin pair, it may be difficult to be certain whether a given pair is truly discordant.

An association has been shown also between Alzheimer's disease and families that produce children with **Down syndrome**. Further support for a link between Down syndrome and Alzheimer's disease is provided by the fact that patients with Down syndrome tend to demonstrate neuropathological findings consistent with Alzheimer-type senile dementia if they live to adult life. Because Down syndrome represents a disorder of chromosome 21, a point of origin for the search for the genetic determinants of Alzheimer's disease is suggested. Recent data favor the hypothesis of a genetically induced overproduction of amyloid protein as a factor in the cause of Alzheimer's disease.

When families request genetic counseling, one can explain only what is known about the genetic factors. In a family with a single Alzheimer victim, the lifetime risk for a close relative also to develop dementia is approximately 10 percent. Because most dementia develops after the age of 70, this is a relatively small probability. In families with dementia occurring over several generations, an autosomal dominant inheritance is probable, and the risk for children of an affected parent may approach 50 percent. In these families, optimum health management indicates the suspicion of dementia in every elderly person with altered environmental-social interactional skills, multiple physical complaints in the absence of objective disease, or vague and unclear history. Autopsy can be suggested to confirm diagnosis to trace the pedigree more accurately.

Environmental causes for Alzheimer's disease have also been suggested. Some investigators have linked focal intranuclear accumulation of aluminum to the presence of neurofibrillary degeneration in hippocampal neurons. The relationship of aluminum to Alzheimer-type senile dementia, however, is not well accepted. General decline of immunologic competence with aging suggests an autoimmune mechanism. Although elevated levels of brain antibody have been demonstrated in Alzheimer's disease, antineuronal antibodies have not been demonstrated in the central nervous system. Serum protein abnormalities have been demonstrated, notably changes in haptoglobin functions. Finally, a viral cause has been proposed but not substantiated.

Alzheimer's disease remains a major challenge not only to modern medicine but also to the health care delivery system and to society at large. Not only is further research necessary in the diagnosis and management of the disease itself, but also major changes are necessary in the health care delivery system if patients afflicted with this illness are to get the care that they need.

History

Although Alzheimer's disease has only recently become widely known, it doubtless has a long history under such rubrics as "senility," "hardening of the arteries," and "dementia," to name but a few. Certainly senility and dementia are conditions that have been recognized for millennia. The Assyrians, Greeks, and Romans all knew and described them. J. Esquirol, however, has been credited for the first modern description, in 1838, of what seems to have been Alzheimer's disease. Esquirol wrote of a "senile dementia" that increases with age. Seven years later, Wilhelm Griesinger published a textbook on mental disease that clearly recognized the condition of "presenile dementia" caused by brain atrophy found at autopsy. Neither of these reports, however, seems to have had much influence on investigators at the time.

It was during the latter half of the nineteenth century that public as well as scientific concern for problems of the elderly increased considerably. With that concern came the birth of the field of geriatrics and increasing attention paid to dementia in the elderly. Much of the effort during these decades focused on whether it was an inevitable product of aging or an actual disease. Emil Kraepelin, one of the founders of modern psychiatry, pointed out the difficulty in separating normal senility from senile dementia. In applying the new technique of silver staining, Alzheimer, his student, identified a new neuropathological marker of dementia in the brain of a patient who had died at age 55 after a 4-year illness. This marker was the neurofibrillary tangle, which he speculated was the marker of a dead cell. Alzheimer thus made the first correlation between clinical characteristics of dementia in a patient and pathological lesions in the brain. Kraepelin later named the

illness "Alzheimer's disease" in honor of his former pupil.

The question then became one of determining if this disease was the same as senile dementia. It revolved around the ancient problem of what pathological changes can be attributed to aging as opposed to other causes. Kraepelin had emphasized the presenile nature of Alzheimer's disease, yet because of its similarity to senile dementia some investigators suggested that Alzheimer's disease might be caused by "a premature onset of the aging process." Also confusing the picture was the nineteenth century notion that extended also into the twentieth century: that cerebral arteriosclerosis might be the cause of senile dementia. By the late 1920s, there had been a sufficient accumulation of case descriptions of dementia among the elderly that statistical analysis could be brought to bear on the problem. It was found that most of the cases did in fact occur between the ages of 50 and 60, sustaining the notion of its presenile nature. In 1955 Martin Roth showed that mental changes could be triggered by a variety of both "functional" and "organic" diseases, and by the 1960s two major groups of researchers were at work on Alzheimer's disease. One, headed by Robert Terry, was based at Albert Einstein University, and the other, headed by Bernard Tomlinson, Gary Blessed, and Roth, was located at Newcastle upon Tyne. From their work and from other studies, it became apparent, among other things, that the changes in the brain found in cases of presenile dementia were the same as those in senile dementia.

The discovery broadened the definition of Alzheimer's disease and thereby increased enormously the number of individuals viewed as victims of it. It also created major semantic problems. Previously, the presenile nature of Alzheimer's disease was a defining factor. Now the illness, shown to be a major affliction of the elderly population, was called senile dementia of the Alzheimer type (SDAT), which psychiatrists call "primary degenerative dementia." Senile dementia has been used to mean either SDAT or Alzheimer's disease, but it may also refer to other forms of dementia in the elderly. In addition, Alzheimer's disease and senile dementia were often lumped together as senility or as cerebral arteriosclerosis. This latter concept proved to be so tenacious that even as late as the middle 1970s it was called "probably the most common medical misdiagnosis" of the cause of mental deterioration in the elderly.

In the early 1980s, Alzheimer's disease was defined as an "age-associated cognitive decline of gradual onset and course, accompanied by Alzheimer-type neuropathologic brain changes" with "no distinction with respect to age of onset," and was thought to be responsible for 50 percent or more of all dementias. Experts at a 1990 conference on the illness believed that Alzheimer's disease is being diagnosed correctly in about 80 percent of cases, even though such diagnoses can be confirmed only after death, and even though the etiology and epidemiology of the disease remain obscure.

It may well be determined that Alzheimer's disease is not a single disease but, rather, many different diseases with multiple causes ranging from genetics to exogenous toxins. The extent to which age and aging will rank among those causes remains a subject of debate. Reports of the condition among individuals in their 30s have been used to support the contention that the disease is unrelated to aging. On the other hand, there is a rising prevalence with age, such that by age 85 and over, some 20 percent or more are demented. If, of course, Alzheimer's disease is a specific disease or diseases (as opposed to an inevitable product of the aging process for some 5–7 percent of the population over age 65), then, of course, there is hope for a cure.

The question, however, of why Alzheimer's disease has been called the disease of this century – one that has only recently burst upon the developed world in epidemic proportions – is certainly bound up with advancing age for many and with the demographic changes that this has wrought. In 1900, there were only 3 million Americans aged 65 or older. Today there are more than 27 million, and it has been estimated that in the year 2030 there will be 50 million. Given the fact that an individual who lives to be 80 has an almost 1:4 chance of developing Alzheimer's disease or a related disorder, estimates suggest that the number of these victims will increase to about 4 million by the turn of the century. As the 1990s began, it was further estimated that fully half of all nursing home patients in the United States were Alzheimer victims.

The implications of the growing number of these victims for health care delivery systems are staggering. In 1967 a White House conference on aging resulted in the creation of the National Institute on Aging, which greatly facilitated research on Alzheimer's disease. In 1983, a Task Force on Alzheimer's Disease was created by the Department of Health and Human Services, which has emphasized the need for increased research and increased research funding, and in 1987 the international journal *Alzheimer's Disease and Associated Disorders* was founded to report such research. As more and more resources are brought to bear, the outlook for breakthroughs in understanding the causes of Alzheimer's disease and treating it are more optimistic than in former times. But it remains a devastating disease whose etiology is unknown.

Joseph A. Kwentus

Postscript

There are now some 4 million Alzheimer's patients in the United States. Around 10 percent of those over age 65 are affected; in the over-85 category, upward of 45 percent have the disease. Typically, death follows diagnosis by 7–10 years, although the range can vary from 3–20 years.

To the discovery in the 1980s of a type of protein in plaques (called amyloid protein) that appeared to be toxic to neurons, scientists have subsequently added another – a protein called "tau" that may be associated with Alzheimer's characteristic tangles. In healthy brains, the tau protein provides neurons with structural support, but in Alzheimer's disease the structural support becomes twisted and tangled.

The cause of the disease remains a mystery, although much promising research has been conducted – especially in the field of genetics, where, it is increasingly believed, lie most of the important solutions to the Alzheimer's mystery. One recent and important finding is that carriers of a fairly uncommon apolipoprotein E gene (APOE4) are far more likely to develop Alzheimer's disease than those who carry the common (APOE3) version. Almost half of late-onset Alzheimer's patients have APOE4. Another discovery, especially in the case of early-onset Alzheimer's, has linked a genetic mutation with the production of the protein amyloid–the protein in plaques that is suspected of neuron destruction. Interestingly, the mutation occurs in genetic territory where Down syndrome is also found, and those afflicted with this genetic disorder also develop plaques and tangles in the brain as they grow older.

Because thus far the only positive diagnosis of Alzheimer's is at autopsy, diagnosis in living patients is a matter of ruling out the possibility of other problems (such as stroke or alcoholism), a physical examination, mental tests, brain scans, and a scrutiny of family medical history. Thus, Alzheimer's disease is (probably inevitably) at times confused with other forms of dementia and misdiagnosed in 10–20 percent of cases or not diagnosed at all in its early stages. In 2000, however, it was announced at the World Congress on Alzheimer's in Washington, D.C., that scientists had located an enzyme that can determine with 95 percent accuracy whether a person has Alzheimer's in its early stages.

In terms of prevention, there is a vaccine that has proven effective with mice, which was recently (in 2000) pronounced safe for humans. Vaccine trials in humans now under way appear promising and have prompted some to optimistically predict the end of "the disease of the [twentieth] century" early in the twenty-first. But there is still no cure for Alzheimer's disease, and much of the treatment remains

supportive. There are, however, a number of pharmacologic interventions mostly aimed at mild-to-moderate Alzheimer's patients to slow the course of the disease. Inflammation of the brain (perhaps associated with amyloid), has been implicated in the etiology of the disease and is now treated with anti-inflammatory drugs. Other drugs (including ginkgo biloba) are administered to help with memory and slow down its loss. Estrogen therapy has proven beneficial for women with Alzheimer's, and vitamin A is frequently administered. However, there is difficulty in determining which medications work best in various patients, and in the absence of a "miracle" drug, at this point prevention in the form of the Alzheimer's vaccine seems far more promising than treatment.

Kenneth F. Kiple

5. Amebic Dysentery

Amebiasis is an infection of the colon caused by a parasitic protozoan, the ameba *Entamoeba histolytica*. Several species of ameba inhabit the large intestine. Most are harmless commensals or minor parasites, usually causing little or no clinical damage. The closely related species *Entamoeba coli* and *Entamoeba hartmanni* are commensals, and infection with *E. histolytica* is also often asymptomatic. Pathogenic amebas cause light to severe intestinal damage (**amebic dysentery**) and sometimes spread to the liver, lungs, brain, and other organs.

Characteristics
The parasite exists in two forms during its life cycle. Active adults, trophozoites, multiply in the lumen of the colon. They frequently live there harmlessly, feeding on the contents of the intestine. Some strains are generally commensal; others are highly pathogenic. Under conditions of stress, lowered host resistance, or when a particularly pathogenic strain is involved, amebas invade the intestinal wall and cause abscesses. As they pass lower into the

large intestine, the drier environment stimulates them to form a cyst wall. The original cell nucleus divides twice, producing four daughter nuclei. Cysts are passed with the feces and are infective when swallowed. Excystation takes place in the small intestine, and the young trophozoites, four from each cyst, are carried in the fecal stream to the large intestine. When dysentery occurs, trophozoites are swept out too rapidly to encyst. Even though huge numbers of amebas may be passed, they die quickly and are not infective. Persons with mild or no symptoms produce infective cysts, and it is they, not the patients with dysentery, who spread the disease.

Infection is by the fecal-oral route. Direct infection can take place in circumstances of extreme crowding, among inmates of institutions, and among male homosexuals. Indirect spread, however, by fecal contamination of food and water, is more common. Waterborne epidemics of amebic dysentery are not so frequent as those of **bacillary dysentery**, but the former do occur when sewage contaminates wells or water pipes. Fruits and vegetables can become covered with cysts when human feces are used as fertilizer, or when fruits are washed in contaminated water or are handled by a carrier. Flies and cockroaches can transmit cysts from feces to food. The disease thus flourishes in poor sanitary conditions but is rare where good personal hygiene is practiced and where water and sewer systems function properly. Dogs, cats, and monkeys can be infected in the laboratory, but there is no evidence that animal reservoirs have an epidemiological significance.

Infection with *E. histolytica* occurs around the world, although both commensal and pathological amebiasis is more common in poor, tropical countries. Prevalence rates vary greatly, as does the proportion of infections that result in clinical disease.

Amebiasis, especially clinical disease, is rare today in developed countries. In the United States, 3,000–4,000 cases were reported annually through the late 1970s. However, a spurt to roughly twice that level occurred in 1979–84. The disease was concentrated in Texas and California and probably resulted from increased immigration from Mexico and Southeast Asia. But annual case rates may be significantly underreported.

Asymptomatic and clinical amebiasis is much more common in Third World countries. Surveys have shown prevalence rates of up to 60 percent, reflecting real differences as well as technical difficulties. It is clearly a major public-health problem in much of South and Southeast Asia, China, Africa, and parts of Latin America. Mexico appears to have an unusually high prevalence. Estimates in the latter part of the twentieth century indicated that about 480 million people were infected throughout the world: 290 million in Asia, 80 million in Africa, 90 million in the Americas, and – remarkably – 20 million in Europe. Serious disease, however, strikes only a small percentage of those infected, and those who die of it constitute a very tiny fraction indeed.

Amebas cause disease when they invade the mucosal and submucosal layers of the large intestine, producing characteristic flask-shaped lesions. In severe cases, the lesions become large and confluent, resulting in substantial tissue destruction, bleeding, loss of fluids, and sloughing of patches of mucosa. Damage to the intestinal wall reduces water absorption, and loose stools with blood and mucous are passed. In addition to severe and perhaps fatal damage to the gut, amebas sometimes penetrate through the muscular coat of the bowel, where they enter the bloodstream and are carried to other organs, especially the liver. Intestinal perforation may result in fatal **peritonitis**. Large abscesses may form in the liver, with grave and sometimes fatal consequences. Amebas may also migrate from the liver through the diaphragm to the lungs and cause new abscesses there. Brain abscesses are rare, but lethal. Very destructive skin ulcerations can also occur, especially around the anus.

Clinical symptoms of intestinal amebiasis range from mild **diarrhea** and abdominal discomfort to frequent loose stools with blood mucus, severe pain, emaciation, and prostration.

Onset is generally insidious. Liver involvement may develop without evidence of intestinal disease. Symptoms include severe, continuous pain, enlarged and tender liver, fever, and weakness. Chronic amebiasis, both intestinal and hepatic, is sometimes very difficult to identify.

Differential diagnosis must rule out bacillary dysentery. Amebic dysentery tends to be a chronic disease with a gradual onset and little or no fever. The stools tend to be more abundant but less frequent and not to be bright red with blood, as is common in bacillary dysentery. Amebic dysentery has a longer incubation period, 20–90 days or more, compared to 7 days or less for the bacillary form. Finally, with its shorter incubation period and greater probability of water transmission, bacillary dysentery is more likely to occur in dramatic epidemics.

History

Amebiasis probably did not become a serious problem until people began to adopt a sedentary, agricultural way of life. Dysentery has been described in early medical writings of Europe and Asia, and outbreaks were frequent in military units, on slave ships, and in prisons. It is generally impossible, however, to determine whether amebic or bacillary dysentery was involved in any particular outbreak of the "flux."

British doctors in India provided good clinical accounts of amebiasis in the early nineteenth century. In 1828, James Annesley clearly linked the intestinal and hepatic aspects of the disease. The pathogen was described in 1875 by Russian physician Fedor Lösch, who noted the clinical course of the disease, identified the ameba, and induced similar lesions in dogs by feeding them ameba-rich stools from his patient. Lösch, however, believed that something else initially caused the disease and that the ameba merely "sustained" it. Technical problems, especially in identifying amebas and determining which were pathogenic and which were harmless, greatly impeded further research.

Stephanos Kartulis kept interest in the subject alive in the 1880s, establishing that an ameba was the probable cause of "tropical" dysentery.

Then in 1890, Canadian Henri Lafleur and American William Councilman published a definitive study of the pathology of the disease. German researchers H. Quincke and E. Roos distinguished between pathogenic and commensal human amebas.

Still, the situation remained confused, as ameba identification and taxonomy was controversial, and many research results could not be replicated. Doubts about the significance of pathogenic amebas were widespread in the early 1900s. Even Patrick Manson, perhaps the most important figure in tropical medicine, expressed skepticism about the role of amebas in dysentery as late as 1909. In 1913, American scientist Ernest Walker established the basic outline of the life cycle of *E. histolytica* and cleared some of the confusion about nonpathogenic forms. The discovery in 1925 of methods to raise amebas in culture has contributed to further clarification. Many mysteries remain, however, as to distinctions between pathogenic and nonpathogenic strains, and factors such as diet, stress, and concomitant infections that trigger invasiveness in longstanding, asymptomatic infections.

K. David Patterson

6. Anemia

Anemia, an insufficiency of red blood cells (RBC) and hemoglobin for oxygen-carrying needs, results from a variety of disease processes, some of which have existed since ancient times. It was defined in quantitative terms in the mid-nineteenth century, but before that the evidence of anemia is found in the descriptions of pallor or in the occurrence of diseases that we now know cause anemia. For example, **lead poisoning** decreases RBC production and was apparently widespread in Rome. Intestinal parasites cause **iron deficiency anemia** and were known to exist in ancient times. Parasites found in paleopathological specimens include many that can cause intestinal blood loss and anemia.

Congenital abnormalities in RBC metabolism (including **glucose 6-phosphate dehydrogenase [G6PD] deficiency** and various forms of **thalassemia** and **sickle-cell anemia**) were probably also present in ancient times. All of these, including thalassemia, protect against **malaria**, and the incidence of the relatively mild, heterozygotic **thalassemia minor** probably increased in the Mediterranean region after the appearance of **falciparum malaria**, the most fatal type of the disease.

Iatrogenic anemia was also common throughout most of recorded history, because bleeding was considered therapeutic from Greek and Roman times until the mid-nineteenth century.

Pernicious Anemia

Awareness of this type of anemia appears in the second half of the nineteenth century. Thomas Addison of Guy's Hospital described a severe, usually fatal form of anemia in 1855. Macrocytes were recognized by George Hayem in 1877; he also noted a greater reduction of hemoglobin than of RBCs in **pernicious anemia** (PA). In 1880, Paul Ehrlich found large nucleated RBCs in the peripheral blood containing dispersed nuclear chromatin; he called them megaloblasts, correctly concluding that they were precursors of Hayem's giant red cells that had escaped from the marrow.

In 1894, T. R. Fraser of Edinburgh became the first physician reported to have fed liver to patients with PA. Although he achieved a remission in one patient, others could not immediately repeat his success. But in 1918, George H. Whipple bled dogs and then fed them canned salmon and bread. After the dogs became anemic, he needed to remove very little blood to keep the hemoglobin low, although when the basal diet was supplemented, he found that he needed to bleed them more often. It turned out that liver was the most potent supplement, but it was not until 1936 that hematologists realized that the potency of liver was due to its iron content.

George Richards Minot of Harvard University became interested in the dietary history of his patients following the first reported syndromes due to deficiency of micronutrients. He focused attention on liver after Whipple's observations in dogs; in trying to increase the iron and purines in the diet of patients with PA, he fed them 100–240 grams of liver a day. He observed that the reticulocytes (an index of bone marrow activity) started to rise 4–5 days after the liver diet was begun. In fact, patients showed a consistent rise in RBC count and hemoglobin levels whenever they consumed liver in adequate amounts. In an attempt to purify the protein in liver, it was found that extracts were effective, and subsequently, cyanocobalamin – vitamin B_{12} – was identified. It was purified in 1948 and synthesized in 1973.

The possible role of the stomach in PA was pointed out by Austin Flint in 1860, only 5 years after Addison's description of the ailment appeared. In 1921, P. Levine and W. S. Ladd established that there was a lack of gastric acid in patients with PA even after stimulation. William B. Castle established that gastric juice plus beef muscle were effective in treating PA, although either alone was not. An autoimmune basis for development of PA has been established in recent years.

Iron Deficiency Anemia

Iron deficiency anemia is by far the most common cause of anemia in every part of the world today. It undoubtedly existed in ancient times as well. In this condition, fingernails develop double concave curvature, giving them a spoon shape (*koilonychia*). A Celtic temple at Nodens, in Gloucestershire, England, built in Ascelpian style after the Romans had left Britain in the fourth century A.D., contains a votive offering of an arm fashioned crudely proximally but with increasing detail distally; it shows characteristic *koilonychia*.

Pallor, the hallmark or cardinal sign of anemia, is seen especially in the face, lips, and nails, often imparting a greenish tint to Caucasians, a presenting sign that led to the diagnosis of

chlorosis or the "green sickness" in the sixteenth century. In the seventeenth century, pallor became associated in the popular mind with purity and femininity, and chlorosis became known as the "virgin's disease." Constantius I, father of Constantine the Great, was called Constantius Chlorus, because of his pale complexion, and it seems most likely that he had a congenital form of chronic anemia. (He came from an area known today to have a relatively high frequency of thalassemia.)

Preparations containing iron were used therapeutically in Egypt around 1500 B.C. and later in Rome, suggesting the existence of iron deficiency. In 1681, Thomas Sydenham mentioned "the effect of steel upon chlorosis. The pulse gains in strength and frequency, the surface warmth, the face (no longer pale and death like) a fresh ruddy coulour ... Next to steel in substance I prefer a syrup ... made by steeping iron or steel filings in cold Rhenish wine." In 1832 P. Blaud described treatment of chlorosis by use of pills of ferrous sulfate and potassium carbonate that "returns to the blood the exciting principle which it has lost, that is to say the coloring substance."

Children have increased needs for iron during growth, as do females during menstruation, pregnancy, and lactation. Chronic **diarrhea**, common in the tropics where it is often associated with **parasitism**, decreases iron absorption whereas parasitism increases iron losses. Estimates indicate that the needs of pregnant and lactating women in tropical climates are about twice those of women in temperate zones. In the tropics, high-maize/low-iron diets are common, and soils are iron deficient in many areas.

Glucose-6-Phosphate Dehydrogenase (G6PD) Deficiency

Favism, or **hemolytic anemia** due to ingestion of fava beans, is now known to occur in individuals deficient in G6PD. The Mediterranean type of G6PD deficiency is found in an area extending from the Mediterranean basin to northern India, an area corresponding to Alexander's empire. Sickness resulting from ingestion of beans was probably recognized in ancient Greece, forming the basis for the myth that Demeter, Greek goddess of harvest, forbade members of her cult to eat beans. Pythagoras, physician and mathematician of the fifth century B.C. who had a great following among the Greek colonists in southern Italy, also seems to have recognized the disorder, since he, too, forbade his followers to eat beans. It is in that area of southern Italy that the incidence of G6PD deficiency is highest.

In 1956, the basis for many instances of this type of anemia was recognized as a hereditary deficiency of the enzyme G6PD within the red cell. Inheritance of G6PD is now recognized to be a sex-linked characteristic with the gene locus residing on the X chromosome.

It is estimated that currently over 100 million people in the world are affected by this deficiency. Nearly 3 million Americans carry the trait for G6PD deficiency, which is also found among Sephardic and Kurdish Jews, Sardinians, Italians, Greeks, Arabs, and in the Orient among Filipinos, Chinese, Thais, Asiatic Indians, and Punjabis. It has not been found among North American Indians, Peruvians, Japanese, or Alaskan Eskimos.

The first documented report of drug-induced (as opposed to fava-bean-induced) hemolytic anemia appeared in 1926 following the administration of the antimalarial drug pamaquine (Plasmoquine). During World War II, after the world's primary sources of quinine were captured by the Japanese, about 16,000 drugs were tested for antimalarial effectiveness. In 1944, an Army Medical Research Unit at the University of Chicago studying these potential antimalarial drugs encountered the problem of drug-induced anemia. Research by this group over the next decade elucidated the basic information on G6PD deficiency.

Pamaquine was found to cause **hemolysis** in 5–10 percent of American blacks (about 10–14 percent of black American males are G6PD-deficient) but only rarely in Caucasians, and the severity of the hemolysis was observed to be dependent on the dose of the drug. Similar sensitivity to the related drug primaquine and many other related drugs was demonstrated, and the term "primaquine sensitivity" came to be used to designate this form of hemolytic anemia. It was subsequently demonstrated that the hemolysis was due to an abnormality in the erythrocytes of susceptible individuals and that it was self-limited even if administration of primaquine was continued. Several biochemical abnormalities of the sensitive red cells, including glutathione instability, were described. In 1956, Paul E. Carson and colleagues reported that G6PD deficiency of red cells was the common denominator in individuals who developed hemolysis after one of these drugs was administered, and the term G6PD deficiency became synonymous with primaquine sensitivity. It was soon found that this deficiency was genetically transmitted.

Sickle-Cell Disorders

Sickle-cell disorders have existed in human populations for thousands of years. However, the discovery of human sickle cells and of sickle-cell anemia was first announced in the form of a case report by James Herrick at the Association of American Physicians in 1910. In 1904, Herrick had examined a young black student from Grenada who was anemic; in the blood film he observed elongated and sickle-cell-shaped RBCs.

By 1922, there had only been three cases of this type of anemia reported. But in that year Verne R. Mason, a resident physician at Johns Hopkins Hospital, described the first patient recognized to have that disease at that institution. Mason introduced the term "sickle cell anemia," which became the standard designation.

In 1923, C. G. Guthrie and John Huck performed the first genetic investigation of this disease and developed a technique that became an indispensable tool for the identification of sickle trait in later investigations, population surveys, and genetic studies.

Virgil P. Sidenstricker, of Georgia, recorded many of the clinical and hematologic features of sickle-cell disease. He introduced the term

"crisis," was the first to suggest that the anemia was hemolytic, and reported the first autopsy describing the typical lesions of the illness including a scarred, atrophic spleen. He was also the first to describe sickle-cell anemia in childhood, noting the peculiar susceptibility of victims to infection, with a high mortality rate.

The first case of sickle-cell anemia to be reported from Africa was described in 1925 in a 10-year-old Arab boy in Omdurman, and the first survey of the frequency of **sickle-cell trait** in the African population was reported in 1944 by R. Winston Evans, a pathologist in the West African Military Hospital. In a study of almost 600 men of Gambia, the Gold Coast, Nigeria, and the Cameroons, he found approximately 20 percent to have the trait, a sickling rate about three times that in the United States.

In East Africa, E. A. Beet found a positive test for sickling in 12.9 percent of patients in the Balovale district of northern Rhodesia. He also reported striking tribal differences in the prevalence of sickle-cell trait. By 1945, H. C. Trowell had concluded that sickle-cell anemia was probably the most common and yet the least frequently diagnosed disease in Africa. He noted that in his own clinic in Uganda no cases had been recognized before 1940, but 21 cases were seen within the first 6 months of 1944 when he began routine testing for sickling.

For many years, it was thought that sickle-cell anemia was rare in Africa in contrast to the greater prevalence observed in the Americas (Especially North America), and some thought that interbreeding with white persons brought out the hemolytic aspect of the disease. It was not until the mid-1950s that it was understood that few homozygous sickle-cell cases came to medical attention because of a high infant mortality rate from that disease. This was demonstrated in Léopoldville when J. and C. Lambotte-Legrand found that only two cases of sickle-cell anemia had been reported among adults in the Belgian Congo, although sickling occurred in about 25 percent of the black population. They subsequently followed 300 infants with sickle-cell anemia. They found that 72 died before the end of the first year of life, and 144 had perished by the age of 5.

Subsequent research by others, however, established the fact that sickle-cell anemia patients who did survive to adolescence came from the higher social groups, and that the standard of living, the prevalence of infection and nutritional deficiency, and the level of general health care were the principal factors affecting the mortality rate from sickle-cell anemia in young children. By 1971, as improved health care became available, the course of the disease was altered; at the Sickle Cell-Hemoglobinopathy Clinic of the University of Ghana, it was reported that 50 percent of the patients with sickle-cell anemia survived past age 10.

Geographic distribution of sickle-cell gene frequency was mainly charted by the mid-twentieth century. The prevalence of sickling in black populations of the United States was well established by 1950. Numerous studies performed in Central Africa and South Africa also revealed that, although the frequency of sickling varied, the occurrence of the gene that caused it was confined mostly to black populations.

In Africa, after World War II, surveys established that across a broad belt of tropical Africa, more than 20 percent of some populations were carriers of the sickle-cell trait. Significantly, a high frequency of sickle trait was also found among whites in some areas of Sicily, southern Italy, Greece, Turkey, Arabia, and southern India. Yet, by contrast, sickling was virtually absent in a large segment of the world extending from northern Europe to Australia. These observations led to several hypotheses about where the mutant gene had had its origin and how such high frequencies of a deleterious gene are maintained.

Hermann Lehmann presented evidence that sickling arose in Neolithic times in Arabia, and that the gene was then distributed by migrations eastward to India and westward to Africa. He and others have speculated that the fre-

quency of the gene increased significantly in the hyperendemic malarial areas of Africa and spread northward across the Sahara along ancient trade routes. Because the eastern and western Arabian types of sickle-cell disease are different, spread must have occurred along sea trade routes, accounting for similarities in sickle-cell anemia in eastern Africa, eastern Arabia, and southern India.

Obviously then, there was much interest generated in the cause of the very high frequency of the sickle-cell gene in Africa. In 1946, Beet in Rhodesia noted that only 9.8 percent of sicklers had malaria, whereas 15.3 percent of nonsicklers were affected. P. Brain, of Southern Rhodesia, suggested that RBCs of sicklers might offer a less favorable environment for survival of malarial parasites. In 1954, J. P. Mackey and F. Vivarelli suggested that "the survival value [of the trait] may lie in there being some advantage to the heterozygous sickle cell individual in respect of decreased susceptibility of a proportion of his RBC to parasitization by *P. falciparum.*"

A relationship between sickle-cell trait and falciparum malaria was reported by A. C. Allison in 1954. He noted that the frequency of heterozygous sickle-cell trait was as high as 40 percent in some African tribes, suggesting some selective advantage or else the gene would be rapidly eliminated because most homozygotes die without reproducing. He decided that a high spontaneous mutation rate could not account for the high but varying frequencies of the gene and postulated that sickle-cell trait occurs as a true polymorphism and that the gene is maintained by selective advantage to the heterozygous. Comparing the distribution of falciparum malaria and sickling, Allison found that high frequencies of the trait were invariably found in hyperendemic malarial areas. He also found that people with sickle-cell trait suffer from malaria not only less frequently but also less severely than other persons, and he concluded that, where malaria is hyperendemic, children with the sickle-cell trait have a survival advantage.

Thalassemia

Thalassemia, an inherited form of anemia, results from the deficient synthesis of a portion of the globin molecule and is also thought by some to have stabilized in the face of malaria. A variety of forms exist, based on the chain and site within a specific chain at which the genetically determined defect exists. It has been suggested that thalassemia originated in Greece and spread to Italy when it was colonized by Greeks between the eighth and sixth century B.C. At present, it is most frequent in areas where ancient Greek immigration was most intense: Sicily, Sardinia, Calabria, Lucania, Apulia, and the mouth of the Po.

Porotic Hyperostosis

Chronic anemia from any cause produces bone changes, which can be recognized in archaeological specimens. These changes, called **porotic hyperostosis** (or symmetrical hyperostosis) result from an overgrowth of bone marrow tissue, which is apparently a compensatory process. Today, porotic hyperostosis is seen classically in X-rays of patients with congenital hemolytic anemias, as well as in children with chronic iron deficiency anemia. This is especially the case when the iron deficiency occurs in premature infants or is associated with **protein malnutrition** or **rickets**.

Porotic hyperostosis has been observed in archaeological specimens from a variety of sites, including areas of Greece, Turkey, Peru, Mexico, the United States, and Canada. In most areas, the findings are considered evidence of iron-deficiency anemia, although thalassemia was apparently responsible in some areas. Around the shores of the Mediterranean, malaria was probably the most frequent cause of chronic anemia at certain times.

Archaeological specimens from the Near East show an incidence of anemia of only 2 percent in early hunters (15,000–8000 B.C.), who ingested a lot of animal protein and thus took in reasonable amounts of dietary iron. By contrast, farming populations of 6500–2000 B.C. showed an anemia incidence of 50 percent.

Many New World natives whose diet consisted primarily of corn (maize) and beans had a diet deficient in iron and protein. Moreover, when cooked in water for long periods of time, the food in the diet was also low in ascorbate and folate. Ascorbate helps convert dietary ferric to ferrous iron, which is more easily absorbed; therefore, deficiency of this vitamin increased the problem of deficient dietary iron. A high incidence of iron deficiency has been demonstrated by modern studies of infants and children in populations living on a diet consisting mostly of maize and beans. It is not surprising then, in North America, that porotic hyperostosis was found in 54 percent of skeletons in the canyons of northern Arizona and northern New Mexico, among a population that ate little meat and subsisted mainly on maize. By contrast, plains dwellers in southern Arizona and southern New Mexico, who used more animal foods, had an incidence of only 14.5 percent. Absence of evidence for malaria or **hemoglobinopathies** in the New World before the arrival of the Europeans argues against these possible causes of porotic hyperostosis.

Alfred Jay Bollet and Audrey K. Brown

7. Anorexia Nervosa

Anorexia nervosa is a psychophysiological disorder especially prevalent among young women and characterized by refusal to eat or maintain normal body weight, intense fear of becoming obese, a disturbed body image in which the emaciated patient feels overweight, and absence of any physical illness accounting for extreme weight loss. The term anorexia is actually a misnomer, because genuine loss of appetite is rare and usually occurs only late in the illness. Most anorectics are actually obsessed with food and constantly deny natural hunger.

Characteristics

In anorexia nervosa, normal dieting escalates into a preoccupation with being thin, profound changes in eating patterns, and weight loss of at least 25 percent, usually accomplished by severe restriction of caloric intake. Anorectics may couple fasting with emetics, laxatives, diuretics, and exercise.

The most consistent medical consequences of anorexia nervosa are **amenorrhea** (ceasing or irregularity of menstruation) and estrogen deficiency. The decrease in estrogens causes many anorectics to develop **osteoporosis**. Further complications arising from severe malnutrition include **bradycardia**, **hypotension**, lethargy, **hypothermia**, constipation, and various other metabolic and systemic changes.

Anorectics also display a relatively consistent cluster of emotional and behavioral characteristics and unusual eating habits that include monotonous or eccentric diets, hoarding or hiding food, and obsessive preoccupation with food and cooking for others. Emotionally, anorexic patients are often described as perfectionistic, dependent, introverted, and overly compliant. Frequently reported neurotic traits include obsessive-compulsive, hysterical, hypochondriacal, and depressive symptoms. A distorted body image is an almost universal characteristic of anorectics, with many patients insisting that they are overweight even when their bodies are extremely emaciated. As a result, most individuals with anorexia nervosa deny or minimize the severity of their illness and are thus resistant to therapy.

Once considered extremely rare, the incidence of anorexia nervosa more than doubled in the late twentieth century. As many as 1 in 250 females 12–18 years old may develop the disorder. Onset occurs almost exclusively during the teens, although some patients have become anorectic as early as age 11 and others as late as the sixth decade of life. Patients are typically from middle- or upper-class families.

Approximately 5–10 percent of anorectics are male, whose clinical picture is much different from that of women. In general, male anorectics tend toward greater psychopathology, are often massively obese before acquiring the disorder, are less likely to be affluent, and are even more resistant to therapy than their female counterparts.

Among North American minorities, there are few reported cases. However, this reflects socioeconomic status rather than ethnic characteristics. Similarly, anorexia nervosa is confined to highly industrialized areas. The absence of the disorder in developing nations and its high incidence among affluent social groups in Westernized countries have led many clinicians to classify anorexia nervosa as a "culture-bound" syndrome.

Although the etiology of anorexia nervosa is an area of intense investigation, researchers have yet to reach a consensus about its origin. The most sophisticated thinking on the subject regards anorexia nervosa as a disorder that involves the interplay of biological, psychological, and cultural factors.

History

Anorexia nervosa's past prevalence has been a subject of much historical debate. Some clinicians and medical historians have postulated that it was first identified in 1689 by Richard Morton, physician to James II. Others have dated the origins of anorexia nervosa even earlier, claiming that certain medieval female saints, who were reputed to live without eating anything except the eucharist, actually suffered from anorexia nervosa. Some historians, however, have argued that attempts to label all historical instances of food refusal and appetite loss as anorexia nervosa are simplistic and maintain that the historical record is insufficient to make conclusive diagnoses of individual cases.

The modern disease classification of anorexia nervosa emerged in the second half of the nineteenth century. In 1859, William Stout Chipley published the first North American description of **sitomania**, a type of insanity characterized by an intense dread or loathing of food. Although Chipley found sitomania in a broad range of social and age groups, he identified a special form of the disease that afflicted adolescent girls. Chipley's work was ignored, however, and not until British physician William Withey Gull and

French alienist Charles Lasègue published two influential studies in the 1870s did physicians begin to pay significant attention to anorexia in girlhood.

Gull's primary accomplishment was to name and establish anorexia nervosa as a coherent disease entity. Despite widespread acclaim for his work with anorectic patients, however, clinicians during the late nineteenth century generally rejected the conception of anorexia nervosa as an independent disease. Instead, they conceptualized it either as a variant of **hysteria** that affected the gastrointestinal system, or as a juvenile form of **neurasthenia**.

Nineteenth century physicians also tended to focus on the physical symptom of not eating and ignored the anorectic patient's psychological reasons for refusing food. An important exception was Lasègue, who was the first to suggest the significance of family dynamics in the genesis and perpetuation of anorexia nervosa. Because of the somatic emphasis of nineteenth century medicine, however, most nineteenth century medical practitioners disregarded Lasègue's therapeutic perspective. Instead, they directed medical intervention toward restoring the anorectic to a reasonable weight and pattern of eating rather than exploring the underlying emotional causes of the patient's alleged lack of appetite.

In the twentieth century, the treatment of anorexia nervosa changed to incorporate new developments within medical and psychiatric practice. Before World War II, two distinct and isolated models dominated medical thinking on anorexia nervosa. The first approach was rooted in late nineteenth century research in organotherapy, a form of treatment based on the principle that disease resulted from the removal or dysfunction of secreting organs and glands. Between 1900 and 1940, a variety of different endocrinologic deficiencies were proposed as the cause of anorexia nervosa. Many clinicians assumed that a pituitary hormone deficiency underlay the conditions; others implicated thyroid insufficiency as the cause. Throughout the 1920s and 1930s, insulin, antuitrin, estrogen, and a host of other hormones were also employed in the treatment of anorexia nervosa.

The second major approach grew out of the field of dynamic psychiatry, which emerged during the 1890s and early 1900s. Practitioners in dynamic psychiatry increasingly focused on the life history of individual patients and the emotional sources of nervous disease. Two of the leading pioneers in this new field – Sigmund Freud and Pierre Janet – were the first to suggest a link between the etiology of anorexia nervosa and the issue of psychosexual development. According to Freud, all appetites were expressions of libido or sexual drive. Thus, not eating represented a repression of normal sexual appetite. Similarly, Janet asserted that anorectic girls refused food in order to retard normal sexual development and forestall adult sexuality.

Because of the enormous popularity of endocrinologic explanations of disease, the idea of anorexia nervosa as a psychosexual disturbance was generally overlooked for more than 30 years. By the 1930s, however, the failure of endocrinologic models to establish either a predictable cure or a definitive cause of anorexia nervosa, the growing reputation of the Freudian psychoanalytic movement, and increased attention to the role of emotions in disease led a number of practitioners to assert the value and importance of psychotherapy in the treatment of anorexia nervosa. Although biomedical treatment of the disorder continued, most clinicians realized that successful, permanent recovery depended on uncovering the psychological basis for the anorectic's behavior.

After World War II, a new psychiatric view of eating disorders, shaped largely by the work of Hilde Bruch, encouraged a more complex interpretation of the psychological underpinnings of anorexia nervosa. Although Bruch agreed that the anorectic was unprepared to cope with the psychological and social consequences of adulthood and sexuality, she also stressed the importance of individual personality formation and factors within the family to the psychogenesis of anorexia nervosa. Here, Bruch revived Lasègue's work on the role of family dynamics in anorexia nervosa. According to Bruch, the families of most anorectic patients were engaged in a dysfunctional style of familial interaction known as "enmeshment": Such families are characterized by extreme parental overprotectiveness, lack of privacy of individual members, and reluctance or inability to confront intrafamilial conflicts. Although superficially these families appeared to be congenial, said Bruch, this harmony was achieved through excessive conformity on the part of the child, which undermined the child's development of an autonomous self. Anorexia nervosa, according to Bruch, was therefore a young woman's attempt to exert control and self-direction in a family environment in which she otherwise felt powerless.

Bruch was also primarily responsible for the tremendous growth in the popular awareness of anorexia nervosa and other eating disorders in the 1970s and 1980s. Through both scholarly and popular writings, Bruch brought anorexia nervosa into common North American parlance. At the same time that the North American public was becoming increasingly aware of anorexia nervosa, the number of reported cases of the disorder grew tremendously. This phenomenon has led some clinicians and social commentators to suggest that the popularization process itself may promote a "sympathetic host environment" for the disorder.

Heather Munro Prescott

8. Anthrax

Anthrax is an acute zoonotic disease, primarily of herbivorous animals, which is transmissible to humans. The causative organism is *Bacillus anthracis*, often referred to in earlier, and especially in French, texts as *bactéridie*, the name first bestowed on it by Casimir Davaine in 1863. Humans are infected only secondarily through contact with animals or animal products, and thus the disease must be considered in relation to anthrax in animals.

The species of domestic animals most commonly affected are cattle, sheep, and goats; pigs, dogs, and cats are less susceptible. An enlarged spleen is a classic observation in animals with anthrax, thus the disease has also been known as "splenic fever" or "splenic apoplexy." In humans, the cutaneous form is known as "malignant pustule," and the pulmonary or intestinal (industrial) type as "woolsorters' disease" or "industrial anthrax." In French, the equivalent of splenic fever is *sang de rate*, in German *Milzbrand*; other French synonyms include *charbon* and *pustule maligne*.

Characteristics

Because *B. anthracis* produces resistant spores in suitable soils, the disease has long been endemic in many areas throughout the world, with most outbreaks occurring in Europe and Asia. Once contaminated with anthrax spores, an area can be extremely difficult to clear, as has been demonstrated on the island of Gruinard off the west coast of Scotland, which was experimentally contaminated during World War II. This is of prime importance for the epidemiology of the disease because it is rarely spread directly from animal to animal, but almost always through ingestion of contaminated food, either by grazing or, in cooler climates, through imported winter foodstuffs. The infectivity of the anthrax bacillus for people is low, and therefore, even where large numbers of spores and bacilli are found in an industrial environment, only relatively few cases occur.

Cutaneous anthrax, the nonindustrial type in humans, affects those in professions such as veterinary surgery, pathology, farming, butchery, and the like and takes the form of malignant pustule – a lesion caused by contamination of skin with material from infected animals. **Pulmonary anthrax**, the industrial type, may present as either malignant pustule or pulmonary disease and is acquired in the woolen industries, especially through contaminated air. The disease approached an epidemic situation during the late-eighteenth and nineteenth centuries in France and England in factories processing imported horsehair and sheep's wool.

Outbreaks in animals in Europe (mainly cattle) and in Asia (sheep and goats) heavily outweigh those in the United States and Africa, whereas Australia and Canada are rarely affected. Extensive enzootic areas with a constant presence of infection include China, Ethiopia, and Iran, and, in the Americas, Mexico and some South American countries. Available data suggest an annual average total of some 10,000 outbreaks throughout the world. Since World War II, fatal cases in humans have been substantially reduced by antibiotic therapy.

The immunogenic behavior of the anthrax bacillus is complex, and it is not certain whether or to what extent immunity develops in cases of recovery from infection. The existence of an extracellular toxin produced by *B. anthracis* (which in part determines its virulence) was demonstrated only during the 1980s. Certain strains of certain animal species possess high natural resistance, which introduced confusion and fed much of the controversy surrounding early work on anthrax. The live attenuated vaccines used by Louis Pasteur have undergone continued development and improvement over the years, but early claims of reductions in incidence and fatality rates following their use were not readily sustained. Thus, the early vaccines have gradually been replaced by spore-based vaccines and prepared antiserum. Until recently, vaccines have not been considered safe for use in humans, but serum treatment has been used extensively for prophylactic and therapeutic purposes. For occupational reasons, women are less liable to exposure than men, but the disease, when established, is more commonly fatal in females.

In its principal animal hosts, anthrax may take one of three forms: a *peracute* type (splenic apoplexy), where sudden death occurs almost simultaneously with the first symptoms; an *acute* type characterized by acute fever, usually followed by death after 2–12 days; and a *subacute* type often followed by recovery. Classical signs include fever, stupor, spasms, convulsions, intestinal disturbances, and respiratory or cardiac distress. Death follows **septicemia** and accompanying severe toxic manifestations.

Anthrax in people may take the form of a malignant pustule (cutaneous anthrax) where the bacilli enter through the skin, producing a primary lesion developing into a characteristic area of inflammation surrounding a dark necrotic center; or it may take the form of the pulmonary or – less commonly – the intestinal type, which follows inhalation of dust containing anthrax spores, as has occurred in the woolen industries. Monkeys exposed to artificially generated aerosols of anthrax spores develop symptoms mimicking woolsorters' disease. Postmodern findings include hemorrhages in the lung, **hemorrhagic mediastinitis** and **lymphadenitis**, and sometimes **hemorrhagic meningitis**.

History

In the past, outbreaks of anthrax (along with other epizootic diseases) among animals have undoubtedly helped to prepare the way for major outbreaks of epidemic disease in humans. When anthrax has decimated herds of cattle or sheep, for example, human populations have faced starvation, which in turn has lowered their ability to resist those epidemics. Anthrax has been known from antiquity, although until relatively recently it was not clearly separated from other diseases with similar manifestations. Possibly, sudden death of animals at pasture, blamed by Aristotle (and subsequently by his followers over the centuries) on the shrew-mouse and its "poisonous bite," may in many cases have resulted from the peracute form of anthrax commonly known as splenic apoplexy.

Nineteenth century authors speculated that the fifth and sixth plagues of the Egyptians (as described in *Exodus*), which struck their herds and the Egyptians themselves, might have been anthrax. Evidence centers on the Israelites, who were installed on sandy ground above the level of the Nile. They escaped the plagues, whereas those who did not lived in areas subject to flooding, which could have provided perfect conditions for growth of the bacillus. Three decades before the birth of Christ, Virgil vividly described an animal plague that had much in common with anthrax and warned against its transmission to people through contact with infected hides.

Through the centuries, there are many records of animal plagues that almost certainly were anthrax but were often confused with other complaints. By 1769, when identification of epidemic diseases of animals and humans had become more precise, Jean Fournier in Dijon, France, classified a number of different lesions as a single disease entity (anthrax), which he called *charbon malin*. More importantly, he recognized the transmission of the disease to people and drew attention to cases occurring in workers who handled raw hair and wool, a theme developed in several French accounts during the following decade. From the mid-nineteenth century, the disease became a problem in English factories as well, and subsequently in Scotland. About the same time, the woolen industries began experiencing the problem as wool and hair from the East were introduced into British trade. Woolsorting, until then considered a particularly healthful occupation, suddenly produced an alarming increase in the number of deaths and extent of disease among workers. The workers themselves suspected an association between the disease and the growing proportion of wool and hair imported from the East. By the late 1870s, concern in Yorkshire factories was acute, but by then the new bacteriology had identified the cause of anthrax: J. Bell demonstrated that both woolsorters' disease and malignant pustule in humans derived from anthrax in animals.

Bell's work was made possible by the work of Davaine and that of Robert Koch in the 1860s and 1870s. During the nineteenth century, the study of anthrax and its use of animal models had become an important part of the framework for the emergence of bacteriology as an academic discipline. In France, Eloy Barthélemy established the transmissibility of anthrax in 1823. From 1850 onward, study of the putative agent was pursued, beginning with the results obtained by Aloys Pollender, then by Pierre Rayer, and finally by Davaine who, during extensive work with guinea pigs in the 1860s, bestowed on it the name of *bactéridie*, which survived in the literature for a long time. From 1876 onward, the anthrax bacillus became a cornerstone of both Koch's theories and his development of pure culture methods; in the late 1870s, W. Greenfield and H. Toussaint reported studies of acquired immunity against anthrax in animals. Pasteur took over the field and in 1881 demonstrated that immunity could be produced through vaccination of sheep.

Lise Wilkinson

9. Apoplexy and Stroke

The old, very popular, and quite international term **apoplexy** (or its equivalents "apoplectic attack," "apoplectic ictus," and "ictus") today generally means **stroke**. The word "apoplexy" comes from the Greek meaning "stroke" and "to strike." To define apoplexy is therefore to relate the history of the word and its different successive significations. This is followed by the medical details of stroke.

History

In the Hippocratic corpus, "apoplexy" appears as an obviously clinical term. For many centuries after Galen's writings of the second century A.D., it was thought that apoplexy involved brain matter, whereas **epilepsy** represented a disturbance of brain function. From the invention of the printing press to the late nineteenth century, several hundred monographs were devoted to apoplexy.

The first autopsies involving examination of the brain were performed in the seventeenth century. In 1761, Giovanni Battista Morgagni reported numerous cases of postmortem examinations of apoplexy, which he separated into "serous apoplexy" (*apoplexia serosa*) and "sanguineous apoplexy" (*apoplexia sanguinea*).

In 1820, John Cooke wrote that he considered hemorrhagic lesions the commonest and that other types of lesions (e.g., tumors, suppuration, cysts) were questionable cases of apoplexy. In a book published in 1812, John Cheyne thought that apoplexy might be "serous" or "sanguineous," but he was skeptical of the former entity. Periodic **apnea**, now known as Cheyne-Stokes respiration, was first described by Cheyne in 1818. For John Abercrombie, writing in 1828, the cerebral lesion of apoplexy might be either a hemorrhage or a serous effusion, but sometimes there seemed to be no apparent anatomic lesions.

Jean Cruveilhier, professor of morbid anatomy in Paris, used the word "apoplexy" as a synonym for "hemorrhage" (in its anatomic, pathological meaning). He distinguished "apoplexy without loss of consciousness" from "apoplexy with loss of consciousness" and wrote of pontine or spinal apoplexies as well as cerebral ones. This pathological point of view was strengthened by Richard Bright, who described and illustrated under the term "apoplexy" several cases of **cerebral hemorrhage**. This association of apoplexy with hemorrhage in the central nervous system led gradually to the use of apoplexy as a synonym for hemorrhage and to the creation of expressions such as "spinal apoplexy" (in place of "spinal hemorrhage"), "pulmonary apoplexy" (in place of "hemorrhagic pulmonary infarct"), "abdominal apoplexy" (in place of "massive abdominal hemorrhage"), "renal apoplexy" (in place of "renal hemorrhage"), "splenic apoplexy" (in place of "hemorrhage of the spleen"), and so forth.

From the second half of the nineteenth century to the early twentieth century, the semantic confusion between apoplexy and hemorrhage continued. Russell Reynolds, for example, in 1866 stated that an apoplectic attack could result from congestion, hemorrhage, tumor, uremia, or vascular obstruction. But A. Trousseau, a professor in Paris, had attacked this problem of confusion in 1865, and French neurologist J. Charcot later emphasized that apoplexy was a clinical syndrome that unfortunately was often used synonymously with cerebral hemorrhage.

Thus, Trousseau and Charcot, along with others, concluded that apoplexy could arise from conditions other than intracerebral hemorrhage, and that the use of the term should be restricted to the clinical syndrome that involved a sudden loss of brain functions. Surprisingly, in 1921 J. Lhermitte nonetheless persisted in the use of apoplexy as a synonym for hemorrhage and opposed "hemiplegy of the apoplexy" and "hemiplegy of the infarctus."

The term "apoplexy" has since become obsolete and disappeared from most contemporary textbooks and from the usual vocabulary of the modern physician. Nevertheless, it remains widely used in popular language and literature. Its proper use, however, should be restricted to the history of medicine, from Hippocrates to the beginning of the twentieth century. In present medical vocabulary, the term "apoplexy" must be replaced by either "stroke" or "hemorrhage," according to the context.

Characteristics of Stroke

According to the World Health Organization, a stroke consists of "rapidly developing clinical signs of focal (at times global) disturbance of cerebral function, lasting more than 24 hours or leading to death with no apparent causes other than that of vascular origin." "Global" refers to patients in deep coma and those with subarachnoid hemorrhage. This definition excludes transient ischemic attacks (TIAs), a condition in which signs last less than 24 hours.

Strokes are the most common life-threatening neurological disease and the third leading cause of death, after heart disease and cancer, in Europe and the United States. Death rates from strokes vary with age and sex; for example, in the United States, the rates for males are 11.9 per 100,000 for those aged 40–44 and 1,217 per 100,000 for those aged 80–84. For females, the respective rates are 10.9 and 1,067. Large differences in **cerebrovascular disease** (CVD) mortality have been noted among races. For example, in the United States, mortality is 344 per 100,000 for nonwhites but 124 per 100,000 for whites. Among countries, differences in mortality from stroke ranged from 70 per 100,000 in Switzerland to 519 per 100,000 in Japan.

Decline in CVD deaths has occurred in all developed countries since 1915, and the decline accelerated in recent decades. The acceleration seems related to a decline in incidence. Strokes, however, are more disabling than lethal: 20–30 percent of survivors become permanently and severely handicapped. Moreover, recurrent strokes are observed in 15–40 percent of stroke survivors.

Apart from age, the most important risk factor for CVD is arterial **hypertension**. Control of severe and moderate, and even mild, hypertension has been shown to reduce stroke occurrence and stroke fatality. Cardiac impairment ranks third, following age and hypertensive disease. At any level of blood pressure, people with **cardiac disease**, occult or overt, have more than twice the risk of stroke. Other risk factors are cigarette smoking, increased total serum cholesterol, blood hemoglobin concentration, **obesity**, and use of oral contraceptives.

Strokes are a heterogeneous entity caused by **cerebral infarction** or, less commonly, cerebral hemorrhage. Cerebral infarction accounts for the majority of strokes. When perfusion pressure falls in a cerebral artery below critical levels, brain **ischemia** (deficiency of blood) develops, progressing to infarction if the effect persists long enough. In most cases, ischemia is caused by occlusion of an intracerebral artery by a thrombus or an embolus arising from extracranial artery disease or a cardiac source. The main cause of ischemic strokes is atherosclerotic brain infarction, the result of either intracerebral artery thrombosis or embolism arising from stenosed (narrowed or restricted) or occluded extracranial arteries.

Lacunar infarction (14 percent of ischemic strokes) is a small, deep infarct in the territory of a single penetrating artery, occluded by the parietal changes caused by hypertensive disease. Cerebral embolism from a cardiac source (15–30 percent of ischemic strokes) is mainly caused by atrial fibrillation related to valvular disease or ischemic heart disease. Other causes of cerebral infarction are multiple, resulting from various diseases, hemopathies, or coagulation abnormalities. However, in 20 percent of cases, the cause of cerebral infarction remains undetermined.

Intracranial hemorrhage (ICH) accounts for 37 percent of strokes. The main cause of ICH is the rupture of miliary aneurysms that have developed in the walls of interior arteries because of hypertensive disease. Nonhypertensive causes of ICH are numerous.

Clinical manifestations of strokes depend on both the nature of the lesion (ischemic or hemorrhagic) and the part of the brain involved. In the 1960s, a classification of strokes according to temporal profile was proposed to promote common terminology in discussion of history and treatment.

The term "incipient stroke" (also TIA) was defined as brief (less than 24 hours), intermittent, and focal neurological deficits from cerebral ischemia, with the patient normal between attacks. The term "reversible ischemic neurological deficit" was coined for entirely reversible deficits occurring over more than 24 hours. The term "progressing stroke" (stroke-in-evolution) is applied to focal cerebral deficits observed by the physician to progress in severity of neurological deficit over a period of hours or, occasionally, a few days.

The term "completed stroke" is used when neurological signs are stable and no progression has been noted over 18–72 hours. "Major stroke" is applied when immediate coma or massive neurological deficit occurs. In these cases, chances of recovery and effective treatment are minimal. "Minor stroke," by contrast, is applied to cases where deficits relate to only a restricted area of a cerebral hemisphere, or where the symptoms experienced are of only moderate intensity. With minor strokes, diagnosis and institution of treatment should be rapidly combined to avoid further deterioration and, if possible, facilitate the regression of deficit.

These definitions contain some obvious uncertainties, particularly in categorizing a stroke during the early hours. However, they underscore the fact that the management of a stroke often depends more on its temporal profile and on the severity of neurological deficit than on the nature of the lesion.

Jacques Poirier and Christian Derouesne

10. Arboviruses

Arbovirus is a truncated term for arthropod-borne viruses, all of which require multiplication in their vectors for transmission. **Arboviral diseases** may be simpler to understand when viewed solely from the position of the end product, which is disease in humans or other vertebrates. The diseases fall into a few recognizable sets: (1) **encephalitides**; (2) diseases with fever and rash, often fairly benign; (3) diseases with hemorrhagic manifestations, often fatal; and (4) mild fevers, quite undiagnosable except through laboratory study. A common feature of all of these is periodic outbreaks, with dozens, hundreds, or thousands of cases. A second common feature is lack of specific treatment. In addition, vaccines exist for only a very few of the diseases. Possibility of disease control is real, however, and is based on a knowledge of the epidemiology of arbovirus infections in general, the role that vectors play, and the particular features in regard to the transmission of the specific disease in question.

General Characteristics

Arboviruses, numbering at latest count 512 separate and identifiable agents, are placed in 11 families, with a few unclassified agents. There is no simple delimiting definition of an arbovirus on a taxonomic basis, or even on a biochemical basis. Viruses must qualify in several important points to be considered arboviruses. The life cycle of an arbovirus involves an arthropod (usually insect, tick, or mite) that is capable of becoming infected itself when it imbibes the virus from an infected host. The arthropods serve as vectors of the virus, from an infected vertebrate host to an uninfected one. The virus must multiply in the arthropod, a process requiring several days, and reach a concentration sufficient to be passed, in a later feeding, to the host, and to induce an infection in that host. The host, in turn, must have a viremic phase in order to pass the virus back to a biting or sucking arthropod.

This rigid definition can give rise to confusion but is uncompromising. The confusion is compounded when it is realized that although an arthropod, with mouth parts freshly contaminated by feeding on an infected host, may possibly transmit virus mechanically, a defined vector must be capable of multiplying the virus internally over a period of several days and of transmitting it by then biting a susceptible host in later feedings. This is referred to as the biological transmission cycle. Mechanical transmission must be quite unusual and with respect to arboviruses has never been observed in nature, but has been achieved in the laboratory under controlled conditions. Again, from the point of view of the virus, it must be capable of multiplying in one or more vertebrate hosts, usually over a period of several days, reaching a level in the bloodstream adequate to infect a foraging vector.

The above considerations define (1) the interval between the arthropod's ingestion of infected blood and the ability to transmit virus biologically, again by biting, to a susceptible host (the extrinsic incubation period); and (2) the period, in the host, before the viremia level rises to a height necessary to infect the biting arthropod (the intrinsic incubation period). The minimum interval between infection in one vertebrate host and acquisition of infection by the next vertebrate host is the sum of the extrinsic and intrinsic incubation periods. It is frequently a week or more, and the maximum interval from one infection to the next may be weeks or months.

Arboviruses that are of importance to humans or other vertebrates are not all alike. Size varies considerably – as does shape – and there are other differential characteristics. Again, the common bond is biological transmission by arthropod to vertebrate. How, in the evolution of viruses, this ability to exploit two phyla of living creatures arose again and again in such widely different taxa, is not known.

When the science of epidemiology of the nineteenth century was applied to the study of **yellow fever**, epidemiologists were hampered by a lack of knowledge of infectious agents and of vector arthropods in the transmission cycle. Consequently, there was great confusion and an endless diatribe surrounding various hypotheses on how infection could travel so mysteriously from place to place, with infections occurring in people who apparently never had contact with a case. With Theobald Smith's demonstration in cattle of transmission of the **Texas redwater fever** organism by ticks, Ronald Ross's demonstration of transmission of the parasite of **malaria** by mosquitoes, and Walter Reed's demonstration of transmission of the virus of yellow fever by mosquitoes, came the dawn of modern epidemiological studies on arthropod-transmitted diseases.

A mysterious specificity exists between certain feeding arthropods and certain viruses; furthermore, a preferential feeding of certain arthropods (mosquitoes, for example) on certain food sources is shown. Some vertebrates react to a specific virus with severe disease. Yellow fever, for example, produces severe illness in humans, laboratory white mice, rhesus monkeys, and Alouatta monkeys. On the other hand, yellow fever may infect dogs, cats, Cebus monkeys, cows, and horses without producing overt disease. Among the encephalitides, **eastern equine encephalitis** (EEE) virus (endemic strains) can produce severe disease and death in humans, laboratory mice, certain other vertebrates, and very specifically equines. But cattle do not develop illness with this agent, nor do sheep, goats, dogs, or cats. By contrast, the South American EEE strain that kills horses produces no illness in humans but does produce detectable antibodies.

The resistance of various vertebrates to various arboviruses can be of use to the investigator because it permits the production of large quantities of immune sera in such vertebrates. Such immune sera are of minimal importance in treating disease in humans, but are of cardinal importance in the design of specific serologic tests for virus identification. Modern techniques, founded on studies carried out over a period of half a century, involving basic laboratory techniques of complement fixation, precipitation, electrophoresis, centrifugation, hemagglutination inhibition, and virus neutralization, have been extended by later advances such as "tagged" antibodies – that is, the use of monoclonal antibodies in combination with "tagged probes" in electron microscopy. Such new techniques, involving the use of specific "probes," are currently a fertile area of research, from which is emerging a more rational and complete knowledge of the virus particle itself and its interactions with vertebrate and invertebrate hosts.

Dengue

Geographic distribution of viruses and disease is determined by the characteristics of the vectors rather than by the characteristics of the viruses. Taking **dengue** viruses (genus *Flavivirus*) as an example, the limits of their distribution are defined by the limits of the distribution of the principal vector, *Aedes aegypti*. This mosquito, originally found in Southeast Asia, spread worldwide, traveling wherever humans traveled and established itself in tropical and subtropical and often temperate regions, but not in Arctic and Antarctic polar extremes. The dengue viruses moved with the vectors and became established worldwide, particularly in tropical and subtropical regions. The viruses may have had, in their original territories of Southeast Asia, cycles involving *A. aegypti* and/or *Aedes albopictus* and subhuman forest primates, but as the viruses left their original home, they adapted to a vector-human-vector cycle, allowing them to exist in endemic form wherever humans exist and to appear in epidemic form at intervals.

The other Southeast Asian vector, *A. albopictus*, has of recent years established itself in other countries such as the United States, with unknown potential for involvement in the life cycles of still other viruses such as yellow fever. There are also other aedine vectors of dengue in Polynesia. The dengues are placed in four serotypes, one or more of which are associated with often-fatal manifestations of **dengue hemorrhagic fever** and **dengue shock syndrome**. These are important causes of mortality in small children in countries of Southeast Asia, with scattered cases being seen elsewhere. It is hypothesized that sequential infections in the same individual by different serotypes of dengue may lead to these serious complications.

Yellow Fever

Yellow fever, a *Flavivirus* serologically related to the dengues, is also capable of being transmitted from human to human by *A. aegypti* and can maintain itself endemically in a human population by such means. The virus is found in Africa south of the Sahara and in the equatorial South American jungle regions. In both Africa and South America (here including Central America, and the West Indies), and in the United States, Spain, France, Gibraltar, and England, periodic outbreaks of the disease have been observed, as *A. aegypti* may establish itself in subtropical and even temperate locales. Although *A. aegypti* (and *A. albopictus*) is prevalent in Asia and Australia, yellow fever has never established itself in these regions. With vectors present, as well as millions of nonimmune humans, there is a continuing threat of its introduction.

A reason yellow fever has been able to maintain itself in tropical South America and Africa is that the virus can utilize a different set of vectors. Using various endemic *Haemagogus* or *Aedes* species, the virus remains established as an endemic virosis in various subhuman primates of these regions. This maintenance cycle is referred to as "sylvan" or "jungle" yellow fever. The sylvan *Haemagogus* or *Aedes* can and often does bite humans, and thus can transfer the virus out of the mosquito-monkey-mosquito cycle into a mosquito-human-mosquito cycle. An infected forest worker in the early stage of illness can migrate to an urban setting infested with *A. aegypti* and establish the dreaded urban mosquito-human-mosquito cycle. Recently, several large outbreaks of this type have occurred in Africa and in South America, some of them involving the deaths of thousands of people such as in the Nigeria epidemic in 1986.

A completely effective attenuated yellow fever vaccine (17D) has been available since 1935, but governments in regions where yellow fever is endemic have failed to react adequately in getting the population at risk immunized. Mosquito-control programs often suffer from a similar bureaucratic inefficiency.

Encephalitides

Another group of arboviruses, the encephalitides, present mechanisms quite different from the dengue or yellow fever models. The vectors in question – mosquitoes and ticks – are themselves geographically delimited, and therefore the specific viruses associated with specific vectors have little chance of spread beyond natural ecological barriers. The viruses themselves have a basic vertebrate cycle in birds and small mammals. Certain of the viruses, such as **Venezuelan equine encephalitis**, **EEE**, and **western equine encephalitis**, can escape from their natural cycle between mosquitoes and small vertebrates and spread like wildfire in one or another of the larger vertebrates, causing widespread mortality, and humans may be thus involved. These epidemics are sporadic and unpredictable.

Other viruses are associated particularly with birds and mosquitoes. These viruses include **St. Louis encephalitis** virus of the Americas, **Japanese encephalitis** virus of the Orient, **Murray Valley encephalitis** of Australia and New Guinea, **Ilheus virus** of South America and Trinidad, **Rocio virus** of southeast Brazil, and **West Nile virus** of Africa, the Middle East, and India (now a threat in the United States). The viruses are often very prevalent in a region, in birds, with the disease usually being uncommon in humans, but sometimes occurring in large epidemics. Heron rookeries and pig farms in the Orient have been shown to be Japanese encephalitis virus-amplifying localities, providing opportunities for infection of large numbers of mosquito vectors and thus facilitating large-scale transmission of virus to humans. Immunity rates in populations are often high (bespeaking inapparent infections), and encephalitis rates low.

In the central United States, a recent arrival on the virus scene, **La Crosse virus**, a member of the California virus group, has established its position as the commonest arboviral cause of encephalitis. This endemic disease has some unusual features. It is transmitted by woodland aedine mosquitoes and has as vertebrate hosts certain small mammals of the region. It has been further established that the virus can be transmitted transovarially (TOT) from mosquito to mosquito, vertically through the egg, and laterally from female to male or from male to female during copulation. This mechanism has been hypothesized to explain the long persistence of virus in a vector, serving to carry it over periods of inclement weather or drought. Similar TOT has been shown for dengue, Japanese encephalitis, and yellow fever.

Tick-borne encephalitis (**Russian spring-summer encephalitis [RSSE]** in the Eurasian continent and **Powassan virus encephalitis** in North America) are delimited by the range of specific tick vectors; these viruses are endemic in small mammals and present themselves in humans as sporadic cases.

Treatment and Control

The early days of onset of most arboviral infections are usually accompanied by fevers, aching, and general malaise and cannot be distinguished from early stages of other very common diseases such as **influenza**, malaria, **measles**, pneumonias, **meningitis**, other respiratory afflictions, and even **Lassa fever** and **smallpox**. As diseases progress in their course, specific later manifestations may provide aid

in differential diagnosis. Such specific manifestations include rashes, eruptions, nausea and vomiting, diarrhea, cough, and encephalitis.

Definitive diagnosis demands the assistance of experienced virologists working in adequate laboratory diagnostic facilities. Only a few dozen such facilities exist in the world, supported by the World Health Organization, governments, military establishments, and, in a few instances, private philanthropy. Such laboratories usually combine laboratory diagnostic methodology and facilities for carrying out field epidemiological studies.

Specific diagnosis rarely benefits the patient but is of vital importance in alerting health departments of the presence of a potentially threatening epidemic. Appropriate control procedures directed at the vectors can then be applied on an emergency basis. In the special case of yellow fever, mass immunization of exposed populations can successfully halt an epidemic in its tracks. Such an immunization campaign is usually combined with emergency mosquito control.

Aside from provision of nursing care, and maintaining nutrition and fluid balance, there are no specific remedies for infections. Nonspecific measures, particularly treatment of shock (maintaining fluid and electrolyte balance), may be lifesaving in dengue shock syndrome cases.

Vector control is applicable in certain situations. Fred Soper and co-workers in the 1930s eradicated *A. aegypti* from all of Brazil, thus eliminating the risk of urban yellow fever. The mosquito, however, has reinvaded much of its former territory, and the threat of yellow fever has returned. Short-term vector control is widely practiced, particularly when epidemics threaten. This may include airplane spraying of insecticides, treatment of interior walls of buildings with residual insecticides, insecticide treatment of mosquito breeding places, destruction or drainage of mosquito breeding places, screening of dwellings, use of insecticidal fogs in and around dwellings, use of insect repellents, and wearing of protective clothing.

The attenuated live yellow fever virus vaccine (17D) has been used for over 50 years in the successful immunization of millions of people. A live attenuated dengue virus vaccine is being tried. A killed Japanese encephalitis virus vaccine is given to millions of people in the Orient. A killed RSSE virus vaccine is used extensively in parts of the former Soviet Union. Killed virus vaccines against EEE, western equine encephalitis, Venezuelan equine encephalitis, and **Rift Valley fever** virus are used primarily to protect livestock. Laboratory workers studying these viruses are routinely immunized.

Wilbur G. Downs

11. Arenaviruses

Several of the Arenaviridae are important human disease viruses. They are not arboviruses but have been discovered largely by arbovirologists. Most of the 14 arenaviruses have rodents as reservoir hosts but occasionally infect humans in contact with rodent-contaminated environments. **Lassa virus**, however, is known to pass directly from person to person, particularly in hospital settings. Others are **Junin virus (Argentine hemorrhagic fever)**, **Machupo virus (Bolivian hemorrhagic fever)**, and the virus that causes **lymphocytic choriomeningitis (LCM)**. Six arenaviruses – Junin, Machupo, **Pichinde**, **Tacaribe**, Lassa, and LCM – have infected laboratory workers.

History

The first arenavirus discovered was that causing LCM in mice and monkeys. It was reported in 1934 by C. Armstrong and R. D. Lillie. Studies showed that it was present in feral *Mus musculus* (the common house mouse) and afflicted a few humans annually in Europe and North America. Usually, such cases involved personnel handling laboratory animals, particularly mice and hamsters. No serologic relatives of the virus were found, and only scattered cases and outbreaks have ever been reported.

In 1957, a virus named Tacaribe was recovered from a fruit-eating bat in Trinidad. This agent remained unclassified. Meanwhile, fieldworkers in Argentina suffered a disease that occurred at harvest and caused considerable mortality. A virus named Junin was recovered from these patients, and the disease was named Argentine hemorrhagic fever. Cases occur annually, and epidemics occasionally.

A particularly virulent infection – later named Bolivian hemorrhagic fever – attacked the small town of San Joaquin, Bolivia. The outbreak was checked after the rodent host of the Machupo virus was implicated and rodent-control mechanisms were instituted. Since then Machupo virus has "gone underground," with no further outbreaks and little research in progress.

In January 1969, another arenavirus attracted attention with an outbreak among medical personnel in Lassa, Nigeria. At least seven more outbreaks of **Lassa fever** have occurred since then. The virus appears to have a natural cycle of transmission in rodents but, as previously mentioned, can spread from human to human.

The other Arenaviridae are apparently nonpathogenic for humans. Epidemiological information about them is scanty, although several – particularly Tacaribe and Pichinde – have been studied intensively in the laboratory.

General Characteristics

A rodent association is usually found. Exceptions are Tacaribe, isolated several times from bats in Trinidad, and two recently associated agents, **Quaranfil** and **Johnston Atoll**, found in birds and tick ectoparasites of birds.

A fascinating feature is the geographic host range of the Arenaviridae. Each rodent species involved has its ecologically determined range, thus delimiting the distribution of its virus. The exception is the house mouse. *M. musculus* is well adapted to human environments and has worldwide distribution, particularly in temperate regions of North America, Europe, and Asia. It moves where humans move, although in the tropics it remains more restricted to coastal and riverine settlements.

Praomys natalensis, the multimammate mouse, is also common and commensal with humans. Widely distributed in Africa, it is associated with Lassa virus and **Mopeia virus**. *Praomys jacksoni* is associated with **Mobala virus** in central Africa. (Currently, *Mastomys*, *Myomys*, and *Myomyscus* are all considered synonymous with *Praomys*.)

New World rodents hosting arenaviruses are all in the family Cricetidae. It is likely that there have been many opportunities for virus dispersal as well as adaptation of viruses to new rodent hosts, and it seems evident that the whole world is at risk for species radiation of Arenaviridae.

Lymphocytic Choriomeningitis (LCM)

LCM has been found in the Americas, Europe, and Asia, but not in Africa and Australia. The disease in humans is usually benign, with symptoms resembling **influenza**. Inapparent cases are frequent during outbreaks. **Meningitis** may occur as a primary symptom or more usually as a relapse several days after apparent recovery. In some cases, meningoencephalitic symptoms occur, with reflex changes, paralyses, **cutaneous anesthesias**, and somnolence. Fatal cases are rare. When infections occur in pregnancy, complications in the fetus and newborn may be seen. Treatment is limited to supportive care. Control is limited to control of residential mouse populations and to vigilant supervision of laboratory colonies of mice and hamsters.

Argentine Hemorrhagic Fever (Junin)

This disease occurs in the heavily agricultural pampas west of Buenos Aires. It is seen in rural regions, mostly in farm workers. Several hundred cases occur annually, mainly in the harvest season between April and July. Infection in humans results from contact with field rodents. The incubation period is 10–14 days, and an insidious onset begins with malaise, fever, chills, head and back pains, nausea, vomiting, and **diarrhea** or constipation. Hemorrhagic manifestations may proceed to death (in about 10 percent of cases). In some cases, neurological symptoms predominate.

Convalescence lasts several weeks after severe illness, and recovery is usually complete. No specific antiviral agents are known but recent reports describe successful treatment with immune plasma. When given before the eighth day of illness, it markedly reduces mortality. Rodent control appears an obvious prevention measure but is impractical given the vast areas of endemicity. A live attenuated vaccine shows promise for preventing the disease in humans. Another possibility being explored utilizes the avirulent Tacaribe virus to induce immunity against Junin.

Bolivian Hemorrhagic Fever (Machupo)

This disease is localized in several provinces of Bolivia in the Amazonian lowlands and is endemic in local rodent (*Calomys*) populations. Exposed humans have an incubation period of about 2 weeks. Patients manifest high fever for at least 5 days, along with **myalgia**, headache, **conjunctivitis**, **cutaneous hyperesthesia**, nausea, and vomiting. Hemorrhagic manifestations occur in some 30 percent of patients; serious bleeding is possible. **Hypotension** in the second week of illness is seen in about 50 percent of patients – in many proceeding to **hypovolemic shock** and death. Symptoms of central nervous system involvement appear in almost half of the cases. The death rate in several epidemics has been about 25 percent. Convalescence is protracted. Pathological findings include generalized adenopathy and focal hemorrhages in various organs. No specific therapy is known. Treatment is limited to supportive measures. Rodent control in homes and villages has proven effective in controlling epidemics as well as sporadic cases.

Wilbur G. Downs

12. Arthritis (Rheumatoid)

Rheumatoid arthritis, the major crippling illness among chronic rheumatic disorders, is a systemic disease affecting joints with an inflammatory reaction lasting months or years. Frequently, the small joints of hands and feet are affected first, although often the larger peripheral joints of the wrists, hips, knees, elbows, and shoulders are involved as well. Some remissions occur, but the illness progresses to damage and deformity. Its etiology is unknown.

Characteristics

The prevalence of rheumatoid arthritis is consistently between 1 and 2 percent of the adult population in all parts of the globe. Females suffer the illness about two and a half times more frequently than males, although prevalence increases for both sexes over age 35, making it normally a disease of the middle years. The number of new cases per year ranges from 0.68 to 2.9 per 1,000 population.

Despite years of intensive study of endocrine, metabolic, and nutritional factors as well as geographic, occupational, and psychological variables, the etiology of rheumatoid arthritis has not been elucidated. A genetic predisposition is suspected; however, bacterial and viral infections are often associated with acute **polyarthritis** in humans, and thus an infection followed by an altered or sustained immunologic response could be instrumental.

Certainly, immunologic abnormalities appear to play a role in both aggravation and perpetuation of the inflammatory process. Immunologic reactions occur at the local site (joints) and often systemically. Production of antiimmunoglobulins or rheumatoid factors occurs initially in the inflammatory tissue of joints and can subsequently be detected in the serum of 80 percent of patients; those who are seropositive for rheumatoid factor show a more marked progression of the disease than do those who are seronegative.

The onset and course of rheumatoid arthritis are particularly variable. Usually, fatigue, weight loss, and generalized aching and stiffness, especially on awakening in the morning, precede localization of symptoms and joint swelling. These symptoms at times develop explosively in one or more joints, but more often there is progression to multiple joint involvement. The disease may remit spontaneously in the first year or diminish in intensity, only to recur in the same or additional joints at intervals.

The more troublesome cases affect many joints with sustained inflammatory reactions for months or years, with marked bone and joint damage, ulna drift, and consequent deviation of fingers, leading to limited function and instability. Signs of systemic involvement may also be seen: nodules at the elbows, **cutaneous degeneration** at the fingertips or elbow, **pulmonary fibrosis**, inflammation of the sac enclosing the heart, **anemia**, fever, rash and peripheral ulcers in the lower limbs, disease of the nervous system, and wrist weakness occasioned by **carpaltunnel syndrome**. In addition, there is usually gradual weight loss as well as loss of muscle volume and power.

Although there is no cure, a number of medical and surgical modalities are available to manage patients over the course of the disease. Drug therapy is an important part of this management as it is directed toward controlling the destructive inflammatory processes within the joint.

History

The clinical term "rheumatoid arthritis" was first introduced in medical literature by A. B. Garrod in 1859. It was not in common usage, however, until "officially recognized" in Britain by the Department of Health in 1922 and by the American Rheumatism Association in 1941. Until recent times, many names were used to describe the condition: "rheumatic gout," "chronic rheumatic arthritis," *goutte asthenique primative, rheumatismus nodosus,* and "rheumatoid osteoarthritis." Broader terms such as **gout**, **arthritis**, and **rheumatism** also encompassed rheumatoid arthritis as well as numerous other conditions.

Evidence for the existence of rheumatoid arthritis in earlier times, however, must be gleaned from literature, from art, and from paleopathological studies of ancient bones; to date that evidence has been far from overwhelming. Indeed, the lack of early descriptions of this disease has led some authors to suggest that it is recent in origin (i.e., since the seventeenth century) and is evolving to develop a peak incidence before ultimately disappearing.

By contrast, other arthritic disorders such as **ankylosing spondylitis**, **osteoarthritis**, and **spinal hyperostosis** have been recognized in skeletons thousands of years old and appear no different from present illnesses. In fact, given the lack of evidence of rheumatoid arthritis until relatively recent times, it has also been suggested that rheumatoid arthritis evolved from ankylosing spondylitis. Uncertainty about the antiquity of rheumatoid arthritis results at least partly from our methods of examining the evidence of a disease whose current definition includes clinical, radiological, and serologic criteria.

European accounts of a disease that was probably rheumatoid arthritis appeared in 1676, 1770, 1800, and 1818. Each described a long-term, chronic, debilitating disease affecting multiple joints, including typical hyperextension deformity of the interphalangeal joints of the fingers.

Before these dates, there are several descriptions of disease that *could* represent phases of rheumatoid arthritis, ranging from acute explosive attack to chronic sustained disability. This is particularly so in the case of Emperor Constantine IX (c. 980–1055), who at age 63 suffered from polyarthritis in the feet and subsequently hands, shoulders, and knees, leading to nodularity and residual deformity in the fingers, and flexion and swelling of the knees. This description does not absolutely exclude **polyarticular gout** or some other erosive joint disease, but it is very suggestive. In the thirteenth century, Bartolemeus Anglicus penned a less complete but also suggestive description.

Perhaps the earliest known description suggestive of rheumatoid arthritis is in the *Caraka Samhita* of India, written about 123 A.D. The disease in question manifested itself as swollen, painful joints – initially in hands and feet and then the whole body. The ailment was reported to be protracted, difficult to cure, and associated with **anorexia**.

In art, attention is drawn to representations of hand deformities in works of Flemish painters (1400–1700), who otherwise painted the ideal unaffected limb with considerable accuracy. Some works of Peter Paul Rubens show changes typical of rheumatoid arthritis, suggesting that Rubens, who himself suffered from rheumatoid arthritis, painted the progressive phases of his own disease in the hands of his subjects during the years 1609–38.

As for paleopathology, thousands of ancient mummies and skeletons have been examined, but surprisingly few show features compatible with rheumatoid arthritis. Of course, determination of the required symmetrical pattern of joint disease is not possible when one or more long bones are missing, and the small bones of hands and feet are frequently lost.

Although rheumatoid arthritis is at present a major cause of **symmetrical erosive polyarthritis**, other causes do exist, and thus it seems appropriate to employ the term **erosive joint disease** (which may or may not have been rheumatoid arthritis) when describing the arthritis seen in ancient bones. Some possible ancient cases of rheumatoid arthritis include reports of an Egyptian mummy 5,500 years old, two or three skeletons in Britain dating from Saxon to Roman and British medieval times, and a well-preserved Eskimo mummy.

More recently, reports of erosive polyarthritis occurring in ancient bones ranging from 5,000 to 1,000 years old in North America have been identified. In fact, the researchers investigating these remains have speculated that rheumatoid arthritis could have had a viral origin in North America and then migrated to Europe in the post-Columbian period, where it manifested itself as a more severe disease in subsequent centuries. This, they argue, might account for the apparent relative infrequency of the disease in Europe prior to the seventeenth century.

Today, the disease afflicts most ethnic groups in all parts of the world. Thus, only detailed studies and precise reports on skeletal remains can establish whether **erosive arthritis**, which may have been rheumatoid arthritis, was more or less prevalent in the past than it is currently. These findings could impact considerably upon our understanding of the disease and perhaps also suggest whether it is likely to disappear, as some have argued.

Howard Duncan and James C. C. Leisen

13. Ascariasis

The giant intestinal roundworm, *Ascaris lumbricoides*, is a common parasite with worldwide distribution. Adult worms are 15–35 cm (6–14 inches) long and reside in the lumen of the small intestine. Sometimes, however, they are passed in the feces and, if vomited into the oral cavity, may exit from the host's mouth or nostrils; thus they have been known to medical observers for millennia. Female worms produce up to 200,000 fertilized eggs daily, which are passed in the feces. Eggs incubate in soil for at least 2–3 weeks to produce an infective larval stage within them. The eggs are resistant to chemicals, desiccation, and extreme temperatures but mature or "embryonate" most rapidly in warm, moist, shady conditions in clay soils. People become infected by eating embryonated eggs in contaminated food or water; or, in the case of toddlers, infection occurs by direct ingestion of eggs with dirt. Poor rural sanitation and the use of human feces for fertilizer obviously favor transmission. Mature eggs hatch in the small intestine, and the larvae then undergo a remarkable migration in the host. They penetrate the intestinal wall and are carried in blood or lymph vessels to the liver and heart, and then the lungs. Here they break out into the air sacs, develop, and molt for about 3 weeks, and then climb up the trachea to the throat, where they are subsequently swallowed to establish themselves as adults in the small intestine.

This nematode was known to ancient writers in China, India, Mesopotamia, and Europe and was present in pre-Columbian America. The World Health Organization has estimated that between 800 and 1,300 million people harbor an average of six worms each. The true figure may be even higher. Surveys have demonstrated infection in more than 50 percent of sampled populations in countries such as Bangladesh, Brazil, China, Colombia, India, Iran, Kenya, Mexico, Tanzania, and Vietnam, and the rate approaches 100 percent in many rural areas. In China, it was estimated that the 1947 *Ascaris* population produced 18,000 tons of eggs a year; they may be even more productive today. The worm is also common in developed countries, although improved sanitation has greatly reduced prevalence in recent decades.

Symptoms of **ascariasis** vary widely. As is often true of helminthic infections, low wormloads may cause few or no symptoms. Large numbers of larvae in the lungs may produce **ascaris pneumonitis**, with symptoms resembling **pneumonia**. Allergic reactions can cause **asthma** attacks. Larvae can reach atypical (ectopic) sites such as the brain, eye, or kidney, where they may produce grave, life-threatening conditions, but such events are fortunately rare. Adult worms in the intestine can cause fever, abdominal discomfort, **diarrhea**, and allergic reactions to their proteins. Fever may induce worms to wander to the larynx, where they can cause suffocation, or to exit the mouth or nostrils. Heavy infection robs the host of nutrients, and tangled masses of worms can result in fatal intestinal obstruction if not treated promptly. **Intestinal ascariasis** is especially serious in young children. In the Third World, ascariasis may produce signs of **protein-energy malnutrition** in many children and often retard their growth. Even if severe effects occur in only a small percentage of cases, the ubiquity of the worm makes it an important cause of morbidity in many countries.

K. David Patterson

14. Bacillary Dysentery

Bacteria from several genera, including *Campylobacter, Salmonella,* and *Yersinia,* as well as some strains of the common intestinal bacillus *Escherichia coli,* can invade mucosa of the large intestine and cause **dysentery**, but members of the genus *Shigella* are by far the most important agents. **Shigellosis** is a common disease that afflicts persons of all races and age groups. In addition, *Campylobacter* appears to be an emerging pathogen, at least in the United States. It lives in the small intestine and produces a dysentery-like condition that is usually self-limiting.

Characteristics

Four species or subgroups of *Shigella* cause human disease. *Shigella dysenteriae,* the first to be discovered, is the most virulent. *Shigella flexneri, Shigella boydii,* and *Shigella sonnei* are less dangerous. More than 40 serotypes are recognized and are useful in tracing the spread of outbreaks.

Shigella organisms are passed in the feces and spread from person to person by the fecal-oral route. Bacteria are excreted during the illness and for about 4 weeks after recovery, but some asymptomatic individuals act as carriers for a year or more. Contaminated food and water are the most common modes of transmission. Direct fecal contamination or mechanical carriage by flies can introduce bacteria into food, milk, or water. Sick, convalescent, or even healthy food handlers with poor hygienic practices are especially dangerous; proper handwashing after defecation is a simple but effective preventive measure. Crowding and poor sanitation favor transmission, and outbreaks are common in jails and institutions. Epizootics have been reported in colonies of primates, and two species have been isolated from dogs, but animal reservoirs have no known epidemiological significance.

Shigellosis occurs worldwide but is especially common in countries with poor water and sewage systems. The virulent *S. dysenteriae* is mostly confined to the tropics and East Asia; a much less pathogenic form, *S. sonnei,* is the most abundant species in the United States. All age groups are vulnerable, but severe disease is most common in children and among the elderly. No racial or ethnic immunity is apparent, although populations can acquire considerable resistance to locally prevalent strains. Travelers may become ill when they encounter unfamiliar strains. Accurate incidence rates are impossible to obtain, but shigellosis is a serious health problem in most underdeveloped countries and a major cause of infant and child mortality. The disease is commonly endemic, but great epidemics also take place. During World War II, acute dysentery, apparently introduced by Japanese and/or Allied troops, attacked indigenous groups in western New Guinea, causing thousands of deaths despite the efforts of Australian authorities. In 1969, an epidemic of *S. dysenteriae* caused 110,000 cases and 8,000 deaths in Guatemala.

Shigellosis is also a constant threat in developed countries, especially when sanitary standards are weakened. For example, two important *S. sonnei* outbreaks occurred in the United States in 1987. One took place among Orthodox Jews in New York, New Jersey, Ohio, and Maryland, with the majority of cases occurring among small children in religious schools. Patterns of spread were consistent with person-to-person transmission among religious communities in the four states. The first outbreak was in New York City, where 132 cases were reported and at least 13,000 were suspected. Smaller epidemics in upstate New York and other states appeared to be linked with Passover visits to relatives in the city. The second epidemic began with the annual meeting of a counter-culture group, the Rainbow Family, in a national forest in North Carolina in early July. Poor hygiene and inadequate latrines allowed infection to spread among the campers, who caused at least four clusters of cases in Missouri and Pennsylvania when they dispersed.

The disease begins when bacteria invade mucosa of the large intestine, where they cause mucus secretion, edema, and, usually, superficial ulceration and bleeding. The watery diarrhea is probably caused by a toxin that increases the secretions of cells of the intestinal wall.

Incubation is from 1 to 4 days. Onset is sudden in children, with fever, drowsiness or irritability, anorexia, nausea, abdominal pain, **tenesmus**, and **diarrhea**. Blood, pus, and mucus appear in diarrheal stools within 3 days. Increasingly frequent watery stools cause dehydration, and death occurs as early as 12 days. If the patient survives, recovery usually begins after about 2 weeks. In adults, there is usually no fever, and the disease resolves itself in 1– 6 weeks. Symptoms in both children and adults may vary from simple, transient diarrhea to acute dysentery and death.

A variety of antibiotics can be effective against various *Shigella* species, but drug resistance is a growing problem. Many strains of *S. sonnei* in the United States have developed such resistance; thus, in cases in which drug therapy is essential, new agents must frequently be employed.

History

Medical writers have described dysentery or "the flux" since ancient times, but the bacterial form of the disease was not clearly distinguished until late in the nineteenth century. Dysentery ravaged Persian armies invading Greece in 480 B.C., and the disease has always been a companion of armies, often proving more destructive than enemy action. This disease was, and remains, common among both rural and urban poor people around the world. An epidemic of what must have been shigellosis swept France in 1779, causing especially severe damage in some rural areas of the western part of the country. Troop movements for a planned invasion of England helped spread the disease. At least 175,000 people died, with some 45,000 deaths in Brittany alone. Children constituted the majority of the fatalities. During the U.S. Civil War, Union soldiers had annual morbidity rates of 876 per 1,000 from dysentery, and annual mortality rates of 10 per 1,000. Dysentery outbreaks were problems for all belligerents in World War I, especially in the Gallipoli and Mesopotamian campaigns.

Bacterial dysenteries took a heavy toll among infants and young children in Western countries until recent times. During the late nineteenth and early twentieth centuries, the decline in breast-feeding and the growing use of cows' milk in European and American cities exposed infants and toddlers to a variety of bacterial and other agents of dysentery and diarrhea. As milk is an excellent growth medium for *Shigella* and many other pathogens, contaminated milk and lack of refrigeration led to especially high death rates in hot weather. Milk-borne shigellosis was a significant contributor to the "summer complaint," which took thousands of young lives annually in cities like Paris and New York. Infant health movements, public-health education, and pasteurization of milk largely eliminated the problem in Western Europe and North America by about 1920. Shigellosis, however, still contributes to the "weanling diarrhea," which afflicts tens of millions of Third World children every year.

Japanese bacteriologist Kiyoshi Shiga isolated *S. dysenteriae* in 1898 and confirmed its role as a pathogen. The other species were discovered early in the twentieth century, and much research has been directed to immunologic studies of various strains. The role of *Campylobacter* species as common human pathogens has been recognized only since the 1970s.

K. David Patterson

15. Beriberi

Beriberi is a disease caused by a deficiency of thiamine that is expressed in three major clusters of symptoms, which vary from person to person. It may involve edema, or swelling, of the legs, arms, and face. The nerves may be affected, causing, first, a loss of sensation in the peripheral nerves and, later, paralysis. The cardiovascular system may be involved, evidenced by enlargement of the heart and extremely low diastolic blood pressure. In its chronic form, beriberi may result in disability for months or years; or it may be acute and produce death in a few weeks. Until major tissue damage occurs, it is curable and reversible by consumption of thiamine.

The name "beriberi" derives from a Sinhalese word, meaning weakness. It has been known in Japan since antiquity and is described in the earliest Chinese medical treatises. The several forms of beriberi have often been considered as separate diseases. In **wet beriberi**, swelling and heart complications occurred, although often with loss of the sense of touch, pain, or temperature. In **dry beriberi**, there was little swelling, but instead a progressive loss of those senses and then of motor control followed by atrophy of the muscles of the paralyzed limbs and a general wasting syndrome. Today it is thought that dry beriberi was partly due to a deficiency of riboflavin. **Shoshin beriberi** was a term used to denote a fulminating, or acute, form with severe heart complications. **Infantile beriberi** was the last form to be recognized; in addition to swelling, heart enlargement, and other cardiovascular complications, suckling infants also had symptoms such as loss of voice and gastrointestinal disturbances, neither of which occurred in adults.

The discovery that beriberi was caused by a nutritional deficiency led to the identification and study of vitamins. The isolation and later synthesis of thiamine resulted in the enrichment of key foods as a public-health intervention. Beriberi was not only a cause of much suffering and death, but also one of the most important diseases in the development of medical science.

Characteristics

Thiamine is vital to every living thing, both plant and animal. It is an essential component of dozens of enzymes that metabolize food. In particular, thiamine is necessary to derive energy from glucose, the preferred food of nerve cells, and from other carbohydrates. It is more indirectly involved in the metabolism of the amino acids isoleucine, leucine, and valine.

Thiamine is a water-soluble vitamin that is found widely in foods. It is most concentrated in whole grains, yeast, and legumes; in liver, heart, and kidneys of most mammals; and in oysters. It is available also in most green vegetables and pork. An antagonistic enzyme produced by bacteria – thiaminase – is found in a few diverse foods such as raw fish and tea. Thiamine deficiency usually results from a shortage of thiamine in the diet, but it can sometimes be exacerbated by the consumption of large amounts of foods high in thiaminase.

The epidemiology of beriberi follows from the role of thiamine in energy metabolism and its deficiency in restricted diets. The populations in which beriberi has been most prevalent have been of two kinds: people confined to institutions, such as prisons, asylums, and naval ships, who are limited to monotonous and restricted diets such as bread and water or fish and rice; and people who derive a large portion of their calories from rice from which milling has removed most of the bran in which thiamine is found.

Beriberi is in large part a disease of rice culture. When rice is the staple food, it is eaten in large quantities and commonly provides 80 percent or more of caloric energy. When the hulls are removed manually, enough bran remains on the rice to provide the necessary thiamine. When the rice is milled in modern plants, however, it is polished into white rice and thiamine is almost entirely eliminated.

Cooking methods are also important in the etiology of the disease. In northern China, Korea, and Japan, the rice hulls were traditionally removed before shipment in order to reduce bulk, and cooking procedures called for the rice to be thoroughly washed several times, removing the thiamine. In Burma and other parts of Southeast Asia, the custom has been to cook rice with excess water that is then discarded with the thiamine it assimilated. By contrast, in the lower

Ganges Valley of India, the custom has been to parboil rice. Steaming the rice before drying and milling it for distribution preserves most of the thiamine in white rice and is protective against beriberi. However, the different taste and texture produced have not been widely acceptable among other peoples in Asia.

Numerous variations in practice are involved in the regional etiology of beriberi. In northeastern Thailand and Laos, for example, people usually steam their glutinous variety of rice – a protective behavior. But, unlike other Thailand natives, they have very limited supplies of fresh fruit or vegetables or meat. They eat fish, most of which is in the form of a fermented raw paste and is high in thiaminase, the destroyer of thiamine.

In eighteenth and nineteenth century Brazil, beriberi was likely endemic among slaves and other workers. The deficiency resulted from a diet of manioc flour and a little dried meat. Manioc flour actually contains less thiamine than does milled rice, and the lean dried meat not only was low in thiamine but also increased the body's need for the vitamin.

Another population at risk has recently been recognized. In urbanized and industrial countries, beriberi occurs most frequently among alcoholics. Chronic alcohol consumption impairs both the absorption of thiamine by the intestine and its storage and utilization in the liver; moreover, relatively enormous amounts of thiamine are required to metabolize the alcohol. When the alcoholic substitutes alcohol for other foods in his diet and curtails consumption of thiamine, **Wernicke's encephalopathy** and other neuropsychiatric disorders associated with beriberi may occur. Other groups at risk of beriberi include individuals undergoing long-term dialysis for renal failure and long-term intravenous feeding.

Beriberi is entirely preventable by the consumption of adequate amounts of thiamine. In the United States, enrichment of white bread with the vitamin virtually eliminated the disease except among alcoholics. More recently, rice enrichment has also proved beneficial.

Beriberi has afflicted poor Americans subsisting mainly on white bread and poor Europeans consuming a monotonous diet of potatoes without meat or vegetables, but the disease is and has been most prevalent among the large Asian populations that consume white rice. In the first decade of the twentieth century, mortality from beriberi was significant in Japan, Malaya, and the Philippines, and even in recent years the disease still occurred throughout Southeast and South Asia as well as in parts of Africa and South America.

The true contemporary incidence of beriberi cannot be determined. As it is so easily treated upon detection by the administration of thiamine, it has almost ceased to be fatal. As a nutritional deficiency, it is rarely reportable at any governmental statistical level. At the subclinical level, however, it probably still occurs widely. In a study in Australia, one in five healthy blood donors and one in three alcoholics were found to be deficient in thiamine.

There was an epidemic of beriberi in the decades following World War II. Before the war, hand-milling of rice was common except in the largest cities. With political and economic development, power-milling spread to the rural hinterland and eventually even to the remote hill country. In the late 1950s, beriberi was thought to be responsible for a quarter or more of the infant mortality in parts of Burma and the Philippines and to be the tenth greatest cause of overall mortality in Thailand. Enrichment of rice has greatly reduced clinical beriberi, but it still occurs.

The complex of symptoms resulting from thiamine deficiency has often been confused by the simultaneous occurrence of other vitamin deficiencies. Thus, some of the symptoms that distinguished dry beriberi were indicative of riboflavin deficiency. A diet deficient in thiamine would usually be deficient in other B vitamins as well. Some of the differences in the manifestation of thiamine deficiency disease among laboring adults, suckling infants, and alcoholics result from such complications.

A person with beriberi classically entered the medical system when he or she developed symptoms of the weakness that gave the disease its name: malaise, heaviness in the lower limbs, loss of strength in the knees and wrists, some loss of sensation, tightness in the chest, palpitations, restlessness, and loss of appetite. Infants also vomited, had diarrhea, and had difficulty breathing.

Edema is one of the important signs and is always present in the early stages. Edema, or **dropsy**, commonly progresses until the lower extremities and the face are swollen. Pain and sensitivity in the calf muscles is an early sign, as muscles begin to swell, degenerate, and atrophy. Swelling of the lining of the intestines can also congest them. Edema of the lungs often causes sudden respiratory distress and, with heart failure, death.

Heart palpitations, even at rest, and a diastolic blood pressure below 60 millimeters of mercury are usually diagnostic. There is an **enlarged heart**, particularly the right ventricle. A **heart murmur** may be heard. An EKG may be normal in a mild case but shows abnormal waves of sinus origin in advanced ones.

First the autonomic, then the sensory, and finally the motor nerves are affected. Chronic cases exhibit progressive degeneration of nerve fibers and loss of coordination, sometimes even of the eyes. Sensibility to tactile stimulation, then to pain, and finally to temperature is lost. When the motor nerves are affected, **paralysis** begins in the lower extremities. Then the fingers weaken, and the hand drops limp at the wrist and contracts into a claw. Eventually, even the intercostal muscles, diaphragm, and speech control muscles are affected.

Other symptoms that commonly occur include a full sensation or cramping of the epigastrium, heartburn, constipation, and mental confusion. Thiamine reverses most of the mental symptoms, but some patients are left permanently with an inability to form new memories (**Korsakoff's psychosis**). In classic beriberi, death results eventually from severe disturbances of the circulatory system and paralysis of the respiratory muscles, ending in heart failure.

History

In the nineteenth century, beriberi was common among troops and institutionalized people around the globe. Apparent epidemics occurred on British ships in the Bay of Bengal, Dutch ships in the East Indies, Norwegian whalers, ships plying the China trade in the Sea of Japan, and ships bringing workers home to India from labor in the French Antilles.

Medical historian August Hirsch noted many contradictions as he described the changing pattern of beriberi in the latter half of the nineteenth century. In a few places, notably Japan, the Malay archipelago, and the state of Minas Gerais in Brazil, the disease was endemic. Beriberi first appeared in Bahia in Brazil in 1866 and then spread – to Sao Paulo and Rio Grande do Sul by 1874, along the Brazilian seacoast, and on into the interior provinces and Paraguay. Similarly, the disease had been known on the coast of Japan but had now spread into interior towns. Earlier opinion had held that a distance of 40–60 miles from a seacoast or great river was enough to give immunity, but the disease now occurred hundreds of miles into the interior of Burma and India as well as Brazil. Its appearance in new places showed that it was not caused by climate, and yet it was associated with the rainy season and hot, humid weather. It also seemed associated with a period of "acclimatization" to an affected area. Beriberi afflicted people of different modes of life, and no particular societal group was spared. Tainted water, however, was contraindicated.

Evidence for a dietary cause was confusing. There seemed to be an association with insufficient diet, especially lack of fat and albumin, and with preponderance of rice and dried fish in the diet. Rice, however, was eaten widely in places where beriberi did not occur, and cases had been observed in Borneo where troops eating beef and eggs contracted the disease whereas laborers on a diet of rice and fish did not.

Hirsch concluded from the global evidence that the cause of beriberi was a peculiar, specific poison and not the climate, weather, soil, manner of living, or diet. The complexity of the disease was not clarified until the twentieth century, when the concept of a nutritional deficiency was developed and replaced the idea of a positive poison. But there were early suspicions that diet was responsible. K. Takaki observed as a student in Europe the low incidence of beriberi among European navies. In 1885, as surgeon general of the Japanese navy, he altered the diet of sailors who had previously been much afflicted with beriberi. The results provided convincing evidence of beriberi's nutritional etiology. He subsequently ordered the protein ration increased for all naval personnel, and barley was added to their diet.

By the late nineteenth century, the Dutch in Indonesia had also become convinced that diet was somehow involved. Experiments were carried out at the penitentiaries of Java in which hand-milled rice was substituted for white rice, and beriberi almost disappeared among the prisoners. In 1890, Christian Eijkman, a Dutch officer in Java, discovered that a paralytic disease with nerve damage characteristic of beriberi could be induced in chickens fed polished rice. He and his successor, Gerrit Grijns, demonstrated in 1900 that this condition could be prevented or cured by feeding rice bran. Later Grijns extracted the water-soluble factor from the bran and used it to treat people.

These Dutch efforts were the first experimental characterization of nutritional deficiencies, and a model essential for later nutritional work had been developed. Its immediate impact was limited, however, because American and Japanese physicians did not read Dutch. In much of the world, the belief continued that beriberi must arise from some toxin or microbe, although none could be found, or from food spoilage.

In 1910 in the Philippines, U.S. Army physician Edward B. Vedder began treating beriberi cases with an extract from rice bran and enrolled the efforts of Robert R. Williams, a scientist at the Bureau of Science in Manila, to isolate the active factor. Soon a Filipino doctor, Jose Albert, identified infantile beriberi and suggested its connection with the poor diets of breast-feeding Filipino mothers.

In 1911, Casimir Funk at the Lister Institute in London isolated a crystalline substance, which he erroneously thought was the antiberiberi factor, and called it a "vitamine." In 1926, two Dutch chemists in Java, B. C. P. Jansen and W. F. Donath, succeeded in isolating and crystallizing the active substance from rice bran. They mischaracterized it, however, by missing its sulfur atom, and other scientists were unable to repeat the isolation.

Williams, then a chemist at Bell Laboratories, continued on his own time and money to try to isolate the antiberiberi factor and succeeded in 1933. He and those working with him characterized it chemically and, finally in 1936, synthesized it. Williams named it "thiamin," later altered to "thiamine." Taking out a patent whose royalties funded the Williams-Waterman Fund for the Combat of Dietary Disease, Williams interested Merck & Company in developing a commercial process. Production of thiamine increased from 100 kilograms in 1937 to 200,000 kilograms in 1967, and synthetic thiamine became cheaper than any that could be extracted from natural sources.

From his position on the Food and Nutrition Board of the National Research Council, Williams pioneered and supported the enrichment of food with synthetic thiamine. Russell M. Wilder led the effort to enrich flour, which General Mills supported, and in 1941 the first definitions and standards for enrichment were established. The principle espoused was to raise thiamine to "high natural levels" in the milled flour. However, enrichment of bread in the United States was not fully accomplished until a popular movement was organized during World War II.

Other methods of preventing beriberi had been practiced for decades in Asia. There was considerable success in both Japan and Indonesia in limiting the extent of milling so that bran remained on the rice. Public-health professionals stressed the importance of educating the public and improving diets. In some nations, however, enrichment was viewed with suspicion as a commercial practice not tending to advance the public good. The result was that even as a beriberi epidemic followed the spread of power rice-milling and development through Southeast Asia, the United Nations Food and Agriculture Organization continued to resist rice enrichment. Finally, in the 1970s the government of Thailand began the process, and others followed this example. The success of these efforts portends that, although marginal and subclinical beriberi may persist forever, the scourge of beriberi as a significant killer is ended.

Melinda S. Meade

16. Black Death

The "Black Death" is the name given to the great pandemic of **plague** that ravaged parts of Asia, the Middle East, North Africa, and Europe in the mid-fourteenth century. Contemporaries knew it by many names, including the "Great Pestilence," the "Great Mortality," and the "Universal Plague." This epidemic was the first and most devastating of the second known cycle of widespread plague, which recurred in waves through the eighteenth century. Some later and milder "plagues" seem to have also involved other diseases, including **influenza**, **smallpox**, and **dysentery**. Nonetheless, most historians agree that the Black Death was a massive epidemic of plague (a disease of rodents – caused by the bacillus *Yersinia pestis* – that is transmitted to humans by fleas). The Black Death manifested itself most commonly as **bubonic plague** but also appeared in the forms of **pneumonic plague** and **septicemic plague**.

The geographic origins and full extent of the Black Death are still unclear. The earliest indisputable evidence locates it in 1346 in cities of the Kipchak Khanate of the Golden Horde, northwest of the Caspian Sea. Until recently, most historians claimed that the epidemic originated somewhere east of the Caspian, in Mongolia, Yunnan, or Tibet, where plague is enzootic in rodents. From there, it supposedly spread along trade routes, east to China, south to India, and west to the Kipchak Khanate, Crimea, and Mediterranean. This account has been contested, however, on the grounds that early sources are too vague to identify the disease(s) in question as plague. Alternative theories notwithstanding, much more work on Chinese and Mongol sources is required before we can say anything definite about the course of the Black Death before 1346 and its eastern geography and chronology after that date.

The epidemic's westward trajectory, however, is well established. It reached Crimea in the winter of 1346–47 and Constantinople shortly afterward. From there it followed two great, roughly circular paths. The first swirled counterclockwise through the eastern Mediterranean and the Middle East. The Black Death reached lower Egypt in the autumn of 1347 and moved slowly up the Nile over the next 2 years. By early 1348, it had also hit Cyprus and Rhodes, and during the late spring and summer it moved through the cities of the Mediterranean littoral – Gaza, Jerusalem, Damascus, Aleppo – and then east to Mecca, Armenia, and Baghdad, where it appeared in 1349.

The second circle described by the plague was greater in length and duration and moved clockwise, west and north and finally east again, through the western Mediterranean and Europe. According to Italian chroniclers, Genoese ships brought the disease to Sicily from the Black Sea in the autumn of 1347, at about the same time it appeared in Alexandria. From there it spread to Tunisia, the Italian mainland, and Provence. By the summer of 1348 it had moved westward into the Iberian Peninsula and as far north as Paris and the ports of southern England. During 1349 it ravaged the rest of the British Isles and northern France, parts of the Low Countries and Norway, and southern and western Germany. In 1350 it was in northern and eastern Germany, Sweden, and the Baltics, and in 1351, in the eastern Baltics and northern Poland. During the following 2 years, it attacked Russia, reaching as far eastward as Moscow in the summer of 1353.

Although the Black Death lasted in all at least 7 years, no single city or region suffered for more than a small fraction of that period. The plague moved like a wave through the Middle East and Europe, and the average duration of the epidemic in any given place seems to have been about 5 to 6 months. The Black Death was above all a disease of spring, summer, and early autumn, typically receding in the last months of the year. For this reason, areas first affected in early spring, like Tunis or the cities of central Italy, in general suffered longer and more severely than those, like northern France and Flanders, affected in August or September.

The disease was clearly propagated by humans; rather than moving slowly across fields and forests from one group of rodents to another, it progressed quickly along major routes of trade and communication, traveling faster by sea than by land. Thus in virtually every area in which its trajectory is known (the Black Sea, the Mediterranean, the North Sea, the Baltic), it appeared first in ports and then spread more slowly along roads and rivers to inland cities and from there into the surrounding countryside. A number of extremely remote areas, including parts of the Pyrenees, the central Balkans, and the sub-Atlas region, seem to have escaped largely or entirely.

It is difficult to judge mortality rates during the Black Death with any precision, except in a few areas. Contemporary chroniclers tended to give impossibly high estimates, whereas other records – necrologies, testaments, hearth taxes, and so forth – are incomplete or reflect only the experience of particular groups or require extensive interpretation. Nonetheless, historians generally agree that death rates most commonly ranged between about 30 and 50 percent in both Europe and the Middle East, with the best records indicating mortality in the upper end of that range. Some areas are known to have suffered more than others. It is frequently claimed that central Italy, southern France, East Anglia, and Scandinavia were most severely affected, although the evidence for this claim is uneven. Clearly, however, certain regions were relatively fortunate; Milan, for example, Bohemia, and parts of the Low Countries seem to have experienced losses of less than 20 percent, whereas Nuremberg, for some reason, escaped entirely. In general, however, the trend in recent research is to move the estimated mortality rates upward.

Some groups also suffered more than others, even within a single city or region. A number of contemporary observers in various parts of Europe commented on the relatively high death rates among the poor. These assertions are plausible; the poor lived in crowded and flimsy houses, which would have allowed the easy transmission of plague from rats to humans and from person to person, and they did not have the luxury of fleeing, like the rich, to plague-free areas or to their country estates. Conversely, death rates seem to have been somewhat lower than average among the high European aristocracy and royalty, who lived in stone buildings and were relatively mobile. People whose occupations brought them into contact with the sick, such as doctors, notaries, and hospital nurses, appear to have suffered disproportionately, at least in some areas, as did people who lived in large communal institutions, such as the Mamluks of Egypt and Syria or members of Christian religious orders. For all these groups, the main factor seems to have been increased exposure rather than susceptibility.

For those who could afford it, the most common reaction sanctioned by established medical authorities was flight; even in the Islamic world, where religious authorities inveighed against the practice and exhorted believers to accept the mortality as a martyrdom and a mark of divine mercy, people abandoned infected cities in search of more healthful territory. Those who remained sought spiritual remedies. In both Islamic and Christian countries, religious leaders organized prayers, processions, and special religious services, supplicating God to lift the epidemic. The European reaction, however, had a unique perspective, which was lacking for the most part among Muslims, for whom the epidemic was a morally neutral event: Drawing on traditional teachings concerning sin and penance, Christians on every level of society interpreted the plague as a mark of divine wrath and punishment for sin and, in some cases, even as a sign of the approaching apocalypse.

The most extreme and shocking example of Christian religious reaction to the Black Death was directed against Jewish communities in Provence, Catalonia, Aragon, Switzerland, southern Germany, and the Rhineland. Jews in these areas were accused of spreading the plague by poisoning Christian springs and wells. This kind of scapegoating was not unprecedented, but the violence of the popular reaction was extraordinary, in some places resisted and in some places abetted by rulers and municipal governments. Despite the protests of the pope, hundreds of Jewish communities were completely destroyed in 1348 and 1349, their members exiled or burned en masse, while the residents of many others were imprisoned and tortured and their property confiscated. The destruction was great enough to shift the center of gravity of the entire European Jewish population significantly eastward. There is no evidence for practices of this sort in Islamic communities, which could boast both a long tradition of religious pluralism and tolerance and a less morally loaded theological interpretation of the epidemic.

A second set of defensive reactions belonged to the realm of medicine and public health. Although both Muslims and Christians identified Divine Will as the ultimate cause of plague, most accepted that God worked through secondary causes belonging to the natural world, and this allowed them to interpret the epidemic within the framework of contemporary medical learning. Both societies shared a common medical tradition based on the works of Greek writers such as Hippocrates and Galen, which explained epidemics as the result of air corrupted by humid weather, decaying corpses, fumes generated by poor sanitation, and particular astrological events. Thus both Muslim and Christian doctors recommended (with some differences in emphasis) a similar set of preventive and curative practices that included a fortifying diet, rest, clean air, and moderate bloodletting for the healthy, together with salves, internal medication, and minor surgery for the sick.

Where Europe and the Islamic world clearly diverged was in their attitudes toward public health. There is little evidence that Islamic communities (where theological teachings combined with the classical medical tradition to deemphasize contagion as a cause of infection) engaged in large-scale social measures to prevent plague, beyond religious ceremonies and occasional public bonfires to purify the air. From the very beginning of the epidemic, however, the populations of a number of European cities – above all, in central and northern Italy, which boasted a highly developed order of municipal and medical institutions – reacted aggressively in a largely futile attempt to protect themselves from the disease. Initially they fell back on existing sanitary legislation, most of it dating from the thirteenth and early fourteenth centuries; this emphasized street cleaning and the control of particularly odoriferous practices like butchery, tannery, dyeing, and the emptying of privies.

As the plague moved closer, however, a number of Italian governments instituted novel measures to fight contagion as well as corrupt and fetid air. They imposed restrictions on travel to and from plague-stricken cities and on the import and sale of cloth from infected regions and individuals. They passed laws against public assemblies and regulated the burial of the dead. They hired doctors to study the disease and treat its victims (many physicians had fled the cities along with others of their class), and they appointed temporary boards of officials to administer these measures. In Milan the ducal government boarded up the houses of plague victims, and in Avignon, the pope created a settlement of wooden huts outside the city walls to receive the sick and isolate them from the rest of the community.

These measures against contagion were unprecedented in the context of both contemporary medical theory and municipal practice; they seem initially to have been a response to the experience of pneumonic plague, which ravaged the cities of Italy and southern France in the winter and spring of 1347–8. The ecology of plague and problems of enforcement made such measures largely ineffective, although it is striking that Milan, which applied anticontagion practices most drastically, was the least affected of all major Italian cities. Nonetheless, such measures represent the beginnings of large-scale public health organizations in Europe; succeeding epidemics saw their elaboration and spread to other parts of the continent, where they eventually became the basis for widespread practices such as quarantines and cordons sanitaires.

Katharine Park

17. Black and Brown Lung Disease

Black lung and **brown lung** are the names given by workers in the coal and textile industries, respectively, and by some physicians and public officials, to symptoms of respiratory distress associated with dusty work. Most physicians and epidemiologists have, however, preferred to categorize these symptoms as they relate to findings at autopsy and studies of pulmonary function and to name their appearance in particular patients as, respectively, **coal workers' pneumoconiosis** and **byssinosis**. The terms "black lung" and "brown lung" are historical legacies of intense negotiations about the causes of respiratory distress and mortality among workers in the coal and textile industries of Europe and North America, especially since the nineteenth century.

History

For many centuries, medical observers, workers, and employers have recognized respiratory distress and its consequences as an occupational hazard among underground miners and employees of industries that generate considerable dust (notably, refineries, foundries, and the manufacturing of cotton, flax, and hemp). Pliny described the inhalation of "fatal dust" in the first century. In the sixteenth century, Agricola indicated that miners, physicians, and engineers were aware of shortness of breath and suffered premature death. In the early nineteenth century, pathologists observed that some miners in Scotland had black lesions on the lung at autopsy. The term pneumoconiosis appears to have been invented in 1867. Brown lung seems to have been named by analogy with black lung, apparently in the 1960s.

The contemporary, imprecise medical synonym for black lung is coal workers' pneumoconiosis (CWP). CWP occurs in two forms: simple CWP and **progressive massive fibrosis**. Both forms have characteristic lesions. Agencies awarding compensation for disability usually use the designation "black lung" as a rough synonym for pathologically defined CWP and for **obstructive airways disease** among coal miners.

Most medical authors, epidemiologists, and compensation agencies usually use "brown lung" as a popular synonym for byssinosis or **chronic dust-induced respiratory disease**. The pathology in these descriptions resembles that of chronic bronchitis.

The rich literature on the history of black and brown lung cannot be summarized in conventional terms. Many authors have attempted to describe the history of these conditions, but they have almost invariably done so on the basis of the precise definition of symptomatology accepted at the time they were writing. The reported geography of the conditions is consistent with the distribution of industries in which dust is a by-product.

Characteristics

Each condition has been described among workers exposed to coal dust (CWP) and cotton dust (byssinosis). Perhaps 1 million workers worldwide are currently exposed to both coal and cotton dust. The incidence of each condition (and of particular diseases defined in different eras) has been influenced by public policy and regulations for dust suppression, by the characteristics of mining and manufacturing processes (and, for black lung, by the type of coal itself), by workers' general state of health, by their exposure to other causes of respiratory disease (notably cigarette smoke), and by the availability of publicly supported programs of disability compensation and medical care.

Opinions about the distribution and incidence of the conditions have been linked to competing views about their clinical manifestations and pathology. For many years and in many communities, physicians did not differentiate the symptoms of black and brown lung from those of other common respiratory disorders. In the early stages of both diseases, workers are frequently asymptomatic and without functional impairment. For black lung defined medically as CWP, the progression of symptoms often includes chronic cough and phlegm, shortness of breath, and then functional impairment; but some workers with lesions of CWP at autopsy remained free of symptoms. The initial symptoms of byssinosis are tightness in the chest, **dyspnea**, and a cough following a return to work after a weekend or holiday. Later symptoms extend to other workdays and include a chronic stage, with severe continuous dyspnea, chronic cough, and permanent ventilatory insufficiency.

Both black and brown lung have been the focus of many studies – and are highly controversial. Early epidemiological studies established an association between occupation and respiratory disease. Studies of both conditions in the United States were, in general, initiated later than those in Britain for reasons that in-clude the political roles of manufacturers and unions and the structure of public regulation as well as different perceptions of the relative importance of silica and coal dust and the amount of dust that constituted a dangerous exposure in textile manufacturing. Moreover, many epidemiological, clinical, and pathological investigations have yielded uncertain results.

Aspects of coal miners' lung distress that remain controversial include the mechanisms by which coal dust acts on the lungs; the significance of the correlation, or lack of it, between clinical evidence of respiratory impairment and X-ray findings; and the absence, in some studies, of strong, independent correlations between respiratory disorders in mining communities and work in the mines. **Caplan's syndrome** is an example of the complexity and controversy surrounding coal miners' lung conditions. This syndrome, first described among Welsh coal miners in 1953, appears to be a consequence of the interaction of characteristics of **rheumatoid arthritis** with a residue of silica in the lungs; yet the syndrome seems extremely rare in the United States, despite the high incidence of both dust exposure and arthritis among miners.

For byssinosis, areas of uncertainty include the substance in cotton dust that causes respiratory distress, lack of clear evidence linking levels of dust exposure to findings indicative of clinically defined disease, and the absence of widely accepted findings sufficiently specific to permit a diagnosis of disease.

Nevertheless, the literature on both conditions is widely regarded as offering considerable guidance for public action. Most investigators agree that the relatively high incidence of respiratory distress in mining and textile workers is evidence of exposure to toxic agents in industrial dust. Many authors have hypothesized mechanisms by which these agents could operate in the lung. There is considerable agreement about clinical manifestations and pathology. And there is overwhelming consensus that reducing dust levels in the workplace contributes to reducing the incidence of both black and brown lung and the findings defined by medical scientists as diseases among workers in dusty industries.

Daniel M. Fox

18. Bleeding Disorders

The existence of a hereditary tendency to excessive bleeding was recognized in the second century A.D. by Rabbi Judah, who exempted from circumcision the son of a woman whose earlier sons had bled to death after this rite. But only in the twentieth century did expanding knowledge of the physiology of **hemostasis** – the arrest of bleeding – make evident the diverse nature of inherited bleeding disorders. In addition, only recently has it been recognized that a tendency to **thrombosis** might likewise be due to an inherited hemostatic defect.

The mechanisms in mammals that stop blood loss after vascular disruption are complex. Small vascular injuries are sealed by platelets that adhere to the site of damage, where they attract other circulating platelets, so as to form an occlusive aggregate or plug that can close small gaps. Larger defects in vessel walls are occluded by coagulation of blood, that is, by its transformation from a fluid to a gel-like state. Uncontrolled bleeding and its antithesis, thrombosis (the formation of a clot within a blood vessel), are important pathogenetic factors for human disease, including a large variety of hereditary disorders. Human disorders arising from functional deficiency of each of the factors needed for the formation of a clot have been recognized and extensively studied.

Classic Hemophilia
The best known of all the bleeding disorders is classic **hemophilia** (hemophilia A, the hereditary functional deficiency of factor VIII), which is the prototype of an X chromosome-linked disease, limited to males but transmitted by female carriers. Necessarily, all daughters of those with the disease are carriers, as are half the daughters of carriers. In turn, half the sons of carriers inherit the disease. A typical family history of bleeding inherited in the manner described is found in about two-thirds of cases; in the rest, the disorder appears to arise *de novo*, either because a fresh mutation has occurred or because cases were unrecognized in earlier generations.

Classic hemophilia varies in severity from family to family. In the most severe cases, in which plasma is essentially devoid of factor VIII, the patients may bruise readily and bleed apparently spontaneously into soft tissues and joints, with the latter resulting in crippling joint disease. Trauma, surgical procedures, and dental extractions may lead to lethal bleeding. The life expectancy of those with severe classic hemophilia is foreshortened, death coming from exsanguination, bleeding into a vital area, or infection. The prognosis of classic hemophilia has been greatly improved by modern therapy in which episodes of bleeding are controlled by transfusion of fractions of normal plasma containing the functionally missing proteins. This therapy is not without hazard, for transfusion of concentrates of factor VIII derived from normal plasma has been complicated by transmission of the viruses of **hepatitis** and the **acquired immune deficiency syndrome (AIDS)**.

In those families in which classic hemophilia is milder, bleeding occurs only after injury, surgery, or dental extraction. The severity of clinical symptoms is paralleled by the degree of the deficiency of antihemophilic factor (factor VIII), as measured in tests of its coagulant function.

Classic hemophilia appears to be distributed worldwide, but geographic differences in incidence have been described. Whether classic hemophilia is less prevalent in blacks than in other groups, as has been suggested, is uncertain.

Christmas Disease
Christmas disease (hemophilia B), the hereditary functional deficiency of Christmas factor

(factor IX), is clinically indistinguishable from classic hemophilia and can be differentiated only by laboratory tests. It is inherited in the same way as an X chromosome-linked disorder and is therefore virtually limited to males. As is true of classic hemophilia, the disorder varies in severity from family to family in proportion to the degree of the clotting factor deficiency. Christmas disease is heterogeneous in nature, for in some families the plasma is deficient in Christmas factor, whereas in others the plasma contains one or another of several nonfunctional variants of this clotting factor. Therapy for hemorrhagic episodes in Christmas disease is currently best carried out by transfusion of normal plasma, which contains the factor deficient in the patient's plasma. An alternative therapy, infusion of concentrates of Christmas factor separated from normal plasma, may be needed in some situations, but its use may be complicated by the transmission of viral diseases as well as by other problems.

Worldwide, Christmas disease is perhaps one-eighth to one-fifth as prevalent as classic hemophilia. Most reported cases have been in individuals of European origin, but, in South Africa and possibly in the United States, Christmas disease is relatively as common in blacks as in whites. The disorder is said to be rare in Japan.

Von Willebrand's Disease

Classic hemophilia is not the only hereditary deficiency of antihemophilic factor. Indeed, **von Willebrand's disease** is a bleeding disorder of both sexes, which in its usual form is present in successive generations; thus, it is inherited as an autosomal dominant trait. The plasma of affected individuals is deficient in both parts of the antihemophilic factor complex, that is, the coagulant portion (factor VIII) and von Willebrand factor. The disorder is usually mild, although variants have been observed in which severe bleeding episodes are frequent. Inheritance in these cases is probably recessive in nature.

The prevalence of von Willebrand's disease is uncertain because mild cases are easily overlooked. In the United States, it is perhaps about one-fourth as prevalent as classic hemophilia, meaning 2 or 3 cases per 100,000 individuals. Prevalence is somewhat higher in certain European countries. The disorder is relatively uncommon in blacks. The severe, autosomal recessive form of von Willebrand's disease is unusual in most individuals of European extraction (perhaps 1 per 1 million) but is particularly prevalent among Israeli Arabs (about 5 per 100,000) and in Scandinavia.

Unusual Disorders of Hemostasis

Functional deficiencies of Hageman factor (**Hageman trait**), plasma prekallikrein (**Fletcher trait**), and high molecular weight kininogen (**Fitzgerald trait**, **Flaujeac trait**, or **Willimas trait**) are all asymptomatic, although in each case a major defect in clotting is found in the laboratory. These disorders occur with equal frequency in both sexes and are recessive traits, meaning that they must be inherited from both parents. All are quite rare, although a disproportionately high number of cases of Hageman trait have been reported from the Netherlands. No racial predilection for Hageman trait or deficiency of high molecular weight kininogen has been described, but deficiency of plasma prekallikrein appears to be more frequent in blacks and in individuals of Mediterranean extraction.

Hageman trait is a heterogeneous disorder; in most families, the plasma appears to be deficient in Hageman factor, but plasma in a few contains a nonfunctional variant of this clotting factor. A similar heterogeneity has been observed in plasma prekallikrein deficiency, with the plasma of Mediterranean-origin patients containing a nonfunctional variant.

The hereditary deficiency of plasma thromboplastin antecedent (PTA or factor XI deficiency) is also inherited in an autosomal recessive manner. The hemorrhagic symptoms are usually mild; in women, excessive menstrual bleeding may be troublesome. Nearly all reported cases have been Ashkenazi Jews or Japanese, although cases in individuals of other heritages have been recognized.

Hereditary deficiencies of factor VII, Stuart factor (factor X), proaccelerin (factor V), and prothrombin are rare, and no racial or geographic distribution is yet apparent. In **factor VII deficiency**, estimates indicate 1 case per 100,000. A still rarer syndrome, the combination of factor VII deficiency and **Dubin–Johnson syndrome** (the latter a disorder of bilirubin metabolism) has been described in Israeli Jews of Sephardic origin.

In each of these disorders, the deficiency appears in both sexes and is inherited as a recessive trait, and in a number of instances the parents have been consanguineous. In general, the basic nature of these functional deficiencies is variable. In some instances, the plasma of the affected individuals appears to be deficient in the factors. In others, the plasma contains an incompetent variant of the supposedly missing factor.

The symptoms of deficiencies of factor VII, Stuart factor, and proaccelerin (the last called **parahemophilia**) are variable; some individuals have hemorrhagic episodes comparable to those of severe hemophilia, whereas others are spared except in the event of severe trauma. In women, excessive menstrual bleeding may be a serious problem.

Disorders of fibrin formation are of peculiar interest. Patients with **congenital afibrinogenemia** (who have no detectable fibrinogen in plasma) may bleed excessively from the umbilicus at birth and thereafter from injuries or surgical procedures. In addition, they may exsanguinate from relatively minor vascular injuries, and menorrhagia may be disastrous; yet they may have little in the way of spontaneous bleeding. Fortunately, cogenital afibrinogenemia is a rare recessive disorder, detected in both sexes, and only about 150 cases have been recorded to date. Often the parents are consanguineous. A milder form, **congenital hypofibrinogenemia** (in which the plasma contains small but measurable amounts of fibrinogen), has also been

described in about 30 families, and some investigators believe that this is the heterozygous state for congenital afibrinogenemia, meaning that these individuals have inherited the abnormality from but one parent. In still other families, the concentration of fibrinogen in plasma is normal or only moderately decreased, but the fibrinogen is qualitatively abnormal. This disorder, **congenital dysfibrinogenemia**, occurs in both sexes and in successive generations; that is, it is inherited as a dominant trait. The affected individuals may be asymptomatic, detected only by chance, or they may suffer mild bleeding problems. Paradoxically, they may also sustain thrombosis. More than 100 families with dysfibrinogenemia have been described, and the molecular defect in each family is almost always unique.

Fibrin-stabilizing factor deficiency is similarly rare; perhaps 100 cases have been described thus far. In some, plasma appears to be deficient in fibrin-stabilizing factor; in others, plasma contains a nonfunctional variant of this agent. Patients with fibrin-stabilizing factor deficiency have severe bleeding problems beginning with the umbilicus at birth. The patients may die of central nervous system hemorrhage, and in women spontaneous abortion is frequent. Some evidence suggests that affected males are sterile.

Another disorder of great interest is the hereditary **alpha-2-antiplasmin deficiency**. In this disease, which is inherited as a recessive trait, patients may have symptoms suggestive of severe classic hemophilia. Bleeding apparently results from the rapid dissolution of clots by plasmin, whose proteolytic activity is unchecked because of the deficiency of alpha-2-plasma inhibitor. Too few cases have been recognized to determine any geographic predilection for this disorder, but it has been reported in Japan, the Netherlands, Norway, the United States, and Argentina.

Hereditary Thrombotic Disorders
In contrast to the deficiency states described to this point, a hereditary deficiency of certain

of the inhibitors of clotting results in an increased tendency to thrombosis. Thus, familial recurrent thrombosis has been observed in individuals of both sexes, with inherited partial deficiencies of antithrombin III, protein C, protein S, or heparin cofactor II. Affected individuals, most of whom are heterozygotes, have about half the concentration of the inhibitory proteins of normal individuals. Only a handful of cases of deficiencies of heparin cofactor II, protein C, or protein S have been recorded, but **antithrombin III deficiency** is relatively common.

Most reported cases of deficiencies of these several inhibitors have been in individuals of European origin. Additional instances of antithrombin III deficiency have been recognized in Japanese, Algerians, and American blacks; **protein C deficiency** has been seen in Jordanian and Israeli Arabs, and in Japanese; and **protein S deficiency** has been reported in Japan.

History

The earliest record of the existence of hereditary hemorrhagic disease is in the Babylonian Talmud. Recurrent descriptions of what was probably hemophilia were recorded thereafter, but it was only in 1803 that John Otto recognized that this disorder was limited to males and transmitted by certain of their asymptomatic female relatives. During the nineteenth century, the mode of inheritance of hemophilia was delineated, and in a 1911 review of all published cases, investigators were unable to find a single authentic case of hemophilia in a female.

The mechanism underlying the defect in classic hemophilia was elucidated in 1936: It was determined that patients were functionally deficient in what is now called antihemophilic factor. Only later was it realized that an essentially identical disorder, inherited in the same way, resulted from a deficiency of Christmas factor. In 1926, E. A. von Willebrand recognized the disease that bears his name. In 1953, several investigators found that the titer of antihemophilic factor was abnormally low in patients with von Willebrand's disease, and some years later, a deficiency in the concentration of von Willebrand factor was also reported.

With few exceptions, the existence of the various clotting factors required for normal coagulation of blood was detected by the study of patients with unusual hemorrhagic disorders. In each instance, a protein extracted from normal plasma corrected the specific defect in the patient's plasma. Thus, current knowledge about the physiology of blood clotting has been derived from the interplay between the clinic and the laboratory.

Oscar D. Ratnoff

19. Botulism

Botulism is a potentially fatal disease caused by neurotoxins produced by the bacterium *Clostridium botulinum.* The disease usually occurs as a food-borne intoxication; however, two other forms have been identified: **wound botulism** and **infant botulism**.

Characteristics

C. botulinum, which exists naturally as a spore, multiplies (and produces its powerful neurotoxins) in anaerobic conditions, such as in canned foods and unclean wounds. The spores occur naturally in soil and marine sediments and are a normal contaminant of many foods. The spores and toxins are inactivated by boiling canned foods according to food-industry specifications. To date, seven distinct botulinum toxins, labeled A through G, have been identified. Botulism in humans is generally associated with toxins A, B, E, or F, whereas the C and D toxins have been identified in outbreaks among animals.

Onset usually occurs 12–36 hours after ingestion of toxin-contaminated food. Botulism typically presents distressing signs of motor-nerve dysfunction, including vision problems and difficulty with speech and swallowing. The unabated disease progresses to generalized paralysis and death from respiratory muscle involvement.

Diagnosis is confirmed by detecting botulinum toxin in the blood, feces, or wound site of the patient. Depending on the toxic dose, untreated botulism carries a high fatality rate. Early treatment with antitoxin, respiratory support, and other intensive care may be lifesaving.

Infant botulism, confined to babies 2 weeks to 9 months old, typically presents with generalized weakness ("floppy baby") and has been implicated as a cause of **sudden infant death syndrome**. It is associated with ingestion of processed infant foods – honey in particular – containing botulinum spores. First described in 1976 in the United States, where most cases are reported, infant botulism has also occurred in Europe, Australia, Asia, and South America.

History

Botulism derives its name from the Latin word *botulus* ("sausage"). In the late 1700s and early 1800s, German physicians noted an unusual but frequently fatal disease following ingestion of spoiled sausage. Justinius Kerner, a district health officer in Württemberg, compiled such reports, with the result that botulism is sometimes called **Kerner's disease**. A similar illness in nineteenth-century Russia was associated with eating smoked or pickled fish and labeled **ichthiosismus**.

In 1896, bacteriologist Emile von Ermengem, investigating a dramatic outbreak at a gathering in a Belgian village, established botulism's cause as a neurotoxin produced by an anaerobic bacterium. In the United States, repeated outbreaks associated with commercially canned foods led to extensive research in the 1920s. Sponsored by the National Canners Association, these studies established safe food-processing practices now widespread in industry.

Although of low incidence and sporadic occurrence, botulism clearly exhibits significant case-fatality rates wherever reported. The foods responsible vary considerably, reflecting regionally different dietary and food-preservation practices. In Poland, Germany, and France, canned meats have accounted for most outbreaks, whereas in Japan and Russia, home-preserved and pickled fish are usually incriminated. In the United States, low-acid canned vegetables, particularly beans, peppers, and mushrooms, have been the most common sources, with relatively few outbreaks traced to meat or fish. Most instances everywhere are associated with improper home canning or pickling, though the more serious public-health problem of outbreaks associated with faulty commercial canning still occasionally occur.

William H. Barker

20. Brucellosis (Malta Fever, Undulant Fever)

Brucellosis or **undulant fever** is a zoonotic infection caused in humans by organisms of the genus *Brucella*: *Brucella melitensis*, *Brucella abortus*, and *Brucella suis*, transmitted, respectively, from goats, cattle, and pigs. Human infections are characterized by intermittent fevers, possibly persisting for weeks, with subsequent relapses and prolonged ill health. The causal relationship between organism and disease was first recorded by David Bruce in Malta in 1887; the name "Malta fever" reflects its prevalence on that island in the nineteenth century.

Characteristics

The type of brucellosis described by Bruce in 1887 is caused by *B. melitensis*, usually transmitted to humans via milk from infected goats. Occasional contamination by touch has also been observed. The mode of transmission was not established until the twentieth century. In Malta and elsewhere in the Mediterranean, the disease was endemic rather than epidemic, its highest incidence occurring during summer months. Military officers and their families appeared more susceptible than the lower ranks; likewise, among civilians the professional classes suffered more than laborers.

Other areas show variations in epidemiological patterns. For example, in southeast France, where sheep and goats vastly outnumber cattle, brucellosis was still widespread in the 1930s but more an occupational than a consumers' disease. Most cases occurred in farming communities, resulting from direct contact with infected animals and manure, although consumption of infected milk and cheese also played some part.

In 1918, Alice Evans suggested that the agent of **contagious abortion** (a disease of cattle) was similar to *B. melitensis* and might cause disease in humans. This was confirmed: brucellosis cases caused by *B. abortus* transmitted via consumption of raw cows' milk have occurred worldwide.

The third major undulant fever is caused by *B. suis*, naturally hosted by pigs. The disease attacks mainly slaughterers and packers infected by contaminated carcasses. Usually, *B. suis* invades humans through skin lesions, although airborne infection may also be possible. The disease is far less common than its counterparts in goats and cattle. Sporadic cases among Alaskan Eskimos have resulted from infected reindeer.

Brucella melitensis follows the distribution of goats about the Mediterranean area (thus another nickname is "Mediterranean fever") as well as in China, India, South Africa, and South America. Pasteurization of milk has substantially reduced its incidence. The same applies to *B. abortus* infections, which have been almost completely eradicated from northern Europe, where incidence is now quite low. In the United States, brucellosis is still extant, caused by, in order of importance, *B. abortus*, *B. suis*, and lastly *B. melitensis*. Most cases occur sporadically, although occasional minor outbreaks have been reported. The situation constantly changes because of various eradication programs.

Bruce's discovery of the causal agent had no immediate impact on incidence; only after identification of the mode of transmission was there a dramatic fall in number of cases, first among British troops, whose consumption of goats' milk was curtailed by 1906. But control of brucellosis among civilians was more difficult. It was achieved, in Malta and elsewhere, only after World War II, when pasteurization became generally accepted.

Neither animal nor human immune systems deal quickly and decisively with *B. melitensis* and *B. abortus*, which accounts for persistent infections and cases of long duration. Evans herself contracted a laboratory infection in 1922 and suffered recurring episodes of debilitating fever for more than 20 years. (Despite this, she finally recovered and lived until the age of 94.)

B. abortus, in particular, can foster latent infection leading to latent immunity, which occurs more frequently with exposure over a period of time than with sudden heavy doses of infective material. This may explain the low rate of disease in veterinarians, who as a group evidence exceptionally high levels of immunologic response.

Vaccination is possible against *B. abortus* in cattle and against *B. melitensis* in sheep and goats, but a human vaccine is still experimental. The animal vaccines are too toxic for use in humans. In 1962, the British Ministry of Agriculture introduced a free calf-vaccination service.

Undulant fever is essentially a **septicemia** (blood poisoning) characterized by irregular temperatures with intermittent waves of fever, usually lasting 10–30 days. Although case-fatality rates are low, it is a protracted and debilitating illness. Its duration varies from only a few days to as long as a year. Subsequent relapses may occur over several years, alternating with periods of apparent recovery. Symptoms include weakness, muscular pain, nocturnal sweats, **anorexia**, chills, and nervous irritability. Recorded postmortem appearances include congestion and enlargement of the liver and hypertrophy of the spleen; cultures from these organs are positive for *B. melitensis* in all cases.

Once established, *B. abortus* – despite its tendency to produce latent infection – seems to develop in similar fashion, lasting an average 13 weeks and possibly becoming chronic. *B. abortus* also causes a short influenza-like illness and a persistent low fever. Undulant fever caused by *B. suis* is clinically similar to the others.

History

In the Mediterranean region, a low fever with regular remissions has been recorded since the time of Hippocrates. Its geographic origins are indicated by many synonyms, of which the best known are "Malta fever" and "Mediterranean fever," although other variants involve Naples, Constantinople, Crete, and Gibraltar.

In 1863, J. A. Marston provided the first differential description of Malta fever; describing several cases, he called it "gastric remittent fever." In 1887, Bruce – surgeon to the Malta garrison like Marston before him – recorded his discovery of a microorganism in the spleens of fatal cases. He established its causal role, calling it *Micrococcus melitensis*, although in the 1920s it was renamed *Brucella melitensis* in his honor.

Returning from Malta, Bruce taught at the Army Medical College at Netley in England; among his students was Matthew Louis Hughes who, posted to Malta in 1890, enthusiastically embraced Bruce's interest in the fever. Hughes wrote several papers on the disease during the next decade, until he died under enemy fire while tending casualties in South Africa in 1899. In 1897, he published a clinical description of Malta fever still quoted today as a model of its kind.

After Bruce's time, brucellosis received particular attention in Malta. The British Mediterranean Fever Commission began work in 1905, during which time Themistocles Zammit established the presence of the disease in goats and the role of goats' milk in transmitting it to humans. His research caused British troops to cease drinking goats' milk; within a year, the disease had all but disappeared from British forces in Malta. As already mentioned, control of the disease among civilians proved far more difficult. Although pasteurization eventually solved this problem, the disease in goats still resists control.

With *B. abortus* infections, the sequence of events was rather different. During the nineteenth century, several authors had described the disease in cattle. Its transmissibility was demonstrated in 1878, and just before the turn of the century Bernhard Bang in Copenhagen isolated and identified the causal agent. Only in 1918, however, did Evans note the similarity between *B. melitensis* and *B. abortus*; within a few years, *B. abortus* was shown to be pathogenic for humans, causing brucellosis in many areas around the world.

Last of the undulant fevers to attract attention was that caused by *B. suis*. The first known case was apparently diagnosed in the United States in 1922, although the agent's identity was not immediately recognized. Clinically and bacteriologically, the disease is similar to the other brucelloses although less extensively distributed in either pigs or humans. *B. suis* infection of swine began to cause concern in hog-raising areas of the American Midwest during the 1930s. It has since been reported in several other countries, but cases are mostly sporadic, with only a few recognized outbreaks.

Lise Wilkinson

21. Bubonic Plague

Plague is often a synonym for pestilence, which refers nonspecifically to any acute epidemic accompanied by high mortality. But the term also refers to the recurrent waves of **bubonic plague** punctuating European history from 1348 to 1720. Bubonic plague epidemics occurred as *Yersinia pestis*, a rodent disease, was communicated to humans through the bite of infected fleas. Humans have exceedingly poor immune defenses to this organism, and within 6 days of infection most victims develop a grossly swollen lymph node, a bubo, signifying the body's attempt to contain and arrest multiplication of *Y. pestis*. On the average, around 60 percent of those infected died within a week after the appearance of the bubo. Thus, bubonic plague brought high and dramatic mortality rates when it extended into human communities.

Characteristics

With the historically ironic exception of Western Europe, *Y. pestis* occurs naturally throughout the world among a wide variety of rodents and lagomorphs (rabbits and related species). Some of the more than 300 rodent species affected are relatively resistant to the disease and can survive and reproduce while technically infected by the organism. *Y. pestis* infects new animals either because fleas transmit it or because the microbe is shed and survives in warm rodent burrows. This part of the plague cycle may be termed "sylvatic" or "enzootic" plague.

The "disease," then, is not always a disease, and it is ecologically complex. Indeed, ecological change or disturbance is what brings susceptible rodents into contact with *Y. pestis*. Historically, the most important of these rodents is *Rattus rattus*, the common black or brown house rat that literally "shares man's table." When infected by *Y. pestis*, these susceptible animals die quickly of overwhelming infection, with blood levels of the microbe so high that rat fleas imbibe large numbers of organisms.

The oriental rat flea (*Xenopsylla cheopis*) and the human flea (*Pulex irritans*) are considered historically important arthropod vectors transmitting "epizootic" plague to humans. *X. cheopis* is an efficient vector because a bend in its feeding tube creates a location for growth of *Y. pestis*, such that the flea becomes "blocked," unable to swallow a full blood meal. Attempting to dislodge this bolus or wad, the flea infects new mammalian hosts. *P. irritans* has an important historical role because it feeds indifferently upon both humans and the common house rat.

Human plague usually arises after an epizootic plague has produced high mortality among susceptible rodents, when infected fleas, deprived of rodent hosts, begin to feed on humans. Humans do not normally carry *Y. pestis* and thus cannot infect fleas or otherwise pass the disease to new hosts. For human communities, plague is an acute infection ultimately derived from infected rodents.

Today, in regions where plague routinely infects resistant rodents, ecologists and public-health officials try to monitor passage of the disease to susceptible species. In such regions – the American Southwest, south-central Eurasia, and Southeast Asia – humans likely to encounter infection must be revaccinated often, for human immunity to *Y. pestis* is short-lived.

Yersinia pestis was once called *Pasteurella pestis*, a name that has persisted from much historical literature about European plagues. In 1971, the name was changed to honor Alexandre Yersin, a French microbiologist and student of Louis Pasteur. Working in Southeast Asia during the late nineteenth century outbreak of plague, Yersin successfully cultured the microorganism.

The antigens (components of the organism that stimulate an immune response) vary in virulence, such that vaccines can be created from mild plague strains. *Y. pestis* causes severe human disease when it contains antigens that facilitate its entry into cells and impede the body's white blood cells' attempts to kill infected cells. *Y. pestis* can liberate both endotoxins and exotoxins, leading to circulatory collapse. These activities stimulate – and can defeat – immune mechanisms, explaining why the disease produces extremely high case-fatality rates. With a typical virulent strain of the bacterium, more than 60 percent of untreated victims die within 10 days of infection. If the organism reaches the lungs, there is even less chance of survival. A victim with infected lungs can cough out highly virulent, encapsulated organisms that are rapidly absorbed by the mucous membranes of any nearby susceptible person. This can lead to "primary" **pneumonic plague**, in which the ordinary mode of transmission by fleas is bypassed, and the disease spreads directly from human to human. When this has occurred, case-fatality rates have been close to 100 percent.

Once a human is infected with *Y. pestis*, the organism rapidly replicates at the site of the fleabite. This area can subsequently become necrotic, and dead tissue blackens to produce a carbuncle or pustule. But in many cases the progress of infection is too rapid for this to happen. The lymphatic system attempts to drain the infection to the regional lymph node, where organisms and infected cells can be ingested by macrophages and white blood cells. That node becomes engorged with blood and cellular debris, creating the grossly swollen "bubo." Because infected fleas usually bite an exposed area of the body, the location of the subsequent bubo is often visible. Frequent sites are the groin, the axilla, and the cervical lymph nodes.

But drainage can occur to an internal lymph node, or the infection can proceed too rapidly for the lymphatic system to effect a defense. In the latter case, blood-borne **septicemic plague** has occurred, seeding the organism quickly in many organs. Victims of septicemic plague become rapidly moribund and often develop neither eschar nor bubos, although the more usual clinical course is the formation of a bubo, described in historical accounts as reaching the size of an egg, orange, or even grapefruit. The area is inflamed, boggy or doughy to the touch, and exquisitely painful. Patients often demanded that a physician or surgeon incise and drain the bubo, a process that could have liberated infective organisms.

The bubo often appears 4–6 days after infection, and because of the multiple ways in which Y. *pestis* is virulent to humans, disease progresses quickly after this point. In 5–15 percent of cases the lungs are infected, but more often a high fever with headache and mental disorientation are characteristic symptoms. Occasionally, circulatory collapse and **hemorrhagic sepsis** occurs, blackening the body's surface. Death typically occurs within another 4–6 days. In the past, a diagnosis of plague might have been made on the basis of this rapid clinical progression from health to death alone, although clearly this could have been caused by countless other conditions. But the acute formation of bubos, visible in 60 percent of bubonic plague victims, is pathognomonic of plague, meaning that no other disease commonly causes this reaction.

History

Most of the historical literature of plague identifies three lengthy time periods when bubonic plague repeatedly assaulted human communities. The first known cycle of widespread human plague occurred during late Greco-Roman antiquity. Byzantine historian Procopius described the devastating epidemic of 542 A.D. in Constantinople, dubbed the "Plague of Justinian" because of his dramatic account. The wave of epidemic reached western Europe by 547, which was also powerfully described by Gregory of Tours. Virulent, epidemic plague recurred throughout the Mediterranean for the next 200 years.

The second cycle, at least in its early stages, is often called the Black Death and is treated in this work as a separate entry, for certainly it is the most heavily studied of the plague cycles. Beginning about 1300, the cycle is generally considered to have ended at about 1800, although the ending date is disputed. This manifestation of the disease took a heavy toll in the Middle East as well as Europe and appears to have also invaded Asia.

The plague has been viewed as pivotal in many areas of historical inquiry. Surely it was to some significant extent responsible for stagnant demographic performance in Europe prior to the mid-eighteenth century, and surely, too, the plague stimulated new and important public-health efforts in European urban centers. The continued presence of the disease in Europe presents a mystery, because at no other time was it able to survive in northern Europe without constant reintroduction from the Middle East.

Historians frequently credit fifteenth through seventeenth century public-health measures devised to combat the plague with some mitigation of the disease and its ultimate disappearance. However, in the light of modern medical knowledge, it is clear that such measures – quarantine of healthy individuals, isolation of the sick and their households, large pesthouses or lazarettoes, and even the elaboration of a theory of contagion – would have had little effect on its course.

Certainly the most important questions about these 500 years of plague in Europe have to do with its disappearance and demographic consequences. In the latter case, much of the mortality credited to the plague resulted from its indirect impact rather than infection. When an epidemic struck, panic ensued, and this alone, by halting normal sanitary and social services while precipitating headlong flight, would have taken a significant number of lives, as would isolating both ill and well in hospitals and pesthouses. Chief among these victims would have been the very young, the very old, and the economically disadvantaged.

Beginning in the early eighteenth century, Europe was increasingly protected against plague invasions from Ottoman lands by a staunch Austrian barrier. Manned by more than 100,000 men and featuring numerous quarantine and checkpoint stations, this famous sanitary cordon limited both trade and human traffic, which may have helped to spare Europe from the third or most recent cycle of the plague that seems to have had its beginning in central Asia about the middle of the eighteenth century. From there, the plague spread to China and India and then, aided by rapid sea transportation, radiated globally from Hong Kong, Bombay, and Calcutta.

But if Europe was bypassed, the Americas were not. Rather, along with Australia and eastern Africa, North and South America were infected for the first time, and by the early years of the nineteenth century some regions of the Western Hemisphere were experiencing relatively minor but nonetheless panic-inspiring epidemics. Those that struck San Francisco are among the best documented in this pandemic cycle, although the disease killed millions in India and Africa.

If the Americas and Australia did not suffer greatly from this third cycle of plague, one consequence was that the disease established itself among the rodents and lagomorphs of the New Worlds. In North America, the geographic extent of plague has subsequently widened each year, and sporadic cases of human plague claim 8–15 victims annually despite effective antibiotic therapy. In the Americas, as elsewhere, smoldering enzootic foci of plague demand a constant global effort in surveillance and control.

Ann G. Carmichael

22. Cancer

In past centuries, people feared epidemic diseases, with ghastly symptoms, agonizing death, and sometimes disfigurement for survivors. Today, especially in the developed world, the dread of epidemic contagion has been replaced by the dread of **cancer**. The basic causes of cancer remain shrouded in mystery.

Cancer is a process whereby uncontrolled cell multiplication produces a tumor that can invade adjacent tissues and metastasize – that is, implant cancerous cells at a noncontiguous site, where abnormal multiplication continues. Cancer in connective tissues (mainly bone or muscle) is called **sarcoma**; cancer in epithelial tissues (lining tissues and organs) is called **carcinoma**. Carcinoma is by far more common. In Egypt, tumors have been found in third-millennium B.C. mummies, and ancient physicians there knew and treated different cancers.

The ancient Greeks, too, were familiar with cancers. Hippocrates is credited with naming the disease "cancer" from *karcinos* (Greek for "crab"), perhaps because some breast cancers appear crablike or perhaps because the pain of cancer resembles the pinching of a crab. The terms neoplasm ("new formation") and oncology ("study of masses") are also derived from Greek, as is the word tumor. Hippocratic medicine attributed tumors – including all sorts of swellings – to abnormal accretion of humors. Galen sought to differentiate cancers from inflammatory lesions and **gangrene**. Cancer was held to be caused by black bile.

Breast cancer was probably the first to be treated by attempting surgical eradication. Some ancient surgeons performed total mastectomies, and although the healing of these terrible procedures was little reported, Rhazes warned in the ninth century that operating on a cancer generally only caused it to worsen unless it was completely removed. It seems likely, however, that few cancers were treated surgically until relatively modern times. Ambroise Paré wrote toward the end of the sixteenth century that those who pretended to cure cancer surgically only transformed a nonulcerous cancer into an ulcerated one. Nevertheless, in the seventeenth century, Wilhelm Fabricius provided adequate descriptions of operations for breast and other cancers.

The discovery of the lymphatic system by Gasparro Aselli in 1622 directed attention toward lymphatic abnormalities in the causation of cancer. Basically, the idea was that cancer was an inflammatory reaction to extravasated lymph. About 150 years later, John Hunter modified the lymph theory by defining "coagulating lymph" (i.e., blood serum). Hunter viewed this substance (when contaminated by "cancerous poison") as the cause of cancer. Quite presciently, he described metastases as "consequent cancers" that traveled via lymphatic channels.

Another hypothesis (advocated particularly by the German Daniel Sennert and the Portuguese Zacutus Lusitanus) early in the seventeenth century was that cancers, at least when ulcerated, were contagious – a popular fear that persisted well into the twentieth century. The first accurate etiologic observation about cancer is attributed to London surgeon Percival Pott, who reported in 1775 that many long-time chimney sweeps suffered **scrotal cancer**. He linked this observation to the men's chronic contact with soot and thereby identified the first occupational cancer.

The impact of microscopy on cancer research came slowly. Robert Hooke, the pioneering seventeenth century microscopist who coined the term "cell," thought that tissues were composed of fibers – a hypothesis that persisted into the nineteenth century. Not until after 1830, when Joseph J. Lister designed the first achromatic microscope lenses, did progress begin. In 1855,

Rudolph Virchow postulated that neoplasms developed from immature cells. In 1867, Edwin Klebs suggested that most cancers originated in epithelial tissues.

Despite its antiquity, cancer is viewed as largely a modern phenomenon. Along with **cardiovascular disease**, it is perceived as the greatest health problem facing the developed world. Thus far, the World Health Organization has classified some 100 kinds of cancer according to sites of origin. Estimates indicate that one-third of the inhabitants of the industrialized world will develop some form of cancer. Cancer cures have largely eluded scientific medicine. Nor has Virchow's observation that irritants could summon forth cancerous cells proved very helpful in cancer prevention – although irritants are among the foci of cancer research today.

The concept of autonomy suggests that once a cell has become truly cancerous it is beyond bodily control. This idea was established around the turn of the twentieth century by Arthur Hanau, Leo Loeb, and Carl Jensen, who transplanted cancer cells into healthy animals and plants, subsequently observing the growth of new cancers in the previously healthy hosts. Yet the fact that established cancers can enter a stage of remission – sometimes permanently – argues that the body can retard or even reverse previously uncontrolled cell proliferation.

The next advances were made when cancer was induced experimentally in plants and animals by various chemical, physical, and biological agents. For example, some 150 different viruses caused tumors, and ultraviolet light, X-rays, radium, uranium, coal tars, certain dyes, and other substances also induced cancer. Even natural bodily compounds such as estrogen have caused cancer in experimental animals.

Cancer is predominantly an illness of middle age and, with a few exceptions, is relatively rare in children. Thus, people in the developed world, having escaped famine and epidemic disease, have extended their life expectancy into the ages in which cancer frequency is increasingly high.

The three most common cancers of men – **prostate cancer**, **lung cancer**, and **colon cancer** – comprise about 50 percent of new cases and 55 percent of cancer deaths. The three most common cancers of women – breast cancer, colon cancer, and lung cancer – also comprise about 50 percent of new cases and account for 50 percent of deaths. Cancer deaths in women peak at 41.0 percent in the 35–54 age group. In contrast, men's average age of cancer death peaks at 30.2 percent in the 55–74 age group. This difference is mostly attributable to the difference in age distribution of women with breast cancer and men with prostate cancer.

Survival has improved variably since the 1960s. The greatest improvements have occurred in **stomach cancer** (both sexes) and female **uterine cancer**. Lung cancer has increased in incidence in both sexes, as has male prostate cancer. The decrease in stomach-cancer deaths has resulted from a decline in incidence rather than any significant improvement in treatment. Survival generally has been and remains poorer for black than for white patients, a difference often attributed to the black population's poorer access to medical care. However, there are no apparent race-related differences in survival of certain common carcinomas (lung cancer, **kidney cancer**, and stomach cancer).

The greatest problem of exogenous carcinogenesis today is not exposure to industrial pollutants, as many believe, but rather the use of tobacco products. Cigarette smoke appears to exert the most potent carcinogenic effect, although cigar smoke and chewing tobacco are also implicated. Historically, the possibility that an increase in lung cancer was related to an increase in cigarette smoking was first raised in Germany in the 1920s. In the United States, interest was stimulated by the 1950 publication of three studies showing that lung-cancer patients were likely to be heavy smokers. Resistance to a causal relationship between smoking and lung cancer was based initially on doubt that lung cancer incidence was actually increasing, and then on a failure to appreciate the long preclinical phase of the disease.

Cigarette smoking is also associated with neoplasms of other organs (such as **bladder cancer**), but this does not obscure the clearly quantitative relationship between smoking and increased probability of lung cancer. Nevertheless, lung cancer occurs in only a small minority of even heavy smokers. This may indicate a predisposition that could warn persons at risk, but investigations have thus far failed to yield useful results. Finally, there have been no reproducible experiments showing tobacco smoke to cause lung cancer in experimental animals.

No potent pulmonary carcinogens have as yet been identified in tobacco smoke, but a 1970s finding appears to clinch the causal relationship between smoking and lung cancer: A 20-year investigation showed that the risk diminishes increasingly after smoking has been discontinued for several years, which cannot be ascribed to genetic or psychological factors. However, even 15 years after cessation, the risk among former smokers remained twice that of similar-aged men who had never smoked.

Smoking has now been common among women long enough to be reflected in an alarming increase in lung-cancer incidence, beginning in the mid-1960s and now half that of men in the United States. By 1986, the lung-cancer death rate of U.S. women equaled that for breast cancer.

Of the half-million women worldwide who develop breast cancer annually, half reside in North America and Europe, which contain less than 20 percent of the world's population. But more localized questions arise as well. For example, why is the breast-cancer death rate in Finland and Denmark more than triple the rate in Sweden, and why is the rate in Scotland quintuple that of England?

A daughter or sister of a woman with breast cancer has a nearly three times greater risk of developing it than a woman without such associations. The risk is greater if the relative's cancer appears at an early age, and greater still if both mother and sister have been affected. This suggests a genetic predisposition, as does the increased risk of a second breast cancer.

However, evidence indicates that environmental factors must also be involved. For example, breast-cancer prevalence in Japan is about one-fourth that in Europe or North America. Nevertheless, among Japanese-descended women in North America, the incidence of breast cancer by the second generation matches that of indigenous whites. But what factors are implicated remains unresolved.

Prostate cancer is the second most frequent cancer among U.S. men and the fifth worldwide. It is more prevalent among U.S. blacks than any other population – about 80 percent more common in black than white men in the United States. It is also common in black Caribbean populations, whereas information from Africa indicates much lower prevalence. The incidence of prostate cancer is more highly correlated with increasing age above 50 than any other neoplasm. It is six to seven times more prevalent in the 75–84 than in the 55–64 age group, and the black/white difference diminishes with age. Increased risk is associated with chronic cigarette smoking, and there is an apparent correlation between above-average sexual drive and susceptibility to **prostatic carcinoma**. This could mean that an alteration in sexual hormones has a predisposing role. Alternatively, a correlation between promiscuity and (male) prostate cancer would suggest an analogy to the better-documented correlation between promiscuity and (female) **cervix cancer**, and the possibility that a sexually transmitted virus is the pathogenetic agent. None of these hypotheses, however, explains the increased incidence of this disease in the late 1900s.

With regard to possible roles of diet in carcinogenesis, both low-fiber and high-fat diets have been proposed to be pathogenetic for **colorectal cancer**. The best evidence now indicates a carcinogenic effect of increased fat consumption, particularly in women. The predominant hypothesis for this association is: Higher fat consumption increases excretion of bile acids and growth of colonic bacteria; therefore, the conversion of bile acids into carcinogenic substances by bacterial metabolism is facilitated.

In the United States, colorectal cancer has remained stable in white men and decreased moderately in white women but increased in the black population.

The ultraviolet component of sunlight is a major cause of **skin cancer**. Susceptibility is related to paleness, poor tanning ability, and chronic exposure. Overall incidence of non-melanoma skin cancers in the white U.S. population is about 165 per 100,000. However, the prevalence in Texas is three times that in Iowa. The incidence of **melanoma** is only about 4 per 100,000, but 65 percent of skin-cancer deaths are caused by this disease. The lesion occurs twice as often on the legs of white women as on those of white men. It occurs nearly twice as frequently on the male trunk than the female trunk. Melanoma is uncommon in blacks, and its location tends to be on palms or soles and within the mouth – less heavily pigmented areas. Melanoma incidence has been increasing everywhere, and mortality has nearly doubled. Whether the increase is attributable to changes in ultraviolet intensity is unknown.

X-rays and related radiation are estimated to cause no more than 3 percent of cancers. Radon gas exposure is clearly a cause of lung cancer in uranium miners. If the concentration of radon in some homes were found to be sufficiently carcinogenic, presumably the proportion of known cases of radiation-caused cancer would increase substantially. **Thyroid cancer** results from small-to-moderate radiation exposure to the neck, with a latency period of about a decade. Bone marrow is another radiosensitive organ. Increased risk of **leukemia** begins as early as 2 years after radiation exposure, reaches peak probability after 6–8 years, and then diminishes.

Suspicion of potential carcinogens in consumer goods led to the 1958 passage of the Delaney amendment to the U.S. Food, Drug, and Cosmetic Act, which bans any food additives that cause cancer in any experimental animals in any dosage. One result has been the forced withdrawal of some products based on dubious and unrealistic experiments.

Worldwide, stomach cancer, now relatively uncommon in the United States, is the most prevalent visceral cancer (second for men, fourth for women). Nevertheless, death rates have declined to about 35 percent of 1930s figures. The decrease has been worldwide and is unexplained. It remains the most prevalent carcinoma in East Asia – the rate in Japan is more than seven times that in the United States, accounting for one-third of all Japanese cancer deaths. Repetitive ingestion of high concentrations of salt has been proposed as a cause of **gastric cancer**; indeed, the decline in incidence has correlated with the decline in salt preservation of foods. In regions where stomach cancer remains common, salted seafood remains a staple. The incidence of gastric cancer among first-generation Japanese immigrants to the West is similar to that in their homeland, but it declines to the incidence of the Western community where the next generation resides. Because this is not a genetic disease, a generation that is not exposed to salt at a critical age presumably will not suffer inordinately from this neoplasm.

Cervix cancer is apparently related not to geography but to cultural sexual practice. Sexual intercourse during adolescence, multiple partners, or partners who have had numerous partners are all risk factors, as is frequent pregnancy. Thus the disease is rare among nuns and common among prostitutes. A sexually transmitted virus is suspected to be a causative factor. In the United States, cervix cancer occurs twice as frequently among black as white women, whereas uterine cancer occurs two to four times as often in white women.

Liver cancer is much more prevalent in developing countries than in the industrialized world. China alone accounts for 45 percent of cases. The liver is subject to two principal types of cancer: one in liver cells, predisposed by a history of **hepatitis B** infection; another in bile-duct cells, predisposed by **liver flukes** and similar infestations. The geographic distribution of such parasites is reflected in the prevalence of this disease.

In summary, the concept of cancer has evolved from the idea of a single illness to one of many diseases with many causes. Most prevalent are carcinomas of the stomach, lungs, breast, cervix, colon and rectum, prostate, and liver. Chief among carcinogens are tobacco, certain metals, radiation, specific chemical compounds, helminthic parasites, and possibly viruses. Various carcinogens constantly bombard everyone, but cancer develops in a minority of people. A few uncommon neoplasms clearly are genetically determined. Resistance to carcinogens also appears to have a genetic basis.

Available treatments are generally drastic, poorly selective, and in many circumstances not curative. Earlier diagnosis improves the cure rate of many but not all cancers. Therefore, public education about cancer and further improvements in diagnostic methods are important. Until our understanding of the fundamental biology of cancer improves, preventive measures, such as minimizing exposure to carcinogens, will constitute the greatest benefit to public health.

Thomas G. Benedek and Kenneth F. Kiple

23. Carrión's Disease (Oroya Fever)

Carrión's disease is an infectious disease caused by microorganisms of the genus *Bartonella*. Two species have been described, the *bacilliformis* and *verrugiformis* types. These bacteria are parasites of human erythrocytes and histiocytic cells. The *bacilliformis* produces two stages of disease, a febrile acute hemolytic **anemia** known as "Oroya fever," followed by a granulomatous mucocutaneous eruption known as **verruga peruana**. The *verrugiformis* produces only the second (verrucose) stage.

Characteristics

Bartonella bacilliformis are pleomorphic bacteria. In red blood cells and histiocytic cells, the bartonella assumes a rodlike or coccoid shape.

It grows well in liquid and semisolid blood media. In 1913, Charles Townsend identified the female sandfly *Phlebotomus verrucarum* as the insect vector of the disease. Transmission occurs at night. Carrión's disease is a rural disease. Like **yellow fever**, it requires no human reservoir because the bartonella lives in small animals as well. However, inoculation of humans with a live germ appears to produce immunity.

The "anemic stage" of Carrión's disease is characterized by acute febrile anemia with bartonellas in the red blood cells, and the "verrucose stage" is characterized by a disseminated verrucous eruption in skin and mucous membranes. In severe infection, erythrocyte levels plummet to less than a million in a few days. The parasitic index in these cells reaches 80–100 percent.

Onset is abrupt, with fever, chills, and osteal pain. Bone-marrow **hyperplasia**, **reticulocytosis**, and **jaundice** present, with increased bilirubin in blood and urine. The blood culture is positive, even in the earliest days of the anemia. The verrucose stage is usually separated from the anemic stage by an asymptomatic interval of several months to over a year. Several types of eruption may occur: "miliary," "nodular," and "mular." The eruption becomes painful only with a secondary infection or increased bleeding.

In the *verrugiformis* type, the clinical picture is that of a diffuse granulomatous eruption similar to the *bacilliformis* type, but less intense. The *verrugiformis*-type eruption can recur two or more times during a lifetime.

The main pathogenic feature is the reproduction of the bartonella inside endothelial cells, which swell with tremendous numbers of bacteria. The resulting pressure ruptures the cell membrane, releasing millions of bacteria, which then colonize other endothelial cells. The bartonellas also parasitize peripheral erythrocytes, inducing the anemia. Severe cases show thrombosis and infarction in the spleen, necrosis of the liver, and lung congestion.

At the end of the anemia stage, immunoresponse occurs against active bartonellas, which are converted into resistant coccoids. This is the most dangerous period of the disease. At least 30 percent of untreated patients die after physical collapse. Another 40 percent die from secondary complications: Most frequent are **salmonellosis**, **tuberculosis**, **malaria**, and **amebiasis**.

From the clinical viewpoint, the patient has recovered, but the bartonellas still live in adventitial cells surrounding subcutaneous capillaries. Blood and bone marrow cultures are still positive. In time, the bartonellas start a new cycle of reproduction in the histiocytes, beginning the second stage of the disease. The histopathology of the granulomatous phase shows a proliferation with large, pale histiocytes and endothelial cells, some filled with coccobacillus bartonellas. The rupture of these cells results in dissemination of the bartonellas through the skin, and new verrucose eruptions appear. The eruptive phase tends to heal spontaneously without scars.

Before antibiotics, mortality from Carrión's disease was high. Antibiotics have a powerful bactericidal effect; the anemia is arrested, and blood regeneration starts immediately. Chloromycetin has been the most effective antibiotic in the anemic stage, and streptomycin is ideal during the eruptive phase.

History

Carrión's disease was probably depicted thousands of years ago in pottery of the ancient Peruvian civilization. The disease flourished in inter-Andean valleys of western South America. The focus of endemic transmission is in Peru, although some cases exist in Colombia and Ecuador. Endemic areas are confined to narrow valleys at elevations of 2,100–7,500 feet.

The disease was probably described during the Spanish conquest but attracted attention only in 1870, when an epidemic of the acute febrile form killed thousands of workers during construction of a railroad from Lima to Oroya. In

1885, Peruvian medical student Daniel Carrión contracted the disease by self-inoculation with verruga and died of Oroya fever, thus establishing the connection between the two conditions. In 1909, Peruvian physician Alberto Barton described organisms in the red blood corpuscles of Oroya-fever victims, and later these findings were confirmed. However, some still felt that Oroya fever and verruga peruana were caused by two distinct agents. H. Noguchi and T. Battistine resolved the controversy, reporting in 1926 that the illnesses were different manifestations of the same disease. In 1942, M. Hertig definitively described both the disease and its vector.

Oscar Urteaga-Ballon

24. Catarrh

Catarrh is now regarded as inflammation of the mucous membranes, especially of the air passages, together with the production of a mucoid exudate. Simple though this definition is, it bears evident traces of the history of the disease.

The name derives from Hippocrates' use of *katarrhoos*, a "flowing down" of humors from the head. In that use, the term was probably not yet technical, and so akin to a Latin word such as *defluxio*. In commenting on Hippocrates, however, Galen distinguishes general "downflowing" from a more precise meaning of "catarrh" – that is, defluxion from head to lungs, producing hoarseness and coughing.

The Greek word became *catarrhus* in Latin and a technical term with, increasingly, Galen's meaning attached to it. Although it is tempting to identify *catarrhus* with catarrh, we have to remember that for Galen and doctors down to the seventeenth century, *catarrhus* could not be defined without reference to Galenic pathology. *Catarrhus* was a process in which the brain, preternaturally affected by cold, produced a qualitatively unbalanced humor in excessive

quantity that passed down through the pores in the palate and by way of the trachea to the lungs. This unspoken assumption behind the name is paralleled by that behind the modern definition: We make the assumption that the "inflammation" of the definition results from infection by an organism. The identity of the organism gives us the ontology of the disease. A similar situation existed in all historical periods; that is to say, definitions of disease have always carried with them some part of a theory of causation. (Purely empirical accounts of disease are descriptions of symptoms.) To put it another way, disease in Western medicine has traditionally been seen as disordered function. But function is a process, and knowledge of it depends on knowledge of how the body works.

In the eighteenth and nineteenth centuries, there were a number of different so-called systems of physiological knowledge, in each of which what was indicated by a single disease name was seen differently. For example Franciscus de Le Boë (F. Sylvius), as an iatrochemist, divided catarrhs into groups distinguished by the chemical qualities of the humor produced. As a hydraulically inclined mechanist, Hermann Boerhaave thought of catarrh in terms of obstruction of the small vessels, which caused swelling. Indeed, his most frequent use of the term was as an adjective to describe **angina**. "Angina" was any difficulty in breathing, and catarrhous angina was the result of swollen membranes. Although membranes also played an important part in the new tissue pathology of early nineteenth century Paris, the Parisian view of the body, and therefore disease, was again different. Marie François Bichat stressed the sympathies between membranes and their ability to secrete and imbibe the fluids of the cavity they lined. To this were added the new techniques of physical diagnosis by percussion and stethoscope.

Catarrh again became a disease of membranes, of excessive secretion, and of fluids moving audibly in their cavities. Some Bichatian sympathy of membranes seems to lie behind the early nineteenth century notion of a catarrh of the urinary bladder. This opinion was recorded by R. Hooper, who also sharply distinguished common catarrh – a **cold**, and particularly a cold in the head – from epidemic catarrh, which is identified with **influenza**. The modern meaning is derived from the former.

Roger K. French

25. Cestode Infection

Cestodes are a class of flatworms in the phylum Platyhelminthes. The adult stages of four species and the larval stages of two are important parasites of humankind. Several other species, most of which normally parasitize other vertebrates, can also cause human disease. See: **Tapeworm Infection**.

K. David Patterson

26. Chagas' Disease

Chagas' disease (also **American trypanosomiasis** or **trypanosomiasis cruzi**) can be either an acute febrile infection or a chronic process. The cause is a protozoan, *Trypanosoma cruzi*, harbored by domestic and wild animals. When transmitted to humans by insects, this essentially untreatable disease presents with fever, edemas, and lymph node enlargement and can cause dilation in the digestive tract, leading to **megacolon** and **megaesophagus** as well as cardiac enlargement and failure. In parts of South America, Chagas' disease is the leading cause of cardiac death in young adults.

Characteristics
Probably originating in Brazil, the disease is limited to the Western Hemisphere, with heavy concentrations in Brazil, Argentina, Chile, and Venezuela. Cases are also reported in Peru, Mexico, and most other American countries, including the Caribbean islands and the United States. *T. cruzi* has over 100 vertebrate hosts, including dogs, cats, armadillos, opossums, monkeys, and humans. Unlike other trypanosomes, which multiply in the bloodstream, it lives within various tissues of the host and reproduces by binary fission. It is transmitted by reduvid bugs that ingest it from a host during a blood meal.

The trypanosomes develop in the intestines of the bug. They neither enter its saliva nor are injected when it bites but do pass out in its feces. Thus the infection is transmitted when the infected insect defecates following its blood meal, thereby contaminating the site of the bite. Infection can also occur when feces are rubbed into the eyes or reach oral mucosa, and possibly via contaminated foods as well. The insect vector flourishes in huts in poor rural areas, where it lives in cracks in the walls and in thatching and mats used as roofing. Cases may be few despite large numbers of infected bugs, if the bugs are not adapted to living in houses.

The disease takes several different forms, but, in all cases, no effective treatment exists. The acute form ends in death in 10 percent of cases, and, although the chronic form may last as long as 40 years, few individuals remain asymptomatic for life. Chronic **cardiac disease**, megacolon, and megaesophagus all can shorten life.

The acute form of the disease, occurring primarily in young children, is usually a febrile illness. When death occurs, it is generally caused by **myocarditis** or a complicating **bronchopneumonia**. The latent form is seen in patients who have recovered from the acute form, as well as others who have harbored the parasite without displaying symptoms. Examinations often reveal changes in esophageal and peristaltic motility as well as electrocardiographic changes. The subacute form is normally seen in young adults, who suffer a rapidly progressive cardiac failure.

The chronic form of the illness is the leading cause of death in endemic areas. The heart becomes tremendously enlarged, and in about 30 percent of cases, parasites are found within pseudocysts in muscle fibers. Although survival may be as long as 5 years, death usually intervenes within 6–12 months.

The digestive form of Chagas' disease presents as megacolon or megaesophagus. Victims suffer degeneration and diminution of nerve cells in the muscular layers of these organs, leading to their enlargement. The condition by itself is normally not fatal, but patients often experience difficulty swallowing because of the enlarged esophagus, and constipation normally accompanies megacolon. These difficulties in turn can promote other illnesses that are life-threatening. The congenital form of the disease has long been known. The fetus is infected transplacentally, resulting in premature fetal death or a newborn with Chagas' disease in its acute stage.

History

Chagas' disease is unusual in that its etiological agent, its vector, and major features of its epidemiology were described before the first human case was ever reported. Brazilian physician Carlos Chagas accomplished this in a series of publications beginning in 1909, and the disease appropriately bears his name. The illness, however, is not new. Studies of mummies from northern Chile have revealed megacardia, megacolon, and megaesophagus in several individuals who lived more than 2,000 years ago. The same area today is endemic for Chagas' disease.

Nineteenth-century visitors to Brazil reported instances of megaesophagus and the presence of the cone-nosed bug vectors of Chagas' disease. Most interesting is the case of Charles Darwin, who wrote that he was bitten by a huge *Triatoma* bug while in South America. It has been suggested that Darwin's mysterious chronic illness dated from this time, and some believe that Darwin was afflicted with Chagas' disease.

Although similar to **African trypanosomiasis** ("sleeping sickness"), Chagas' disease most likely evolved independently. Its cradle is believed to be the Bahia-Minas-Gerais area of Brazil, although it has subsequently spread throughout the Americas and has a notable presence in Argentina. In fact, a mid-twentieth century Argentine study established that the disease was much more widespread than previously believed and stimulated other studies, leading to recognition that Chagas' disease was a serious health threat in South America. Indeed, since the 1950s, it has become increasingly common in southern Peru, although the vector (called *chirimacha*) is known throughout all of Peru.

Marvin J. Allison

27. Chlorosis

Diseases are categorized as degenerative, malignant, genetic, endocrine, and so on in current nosology. For the *history* of disease, we must add a category that we might term "ephemeral." This requires some license, because many "ephemeral diseases" lasted longer than that term usually implies. Ephemeral diseases comprise a large number of entities that bore working diagnostic names (e.g., **typhomalarial fever**) for earlier physicians but that are no longer recognized, at least by their previous names.

A historical example of such a disease is the "green sickness," **chlorosis**. Although noted in two Hippocratic treatises, the condition received its classic description from Johann Lange in 1554; he called it *morbus virgineus*. His description contains many elements from the Hippocratic texts, as do accounts by Ambroise Paré in 1561 and by Jean Varandal (credited with first using the word "chlorosis") in 1615. For Varandal, chlorosis was a class of syndromes. Reflecting a different approach, Thomas Sydenham in 1683 described many clinical features relied upon two centuries later. Friedrich Hoffmann defined the actual clinical entity in 1731.

Characteristics

Chlorosis was associated almost entirely with Caucasian girls encountering puberty. Still, from clinical observations alone, the etiology remained obscure. Inconsistencies abounded. Not all young women developed the disease at the age of menarche. It struck rich as well as poor. Some, but not all, suffered a morbid appetite termed **pica** (consumption of stones, clay, chalk, and other substances of no nutritional value). Even into the nineteenth century, confusion permeated medical thinking about chlorosis. But by the time of William Osler toward the end of that century, medical opinion had become far more confident. The clinical features of chlorosis had been distilled to the point that in many instances the condition could be "recognized at a glance."

Developments in laboratory medicine brought physicians to something approaching consensus regarding the pathophysiology of chlorosis. By the mid-nineteenth century, reasonably accurate methods were available to determine red-blood-cell counts and hemoglobin content. With this, it became apparent that the essential condition of chlorosis was **iron deficiency anemia**. In the minds of many physicians, chlorosis could now be separated from earlier mimics such as lovesickness, **hypochondriasis**, and **neurasthenia**.

The natural history of chlorosis, whether treated with iron or not, remained a matter of dispute. In part, this undoubtedly related to frequent misdiagnoses. Using iron, some physicians reported that a single cure was lasting. For others, the disease progressed to **phthisis**, many cases of which probably were **tuberculosis** rather than chlorosis. After iron became a standard treatment, there was general agreement that the disease recurred when treatment was stopped, but responded when iron was reinstituted and continued. If patients remained on the prescribed iron long enough, chronic cases responded as well as those newly diagnosed.

Some observers might look on the use of iron in treating chlorosis before an iron deficiency had been demonstrated as sheer luck, and one more example in the history of medicine where physicians did the right thing for the wrong reason. Yet, although there are many examples

of right-thing/wrong-reason in medicine's past, iron for chlorosis probably is not one of them. When physicians employed proper iron compounds in correct doses, the clinical results were dramatic and altogether convincing.

Even if it was correct that the central feature of chlorosis was iron deficiency anemia, a good deal of confusion remained. Still to be elucidated were a host of diseases marked by pallor, wasting, and lassitude, some of which had anemia as a secondary manifestation. These included **nephritis**, **hypothyroidism**, subacute bacterial **endocarditis**, **mitral stenosis**, and tuberculosis. What did subside was the focus on many factors once considered central but now relegated to a contributory role at most, including lack of fresh air and exercise, corsets, lovesickness with its related sexual frustration, and a variety of uterine disorders.

Chlorosis reminds us of the complex interaction between physiology and social elements in the genesis of human disease. This interplay is better understood in light of current notions of iron metabolism. To protect the body against the destructive effects of excessive iron, intestinal absorption is fixed at a rate that barely replaces the small amount lost normally. This balance is so exquisite that the prolonged loss of 2 teaspoons of blood daily exceeds the body's ability to absorb iron from a normal diet, and anemia follows. Iron deficiency anemia can result from decreased dietary iron, increased bodily demand for iron, or loss of blood.

In chlorosis, decreased iron intake came about either from poverty that precluded the intake of iron-rich foods or from cultural influences encouraging young women to avoid meat, eggs, and even milk because of a belief that animal foods increased sexual drive, an undesirable result in Victorian times. The increase in bodily demands for iron resulted simply from the rapid growth associated with adolescence.

The green skin-color of chlorosis, from which it may have derived its name, remains, like the origin of syphilis, one of the fascinating problems in the history of disease. The conundrum appeared when chlorosis was equated with iron deficiency; yet greenish skin in Caucasians was rarely observed in the many cases of **hypochromic anemia** then being diagnosed. Another possibility is that chlorosis was a misnomer, that the word "green" was used metaphorically to mean immature, raw, or inexperienced.

Significantly, green skin was included only sporadically in clinical descriptions of chlorosis over the years. Lange made no mention of it in his original description. In one study of 27 authors who listed signs of chlorosis, only 16 mentioned greenish skin as characteristic. In another analysis of 19 descriptions, only 3 seemed definitely green, 3 possibly so, and 2 yellowish-green. At least it is now reasonable to remove green skin as *the* outstanding characteristic implied by the designation chlorosis.

History

The incidence of chlorosis in earlier times is impossible to determine. From the attention it received in literature as well as art, one may infer that the condition was not rare. By the end of the nineteenth century, it was viewed as extremely common. This conclusion is all the more striking in light of the rapid exit of chlorosis from center stage. By 1915, medical observers were commenting on the disappearance of the green disease. Some concluded that chlorosis had never been anything but a simple iron deficiency anemia brought on by inadequate diet and loss of menstrual blood.

But the condition was not that easily dismissed, as physicians continued to find chlorosis very much alive. In 1969, it was listed as one of five major categories of hypochromic anemia considered diseases *sui generis*. In 1980, one student of the illness concluded that chlorosis was a functional disease intimately related to **anorexia nervosa**. Current medical dictionaries still carry the term and define it as an iron deficiency anemia of young women.

Recent revisionist historical work has emphasized the importance of general perceptions of women and their role in what physicians thought and did about disease, although there is surprisingly little about chlorosis as such in this literature. Marxist and social historians have become interested in chlorosis. These revisionist approaches, to varying degrees, tend generally to diminish the importance of pathological physiology in explaining the rise and decline of chlorosis. The more committed the revisionists are to their historical biases, the more difficulty they have squaring their interpretations with those of others as well as with more purely medical explanations. The Marxist, for example, must construct social and political conditions that produced chlorosis in young women of the capitalist class as well as the oppressed poor, because the evidence is incontrovertible that the condition affected both.

The feminists who would argue that nineteenth century physicians mistreated women consciously on the basis of gender must account for the fact that many of the treatments accorded women by male physicians at the time derived from an inadequate understanding of reproductive physiology and that masculine sexual conditions were also mistreated. The historian who argues that chlorosis was nothing more than a cultural construction of Victorian family life, that physicians diagnosed the condition simply because they expected to encounter it, and that young women simply learned to manifest the clinical picture of chlorosis must explain the well-documented existence of the disease in young men as well.

Enthusiasm for new historical approaches to disease should not obscure the importance of the final common pathway of social, political, and cultural forces. And that common denominator for chlorosis in the nineteenth and early twentieth centuries was an iron deficiency anemia. Social and cultural factors certainly predisposed individuals to chlorosis, but persons became patients ultimately because they had red blood cells that were too small and lacked the normal amount of hemoglobin. Poor nutrition – whether from poverty or cultural preferences – certainly contributed. Physicians, with their heavy reliance on bloodletting, even prophylactically in pregnant women, undoubtedly played a part as well. Chlorotic women gave birth to iron-deficient children – "larval chlorotics" they were called. Chlorosis, at bottom, was a deficiency disease. Explaining it historically demands an eclectic historiography. The biopsychosocial model emerging as the proper paradigm for health professionals dealing with disease in our time has always operated historically. Ockham's razor may be useful in logic, but it may slice too narrowly in history. Plethora rather than parsimony more often illuminates the complexities of humanity's interaction with society at any given time and place. Chlorosis is a case in point.

Robert P. Hudson

28. Cholera

Cholera is an acute diarrheal disease usually accompanied by vomiting and resulting in severe dehydration or water loss and its consequences. The disease is caused by a comma-shaped bacterium, *Vibrio cholerae,* first isolated in Egypt and Calcutta in 1883. Mortality rates have reached up to 70 percent of infected individuals during epidemics. Cholera has long been endemic in India and Bangladesh, from where it has spread in periodic epidemics to other parts of Asia and eventually to much of the rest of the world. Most of this spread has occurred since 1817, when the modern history of the disease outside India begins; it is now generally agreed that some seven pandemics have occurred since its initial spread. The most recent began in 1961 and is only now receding. The bacterium is disseminated by the so-called fecal-oral route as a consequence of sewage and fecal contamination of water supplies and foodstuffs. This indirect transmission long made its spread difficult to understand.

In the course of history, the term "cholera" has been variously applied. The word first appears in the Hippocratic corpus and there refers to sporadic **diarrheal disease**. Later classical writers

including Celsus, Aretaeus, and Caelius Aurelianus used the term as well. By 1669, Thomas Sydenham employed it in describing an epidemic in London. "Cholera" was also widely used to describe endemic or sporadic diarrhea throughout the nineteenth century and earlier in Western Europe and the Americas. This is sometimes specifically designated as *cholera nostras.*

The term *cholera morbus,* today limited to the disease caused by *V. cholerae,* can cause confusion because in the past it meant either epidemic or endemic forms of such illness. Synonyms include *cholera asiatica, cholera epidemica,* malignant cholera, *cholera asphyxia,* and *cholera spasmodica.* It is now generally accepted that all cholera in the West prior to the nineteenth century epidemics was endemic or sporadic and not caused by *V. cholerae.*

Characteristics

The cholera bacterium, *V. cholerae,* was seen in the excreta and intestinal contents of cholera victims by Filippo Pacini and described and named by him in a report published in Florence in 1854. The bacterium can be grown in the laboratory in an alkalinity greater than that tolerated by most other bacteria. This characteristic is of significance for its growth in the human small intestine. *V. cholerae* survives and multiplies outside the human body in any relatively uncontaminated alkaline environment. It does not regularly infect animals; its host range is limited to humans, who can also act as asymptomatic carriers. The bacteria produce a toxin, which causes the symptoms of the disease.

Cholera is spread solely by infected humans, whose excreta may contaminate drinking water and food. This is not a direct-contact infection as expected from such diseases as smallpox, and communicability was initially a highly controversial matter.

The spread of cholera in a community depends first on the appearance of a person, either ill or well, who is discharging the cholera vibrio from his or her intestinal tract, and second on the state of hygiene, water supply, and sewage disposal in promoting or impeding the transmission of the bacteria to potential victims. Unsatisfactory sanitary facilities were a necessary condition for cholera outbreaks in Europe and the Americas. Indeed, the history of the control of cholera is the history of improved sanitation.

Current distribution of epidemic cholera is largely limited to areas in India and the tropical Far East, where it persists and occasionally breaks out in areas with contaminated water and sewage. Since World War II, it has made sporadic forays into the Middle East and other Asian regions. In the 1970s, cholera appeared briefly in Europe, with outbreaks in Naples (more than 30 deaths), Barcelona, and Lisbon (more than 2,000 cases). One small area of persistent infection appears to be the lower bayou country outside of New Orleans.

The bacterial infection is limited to the intestinal tract; no microbes are found to invade the body tissues. The low bacterial population normally in the small intestine as well as its high alkalinity contribute to the cholera vibrio's ability to survive and grow there, usually in massive numbers. The bacteria adhere to the intestinal wall and secrete a toxin that inhibits the absorption of water and electrolytes (salts) from the intestine into the circulation. Failure of this absorption results in the loss and excretion of many liters of fluid in the course of a single day. This loss presents as a massive, debilitating diarrhea, which is the major clinical feature of cholera. All other symptoms of the disease are attributable to water and salt depletion. These include weakening and finally loss of pulse, thickening of the blood, suppression of urination, loss of tissue fluids giving the face a sunken appearance, **cyanosis**, muscular spasms, and a disastrous fall in blood pressure leading to profound shock, which represents the fatal conclusion of the disease.

Modern therapy consists simply of replacing the lost water and salts. Thus cholera is essentially curable. Antibiotics play only a minor role, in that they may shorten the duration of disease and reduce the massive amounts of necessary fluid replacement.

History

In India, a relatively sparse literature on the disease serves as a prelude to the modern history of true cholera. Modern literature on cholera starts slowly in 1817 and accelerates with its appearance in Russia in 1829, Eastern Europe in 1831, and Western Europe and North America in 1832.

Portuguese explorer Gaspar Correia stated that in the spring of 1503, many soldiers of Calicut died of a "disease, sudden-like, which struck with pain in the belly, so that a man did not last out eight hours time." Correia also met cholera in an epidemic form in the spring of 1543 in Goa, where the mortality was so great that it was difficult to bury all of the dead. The disease was marked "by vomiting, with drought of water accompanying it, as if the stomach were parched up, and cramps that fixed the sinews of the joints."

The disease was repeatedly described by Europeans in Goa in 1563, 1584, and 1585. Reports followed through the rest of the 1500s and 1600s, including that of the well-known physician Jacobus Bontius in the earlier 1600s, who extended his observations to Indonesia. Notices of the disease continued to appear into the eighteenth century, when they were supplemented by reports by English medical men (including famed naval doctor James Lind), who provided good descriptions of cholera cases and symptoms in the 1750s and 1760s.

In 1781, cholera ravaged British troops in the Ganjam district of India, requiring the hospitalization on March 22 alone of no less than 500 men of a division of 5,000. A report of the incident calls the disease a "pestilential disorder" and does not name it cholera, although later writers assumed that it was. This outbreak is reported to have reached Calcutta. In April of 1783, "cholera burst out at Hurdwar, and in less than eight days is supposed to have cut off 20,000 pilgrims." Fragmentary observations continued to appear, depicting the "terrible ferocity" of the disease, which "destroyed an enormous number of people," and further ravages occurred at Arcot and Vellore in October 1787.

Cholera, or cholera-like disease, continued to be observed during the rest of the eighteenth and into the nineteenth century. Then, in the year 1814, outbreaks of cholera occurred in a number of Indian provinces, including the crowded barracks of Fort William at Calcutta among recruits just arrived from England.

It may well be that "it was nothing new for cholera to spread over India in an epidemic form prior to 1817 and 1819." But at this point, something drastically "new" did occur, as cholera escaped the bounds of India and initiated the waves of pandemics that were to engulf the world. This change in cholera's pattern of activity has led a few to conclude that a new disease arose in Bengal in 1817, a contention that was much debated. More recently, it has also been suggested that a genetic modification in the microbe was responsible for this supposed change in cholera's nature.

In any event, in March 1817, a death from cholera took place in Fort William, but because it was a solitary case no notice was taken of it. By July, however, outbreaks occurred in several districts in the Province of Bengal. In July and the following months, Calcutta was affected; 25,000 of its inhabitants were under medical treatment for the disease, of whom 4,000 died. Thus begins the modern history of Asiatic or epidemic cholera, although none of the documents immediately surrounding the event makes reference to the name "cholera," until a letter dated September 16 specifically refers to *cholera morbus.*

Within 3 months the disease had spread throughout the Province of Bengal, and in November it reached the camp of the Marquis of Hastings in Bundelcund. During 1818, it moved over the greater part of India including Delhi and Bombay, with estimated attack rates of up to 7.5 percent of the exposed population. It continued to rage through 1819 and 1820, extending into Ceylon and Burma, Siam, Malacca and Singapore, and the Philippines. By 1821, it had invaded Java, Batavia, and China to the east and Persia to the west, reaching Baghdad with a besieging Persian army, and extending from there

to Aleppo. By 1823, it was in Egypt, Astrakhan, and the Caspian shores and throughout Syria along the shores of the Mediterranean. But it receded for a number of years, thereby terminating the First Pandemic.

By 1824, cholera had retreated to its endemic area in Bengal, where it remained active in the Ganges Delta through 1826. But in 1827, it spread out again in the so-called Second Pandemic into the Punjab, and by 1829 extended through Persia to the shores of the Caspian Sea. Reaching Orenburg in August 1829, it soon expanded north and west into Russia. By September of 1830, cholera was in Kharkov and Moscow, and began spreading west into Bulgaria. During the winter of 1830–31, it persisted in the Russian army in Poland, and then in the spring invaded Warsaw and, soon after, Riga. Meanwhile, cholera was also raging through Mecca and Turkey, reaching Constantinople and Alexandria by July and August. On August 3, it entered Berlin and Vienna, and reached Hamburg by the beginning of October. Around the end of October, if not before, it appeared in England at Sunderland, supposedly imported from Hamburg or Riga. Late fall and early winter brought a brief respite; observers were sent to infected areas, and efforts were made to prepare for the coming onslaught amid much argument about such matters as quarantine, sanitation, contagiousness, and treatment.

The opening of the year 1832 was soon followed by a reawakening of cholera. In February, it appeared in Newcastle, Edinburgh, and London, as well as places in between. Next it reached France, bursting on Paris on March 24, and soon engulfing all districts of the city. Within 18 days no fewer than 7,000 persons were dead. Next, cholera hurdled the Atlantic Ocean to appear on June 8 in Quebec and on June 19 in Montreal. Presumably, it arrived with emigrants on the brig *Carricks,* which left infected Dublin in April and lost 42 of its 173 passengers before reaching Quebec on June 3. On June 23, cholera invaded the United States, appearing in New York on that date and in Philadelphia on July 5. From these ports of entry, it marched westward across both North American countries.

Entry into Spain, Portugal, the Caribbean, and Latin America was delayed until 1833, and into Italy until 1835. Havana lost 8,253 persons in a population of 65,000 between February 26 and April 20, 1833, and by August no less than 15,000 had perished in Mexico.

Yet by 1834, the disease was beginning to recede, and while it persisted in a number of Mediterranean and Central American areas for a few more years, it retreated once again in 1837 to its Indian homeland. For much of the world, this pandemic was the first modern experience with the disease, and subsequent epidemics or pandemics were to follow much the same route. Popular and governmental response to subsequent appearances was largely based on experience gained during this pandemic.

During the following decade, cholera continued to plague India, and it entered with British troops into Afghanistan in 1839 and China in 1840, where it remained into 1841 and 1842. In 1844–45, it extended into Persia and Central Asia, reaching the Arabian coast as well as the Caspian and Black seas in 1846–47. Constantinople was attacked on October 24, 1847. In the spring of 1848, it broke out with renewed vigor, advancing as far as a line drawn through Arabia, Poland, and Sweden, reaching Berlin in July and Hamburg and Holland by September, and then London and Edinburgh in short order. After a short period of comparative rest, it renewed its activity in the spring, reaching Paris in March and by now covering much the same ground as the earlier epidemic. Meanwhile, in December 1848 cholera had crossed the Atlantic to invade New York and New Orleans, and spread rapidly across the continent from these centers. In 1850, it reached California with wagon trains as well as by ship from Panama. In that year it was reported in North Africa, Europe, and both North and South America. In many of these regions, it continued through 1851 and 1852.

The year 1854 found cholera widely spread in Europe, the Near East, and the Americas to pro-

duce one of the worst cholera years on record. It was during this pandemic that John Snow made his observations in London that in 1855 led to the publication of his critical, if not immediately appreciated, study on cholera transmission by contaminated water. In 1855 and after, the disease died down in much of the West, but it continued in a few spots there as well as in much of the East.

The Fourth Pandemic is generally dated from 1863 and lasted 10–12 years. In 1865, an estimated one-third of 90,000 pilgrims at Mecca succumbed. As before, cholera reached Constantinople and spread around the Mediterranean, reaching northern Europe in 1866 and 1867, and the United States and Latin America in 1866. It raged over its old grounds until 1874.

The Fifth Pandemic is said by many to have begun in 1881 and lasted until 1896. It was during this epidemic that the studies of Robert Koch in Alexandria and Calcutta in 1883-84 led to the isolation and identification of the causative microbe. The epidemic was at first largely limited to the Mediterranean shores of Africa and Europe, although it later became widespread in Russia and in Germany, where it was marked by the explosive outbreak in Hamburg in 1892. Importation into New York in 1887 was arrested, but outbreaks did occur in Latin America. The disease was also widely prevalent in the Far East – in China and Japan.

The Sixth Pandemic ran from 1899 through 1923. It followed much the pattern of the fifth – largely affecting India, the Near and Far East, Egypt, western Russia, and the Balkan Peninsula. Sporadic outbreaks occurred in southern Europe and Hungary in the West and China, Japan, Korea, and the Philippines in the East. But this time cholera did not reach the Western Hemisphere.

The Seventh Pandemic dates from about 1961 and followed much the pattern of the previous epidemic. It was particularly important in providing an opportunity for significant advances in cholera pathogenicity and therapy in studies carried out in Egypt, India, Bangladesh, and the Philippines by several U.S. teams.

This brief sketch provides only the barest outline of the history of cholera. Historians do not always agree on the chronology of the pandemics. In fact, it is sometimes not entirely clear why or when one pandemic is said to have terminated and another to have begun.

Earlier, thoughts on the causes of cholera were embedded in notions of disease causation going back to Hippocrates, such as weather, seasons, geographic environment, bad air and miasmas, and dietary indiscretions. If an infecting agent was even envisioned, it was as a vague poison or miasma.

By the middle of the nineteenth century, however, ideas of a microbial etiology were gaining ground. In 1849, William Budd and two associates described microscopic bodies in cholera excreta and published their findings with illustrations. French botanist Charles Robin reproduced the illustrations in 1853. These were seen by the German botanist Ernst Hallier, who attempted to grow microbes from cholera excreta. He published his findings in 1867.

T. R. Lewis tried to confirm Hallier's work in Calcutta in 1870, but failed. In the meantime, as already described, Pacini made his correct but at the time largely ignored observations of the actual *V. cholerae* in 1854. Thus it was left to the genius, persistence, and technical elegance of Koch in 1883 to isolate and identify the microbe and to introduce the modern phase of understanding of the disease. It was not, however, until 1959 that the toxin produced by the microbe was discovered, along with its role in disease causation.

The question of the "contagiousness" of cholera was a matter of heated debate throughout most of the nineteenth century. The contagionists were viewed by contemporaries as archaic, conservative, and even antisocial, whereas the anticontagionists were seen as modern, bourgeois, mercantile, and socially responsible. Most of the debate focused on the question of quarantine which, of course, was anathema to mercantile interests, and the anticontagionists gained ground as the nineteenth century progressed. The demonstration by Snow of the waterborne nature of cholera was slow to gain acceptance, but this development, coupled with Koch's discoveries, finally proved the "contagion" of the disease, albeit allowing for the intermediary roles of infected excreta, water or food, and of individuals who can act as carriers but do not develop the disease.

Sanitation has always played a major role in efforts to understand and control the propagation of cholera. As a consequence, a large body of literature has been generated on the role and influences of cholera epidemics on the development of public-health policies, public-health organizations, and sanitation procedures and techniques.

The definitive treatment – intravenous fluid and salt replacement – was a long time in developing. As early as 1830, German chemist R. Hermann demonstrated that the change in the blood's fluid balance was reflected in the contents of the cholera excreta. A colleague injected 6 ounces of water into his terminally ill patients, a treatment that produced a quick, temporary return of the pulse, although death nonetheless occurred 2 hours later. In October 1831, Berlin surgeon J. F. Dieffenback took the premature step of injecting several ounces of whole blood into three patients. They died 6 minutes, 2 hours, and 6 hours later, respectively, the first during violent convulsions. In Britain in late 1831 and early 1832, W. B. O'Shaughnessy published papers suggesting the intravenous replacement of salt and water. This led Thomas Latta to try the treatment on patients; he subsequently reported that 5 of 15 survived. Other attempts followed, with some success, during the 1830s. Sporadic trials continued through the century, but the treatment was not successful until Leonard Rogers perfected it in Calcutta in the early 1900s. There were a number of technical problems to be solved first, such as effective sterilization. But with these difficulties resolved, the definitive treatment of cholera was established.

Reinhard S. Speck

29. Cirrhosis

Cirrhosis is a chronic disorder characterized by liver fibrosis and nodule formation, which produce portal hypertension and hepatocellular failure. Cirrhosis is the end product of progressive liver injury resulting from diverse causes including toxins, drugs, viruses, and parasites. Clinical manifestations of cirrhosis vary with the underlying disease. In the West, cirrhosis is a cause of disability and death among middle-aged alcoholic males. Elsewhere, cirrhosis is predominantly an intermediate lesion in the evolution from chronic **hepatitis B** infection to primary **hepatocellular carcinoma**.

Characteristics

Cirrhosis is classified depending on morphology and etiology. Morphologically, there are three types based on the size of nodules on the liver: macronodular (greater than 3 millimeters in diameter), micronodular (less than 3 millimeters), and mixed micro/macronodular (a mixture of small and large nodules). The appearance of the liver cannot alone differentiate among the many causes of cirrhosis. Indeed, the etiology is often unknown. Alcohol injury is most frequently associated with **micronodular cirrhosis**; other causes in this category include primary **biliary cirrhosis**, primary **hemochromatosis**, and chronic **right heart failure. Macronodular cirrhosis** arises from viral, drug, and cryptogenic origins and appears in any end-stage cirrhosis.

Cirrhosis is distributed worldwide, affecting all races, nationalities, ages, and both sexes. Well over 300,000 persons (probably underestimated) die of it annually. The incidence of cirrhosis chiefly depends on per capita consumption of alcohol and prevalence of hepatitis viruses. The increase in cirrhosis cases is attributable to an increase in one or both of these factors. Based on mortality statistics, the incidence of cirrhosis is low (less than 10 deaths per 100,000 population) in countries such as Canada, England, and Australia; intermediate (11–23 per 100,000) in Mexico, the United States, and Japan; and high (more than 24 per 100,000) in Italy, France, and Germany. Statistics on cirrhosis suffer from uncertain diagnoses, which are confirmed only by autopsy or liver biopsy. The prevalence rate of cirrhosis in autopsies averages 3–4 percent in Europe, 5–8 percent in the Americas, and 1–2 percent in Japan.

In the United States, deaths from cirrhosis rose 71.7 percent from 1950 to 1974. This increase was marked for nonwhite males, moderate for nonwhite females, and only slight for white males and females. Among U.S. blacks, cirrhosis mortality was similar to or slightly lower than that of the white population before 1955. Then the pattern changed rapidly, with blacks experiencing an epidemic of cirrhosis compared to the increase in whites. In urban America, cirrhosis mortality in the nonwhite population is at least double that of the white population.

Steadily increasing cirrhosis mortality in industrialized nations is linked to increased per capita consumption of alcohol. During the twentieth century, mortality in the United States, England, and France dropped whenever alcohol was prohibited or restricted. A national doubling of alcohol intake produces a fourfold increase in alcohol-induced disease. Risk of cirrhosis increases with daily alcohol intake much faster in females than in males, and progression to severe liver injury is accelerated in women. However, the male/female ratio remains at least 2:1 for most groups, with some notable exceptions.

In the West, alcoholic damage comprises the majority of all cirrhosis. An estimated 75 percent of cirrhosis in the United States is alcoholic in origin; 15 percent is viral, and 10 percent is cryptogenic. In Britain, 50 percent is alcoholic, 25 percent cryptogenic, and 25 percent viral. In Asia and Africa, where the prevalence of hepatitis B virus is high and per capita consumption of alcohol is low, the proportion of virus-related cirrhosis to alcoholic cirrhosis is reversed from that of the West. However, the incidence of hepatitis B viral cirrhosis is uncertain. Studies strongly support an association between chronic hepatitis B infection and primary hepatocellular carcinoma. Infection at birth results in chronic hepatitis, cirrhosis, and carcinoma 20–30 years later. How the virus causes the carcinoma is unknown, but cirrhosis is involved, especially among males. Like hepatocellular carcinoma, cirrhosis is common where hepatitis B virus is endemic.

Diagnosis of cirrhosis depends primarily on the two cardinal manifestations; portal hypertension and hepatocellular failure. As cirrhosis usually evolves over years, the course may be intermittent with therapeutic intervention or temporary cessation of injury. During the early phase, patients often present with nonspecific signs including malaise, anorexia, or weight gain. As the disease progresses, portal hypertension and hepatocellular failure invariably supervene. These complications are interrelated and often represent the initial presentation of many cirrhotics. Cirrhosis can be checked – for example, in the alcoholic who abstains. Treatment can reverse hepatic **fibrosis** and improve the outlook for patients with chronic active hepatitis, primary hemochromatosis, or **Wilson's disease**. After **ascites** develops, however, the 5-year survival rate falls below 50 percent.

History

The ancient Greeks recognized clinical features of cirrhosis. About 300 B.C., Erasistratus associated ascites with liver disease. Centuries later, Galen discussed the physical diagnosis and noted the danger of heavy wine consumption for those already afflicted. His contemporary Aretaeus suggested that cirrhosis evolved from hepatitis, and carcinoma from cirrhosis. The Greeks' clinical descriptions remained unexcelled until recent times.

In the sixteenth century, Vesalius described rupture of the portal vein in a patient with an indurated nodular liver. When pathological anatomy became a discipline in the seventeenth century, sporadic reports of cirrhotic livers appeared. In 1616, William Harvey discussed two cases of cirrhosis, antedating John Browne, whose 1685 description was long considered the first in English. Among the earli-

est illustrations of cirrhosis was that by Frederik Ruysch in the early eighteenth century. In 1716, Giovanni Morgagni introduced the term "tubercle" for any hepatic nodule, which sowed confusion between carcinoma and cirrhosis for decades. Matthew Baillie's accurate description in 1793 established cirrhosis as a nosological entity; he also strongly associated it with alcohol intake.

During the eighteenth century, corn surpluses led England's Parliament to promote spirits in an effort to stabilize grain prices. Excessive consumption of cheap spirits produced an epidemic of cirrhosis, popularly known as "gin liver" in England and "brandy liver" elsewhere.

Twenty-five years after Baillie, René Laennec introduced the name "cirrhosis." In 1829, Gabriel Andral suggested that hypertrophy of the liver's yellow substance accounted for the nodules, whereas atrophy of the red substance represented the depressed areas of cirrhosis. This concept, relating cirrhogenesis to the dual substance of the liver, influenced thinking on the subject for two decades. In 1838, Robert Carswell conjectured that cirrhosis depended on the growth of interlobular connective tissue. Gottlieb Gluge and Dominique Lereboullet argued that hepatic fat was the basic lesion of cirrhosis. Karl von Rokitansky attributed cirrhotic "granulations" to chronic inflammation.

During the mid-nineteenth century, interest in vascular studies gathered momentum, and the vascular alterations in cirrhosis came under scrutiny. Some researchers, such as Karl von Liebermeister in 1864 and J. M. Legg in 1872, continued to focus on interlobular connective tissue. Others emphasized the regenerative aspects of cirrhosis, which represented the end product of many injurious episodes. In 1911, Frank B. Mallory introduced the entity of "alcoholic hepatitis," identifying it as a precursor lesion of cirrhosis. Mallory's concept was recently revived after decades of dormancy.

Earlier it had been suggested that **alcoholic fatty liver** was the precursor of cirrhosis. By the second half of the nineteenth century, most physicians accepted this thesis, believing that alcohol intake increased hepatic fat, which in turn was converted into cirrhosis. However, experiments failed to demonstrate the cirrhogenic effect of alcohol in animals. This led to the notion that not alcohol but some contaminant in it, such as copper, damaged the liver. Other theories stressed that gastric malfunction was the underlying cause in that it produced – or allowed absorption of – hepatotoxins. Hypotheses of nutritional deficiency were bruited when 1930s experiments showed that the fatty liver condition caused by insulin deficiency was preventable with choline and other agents. Other dietary models of cirrhosis soon followed, including lipotroph deficiency, low-fat diet, and vitamin-E deficiency. However, nutritional theories declined in popularity when Charles S. Lieber (and others) showed in 1968 that alcohol was directly hepatotoxic in humans and cirrhogenic in baboons.

Another technical innovation has advanced understanding of cirrhosis. Introduced by Paul Ehrlich in 1884, the liver biopsy later achieved wide use as a diagnostic method. Studies clarified the relationships among hepatitis, cirrhosis, and hepatocellular carcinoma. They also helped consolidate the various cirrhosis classifications proposed in the past. The recent standardization of nomenclature was proposed by the Fogarty International Center in 1976 and the World Health Organization in 1977.

Thomas S. N. Chen and Peter S. Y. Chen

30. Clonorchiasis

The **Chinese liver fluke**, discovered in 1875, is a small worm that parasitizes the bile ducts and livers of humans, dogs, cats, pigs, and several wild animals in China, Japan, Korea, and Indochina. Estimates indicate that 20 million individuals in China alone are infected. Eggs are laid in the bile ducts, pass in the feces, and, if they reach the proper freshwater snail, undergo a series of stages in this intermediate host. Eventually, free-swimming larvae are formed, which penetrate and encyst the skin or muscles of fish, expecially those of the carp family. Humans and other definitive hosts become infected by eating the cysts (metacercariae) in raw or poorly cooked fish. Raw fish are a delicacy in many Asian countries, and fish are sometimes raised in ponds fertilized with human feces. Encysted metacercaria larvae are resistant to smoking, pickling, salting, and drying. Imported fish have caused human cases in Hawaii, and the popularity of Asian cuisine poses a potential danger to gourmets far beyond Asia.

Light infections are often asymptomatic. Heavy infections may produce **diarrhea**, fever, **jaundice**, and abdominal pain. Bile duct blockage and liver abscesses occur in chronic cases, and *Clonorchis sinensis* has been tentatively linked to **liver cancer**.

K. David Patterson

31. Croup

The term **croup** identifies several respiratory illnesses of children manifested by inspiratory stridor, cough, and hoarseness from upper-airway obstruction. Classically, croup was a manifestation of **diphtheria**, but nowadays, many infectious and noninfectious causes of croup syndromes are recognized. Although long-term obstruction in the glottic and subglottic regions can lead to chronic illness, croup syndromes are described here as acute diseases. Most cases of croup today are either **laryngotracheitis** or **spasmodic croup**.

General Characteristics

Acute epiglottitis (inflammation of the epiglottis) is virtually always caused by *Haemophilus influenzae* type B; rare cases are caused by *Streptococcus pneumoniae* and *Staphylococcus aureus*. **Laryngitis** usually arises from viral agents, most importantly adenoviruses and **influenza** viruses. Laryngotracheitis and spasmodic croup are common childhood illnesses caused by viruses or *Mycoplasma pneumoniae*. The most important agent is parainfluenza virus type 1, which, along with parainfluenza type 2 and influenzas A and B, causes outbreaks of disease. In areas without diphtheria immunization, laryngotracheitis is also caused by *Corynebacterium diphtheria*.

The same viruses that cause laryngotracheitis also frequently cause **laryngotracheobronchitis** and **laryngotracheobronchiopneumonitis**. Other causes of the latter two include *S. aureus*, *Streptococcus pyogenes*, *S. pneumoniae*, and *H. influenzae*.

Croup syndromes occur worldwide, most caused by common "croup viruses": parainfluenzas 1 and 2 and influenza viruses. Outbreaks occur during cold-weather months, and in the tropics during rainy seasons. The highest attack rate occurs in children 7–36 months old; few cases occur after the sixth birthday. During their second year, about 5 percent of children experience an episode of croup. Croup is more common in boys than in girls and also tends to be more severe in boys. A parainfluenza infection in an adult is manifested by a **cold**; older persons suffering trivial illnesses may be the source of severe croup in young children.

Acute Epiglottitis

This is a disease of abrupt onset, which if untreated causes death from airway obstruction. Illness is characterized by fever, severe sore throat, dysphasia, and drooling. Airway obstruction is rapidly progressive and associated with inspiratory distress, a choking sensation, irritability, restlessness, and anxiety. The child with epiglottitis insists on sitting up and exhibits great anxiety if forced to lie down.

Acute Laryngotracheitis

Initial symptoms usually include nasal dryness, irritation, and **coryza** (profuse nasal discharge). Cough, sore throat, and fever occur. After 12–48 hours, signs of upper-airway obstruction develop. The cough becomes "croupy" (sounding like a sea lion), and respiratory stridor increases. Severe disease is manifested by marked respira-

tory distress. **Hypoxia** can occur, and, with no intervention, asphyxial death will occur in some children.

Spasmodic Croup

Unlike laryngotracheitis, in which obstruction results from inflammatory exudate and cellular damage, obstruction in spasmodic croup is caused by noninflammatory edema. Onset is always at night and occurs in children thought to be well or to have a mild cold. The child awakens with sudden **dyspnea**, croupy cough, and inspiratory stridor. There is no fever. Spasmodic croup tends to run in families; affected children often have repeated attacks.

Acute Laryngotracheobronchitis and Laryngotracheobronchiopneumonitis

These illnesses are less common than those discussed previously but are more serious. Initial symptoms are similar to laryngotracheitis. Signs of lower respiratory involvement develop 2–7 days into the illness; occasionally, upper- and lower-airway obstructions occur simultaneously. Along with the usual croup symptoms, laryngotracheobronchiopneumonitis patients have **rales**, air trapping, wheezing, and increased respiratory rate.

History

The word "croup" is derived from the Anglo-Saxon *kropan* ("cry aloud") and was first used in medical writing in 1765 by Scottish physician Francis Home. Until the twentieth century, virtually all croup-like illnesses were confused with diphtheria.

The clinical history of diphtheria has been traced to the time of Homer, and some experts believe that the Hippocratic texts demonstrate knowledge of it. In the second century A.D., Aretaeus noted extension of the disease to the lower respiratory tract, resulting in death by suffocation. Galen noted expectoration of the pseudomembrane. In the fifth century, Aetius added his experience. Although both Aretaeus and Aetius were describing **diphtheritic croup**, confusion with other illnesses – such as **Ludwig's**

angina and **streptococcal tonsillitis** – clearly existed.

The historical trail of diphtheria disappeared in the fifth century and failed to reappear until the sixteenth. In 1557, Peter Forest described an epidemic in Holland. In 1576, Guillaume de Baillou reported an epidemic in Paris and specifically mentioned false membrane. In 1771, Samuel Bard published the first U.S. report on **suffocative angina**. In 1826, Pierre Bretonneau named diphtheria and recognized its infectious nature. In 1883, Edwin Klebs observed the diphtheria bacillus, and a year later Friedrich Löffler established it as the etiologic agent.

From 1920 to 1940, the incidence of diphtheria in the United States fell steeply because of the use of first toxin-antitoxin and then toxoid. In association with and also predating this decline, a general realization of other cases of croup occurred. Prior to 1900, only occasionally were illnesses suggesting nondiphtheritic croup specified. For example, in 1852 E. Bouchut described **false croup** (possibly spasmodic croup). In 1887, A. Sanné mentioned an epidemic of simple croup in Germany, and in 1765 Home noted two forms of croup. Bretonneau differentiated diphtheria from spasmodic croup in 1826.

During the first half of the twentieth century in the United States, severe croup was called laryngotracheal-bronchitis and understood to be caused by *C. diphtheria* – and by other bacteria as well. In 1948, Edward Rabe described three forms: diphtheritic croup, *H. influenzae* type B croup (epiglottitis), and **virus croup**. Soon, the viral etiology of croup was confirmed. But croup resulting from bacteria other than *C. diphtheria* was overlooked. In 1976, nondiphtheria/bacterial croup was rediscovered and has since received considerable attention.

The history of spasmodic croup is unclear because its clinical and pathological aspects are poorly defined. In the 1940s, Francis Davison distinguished it from other forms; since then, however, this entity has received little attention.

James D. Cherry

32. Cystic Fibrosis

Cystic fibrosis, also called "fibrocystic disease of the pancreas" and **mucoviscidosis**, is a genetically determined disease of infants, children, and young adults. Most of its many manifestations result from abnormally viscous mucus, which interferes with pulmonary function, and insufficient production of pancreatic digestive enzymes, which causes nutritional deficiencies and developmental retardation.

Characteristics

Among Caucasians, cystic fibrosis (CF) is the most common fatal disease having an autosomal recessive inheritance. Despite the primary involvement of several organs, the disease is caused by a single defective gene that is located on chromosome 7 and is carried by about 4 percent of the Caucasian population. Its expression is similar in both sexes.

CF manifests itself at birth in about 8 percent of cases through mechanical obstruction of the small intestine by the secretion of abnormally viscous mucus (**meconium ileus**). Symptoms of insufficient secretion of exocrine (noninsulin) digestive enzymes by the pancreas appear during the first year of life in 90 percent of cases. The development of such symptoms indicates that pancreatic function is less than 10 percent of normal; and the more severe the deficiency of pancreatic enzymes, the more severe the fecal excretion of undigested fat, usually as **diarrhea**. As much as 80 percent of dietary fat may be lost. Loss of undigested nutrients can be corrected only partially by treatment with pancreatic enzyme tablets.

Pulmonary disease is responsible for most debility and mortality. Onset occurs during the first 2 years of life in at least 75 percent of cases, and by age 6 in most others. The initial pulmonary abnormality is obstruction of the small bronchi by abnormally thick mucus. Structural deterioration of the lungs results and is exacerbated by an increased susceptibility to infections. A few patients retain sufficient pancreatic function to maintain nearly normal digestion;

such patients also tend to have fewer respiratory difficulties. The variability in severity results from different mutations on the pathogenetic gene.

The sweat of a child with CF contains a concentration of sodium chloride about five times greater than normal, although salt is not lost excessively by other routes. Determining the salt content of perspiration has become a basic diagnostic test. The propensity to become salt-depleted makes persons with CF particularly intolerant to heat. As a result of pulmonary and metabolic therapy, many CF patients are now living into reproductive age, and thus it has been found that CF men, but not CF women, are sterile. In spite of all efforts, few patients survive to age 40.

History

According to a medieval German saying, "The infant who when kissed leaves a taste of salt will not reach the first year of life." Hence, CF was probably recognized many centuries ago. However, it was first identified in 1936 by Swiss pediatrician Guido Fanconi and associates and further delineated in 1938 by Dorothy Andersen. The diagnostic perspirational salt loss was quantified by Paul di Sant'Agnese and associates in 1953.

CF is most prevalent among people of central European ancestry (1 in 2,000 to 3,000 births) and is somewhat less common in Scandinavia. Inbreeding explains incidences of greater than 1 per 1,000 in small areas. For example, the prevalence of CF among nearly 11,000 Amish in one Ohio county was more than 1 per 600 (all cases within six families), whereas there were no cases in another Amish community in a nearby county. Similar results of inbreeding have been reported from Brittany and from Afrikaners in Namibia. CF has been reported in about 1 in 17,000 black Americans, and in 1 in 90,000 Orientals (mainly Japanese) in Hawaii. The prevalence of CF has not been investigated adequately in Asia and Africa. It is possible that its true prevalence is masked by high infant mortality in large portions of these continents.

The CF gene was identified in 1989. With the rapid advances in gene-transfer therapy, it may soon become possible to correct the defect. Then, instead of merely prolonging life by treating the symptoms, physicians may give CF infants a normal future.

Thomas G. Benedek

33. Cytomegalovirus Infection

Cytomegalic inclusion disease (CID) usually occurs as a subclinical infection with periodic reactivation revealed by shedding of the virus. It may be serious in the neonate when infection is transmitted to the fetus in utero. Cytomegalic infection is characterized histologically by the presence of large cells containing inclusion bodies in the midst of an infiltration of mononuclear cells in any of the body organs.

Characteristics

In prenatal infections, most infants are born without clinical evidence of disease, although some 10–15 percent may show **microcephaly**, mental/physical retardation, **hepatosplenomegaly**, **jaundice**, and calcifications in the brain. There may be abnormalities in liver function tests and **hematopoiesis**. Some 10–30 percent of infants with symptomatic disease die in early life. Central nervous system involvement can develop early – even though the child appears normal – and is manifested as impaired intellect, neuromuscular abnormalities, **chorioretinitis**, optic atrophy, or hearing loss.

Neonatal infection acquired at birth from an infected cervix or later from mother's milk usually goes unnoticed but can be identified by the development of antibodies. Respiratory symptoms including pneumonia, as well as **petechial rash** and enlargement of the liver and the spleen, may occur. In these cases, however, acute involvement of the central nervous system is rare.

Infection in children is generally asymptomatic and evidenced only by development of antibodies and shedding of virus. Occasionally, hepatosplenomegaly and abnormal liver function are found. There is no proof that **pharyngitis** occurs at the presumed portal of entry.

When infection occurs in adults, the clinical picture is similar to **infectious mononucleosis**: pharyngitis; **lymphadenopathy**; systemic symptoms of fever, chills, and headaches; and occasionally a **maculopapular rash** are primary symptoms. Atypical **lymphocytosis** is usual, and there may be abnormal liver function.

In instances where the disease is transmitted by transfusion of blood or its products, the infectious mononucleosis syndrome usually appears as a posttransfusion episode in 2–4 weeks. Immunocompromised patients are at special risk of exogenous infection by transplanted organs or transfusions, or of activation of the latent state. Death may occur from **interstitial pneumonia**, often complicated by superinfection with gram-negative organisms, fungi, or other unusual invaders.

Studies show that CID has worldwide distribution. It remains asymptomatic despite prolonged shedding at periodic reactivation and is not highly communicable. Presumably, the virus is spread mainly by oral secretions, because it is shed from the salivary glands. The virus has been isolated from urine, breast milk, semen, and cervix uteri: It may therefore be sexually transmitted.

The most serious aspect of CID is as a prenatal disease. Even though the mother is asymptomatic and immune, transmission of virus to the fetus occurs. Recurrence in the mother is the most probable explanation for prenatal infection, although, of course, primary infection may occur during pregnancy. Evidence suggests that infection in the offspring is more serious in the latter case than the former. One study has shown that children infected in daycare centers may be the source of infection for pregnant mothers.

With a disease spread mainly by oral secretions, higher incidence is anticipated in crowded and unhygienic surroundings. For example, 100 percent of Tanzanian women have antibodies by childbearing age. In England, studies show seropositivity in 50–80 percent of children in boarding schools and orphanages compared to 10–20 percent of children attending day schools. In Puerto Rico, 70–80 percent of adults have antibodies, whereas in London the figure is only 50–60 percent. Studies in the United States and Britain show that from 0.2 to 7.5 percent of newborns are virus positive, making this disease the most common fetal infection.

Antibodies develop upon infection to last for life. Nevertheless, as in other diseases caused by the **herpesviruses**, the presence of circulating antibodies – even in large amounts – does not forestall recrudescences of infection.

History

Early in the twentieth century, pathologists noted enlarged cells with inclusion bodies in organs of children dying of presumed **congenital syphilis**. The inclusions were thought to be amebas. In 1921, noting a similarity to changes found in **varicella**, researchers guessed the inclusions represented viral infection and described the cellular enlargement as "cytomegaly." The virus was isolated in 1956 by investigators working independently in St. Louis, Boston, and Bethesda. Epidemiological studies became feasible with the recognition of antibodies in 1968. Rapid expansion of knowledge of its epidemiology, incidence, and clinical manifestations continues.

R. H. Kampmeier

34. Dengue

Dengue is an acute disease caused by infection with an arbovirus of four serotypes, transmitted by infected *Aedes aegypti* and *Aedes albopictus* mosquitoes. Endemic throughout the tropics and subtropics, uncomplicated dengue is rarely fatal, although convalescence may take several weeks. Sometimes, however, it is complicated by hemorrhagic manifestations (**hemorrhagic dengue**) and circulatory collapse (**dengue shock**

syndrome) with a potentially fatal outcome unless medical facilities are available.

Characteristics

Typical uncomplicated dengue incubates for 3–15 days and is characterized by abrupt onset of chills, headache, lumbar backache, and severe prostration. Body temperature rises rapidly, as high as 40°C; **bradycardia** and **hypotension** accompany the fever. Conjunctival infection, lymph-node enlargement, and a pale rash, especially on the face, are usually present during this phase. In classical dengue, the fever lasts 48–96 hours initially, subsides for 24 hours or so, and then returns ("saddle-back" fever), although the peak temperature is usually lower in the second phase. A characteristic red rash appears, usually covering trunk and extremities but sparing the face. The fever, rash, and headache are known as the **dengue triad**.

Hemorrhagic dengue usually strikes children under 10 and has its highest mortality in infants under 1. It is more likely to occur when type 2 dengue virus infection follows an earlier type 1 infection or when subgroup-specific antibodies have been acquired transplacentally from an immune mother. Signs of this complication include sudden collapse with a rapid pulse of low volume; **cyanosis** of lips, ears, and nail beds; and cold, clammy extremities while the trunk remains warm. Nosebleeds, spontaneous bruising, prolonged bleeding from injection sites, and bleeding from both upper and lower gastrointestinal tract signals gross disturbance of blood-coagulation mechanisms.

The word dengue comes from the Spanish, a homonym for the Swahili *Ki denga pepo* (a sudden cramplike seizure caused by an evil spirit); it was introduced into English medical usage during the Spanish West Indies epidemic of 1827–28. The synonym "breakbone fever" dates from Philadelphia in 1780, and the term *knokkelkoorts* comes from Batavia about the same year.

Dengue viruses belong to the family of flaviviridae (from Latin *flavus* or "yellow," referring to **yellow fever**). The family consists of the genus *Flavivirus*, which has 65 related species and two possible members. Most flaviviruses are arboviruses, and all are serologically interrelated. They infect a wide range of vertebrate hosts, causing asymptomatic infections and diseases such as yellow fever, dengue, and numerous **encephalitides**.

A. aegypti and *A. albopictus* are responsible for dengue transmission in Asia. *A. albopictus* has recently been discovered in the United States and Brazil, but it has not yet been implicated in the transmission of disease. It is an aggressive, human-biting mosquito with both urban and rural habitats and transmits dengue viruses transovarially (from female mosquitoes to their offspring through infection of the eggs) and from person to person. Populations of *A. albopictus* found in the United States are capable of overwinter survival in northern latitudes. Although recent outbreaks of dengue in Brazil have been atrributed to *A. aegypti*, the presence of *A. albopictus* gives rise to serious concern that it may become an important vector for the introduction of flaviviruses into areas previously free of them.

Infection with one dengue serotype confers long-lasting type-specific protection, a benefit that may be more apparent than real because the type-specific protection also brings a greatly increased susceptibility to severe dengue disease in the event of infection with dengue virus of another serotype. Epidemiological studies clearly link the severe forms of dengue disease to previous dengue infection and to transplacental acquisition of maternal dengue antibody. This phenomenon has important implications for the development of dengue vaccine, which carries a serious risk of predisposing partially immune populations to further and more serious disease.

Dengue literally girdles the globe, with a distribution approximately equal to that of *A. aegypti*. Areas of dengue endemicity include tropical and subtropical regions of the Americas, Africa, Asia, and Australia. There are areas of *A. aegypti* infestation in Europe and the southern United States, where dengue has caused epidemics in the fairly distant past, but which have no current dengue activity although they remain susceptible to its reintroduction.

Dengue fever epidemics typically involve large numbers of people and have high attack rates. Up to 75 percent of susceptible persons exposed will acquire the disease. Mosquitoes remain infectious for life; therefore, a single mosquito can infect a number of people. Recurrent outbreaks of dengue in the same geographic region indicate either that new dengue virus types have been introduced or that endemic types are now affecting groups of the population lacking immunity – generally those born since the last epidemic.

Dengue hemorrhagic fever is especially frequent in Southeast Asia, where it is among the leading causes of hospital admissions in children and the commonest cause of death from communicable disease at any age. Its first reported appearance in epidemic form in the Western Hemisphere came in 1981.

Worldwide increase in dengue activity appears to be directly related to a failure to control mosquito populations effectively, to overpopulation, to progressive urbanization, and to the social and political disruptions caused by wars. Although a jungle cycle (involving forest mosquitoes and wild monkeys) similar to that of yellow fever has been demonstrated, zoonotic acquisition of dengue does not appear to be a factor in the general pattern of increasing prevalence.

History

Dengue has been known as a distinct disease entity for several centuries. Benjamin Rush is traditionally given credit for historical priority with his account of "breakbone fever," the epidemic that afflicted Philadelphia in 1780. Although his work is generally accepted as the first modern medical account of dengue, claims have also been made on behalf of David Bylon, a Dutch physician who described an epidemic of *knokkel-koorts* ("knuckle-fever") in the Dutch East Indies in 1779.

Bylon, state surgeon to the city of Batavia, treated 89 patients for *knokkel-koorts* and then

caught it himself. His illness began with pain in the joints of his right hand and arm and rapidly progressed to include high fever within a few hours. He concluded his account by remarking that the disease was well known in Batavia but had never before reached epidemic proportions. That alone would serve to distinguish *knokkel-koorts* from dengue, given what we know of the epidemiology of the latter.

Patrick Macdowall participated in the Darien Scheme, an attempt to found a Scottish colony in 1699 on the Isthmus of Panama, then known as Darien. The colonists were ravaged by disease, and Macdowall, who kept a journal that is still preserved in the National Library of Scotland, gave an excellent description of his own illness, which could well have been dengue. Macdowall survived an acute febrile illness lasting 4–5 days that was characterized by nausea, vomiting, prostration, headache, disordered sensation of taste, bone and joint pain, generalized rash, and faintness. His convalescence was prolonged and marked by general weakness and a continual tendency to faintness.

Was Macdowall's illness dengue? Classical saddleback fever occurs in only 50 percent of cases, and even lymphadenopathy is not an invariable finding. Macdowall's personal case history may well be the earliest recorded description of dengue.

The importance of mosquitoes in the transmission of dengue was recognized early in the twentieth century when T. Bancroft, using human volunteers, proved that dengue could be transmitted via the bite of infected mosquitoes and that the infecting agent was neither an intracorpuscular parasite nor a bacterium, but an ultramicroscopic organism. His observations also incriminated *A. aegypti* as the likely vector, but he erroneously concluded that the dengue organism lives only for a few days in infected mosquitoes. This, however, should not detract from the credit due him for recognizing the viral etiology and mosquito transmission of dengue long before Albert Sabin cultivated the virus in his late-1940s laboratory. Proof that *A. albopictus* is a vector of dengue came in 1931 when

James S. Simmons published experimental studies on dengue in the Philippines.

The general pattern of dengue since World War II has been of increasing prevalence and severity within the context of unrestrained proliferation of its vectors. Today those vectors that spread yellow fever as well as dengue pose a real threat to humanity.

James McSherry

35. Diabetes

Diabetes mellitus (DM) is an endocrine disorder characterized by the lack or insufficient production of insulin by the pancreas. DM has been recognized as a disease for at least two millennia, but only since the mid-1970s has there been a consensus on its classification and diagnosis.

The primary diagnostic criterion for DM is elevation of blood glucose levels during fasting or at 2 hours following a meal. Normal plasma glucose values for adults in the fasting state are 80–120 milligrams per deciliter (mg/dL). Definition of unequivocal DM requires a 2-hour postingestion plasma glucose level equal to or greater than 200 mg/dL for the appearance of classical symptoms of diabetes. These symptoms, which include excessive urination, urine containing sugar, hunger, thirst, fatigue, and weight loss, are common to all types of DM.

Despite the use of a plethora of different terms in the past, diabetes is now generally classified as type I DM (**insulin-dependent diabetes**) and type II DM (**non-insulin-dependent diabetes**). Other variants of DM include **maturity-onset diabetes of youth**, **tropical diabetes**, which shows characteristics of both insulin dependence and nondependence, and **gestational diabetes**, which occurs during the latter part of pregnancy.

Approximately 90–95 percent of all diabetics may be classified as type II, and about 5 percent as type I. Some 2 percent of diabetics have DM as a secondary result of other disease or injury.

History

As early as the sixth century, Hindu physicians recognized diabetes and attributed it to dietary indiscretion. Early descriptions of the classic symptoms of diabetes included the most salient – excessive urination. The term diabetes, meaning "to run through," was first used by Aretaeus.

In 1679 Thomas Willis noted the sweet taste of urine from diabetics, and in 1776 Matthew Dobson measured the amount of sugar in the urine by evaporating it and weighing the dried residue. Dobson stated that this residue looked and tasted like "ground sugar." Subsequently, **glycosuria** (sugar in the urine) became diagnostically important and was used to measure the effectiveness of treatment of DM. In 1815, M. D. Eugène Chevreul published his discovery that glucose is present also in the blood of diabetics.

From the mid-1700s until the 1970s, many types of diabetes were described. Observations by Apollinaire Bouchardat, culminating in his 1875 book on glycosuria, clearly distinguished two types of diabetes: In type I, the patients were relatively young; the onset was acute, weight loss was striking, and death ensued rapidly. In type II, the patients were older and tended to be overweight, and the onset was slower. Some of these individuals could control their glycosuria with a low-carbohydrate diet.

Much of the early work focused on elucidating the causes of polyuria. John Rollo, in the late 1790s, studied an obese diabetic patient at the Greenwich Naval Hospital. He noted that the amount of urine excreted depended upon the food consumed. Urinary production increased after ingestion of vegetables and decreased when the diet was high in animal fat and protein. These findings shifted the focus from the kidneys to the gastrointestinal tract and provided a scientific basis for therapeutic diets high in fat and protein and low in carbohydrates.

Mid-nineteenth century autopsies revealed no abnormalities in the pancreata of diabetics. In 1855 French physiologist Claude Bernard discovered that the liver secretes glucose. Such findings led some to believe that a liver disease caused diabetes. Attention was redirected to the pancreas in 1889 when it was demonstrated that complete removal of the pancreas did cause diabetes in dogs.

Specialized "heaps of cells" had been identified in the pancreas by Paul Langerhans in 1869. Continued research in the 1890s demonstrated that these "islets of Langerhans" were the source of an "internal secretion" that regulated glycosuria. This work suggested convincingly that DM is caused by a disorder of the endocrine portion of the pancreas. In 1921, the internal secretion was isolated and named insulin. Insulin is largely responsible for the control of blood glucose levels.

Although insulin was first used in 1922, it was not until the 1950s that appropriate bioassays of human insulin were developed. These measurements clearly showed that type I diabetics produced no insulin at all, whereas type II diabetics produced varying amounts of insulin. Thus insulin therapy against type I DM was vindicated. Diet, exercise, and – after 1955 – oral hypoglycemic agents were prescribed against type II diabetes.

Insulin-Dependent Diabetes Mellitus (Type I) Insulin-dependent DM is characterized by clinically acute onset, usually at an early age, reduction in the production and excretion of insulin, weight loss, thirst, frequent urination, and high levels of blood sugar. After the onset, remission may occur in some cases for up to 15 months. After this period, all patients require insulin therapy to prevent the profound biochemical aberrations that can lead to death.

Typical type I diabetes is uncommon, affecting less than 0.5 percent of the world's population. There is strong evidence for a genetic susceptibility, but of those individuals who carry the suspected antigens, only 30–50 percent develop DM; thus, environmental factors also appear to have a role. Other possible causative factors include infectious viruses such as **mumps**, **rubella**, and **meningitis**.

A number of studies indicate an increased prevalence of type I diabetes among populations that previously showed low rates. Increases are particularly marked among Japanese, black Africans, and black Americans. In general, these increases are associated with a "Westernization" of lifestyle since World War II.

Some nutritional factors have been suspected of being involved in the etiology of type I diabetes, although there is no consistent picture. Excess caloric intake does not seem to be the important factor it is in type II diabetes. The range of nutritional factors implicated in type II diabetes is much greater and is discussed below.

Non-Insulin-Dependent Diabetes (Type II) Between 90 and 95 percent of all diabetics have type II diabetes and are over the age of 35 years. In contrast to type I, many cases (up to 50 percent) remain undiagnosed. Type II diabetics produce insulin but may require more than they produce themselves. The majority of patients are treated with dietary modifications, often with caloric reductions for weight loss, and with oral hypoglycemic tablets. Many causative factors have been implicated in type II diabetes.

Genetic mechanisms interacting in complex ways with environmental factors are involved in the risk for type II diabetes. Type II DM occurs more frequently in families in which one or more members have DM than in the general population. Yet family studies have not supported a simple mode of inheritance.

Both age and sex are risk factors for type II diabetes. In most affluent societies, the rate of diagnosed type II diabetes increases steadily from 30 to 60 years of age. The extent to which physiological aging is a risk factor is unknown. Many observations have been made on sex differences in the frequency of type II diabetes. Before 1900, diabetes was observed to be more frequent in men in both Europe and the United States. Since 1930, however, clinicians in both America and Europe have repeatedly observed a greater frequency in female diabetics. Nonetheless, many developing nations show a male predominance. Groups with a high male/female ratio include rural Africans, Hong Kong Chinese, and populations in Iraq, Jordan, Japan, Korea, India, and Pakistan. Populations with predominance of females include the United States, the Caribbean countries, Sweden, Belgium, the former Soviet Union, Thailand, and South Pacific countries.

Exercise seems to be a potent protective factor in diabetes. It enhances both carbohydrate metabolism and the efficient use of insulin. As early as 1893, it was noted that active men in India had a lower rate of diabetes than their more sedentary counterparts. Overall, a decrease in energy expenditure has been related to changes in lifestyle, a relationship that has been particularly well documented in the South Pacific. Unfortunately, quantitative data on exercise are limited, and the short- and long-term effects of exercise on carbohydrate metabolism are incompletely understood.

Abundant worldwide evidence associates **obesity** with type II diabetes, and experts have concluded that it is the most powerful risk factor for non-insulin-dependent DM. Between two-thirds and nine-tenths of individuals may be classified as obese at the time of diagnosis of DM. The association between obesity and diabetes was noted long ago, but modern concern with obesity began in 1921. Overwhelming data showed diabetes rates to be 6–12 times greater in obese than in lean individuals. More recent studies documented high frequencies of both obesity and diabetes among a number of Amerindian tribes in Oklahoma and in Latin American populations. Yet it does not hold true for all peoples.

High caloric intake and low caloric expenditure are both related to obesity. Diabetes rates have increased in a number of countries, such as Japan, Taiwan, Haiti, New Guinea, and parts of Africa, where caloric consumption per capita has also increased. Conversely, during World War I and II in Europe and during World War II in Japan, when caloric intake was markedly decreased, obesity and diabetes both declined.

Most researchers agree that there is no convincing evidence that a single dietary component increases the risk of diabetes. Furthermore, the distinction between simple and complex carbohydrates has been questioned recently.

Researchers focusing on complex carbohydrates (such as potato and wheat bread) have shown that these starches engender production of high levels of insulin and glucose. In fact, the glucose response to white potatoes and dextrose sugar was approximately the same.

It has been suggested that dietary fiber decreases the risk for diabetes, and different forms of fiber are being investigated in this connection. However, it is difficult to disentangle the effects of decreased fiber consumption from increased sugar and carbohydrate intake, increased total calories, total fat, decreased caloric expenditure, and stresses associated with rapid dietary change and modernization. Thus, there remain many unanswered questions.

Dietary fats have also been viewed as risk factors, although studies investigating fat intake are often inconclusive. Fats are denser in calories than other nutrients, and high fat intake is generally associated with low fiber intake. An important 1930s study presented evidence positively linking fat consumption to diabetes. Yet other observations have not supported this relationship. Furthermore, evidence challenging any such relationship is found among Eskimos living a traditional lifestyle with diets high in fat and protein yet suffering little from DM. Alternatively, protein deficiency in the tropics has been implicated in certain types of diabetes.

Tropical Diabetes

A type of diabetes found primarily in many tropical areas of the world has characteristics of both type I and type II. The clinical profile involves the following: (1) a different genetic pattern of diabetes than in temperate regions; (2) a low prevalence rate of type I DM; (3) a younger age of onset of type II; (4) a sex ratio with male predominance in India and Africa, but female predominance in the West Indies; (5) an association of low calorie and protein intake with underweight diabetic individuals in Old World areas but overweight individuals in the Western Hemisphere; (6) the predominance of diabetes in urban areas, with the exception of rural populations in the West Indies; and (7) intermittent need for insulin therapy.

Information is relatively sparse on the genetics of diabetes in tropical countries. Recent studies have shown great population variability in increased susceptibility to diabetes. Genetic studies of Indian populations suggest a stronger familial factor among them compared to diabetics in other populations.

Risk factors for tropical diabetes involve unique dietary items. For example, some types of cassava (manioc) may be toxic and produce pancreatic damage. However, many areas show high rates of diabetes in populations that do not consume cassava, and some populations have high cassava consumption and low rates of diabetes. In Kenya, a local alcohol called *changaa* is implicated in causing the disease. Finally, in most tropical areas carbohydrates constitute 70–80 percent of total calories, and such a diet is implicated in classic **malnutrition diabetes** because of low nutrient density and high fiber content.

Gestational Diabetes

A type of diabetes present only during pregnancy was noted in 1882. However, it was not until the 1940s that the term "gestational diabetes" appeared in medical literature. This form of the disease is difficult to distinguish from type II diabetes because a woman could have diabetes before pregnancy but not have it diagnosed until pregnancy. Babies born to diabetic mothers usually are large but may have immature organ systems, in which case they may not survive.

In general, cities in the United States report a higher prevalence of gestational diabetes than do European cities. The highest reported rate of gestational diabetes occurs among the Pima Indians of Arizona, who also have the highest prevalence of type II diabetes of any known population.

General Characteristics

Because of its acute onset and obvious symptoms, type I diabetes is readily identified and, therefore, permits a more accurate picture of worldwide prevalence. Type II DM is a chronic disease with generalized symptoms; therefore, many cases are not diagnosed. However, rates of type II do appear to be increasing in developing nations. Generally, investigators have been cautious in interpreting an actual increase in the incidence of insulin-dependent DM. Prevalence rates continue to rise because of increased longevity of individuals with type I diabetes. Incidence rates for type II diabetes vary extensively by age and sex for different populations. In general, the incidence increases with age for both males and females until the sixth or seventh decade of life.

Diabetes is among the top 10 causes of death in developed countries. In Western countries, DM ranks seventh as a cause of death. Data since the early twentieth century document a decrease in early diabetes mortality because of increasing sophistication in therapeutic approaches, particularly the wide-scale use of insulin.

Migrant populations have been prone to high rates of diabetes. For example, Jews have shown increased susceptibility to diabetes in European enclaves as well as in migrant groups. Jews in New York City had rates 10 times higher than other U.S. ethnic groups. Studies from the early 1900s show high rates of diabetes among Jews in Budapest, Bengal, Boston, and Cairo. Others have shown that Sephardic Jews in Zimbabwe and Turkey have high rates of diabetes.

Early reports for Chinese populations indicate a very low prevalence of diabetes, and one researcher in 1908 observed that none of his colleagues had ever seen a case of diabetes in a Chinese patient. In modern China, rates remain very low. Most authors conclude that the Chinese have a reduced susceptibility to diabetes, although rates are somewhat higher in immigrant Chinese populations outside China. The Japanese also show a very low prevalence of diabetes in their native country, but their rates of DM increase with migration.

Amerindians, in particular, have very high rates of diabetes. The highest rates occur among the southwestern Indian groups. Yet high rates among Amerindians appear to be recent. Early reports indicated very low prevalence of diabetes among North American Indian groups at the turn of this century. Moreover, rates among South American Indian groups still tend to be low.

Other aboriginal groups also seem to be particularly prone to diabetes, among them Polynesians and Micronesians. Rates are somewhat lower among Melanesians. Hawaiians have a diabetes rate seven times higher than Caucasians in Hawaii. Among New World black populations in the West Indies and in the United States, there is a high prevalence of type II diabetes, particularly among women. Studies have also found high rates of diabetes among Mexican Americans.

One explanation of the high frequency of type II DM among these populations is that they developed a highly efficient carbohydrate metabolism under traditional lifestyles of a feast and famine cycle. The thrifty mechanisms of carbohydrate metabolism, however, became detrimental with rapidly changing lifestyles associated with a decrease in physical activity, an increase in energy in the diet, a reduction of dietary fiber, an increase of refined carbohydrates, and an increase in psychosocial stress.

Among Asian Indians, diabetes rates are low. Diabetes is more prevalent among urban populations, the rich, and the professional classes. In Indian men there also is a north-to-south gradient of diabetes prevalence, with thrice the prevalence in the south. Yet like other migrants, Asian Indians migrating to other countries show high prevalence rates compared to indigenous populations. Indians in South Africa, in particular, were brought over as indentured servants and had a lifestyle not dissimilar to that of New World black populations. A diabetes-thrifty genotype may have developed in these populations as well.

Among black Africans, DM is still comparatively rare. Nevertheless, increased prevalence has been noted for urban Africans. Apparently, for susceptible genotypes, the lifestyle changes associated with rural-to-urban migration result in higher relative risks for type II diabetes.

The foregoing data indicate that we may anticipate an increase in the worldwide prevalence of DM. The focus has been and remains on treatment of **hyperglycemia** and the vascular complications of long-term diabetes. Using epidemiological data and historical perspectives, we are beginning to develop better programs aimed at early intervention and prevention.

Leslie Sue Lieberman

36. Diarrheal Diseases (Acute)

Acute diarrhea is the sudden onset of passage of a greater than usual number of stools with decreased form. It is generally accompanied by other symptoms such as fecal urgency, **tenesmus**, abdominal cramps, pain, nausea, and vomiting. In most cases, the symptom complex results from intestinal infection by a viral, bacterial, or parasitic enteropathogen; occasionally it is secondary to ingestion of a microbial exotoxin.

Characteristics

Acute diarrhea is hyperendemic in certain populations: youngsters in developing countries; visitors to developing regions; military populations in tropical areas; and toddlers who are not toilet trained and are attending day-care centers. Diarrhea rates in children less than 5 years of age in developing countries range between three and seven episodes per child each year. The rate for non-toilet-trained infants in day-care centers in urban areas of the United States is comparable to rates seen in developing countries. "Travelers' diarrhea" occurs in 20–40 percent of persons visiting high-risk areas. In all populations, acute diarrhea occurs less commonly in older children and adults than in infants.

The ultimate source of most enteric pathogens is infected humans, yet for selected organisms, animals may serve as a reservoir.

Environmental factors play an important role in disease endemicity. Although microbial contamination of water may be responsible for exposure to diarrhea-producing organisms, the availability of adequate water for personal and environmental cleansing, even if it is contaminated, may be beneficial. Sewage removal is a prerequisite for clean water and a healthful environment.

Personal and food hygiene standards are important, too. Effective handwashing is not routinely practiced in many developing areas. Food is often improperly handled. Vegetables and fruits rarely are washed properly prior to preparation. Foods may be contaminated by unclean kitchen surfaces or hands. Among the most important errors is storage of foods containing moisture at ambient temperatures between meals, which encourages microbial replication. Medical care is often inadequate. Finally, medical conditions contribute to both diarrhea incidence and its severity. **Measles** and **malnutrition** are two important examples. Flies also can play a role in transmitting enteric infections.

A basic prerequisite for infection by enteric pathogens is attachment to the intestinal lining by the microorganism. The mechanism of the attachment varies from a highly specific receptor-ligand interaction, as with enterotoxigenic *Escherichia coli*, to a nonspecific type of attachment, as with the protozoan *Giardia*, which possesses sucking disks. Variable degrees of intestinal damage can be seen in **enteric infection**. No anatomic or structural alterations are found in infection by enterotoxigenic *E. coli* or *Vibrio cholerae*; intestinal secretion and watery diarrhea occur secondary to cyclic nucleotide stimulation.

In **shigellosis** and **campylobacteriosis**, extensive inflammation with microabscess formation is seen. Small-bowel pathogens (rotavirus, Norwalk viruses, and *Giardia*) may deplete intestinal disaccharidases and cause **lactose intolerance**. Malnutrition, common in areas of diarrhea endemicity, prolongs and worsens the disease, although malnutrition does not predispose to its occurrence.

The synergy between malnutrition and diarrhea is an important reason why death from diarrhea is so common in developing countries. Diarrheal illnesses contribute to malnutrition: A 20–60 percent decrease in caloric intake occurs during a bout of diarrhea. Malnutrition contributes to more severe or prolonged diarrhea in several ways. The agents producing the greatest frequency of dehydration are *V. cholerae*, enterotoxigenic *E. coli*, and rotavirus. Rotavirus is the major cause of death in infants with diarrhea.

History

Diarrheal diseases have been important in all societies since the beginning of recorded history. Hippocrates used the term "dysentery" to denote a condition wherein the affected person passed many stools containing blood and mucus. Through World War I, outbreaks of diarrhea and **dysentery** were as important in deciding the outcome of many military campaigns as were war-related injuries.

The modern era of diarrheal diseases, as with other infectious disorders, began with identification of the agents involved. During the mid-1800s, *Giardia lamblia* and *Entamoeba histolytica* were identified. Then during the later nineteenth century, *Shigella* and *Salmonella* organisms were characterized, and the two forms of dysentery (**bacillary dysentery** and **amebic dysentery**) were distinguished.

During the 1960s, studies elucidated the mechanisms of disease production when **cholera** toxin was purified. As an extension of research with *V. cholerae* during the 1970s, enterotoxigenic *E. coli* were identified as important causes of diarrhea. Soon, other enterotoxin- or cytotoxin-producing bacteria were discovered: *Salmonella, Aeromonas, Yersinia, Clostridium perfrigens, Clostridium difficile*, enterohemorrhagic *E. coli*, noncholera vibrios, and *Staphylococcus aureus*.

Also during the 1970s, viruses were clearly implicated as causes of human diarrhea. Norwalk virus was shown to produce **gastroenteritis** in volunteers, and the viral particle was visualized by electron microscopy. Soon, larger particles were observed in the duodenal mucosa of diarrhea patients, and within a few years rotaviruses were established as a cause of **infantile gastroenteritis**. Additional pathogens are identified as the research laboratory discovers novel mechanisms of pathogenesis or as new microbiological techniques are developed. The future will bring studies of organism-specific epidemiology, therapy, and disease prevention.

Herbert L. DuPont

37. Diphtheria

Diphtheria is caused by *Corynebacterium diphtheriae*, named from the Greek: *koryne* ("club") for its clubbed shape, and *diphtheria* ("shield" or "membrane") for the hide-like pseudomembrane that forms on tonsils, palate, or pharynx in severe infections. Although this bacillus may cause only subclinical infections, its more virulent strains cause epidemics with case-fatality rates ranging up to 50 percent of affected children. In such circumstances, the bacterium is itself infected by a phage virus that inspires elaboration of a potent exotoxin, which can cause rapid **fatty degeneration of the heart** muscle and peripheral nervous-system damage resulting in **paralysis**. Children, however, often die because the airway is occluded.

Also called the Klebs-Löffler bacillus, the organism usually spreads by respiratory secretions and droplet infection. After an incubation period of 2–4 days, it multiplies in the upper respiratory tract, creating a membranous exudate on pharyngeal tissues. The bacillus invades local tissues and kills cells, causing necrosis and, often, discoloration of the membrane. The greenish or blackened membrane is a hallmark of the disease. The organism rarely causes a systemic infection, although skin infections are common in tropical regions. Most damage is produced by the powerful toxin disseminated through the bloodstream.

Characteristics

Corynebacteria are distributed throughout the world. *C. diphtheriae* occurs naturally only in humans, although many animals can be infected with it. Indeed, diphtheria's wide host range helped in studying the organism during the early bacteriologic revolution.

In historical accounts, it is often described as a malignant sore throat, and among its puzzling features was the sudden appearance of epidemics. In the "throat distemper" epidemic of colonial New England, Boston avoided the high mortality experienced elsewhere, illustrating the patchy distribution of severe cases that could be observed even during epidemics.

A phage virus is associated with the virulence of the diphtheria bacilli in that the *tox* gene either elaborates toxin (*tox*[+]) or not (*tox*[−]). In both cases, the presence of this gene stimulates immunity. A mixture of organisms during epidemics may have influenced diphtheritic virulence. In the 1735 Boston epidemic, for example, a rash accompanied "sore throats," suggesting coinfection with streptococcus, which is common enough. It is unknown, however, what influence – if any – a copathogen has in the elaboration of toxin.

In addition to respiratory transmission, the disease can be spread by touch and by fomites, such as schoolchildren's pencils. Thus, an infection can be transmitted to a cow's udders from an infected milker's fingers. Unpasteurized milk can also transmit the infection. Even dust around the bed of a diphtheria patient can remain infective for weeks.

Early in the twentieth century, diphtheria was still a leading cause of death for young children, but case-fatality rates declined dramatically with speedier diagnosis and therapeutic interventions such as antitoxin and tracheostomy. After World War II, mass immunization effected a rapid decline in overall incidence, and age of incidence rose. In virulent cases, mortality remains today around 5 percent, which may mean that antitoxin alone is not always sufficient treatment. The organism itself is sensitive to penicillin.

In temperate climates, diphtheria usually peaks in autumn and early winter. Most cases during the last 200 years were individuals under 15 years old. Crowded conditions facilitate passage of the organism, and so accounts prior to the acceptance of germ theory often described diphtheria as a filth disease naturally favoring the poor. In tropical regions, **cutaneous diphtheria** is more common, causing ulcers sometimes called "desert sores." Contact with these lesions is probably important in spreading the disease.

Even virulent diphtheria begins quietly. Victims rarely suffer the fever, vomiting, or myalgias common in acute viral illnesses, and the sore throat is less pronounced than in **streptococcal pharyngitis**. As the organism multiplies, however, the neck can swell dramatically, and respiration becomes difficult. If the victim's mouth can open, observers usually see a membrane 1–3 millimeters thick, its rough edge curling away from tonsils, palate, uvula, or pharynx. Depending upon the amount of destruction of local blood vessels, this "shield" ranges from yellowish-white to green or even black.

German pathologist Edwin Klebs first identified *C. diphtheriae* in 1883 by peeling off the membrane and culturing the bleeding surface underneath. The following year, Friedrich Löffler developed a medium on which to grow the bacillus. Both noted the absence of other affected organs: The bacillus is not distributed through the body. The toxin alone seems to produce the lethal effect. Most perplexing is the characteristic progressive paralysis: first the palate, then eyes, heart, pharynx and larynx (respiratory muscles), and finally the limbs. Penicillin, antitoxin, and maintenance of the airway are the usual means of clinical intervention.

History

It is unknown whether diphtheria was at any historical point a "new" disease, though it was so described during the early modern period. Diseases resembling diphtheria were discussed in ancient Greek literature, and from the sixteenth through eighteenth centuries. Historical interest, however, has been confined largely to the major role diphtheria played in the emergence and confirmation of the germ theory of disease.

French clinician Pierre Bretonneau first described and named the disease. Witnessing epidemics in the mid-1820s, he noted the pseudomembrane and used diphtheria in particular to elaborate his concept of disease specificity. Diphtheria was usually viewed as a disease of poverty but not an exceptional threat to human survival, as were **cholera** and **yellow fever**. Periodic peaks in diphtheria mortality received no attention among clinicians.

Immediately after Robert Koch articulated a germ theory based on his 1882 work with **tuberculosis**, Klebs and Löffler demonstrated the connection between diphtheritic organisms and membranous sore throat. Löffler's 1884 paper also introduced some basic research problems for germ theorists. He speculated that an "extraordinarily deleterious" poison was disseminated through the bloodstream. Moreover, his work illustrated that the organism could not always be cultured from typical cases and that healthy individuals could carry it. The latter phenomenon led Löffler to an 1887 description of nonvirulent diphtheria strains.

Emile Roux and Alexandre Yersin demonstrated the probability that a toxin was involved in lethal cases of diphtheria. In 1888, they showed that bacteria-free filtrates reproduced all features of the disease in experimental animals except the membrane. In 1890, Emil Behring and Shibasaburo Kitasato used serum from convalescing individuals to treat diphtheria patients (and experimental animals). Thus, before the twentieth century, diphtheria had provided the best model for proving the germ theory of disease and suggested the concept of the healthy carrier, the possibility of nonbacterial disease agents, and the general usefulness of serology in diagnosis and treatment.

After a dramatic cure of a diphtheritic child with the Kitasato-Behring serum, Behring escalated his study of "antitoxin," standardizing and popularizing procedures for harvesting immune serum from toxin-inoculated horses. Diphtheria rapidly became largely curable. Behring was acclaimed and elevated to the hereditary nobility of Germany. Simultaneously, however, diphtheria became known as a classic contagious disease and (unlike many such diseases) as a widespread, merciless killer of children.

Diphtheria was involved in two further stages of research on germ theory and its applications. First, the Schick test helped identify individuals lacking immune response to small doses of toxin. In testing immunity and **anaphylactic reaction** to foreign sera of people with "serum sickness" (a considerable problem with Behring's method), clinicians used diphtheria throughout the early twentieth century to delineate research problems in human immunity. Second, in the 1950s, isolation of the phage virus infecting diphtheria bacilli greatly aided research into phage-bacterial relationships and, in the process, the fields of bacterial genetics and molecular biology.

Ann G. Carmichael

38. Down Syndrome

Down syndrome, previously called "mongolism," is a relatively common condition resulting from the presence of an extra chromosome, number 21, in the cells of the body. In each human cell, 23 chromosome pairs contain basic genetic material that organizes the body's development and physiological functioning. Each pair has a distinctive size and conformation and can be readily identified on examination. Chromosome pair number 21 is one of the smaller chromosomes. In Down syndrome there are usually three (**trisomy**) rather than two number 21 chromosomes (**trisomy 21** – 95–98 percent of cases). In some cases, the extra number 21 chromosome is attached to chromosome 13, 14, or 15 (**translocation Down syndrome** – about 2 percent of cases). In others, the extra chromosome is present in less

than 90 percent of cells (**mosaic Down syndrome** – 2–4 percent of cases). Down syndrome is the most frequent chromosome abnormality in live-born humans and is also among the most frequently identified chromosomal abnormalities, representing about 4 percent of all aborted fetuses. Down syndrome is usually recognizable at birth as a cluster of physical and neurological abnormalities that develop in a characteristic fashion during the life cycle.

Characteristics

Recent estimates of overall worldwide incidence of Down syndrome are around 0.8 per 1,000 live births. Figures evidence a decline from previous decades in Western countries, where incidence was about 1.7 per 1,000. This change has probably resulted from more frequent prenatal diagnosis.

Down syndrome occurs in all races and ethnic groups, though good documentation of specific incidence in many groups and geographic areas is lacking. There is some evidence for spatial aggregation, such as in northern Finland and British Columbia, but these instances appear to be sporadic and are probably related to environmental sources.

The presence of the additional number 21 chromosome in all cells of the individual with Down syndrome is usually the result of an error in cell division called **nondisjunction**. In normal cell division, the two members of each of the 23 chromosome pairs separate and move into one of the two resulting cells, whereas in nondisjunction, both members of the chromosome pair end up in a single cell. In Down syndrome, the nondisjunction has usually occurred during meiosis (sex cell division) usually of the female sex cell (the ovum). Thus, when an ovum with two number 21 chromosomes is fertilized, three number 21 chromosomes (two from the mother and one from the father) will be passed on to all the cells in the developing fetus.

The occurrence of Down syndrome is most consistently associated with advanced maternal age: Incidence increases from 0.45 per 1,000 live births for women ages 20–24 years to 9.4 per 1,000 for women ages 40–44 years. The largest risk increase occurs between the 30–34 and 34–39 age groups. Possible causes of the maternal-age association include: (1) The older uterus is less selective in rejecting the Down syndrome conceptus; (2) longer delays between intercourse result in a relatively "aged ovum," more likely to experience nondisjunction; (3) in older women, the ova themselves have aged longer and have an increased rate of nondisjunction; (4) long-term exposure to environmental agents has resulted in damage to the spindle mechanism that in turn produces meiotic nondisjunction.

About 30–60 percent of Down syndrome births, however, are not age dependent, occurring in mothers under 30 years old. Indeed, a high incidence of Down syndrome births has been reported in women under 15. Younger mothers are more likely to have a second Down syndrome birth than are older mothers. The recurrence risk is 1 in 3 for mothers who are translocation carriers.

Possible environmental and metabolic mechanisms for Down syndrome have been evaluated, among them maternal drug, tobacco, alcohol, and caffeine use; use of hormonal and nonhormonal contraceptives; fluoridated water; and radiation exposure. However, findings from such studies have been inconsistent. Some investigators have suggested that a recessive gene producing nondisjunction might explain up to 10 percent of cases. However, studies of consanguineous marriages fail to support this suggestion. The association with elevated maternal age is undoubtedly a surrogate variable for other underlying factors, the most important of which are probably endocrine changes associated with aging.

The most easily recognizable features of Down syndrome derive from abnormalities in growth of the cranium and face. These include a short, relatively broad head (brachycephaly), hypoplastic maxilla, upslanting palpebral fissures, epicanthal folds, increased neck skin, small ears, and flattened nasal bridge. Common postcranial anomalies include wide spacing between first and second toes, abnormal finger and palm dermatoglyphs, and shortened distal long bones. About 80 percent of Down syndrome patients are hypotonic and 90 percent are hyperflexible. There are also various major organ anomalies, most importantly **congenital heart disease**, which occurs in 30–50 percent of patients. Metabolic and hormonal systems are variably affected, including deficient vitamin A absorption, elevated serum uric acid, and abnormal serotonin metabolism.

Down syndrome patients experience abnormal physical and cognitive development. Birth weight and length are near normal, but growth in the first 3 years of life is significantly slower than normal, and most children are less than the fifth percentile in height by the time they reach age 3. Growth rate during childhood is near normal, but the adolescent growth spurt is often absent. Some early developmental milestones are normal, but marked delays in walking, talking, and other motor and cognitive skills usually become apparent by the end of the first year of life. Mild to moderate mental retardation (I.Q. 30–67) is commonly present by childhood. Early intervention and special-education programs allow adults with Down syndrome to hold jobs in sheltered work situations.

History

Probably the earliest record of Down syndrome is a seventh century Saxon skull showing osteological changes consistent with the condition. Sixteenth century paintings depict children with features of the syndrome. Not until the nineteenth century, however, did the first accounts of Down syndrome appear. In 1846, E. Sequin noted a specific type of mental retardation case with associated physical features. In 1866, J. Langdon Down described a congenital defect resembling the Tartar race, which he called Kalmuc or Mongolian. Down, influenced by racial theory and the writings of Charles Darwin, suggested that the entity represented a reversion to an earlier phylogenetic type. This hypothesis never gained wide acceptance, however; in fact, Down's son (also a doctor) disagreed, suggesting that the features of the syndrome were accidental and superficial.

The next important reports, in the 1870s and 1880s, noted similarities between the syndrome and "cretinism" (**congenital hypothyroidism**), and suggested that children with the condition were actually "unfinished," representing a persistence of anatomical characteristics from a particular phase of fetal development. The association between the syndrome and advanced maternal age was already recognized, and many Down syndrome children were the lastborn of large families. During the end of the nineteenth and beginning of the twentieth centuries, many reports appeared, expanding the description of the syndrome's phenotypic manifestations. Important among these were extensive neuropathological descriptions.

From the mid-nineteenth century to 1959, many etiologic hypotheses were advanced, including maternal **syphilis**, familial **tuberculosis**, familial incidence of **epilepsy**, insanity, instability, and mental retardation. Once the increased incidence of congenital heart disease in the syndrome was recognized (in 1898), a cause in early fetal existence was sought. Among theories advanced were maternal alcoholism, fetal **hyperthyroidism**, maternal **dysthyroidism**, **adrenal hypoplasia**, pituitary dysfunction, abnormality of the thymus, chemical contraceptives, curettage, faulty implantation, degeneration of the ovum, and emotional shock in early pregnancy.

As early as 1932, a chromosomal anomaly was suggested as a possible cause of the disorder. In 1959, shortly after the number of chromosomes in the human cell was established, a sample of Down syndrome children were demonstrated to have an extra chromosome and a total chromosome number of 47. Later the same year, researchers concluded that the extra chromosome was most similar to number 21. In 1960, other investigators reported a case of Down syndrome with only 46 chromosomes, and postulated reciprocal translocation occurring between two chromosome groups.

Initially, Down syndrome was thought to occur only in the Caucasian race. Subsequent reports have shown that it occurs in every racial group and country, although studies have not yet provided an accurate picture of its distribution across racial and ethnic groups. Early reports indicated low incidence in Africans and black Americans. However, investigations in Ibadan, Nigeria, and Memphis, Tennessee, found black incidence much the same as that of whites. Similarly, although detection in Oriental populations is thought to be inhibited by sameness of features, studies in Japan reveal rates much like those in the United States.

A number of studies have attempted to indicate spatial and temporal clustering of the syndrome, but all have failed to give satisfactory statistical proof for clustering. A 1983 report describes a cluster of Down syndrome children born to women who attended the same boarding school in their youth. This suggests that, in some instances, an environmental agent may influence the incidence of Down syndrome.

Christine E. Cronk

39. Dracunculiasis

Dracunculiasis results from infection with the parasite *Dracunculus medinensis*. The adult worms – about 1 meter long – are usually quite evident as they slowly emerge through the skin of their victims.

Characteristics

Dracunculiasis is found mainly in India, Pakistan, and several African countries, from Senegal in the west to Ethiopia in the east. Formerly, this disease was much more widespread in the Middle East and Africa, and it occurred for some years in the Americas after introduction by infected Africans during the slave trade.

Incidence of dracunculiasis is significantly higher in endemic African communities than in endemic Asian villages. In West Africa especially, rates of infection in affected areas sometimes exceed 50 percent, whereas in Asia, rates usually are below 20 percent. In rural areas, the disease occurs sporadically, with incidence rates sometimes differing greatly in adjacent villages. Persons at risk of this infection number an estimated 120 million in Africa, with another 20 million at risk in India and Pakistan. The number of persons affected annually is unknown. Diseases are often underreported in the countries affected, and reporting of dracunculiasis is especially poor. Generally, it is found only in impoverished rural communities where medical facilities are rare. Many victims cannot walk and have little incentive to seek treatment, because no curative drug exists.

Dracunculiasis is seasonal, usually occurring just when rural villagers plant or harvest their crops. People are infected by water containing copepods – tiny crustaceans of the genus *Cyclops* that harbor the infective larvae of the parasite. A year later, adult worms emerge through the skin to discharge larvae into freshwater to be ingested by copepods, thus completing the cycle. In drier areas, the infection appears during rainy seasons (summer). In areas with more rainfall, the infection is transmitted during dry seasons (winter).

Most commonly affected are people 15–45 years of age – that is, working adults. Younger children are affected, but not infants under 1 year, and not many under 5 years. Farmers are particularly liable to infection, apparently because they drink large volumes of contaminated water while laboring on their farms. In some areas, schoolchildren also suffer high rates of infection.

No drug is suitable for effective mass treatment of dracunculiasis, and from time immemorial the disease has been treated by slowly winding the emerging worm around a stick. The disease can, however, be prevented by boiling or filtering drinking water, by chemical treatment of contaminated water sources, and by protecting water sources from contamination in the first place.

Usually the first clinical sign of infection is a blister and severe burning sensation where the worm is about to emerge. The blister ruptures when the affected part of the body is immersed in water, leaving a small ulcer with the worm at the center. Most worms emerge on the foot or lower leg, but they can emerge through the skin at any point. Sometimes the worm first appears as a line beneath the skin, or at the center of a painful abscess or nodule.

Worms failing to emerge from the body die and are absorbed or calcified, in which case they appear as characteristic curled lines in X-rays. Worms may invade a major joint, the central nervous system, or another vital area, producing more serious manifestations, but this rarely happens. More common complications are secondary infections of the wound, leading to abscesses, local **arthritis**, or **tetanus**. In most patients, only one worm emerges at a time, although two dozen or more may present themselves simultaneously in one person.

Affected persons may be crippled for several weeks or months by the pain of the worm's slow emergence and secondary infections. Because the infection appears at a critical time for food production and cripples many people simultaneously, it has an enormous economic impact. Moreover, people who are infected develop no immunity, so they may be and often are infected year after year.

History

Dracunculiasis is an old infection, which many believe was the "fiery serpent" said to have attacked the Israelites on the shores of the Red Sea. A calcified *Dracunculus* worm was discovered in an Egyptian mummy from around 1000 B.C., and a treatment for the condition may be contained in the *Ebers Papyrus*.

Greek and Roman writers described the infection, and Galen named it "dracontiasis." The ancient treatment of winding the worm slowly around a stick is thought by some to be the origin of the Staff of Aesculapius. Several medieval Arabian physicians described dracunculiasis, and one of them, Avicenna, gave the first detailed description of what he called "Medina sickness" (because it was common in Medina).

Shortly before, Rhazes showed that the associated swelling was caused by a parasite.

Sixteenth century Europeans mentioned cases of dracunculiasis in Persia and Congo. It may first have been called "Guinea worm" by a European who saw it on the Guinea Coast (west Africa) early in the seventeenth century. The disease is mentioned in the traditional legend of the founding of the Dahomeyans' ancestral cult. Although G. H. Velschius described the parasite clearly in 1674, it was left to Linnaeus to provide its scientific name in 1758.

During the nineteenth century, medical officers reported dracunculiasis among British troops in India, and an English expedition that invaded Ethiopia in 1868 suffered greatly from the disease. The role of the copepod as intermediate host in the parasite's life cycle was discovered in the 1870s by Aleksei Fedchenko.

The distribution of dracunculiasis shrank considerably during the early twentieth century – largely because of improving standards of living, especially improved water supplies. The disease was eliminated from the southern Soviet Union in the 1930s by a deliberate campaign, and from Iran in the 1970s. In the 1980s, India and other endemic countries began campaigns to eradicate dracunculiasis. It appears likely that this ancient disease will soon cease to exist.

Donald R. Hopkins

40. Dropsy

The historical diagnosis of **dropsy** – now obsolete – indicated an abnormal accumulation of fluid; the word derives from the Greek *hydrops* ("water"). Alternative terms included **hydrothorax** (fluid in the chest cavity), **ascites** (excess fluid in the abdominal cavity), **anasarca** (generalized **edema** throughout the body), **hydrocephalus** (used until the nineteenth century to indicate excess fluid within the skull), and **ovarian dropsy** (large ovarian cysts filled with fluid). Edema was often a synonym for dropsy

but now has additional connotations, and **pulmonary edema** has been differentiated from hydrothorax. Since the mid-nineteenth century, dropsy has been recognized as a sign of underlying disease of the heart, liver, or kidneys, or of malnutrition. Untreated dropsy was, eventually, always fatal.

Characteristics

The major causes of dropsy are **congestive heart failure**, liver failure, kidney failure, and **malnutrition**. Because these were not clearly differentiated before the nineteenth century, a historical diagnosis of dropsy cannot be taken to indicate any one of these alone in the absence of unequivocal supporting evidence, as from an autopsy; however, heart failure was probably the most frequent of the four.

Dropsy can be explained most conveniently in terms of fluid balance. One principal force in the maintenance of normal fluid balance is the hydrostatic pressure within capillaries. The other major force is oncotic pressure, the normal tendency for sodium or large particles in capillary blood to draw water out of tissues. Thus, fluid accumulates in tissues when either intracapillary pressure increases or the blood's ability to remove water from tissues decreases. In both cases, fluid that has moved out of the capillaries is poorly reabsorbed. Most hydrostatic defects are primary heart diseases, whereas most oncotic defects result from renal and hepatic disease.

Congestive heart failure produces dropsy, or edema, when the heart becomes too weak to maintain the normal pressure of blood flow in the capillaries, facilitating the leakage of water from capillary blood into surrounding tissues. "Congestive" refers to the accumulation and stagnation of blood in organs, especially the lungs, when they are not adequately emptied.

The other major causes of dropsy, which follow, are discussed here only in relation to heart failure. Liver failure, producing ascites, most often occurs in advanced **cirrhosis** because the diseased liver cannot manufacture sufficient albumin to maintain the oncotic pressure of the blood. **Right ventricular failure** can also produce hepatic congestion and failure. Renal failure causes dropsy when the filtering units become so diseased that large molecules are lost from the blood into the urine, resulting in decreased oncotic pressure. Malnutrition results in ascites when protein intake is so low that the liver is unable to manufacture its own. **Beriberi**, caused by a B-vitamin deficiency, can also weaken the heart.

Heart failure occurs more often in men than in women, inasmuch as men are at greater risk for most forms of cardiovascular disease. The risk is greater for older than younger patients: three-quarters of heart failure patients are over 50 years of age. Risk factors for hepatic cirrhosis include chronic alcoholism and **hepatitis**, just as renal causes of dropsy may be associated with **rheumatic fever** or the **nephrotic syndrome**.

The distribution of dropsy within or among populations parallels the distributions of its underlying causes, such as **hypertension, myocardial insufficiency**, **coronary artery disease**, **hypercholesterolemia, valvular disease, streptococcal diseases**, cirrhosis, and renal **glomerular disease**. Risk factors for these conditions are still being identified and their clinical implications evaluated. Only for malnutrition are geographic distinctions clear-cut.

Historically, the diagnosis of dropsy was so familiar that artists could portray it in popular prints with the expectation that it would be recognized immediately. Consequently, it is not surprising that the reported incidence of dropsy has not changed substantially over the 400 years for which records are available. That is, dropsy was diagnosed in about 3–5 percent of deaths, hospital admissions, or adult patients in London in 1583–1849, and in American villages and cities in 1735–1839. Typical modern incidences of congestive heart failure exhibit similar percentages.

This discussion focuses on congestive heart failure because it was probably the major underlying cause of dropsy. The heart is able to compensate, up to a point, for diminished strength of contraction, for increased resistance to arterial outflow, and for accumulations of blood that cannot be completely removed from the ventricles at each contraction. Symptoms of heart failure begin to occur when no further compensations can be made. "Forward failure" symptoms occur when the heart can no longer empty the left ventricle completely because of reasons such as myocardial weakness or obstruction to aortic outflow. Symptoms of "backward failure" occur when the heart chambers become incapable of complete filling, due to incomplete relaxation of the heart between beats, or to obstructions to venous inflow into the right atrium.

Heart failure can be produced by several underlying pathological causes, such as myocardial insufficiency, failure of the left or right (or both) ventricles, chronic or acute **cor pulmonale** (pulmonary heart disease), and diminished arterial blood flow to the kidneys, although seldom does any one of them occur alone. Whatever the underlying cause, the major manifestation of heart failure is reduced cardiac output in terms of the amount of blood ejected from the left ventricle. The associated symptoms are usually clearly recognizable.

For instance, important symptoms of heart failure include shortness of breath (**dyspnea**), due to insufficient delivery of oxygen to the body's tissues, and rapid breathing (**tachypnea**) as the respiratory system attempts to compensate for the lack of oxygen. Both dyspnea and tachypnea increase as fluid from the pulmonary capillaries begins to flood the lungs. When the lungs become sufficiently congested (pulmonary edema), the patient coughs up copious sputum. A more serious form of dyspnea is **orthopnea**. This term is applied to shortness of breath that prevents the patient from sleeping horizontally because venous blood further congests the lungs, causing dyspnea. An exaggerated form of orthopnea called **paroxysmal nocturnal dyspnea** may waken the patient suddenly at night; it is sometimes called "cardiac asthma" because it produces wheezing and labored breathing.

Other distinctive symptoms may occur in addition to the usual dyspnea and tachypnea. **Pedal edema** occurs, accompanied by hydrothorax. Ascites is a late sign and may be followed by anasarca and **oliguria**. The skin becomes bluish, because the sluggishly moving red cells are not adequately oxygenated in the lungs. The jugular veins distend because increased pressure in the right heart prevents them from emptying completely into the superior vena cava. Other evidence of increased venous pressure includes congestive enlargement of the liver and sometimes the spleen.

History

The symptoms of dropsy have not changed over the centuries. Its history is the story of evolving interpretations of its clinical features over 2,000 years as the relationships of dyspnea, "suffocative catarrh," pulmonary edema, hydrothorax, ascites, **syncope**, and "fever" to heart failure were elucidated.

The first known mention of dropsy is in the *Ebers Papyrus*, an Egyptian medical text of about 1550 B.C. It associates dropsy with increased abdominal girth and possibly with a weak pulse. A Hippocratic text correctly prognosticates that there "is no hope when a patient suffering from dropsy develops a cough." And Jesus defied the Pharisees by healing a man with dropsy on the Sabbath.

Soon after, Aulus Cornelius Celsus described two forms of dropsy: (1) generalized edema, which could be drained through small skin incisions above the ankle; and (2) ascites, in which the excess fluid could be removed by paracentesis, or "tapping" (drainage via a tube inserted through an incision in the abdominal wall).

Galen listed several causes of dropsy in the first century A.D., including a hardened liver, as well as inadequate blood formation (which he thought occurred in the liver), **hemorrhoids**, and both **amenorrhea** and **uterine hemorrhage**. Virtually all writers on dropsy until the mid-seventeenth century cited the teachings of Hippocrates, Celsus, and Galen. In the eleventh century, Avicenna of Baghdad thought that the

tachycardia, palpitations, pulmonary edema, dyspnea, and syncope (fainting or shock, which he postulated was a sign of a weak heart) that accompanied dropsy were related to one another.

Five centuries later, the French surgeon Ambroise Paré described dropsy identically. His countryman Jean Fernel relied on similar theories in associating heart disease with palpitations, syncope, and the pallor, cold sweat, and weak pulse observed in **cardiogenic shock**. Also in the sixteenth century, Paracelsus theorized that dropsy occurred when the body's tissues dissolved. He recommended that dropsy be treated with mercuric oxide to remove superfluous water, with other metallic oxides to dry the patient's body, and with sulfur, because its drying action was analogous to that of the sun in dispelling rain.

Girolamo Capivaccio of Italy agreed with Galen that dropsy was due to liver disease and impaired blood formation, so that fluid was released into the abdominal cavity to form ascites, which he detected by percussion, as Celsus had. Capivaccio also attributed dropsy to disease in other organs, such as obstruction of the pathways to the kidneys. He surmised that dyspnea was caused by pressure from a pathologically enlarged liver on the diaphragm.

The sixteenth-century physician Ludovicus Mercatus of Valladolid defined dyspnea as rapid, difficult breathing caused by constricted airways or excess heat in the heart and lungs; he thought that respiration was for cooling the heart. Mercatus believed that hydrothorax fluid descended from the brain to produce the "suffocative catarrh" described by Galen, and that its associated dyspnea was caused by fluid in the lungs, or even by heart disease. He theorized that hydrothorax fluid was overflow from ascites or from obstructed urinary passages.

Throughout the seventeenth century, it became increasingly clear that dropsy was associated with altered fluid dynamics. Carolus Piso of Lorraine detected hydrothorax as "bubbling" when he applied his ear to the chest. Coupling clinical observations with autopsy findings, he attributed paroxysmal nocturnal dyspnea to fluid in the chest cavity. Fabrizio Bartoletti of Italy used observations like Piso's to hypothesize that hydrothorax fluid came from the lungs. He noted that the first clue to its presence was dyspnea, followed by "fever," tachypnea, orthopnea, dry cough, thirst, syncope, leg and scrotal edema, and finally ascites. Bartoletti thought that hydrothorax was always fatal because it suffocated its victims.

William Harvey postulated that if the venous system were maximally distended, the heart would stop and suffocation would follow. In 1628, he described the heart and lungs as "storehouses" for the blood, a metaphor that may have led to the concepts of pulmonary engorgement and passive congestion, which would be critical to further understanding of dropsy in the chest.

In 1669, Richard Lower of Oxford produced edema and ascites in dogs by ligating the jugular veins and the superior vena cava. He also found that excess fluid in the pericardial sac restricted cardiac expansion. Lower postulated that the two sides of the heart should be of equal strength, while noting that the left side alone may be weakened. He also perceived that excessive pressure or flow rate of blood adversely affected health. He recognized Galen's "suffocative catarrh" as pulmonary edema, although they were considered separate clinical entities for many years afterward.

In 1681, Marcello Malpighi of Bologna noted the increased weight (from the stagnant blood within them) of dyspneic lungs. He had discovered capillaries 20 years earlier and hypothesized that blood escaped from them into the lungs. Malpighi thought that stagnant blood in the pulmonary vessels produced palpitations because it precluded an orderly blood supply to the heart. He reasoned that an imbalance between arterial outflow and venous resorption of water from the blood caused dropsy, but he attributed the imbalance to chemicals that constricted blood vessels or irritated the nerves that controlled the heart and the respiratory muscles. One of Malpighi's students, Giorgio Baglivi,

finally made it clear that suffocative catarrh and acute pulmonary edema (not the result of fluid falling from the head) were the same.

Physicians were slow to understand that the heart could be diseased, probably because it was essential to life. Raymond Vieussens of Montpellier, however, had concluded by 1705 that structural disease of the heart could result in dropsy. At almost the same time, Giovanni Maria Lancisi in Rome recognized that edema, hydrothorax, and ascites could be related to failure of the heart's propulsive force. Explicitly recognizing the importance of hydrostatic principles in cardiovascular physiology, Lancisi went on to explain how stagnation of blood within the pulmonary vasculature could result in dyspnea. He concluded that right heart failure could produce engorgement and pulsation of the jugular vein. Thus Lancisi and Vieussens uncovered the cardiac basis of dropsies of the lungs and thorax.

Another interpretation of dropsy arose from Harvey's demonstration that the blood circulates within a closed system. Dropsy could be seen as a febrile disease, because it was usually accompanied by a fast pulse, which for centuries was regarded as a cardinal sign of fever. Thus Thomas Willis defined fever as an "intestine motion or commotion of the blood" arising in chemical disturbances like those described over a century earlier by Paracelsus.

Hermann Boerhaave of Leyden believed that dropsy was a fever and should be treated accordingly. He argued that in dropsy, fever is the result of increased cardiac work and increased vascular resistance to blood flow. Therefore dropsy was a fever because it was associated with a fast pulse. Boerhaave postulated that dropsical fluid accumulated because defective veins released more fluid into body tissues than the vessels could reabsorb. In Italy, Luca Tozzi differentiated hydrothorax, pulmonary edema, and **pneumonia** at autopsy, which permitted him to differentiate pulmonary and thoracic dropsies ante mortem.

In 1761, Leopold Auenbrugger of Vienna described how to strike the chest with the fingers to estimate, by the resonance produced, the amount and nature of fluid in the pleural cavity and lungs. However, his discovery of percussion was neglected until it was reintroduced in France in 1808.

The first book devoted to dropsy alone was published in 1706 by the Leopoldine Academy of Sciences in Breslau; its principal author was probably Christianus Helwich. The Academicians described the features of dropsy much as previous works had done but attributed the escape of fluid to diminished blood viscosity and to defective vessel walls.

In 1733, Stephen Hales, a rural English clergyman, concluded that dropsy could result from decreased numbers of red blood cells. He thought that the body would compensate for the lack of "red Globules" by heating the blood into a feverish state that caused dropsy. He recognized that inadequate venous return to the heart in dropsy could lead to compensatory tachycardia.

Donald Monro of Edinburgh published the second book devoted to dropsy in 1755, ascribing it to "a weakness and laxity of the fibers . . . when the vessels do not act with sufficient force," and listed causes of weakened blood vessels: a watery diet, "any great evacuation," kidney disease, obstruction of small or large vessels, or any debilitating disease.

In 1763, Samuel Clossey of Dublin realized that the development of hydrothorax is a long process. He computed that it would take about 2 years to accumulate 3 pints of hydrothorax fluid. He associated dropsy with weakness of the heart but postulated that cardiac strength derived from the blood vessels.

Thus, regardless of how they were interpreted, the major clinical manifestations of dropsy had been identified by the mid-eighteenth century. Some physicians thought that dropsy was caused by weak blood vessels, whereas others attributed the dyspnea to weakened cardiac contraction, as did Robert James of London in 1745. By the end of the century, theories of dropsy based on fever, chemical disturbances, blood viscosity, and fiber tone began to fade, and the role of the diseased heart came into sharper focus.

In 1806, Jean-Nicholas Corvisart of France showed how heart disease could produce dropsy, dyspnea, and orthopnea when venous return was slowed. Three years later Allan Burns of Glasgow demonstrated that ossification of the mitral and pulmonary valves leads to right heart dilation and dropsy. And in 1835, James Hope of Cheshire showed how **myocardial failure** results in dyspnea.

In 1813, John Blackall of London suggested that dropsy can result from noncardiac conditions such as liver and kidney disease. He demonstrated that the albumin content of urine can help differentiate among the underlying causes of dropsy. Renal causes of dropsy were confirmed by Richard Bright, whose careful autopsies at Guy's Hospital in London led him to report, in 1827, that albumin could be found in the urine of **glomerulonephritis** patients who died of dropsy. Later, Bright showed that renal disease could be associated with **left ventricular hypertrophy**. In 1909, C. J. Rothberger and H. Winterberg in Austria, and Thomas Lewis in London, independently showed that **atrial fibrillation** could produce heart failure, and in 1935 Paul Dudley White and Sylvester McGinn of Boston described acute cor pulmonale.

All investigators continue to exploit the relationships discovered around the turn of the twentieth century by Ernest Henry Starling and incorporated into his "Law of the Heart." In 1936, Tinsley R. Harrison of Vanderbilt University consolidated Starling's and other concepts of heart failure to explain the phenomenon more or less as we understand it today, although heart failure remains the subject of increasingly detailed investigations.

Until the late eighteenth century, dropsy was treated primarily with a selection of mostly ineffective drugs. In 1785, the most influential – and perhaps most immediately accepted – book in the history of dropsy appeared. *An Account of the Foxglove*, by William Withering of Birmingham, England, was the first prospective study of the efficacy and safety of any drug in the treatment of disease. Withering demonstrated the therapeutic benefit of digitalis (extracted from the purple foxglove, *Digitalis purpurea*, or the white species, *Digitalis lanata*) in patients with dropsies unrelated to primary disease of other organs. Although he noted that the pulse rate fell in patients treated with the new drug, he did not recognize its tonic effect on the heart.

Some physicians who followed Withering concluded that digitalis stimulated the "system," whereas others concluded that it was a depressant because it reduced fast heart rates. In 1813, Blackall first suggested that digitalis actually strengthens the heart. This concept resurfaced in the early twentieth century and was verified in 1938–44, by H. J. Stewart and John McMichael.

The two major goals of treatment in congestive heart failure today are improved oxygenation of the tissues and reduction of hydrostatic pressures in the veins. Digitalis glycosides (chiefly digoxin and digitoxin) increase cardiac output by strengthening the force with which the heart contracts; diuresis occurs secondarily, because the increase in the amount of blood that is circulated to the kidneys permits increased removal of water. True diuretics, which act on the kidneys alone, relieve pressure in the venous system by removing excess fluid from the body via the urine.

Oxygen and rest are important adjuncts to drug therapy. Paracentesis and thoracentesis may occasionally still be required, but the subcutaneous leg drainage tubes described by R. Southey of France in 1871 were abandoned with the advent of true diuretic drugs.

J. Worth Estes

41. Dysentery

Dysentery is inflammation of the large intestine characterized by loose stools containing blood and mucus, and by **tenesmus** – painful and unproductive attempts to defecate.

Diarrhea, marked by frequent production of watery stools, may be confused with dysentery in historical accounts, but references to "bloody flux" refer to true dysentery. The condition may be caused by an ameba, *Entamoeba histolytica*, or by several species of bacteria, especially in the genus *Shigella*. See: **Amebic Dysentery**, **Bacillary Dysentery**, and **Diarrheal Diseases (Acute)**.

K. David Patterson

42. Dyspepsia

Derived from Greek roots meaning "difficult digestion," **dyspepsia** has long served as a synonym for **indigestion**, one of the most common – and etiologically varied – of human miseries. It has also been regularly employed to label symptoms of diverse organic disorders, with the result that some gastroenterologists find the word uselessly elastic. Most practitioners, however, have reached a consensus to use dyspepsia to denote either the ailment of **functional indigestion** or the symptoms of **peptic ulcer**.

Characteristics

Peptic ulcer dyspepsia is rare in people under age 20, but by age 30, 2 percent of males and 0.5 percent of females in a population have developed the condition. For men, incidence increases steadily with age, reaching a peak of around 20 percent in the sixth decade of life. Incidence for women remains low, about 1 percent, until menopause, after which it climbs as rapidly as in men. Death from peptic ulcer occurs three times as often in men as in women.

The prevalence of **functional dyspepsia**, by contrast, is uncertain. Having no distinct pathology, being neither communicable nor reportable, and only occasionally motivating its victims to seek medical help, it generates no statistics. The widely shared clinical impression is that women are affected more than men, and people under age 40 more than their elders.

Functional dyspepsia is also believed to be more prevalent in developed countries.

Although the most common, peptic ulcer is hardly the only organic source of dyspepsia. **Esophagitis**; **hiatus hernia**; **gastritis**; **carcinoma** of the stomach, colon, or pancreas; **Crohn's disease**; **biliary tract disease**; chronic **nephritis**; or any of several other conditions, including pregnancy, can produce indigestion. In approximately half of dyspepsia cases, however, no lesion can be found, and symptoms arise from derangements of motor, secretory, or absorptive functions, especially delayed gastric motility, esophageal reflux, and hyperacidity. This functional indigestion has been related to physical stress (aerophagia, fatigue, dietary indiscretion) and, more commonly, to **nervous stress**. Anxiety, anger, frustration, and other indications of emotional turmoil can significantly impair digestive function in sensitive or tense individuals (a similar psychic component − chronic tension and repression of emotion − has been implicated in peptic ulcer). Because the symptoms of functional dyspepsia are virtually identical to those of peptic ulceration, the condition has also been termed "X-ray-negative" dyspepsia and "nonulcerative" dyspepsia; the term "endoscopy-negative" dyspepsia has been proposed as well in recent years.

Dyspepsia's victims complain of gastric pain, along with fullness or heaviness in the stomach, nausea and vomiting, belching, flatulence, and/or acid eructations. Finally, dyspeptics may suffer **heartburn**, a caustic pain behind the sternum that sometimes climbs into the throat, resulting from esophageal reflux. Heartburn is the special affliction of those with **sliding hiatus hernia** when they bend or recline.

History

If indigestion has plagued the human race for as long as it has eaten − and no less hoary an expert than Hippocrates described its tortures − not until the nineteenth century did dyspepsia attain a prominent standing in pathology. Previously, it was regarded as a too common but predictable and temporary discomfort brought on by immoderacy in diet.

The sources of intestinal turbulence came to appear more numerous during the nineteenth century. The distrust of sensuality that marked the Victorian ethos more than once expressed itself in blaming physical decline on moral perversion. Because dyspepsia was often found in patients guilty of some excess and just as often lacked any apparent organic basis, physicians found it easy to explain the condition with reference to any aberrant behavior that might plausibly have upset the patient's system. Gluttony, of course, was still a sin, and doctors generally added to gluttony the bolting of inadequately chewed food, a practice that many charged was epidemic in the dining rooms of ever-in-a-hurry America. Nevertheless, a nineteenth century attack of dyspepsia was just as likely to be blamed on abuse of spirits or tobacco, reading French novels, or masturbation or "excessive venery."

The nineteenth century's list of dyspepsia's causes was also lengthened by examples of fast living of a second type, that of the mental and emotional excitation accompanying the bustling anxiety-filled life of the industrial city. An 1825 treatise on indigestion, which recommended against excessive venery, also warned in the same breath of the dangers of excessive work and attention to "business." Such caveats appeared with increasing regularity in medical texts and health guides alike until finally becoming mandatory with the ascension of **neurasthenia** (nervous exhaustion) to the position of *the* disease of modern society during the last quarter of the century. Neurasthenia prophet George Beard's message that dyspepsia was on the rise as the special complaint of the modern brainworker and risk-taker met with universal acceptance. The neurasthenia era, furthermore, defined "modern dyspepsia" as a nervous complaint that gave as good as it got, one that having originated in anxiety then generated more anxiety as well as irritability, depression, and other neurotic suffering in addition to mundane heartburn. This virtual equation of dyspepsia with nervousness led to its almost exclusive definition as a functional condition produced by stress.

During the first half of the twentieth century, that same stress of coping with civilization seems to have engendered an abrupt increase in dyspepsia of organic origin as well. Between the two world wars, peptic ulcer (particularly **duodenal ulcer**) grew from a rarely encountered condition to a significant cause of disability, reaching a high point in the 1950s, then declining sharply to the present. This pattern suggests that ulcer dyspepsia is less a disease of civilization than a condition of adjustment to civilization; the first generations to confront the pressures of urban-industrial life are buffeted more heavily than those born after the turbulent transition period. Functional dyspepsia, of course, might be expected to decrease for the same reason, yet its domain has been diminished still more rapidly by the X-ray and the endoscope, improved diagnostic techniques having transferred many cases of "nervous indigestion" to peptic ulcer's column. Advances in understanding the neurohumoral mechanisms that regulate the digestive tract and the biochemical basis of emotion, furthermore, promise to provide organic interpretations for dyspepsias now identified as functional. As a consequence, the very term "dyspepsia," historically associated with nervous, nonorganic illness, is becoming antiquated. In recent decades, medical writers have begun encapsulating the word in quotation marks to call attention to its quaintness, and inserting it into the index only to be followed with "see indigestion."

James Whorton

43. Ebola Virus Disease

With recognition of new, deadly viral infections – such as **Lassa fever**, **Marburg**, **Ebola**, **Congo-Crimean hemorrhagic fever**, **Rift Valley fever**, and **AIDS** – the classic descriptions of diseases such as **malaria** and **yellow fever** must be thoroughly revised. To the roster of lesser ailments can be added **dengue**, **Chikungunya**, **O'Nyong Nyong**, **West Nile fever**, and others. The new knowledge challenges earlier descriptions of African fevers in general.

After the discoveries of Marburg virus in 1967 and Lassa virus in 1969 had jolted medical complacency, the Ebola virus in 1976 provoked convulsive shudders. Almost simultaneous outbreaks of a deadly infection occurred in neighboring regions of southern Sudan and northern Zaire, and along the Ebola River. The Sudan and Zaire foci are about 150 kilometers apart, and continual traffic passes between them.

History

The Sudan epidemic of **Ebola virus disease** began in June 1976. An infected patient went to a hospital in Maridi, where the disease spread rapidly among patients and staff. The epidemic terminated by November, with 148 deaths in 284 cases (52 percent mortality). In 1979, another outbreak occurred with fewer cases and a small number of deaths.

The epidemic in Zaire was traced to an index case seen in September 1976. This individual received an injection of chloroquine for presumptive malaria at the Yambuku Mission Hospital, Bumba District. He recovered, but within a week an epidemic of fever began in hospital patients and staff. There were 318 cases with 288 deaths (90.5 percent mortality). As in Sudan, the epidemic ended by early November. The first epidemiological team sent to the area diagnosed a "fulminating" epidemic of **typhoid fever** in a vulnerable population. Fatalities, however, occurred in a hospital in Kinshasa among three nurses who had been transferred from the infected area, and as investigations continued, it became clear that the virus had passed from human to human via contaminated syringes. Strict needle discipline and isolation of patients were reestablished and maintained.

In 1979, another hospital-centered outbreak occurred in Zaire, 300 kilometers from the original epidemic. Twenty-two of 33 patients died (66 percent mortality).

In 1989, an epidemic – confirmed as Ebola virus disease – erupted among *Macaca cynomolgus* monkeys shipped from the Philippines to a laboratory in Reston, Virginia, via Amsterdam and Kennedy airports. Sixty of 100 monkeys died. Soon, a second shipment arrived including two infected monkeys. Extensive international epidemiological investigation focused on this frightening episode. No human cases were reported and no satisfactory explanations advanced. All exposed individuals were monitored.

Epidemiologists have attempted to trace the origins of the Ebola virus and its distribution, locate host vertebrates, and learn its patterns of maintenance, propagation, and transmission. But efforts have been limited to a handful of dedicated investigators and a spotty sampling of the vast expanse of sub-Saharan Africa. Primate sampling has revealed at best minimal involvement. Associated with the 1979 Zaire outbreak is the unexpected finding of guinea pig immunes. Guinea pigs are South American rodents, raised there as pets and for food. They were introduced into Africa decades ago and in some regions are established as inquilines in houses. In this respect, their behavior resembles that of the multimammate rat (*Mastomys natalensis*), already known to be involved in the maintenance and transmission of Lassa virus. Guinea pig immune rates up to 26.1 percent were found in some locations, but studies failed to indicate transmission among guinea pigs or between guinea pigs and humans.

Characteristics

The Ebola agent consists of long filamentous rods, sometimes branched, often intertwined. The virion contains one molecule of single-stranded RNA. The particles resemble those of the Marburg agent but with differences: For example, Ebola has more branching than Marburg. Serologically, no relationship has been demonstrated, either to Marburg or Lassa or any other

viruses. A distinguishing characteristic between Ebola-Sudan and Ebola-Zaire is pathogenicity. Both cause excessive mortality, but less so for the Sudan strain than for the Zaire strain. A new family, Filoviridae, has been created for Marburg and Ebola.

Onset was usually sudden, with progressively severe frontal headache as seen with *Plasmodium falciparum* malaria, spreading occipitally. Fever and weakness were always present. **Myalgia** appeared early. **Arthralgia** of the large joints was common. Severe generalized disease followed in days. Patients were lethargic, their faces expressionless with deep-set eyes. Loss of appetite, sometimes accompanied by vomiting and weight loss, was nearly constant. Gastrointestinal symptoms developed, frequently accompanied by cramping.

In later stages, particularly in patients with hemorrhagic manifestations, red blood appeared in the stools. Vomiting continued in nearly half of patients with hemorrhagic signs; vomitus was often of red or changed blood. Other common manifestations included sore throat and **dysphagia**, fissures and sores on the lips, **conjunctivitis** and subconjunctival bleeding, and coughing. **Jaundice** occurred in some. **Pancreatitis** was also frequent, and abortion occurred in 23 percent of pregnant women. Hemorrhagic manifestations, seen in many patients (including more than half of fatal cases), probably resulted from disseminated intravascular coagulation. Death occurred as early as the fourth day, more usually on the fifth or sixth day, and occasionally as late as the twentieth day.

Several pathologists deemed differential diagnosis of Ebola infection to be extremely difficult in settings where there might be malaria, Lassa fever, Marburg disease, yellow fever, Congo-Crimean hemorrhagic fever, typhoid, **infectious hepatitis**, **leptospirosis**, **brucellosis**, and other fevers. Others felt the lesions observed were adequately specific to permit an Ebola diagnosis.

Plasmapheresis with plasma from recovered patients was tried as treatment, but indications offered little hope of effective therapy. No drugs have been effective. A possible vaccine remains a dream.

Wilbur G. Downs

Postscript

Thanks to best-selling books, a motion picture, and newspaper and magazine articles, during the 1990s Ebola virus scared the wits out of a public unlikely ever to be called upon to face the explosive disease it generates. The same, however, cannot be said for many tropical African populations who live in peril of what have become the Ebola viruses. This is because the family Filoviridae, created for the Marburg and Ebola viruses, now breaks down Ebola into Ebola-Zaire, Ebola-Sudan, Ebola-Tai Forest (or Ivory Coast), and Ebola-Reston – all of which reveal slight serological differences. Ebola-Zaire and Ebola-Sudan were the first to appear, whereas Ebola-Reston is named for the Virginia town where a form of Ebola broke out in a laboratory among experimental monkeys in 1989. But although the virus spread from monkey to monkey and proved deadly for many of them, no human cases developed. Indeed, it has been suggested that, unlike the other Ebola strains, Ebola-Reston may not be capable of producing serious disease in humans, as four laboratory technicians were infected with the virus, but none became ill.

In 1992, there was a repeat of the Reston episode in Siena, Italy, showing the wisdom of the U.S. Centers for Disease Control and Prevention (CDC) policy – developed in response to Reston – that embargoed importation of experimental monkeys into the United States. This lasted about a year, after which the CDC began to re-license importers, but only those with approved facilities and properly trained staffs. However, safety concerns have created a trend away from wild monkeys toward the use of captive-bred monkeys raised especially for the medical experimentation market.

Because the Reston monkeys (and those at Siena) came from the Philippines (indicating that the Filoviridae are not exclusive to Africa), attempts have been made to find the virus there, although so far without success. As with the other Ebola strains, researchers have no idea where it lives in nature.

The other form of the virus, Ebola-Tai Forest (or Ivory Coast) derived its name from a single nonfatal case in the Tai forest of the Côte d'Ivoire developed in 1994 by a Swiss researcher after performing an autopsy on an infected chimpanzee. The case was important because it was the first evidence that Ebola existed in West Africa; since then, however, West African cases and fatalities have been reported in the Côte d'Ivoire, Liberia, and Gabon. The latter experienced three outbreaks in remote areas during a 20-month period spanning the years 1994–97, involving the deaths of nonhuman as well as human primates.

In the laboratory, a major difficulty with studying Ebola viruses is their high pathogenicity (classified by the CDC as Biosafety Level 4). In the field, the major difficulty in tracking what is now called **Ebola hemorrhagic fever** (EHF) is that, as in Gabon, it often strikes humans in remote areas. But not always: In the summer of 1995, Ebola-Zaire made a third large-scale appearance when it struck the town of Kikwit, in western Zaire (now the Democratic Republic of the Congo). It infected 315 persons and killed 242 of them (77 percent). Interestingly, the virus proved to be virtually identical to that of 1976 in northern Zaire.

Similarly, Ebola-Sudan recently (between October 2000 and January 2001) resurfaced in three widely separated areas of Uganda, where it triggered 425 presumptive cases and caused 224 deaths (53 percent). One is immediately struck by the consistently lower case-fatality rates generated by Ebola-Sudan (50–60 percent) than by Ebola-Zaire (77–88 percent) throughout each of their appearances.

No hosts for the Ebola viruses have been discovered, although mammals (including nonhuman primates), birds, reptiles, and insects all remain suspects. Nor has new light been shed on EHF transmission; as in the 1970s, the blame still rests on dirty needles and close contact with victims or objects they touched. Moreover, there has been no breakthrough in drug therapy and, for the moment at least, there is little hope of a vaccine. Treatment of victims consists of shock prevention and supportive care, both complicated by the need to protect medical personnel. However, studies comparing the RNA sequences of the different viral strains are under way, which ultimately may help to unravel the etiology and epidemiology of EHF – a disease as mysterious as it is deadly.

Kenneth F. Kiple

44. Echinococcosis (Hydatidosis)

The larval stages of three **tapeworms** of the genus *Echinococcus* cause severe disease in humans. All three normally become adults in the intestines of dogs or other canids. Eggs are passed in the feces and, if ingested by a herbivore, develop in the liver or other organs into a sac-like container of larvae, the **hydatid cyst**. Carnivores become infected by eating cysts with the flesh of the herbivore.

Echinococcus granulosus commonly has a dog/sheep cycle but may also infect goats, cattle, swine, and camels and is the most likely to infect humans. Human **echinococcosis** occurs primarily in sheep-rearing areas. Dogs ingest cysts in the offal of dead sheep and pass eggs in their feces. Humans acquire the eggs from a dog's fur or from contaminated food or water. Cysts holding 2 or more liters of fluid and larvae can grow for years in the liver, lungs, brain, or other organs and exert enough mechanical pressure to cause grave or fatal consequences. Rupture of a cyst by trauma or surgery releases daughter cysts, which may grow elsewhere in the victim; the hydatid fluid can cause fatal **anaphylactic shock**.

Hydatid cysts in humans and animals have been known since the ancient Romans, but as with other tapeworms, the relationship between the larval cyst and the adult worm was not suspected until modern times. *E. granulosus* was described as a species in 1850, and its life cycle was understood by 1863.

The parasite first became a serious danger to humans when animals were domesticated. The expansion of European settlement spread infection to the Americas and Australasia. Echinococcosis is also found in North Africa, the Middle East, northern and central Asia, and most of sub-Saharan Africa. Iceland was a major focus in the mid-nineteenth century, but education, dog control, and sanitary slaughtering have eliminated the disease. Similar methods, including mass treatment of dogs, have greatly reduced its incidence in Australia and New Zealand. The highest known prevalence of echinococcosis is among the stock-raising Turkana of Kenya. Colonial medical authorities failed to recognize the disease until the 1950s, and an incidence of 96 per 100,000 has been estimated – over seven times the previous record rate in Cyprus. The Turkana problem is linked to a close association between children and dogs.

Echinococcosis is often difficult to diagnose. Cysts can be detected by X-rays or surgery; several serologic tests are also used. Surgery was the only effective therapy until the 1980s, when the drug mebendazole was employed with some success.

K. David Patterson

45. Eclampsia

Eclampsia is a puzzling hypertensive disorder affecting only women. Associated with pregnancy and childbirth, it is an epileptic form of convulsions that develops during the second half of pregnancy. Eclampsia is associated with **hypertension**, **edema**, and **toxemia**, and all three can cause the symptoms of the disease to vary widely. **Preeclampsia** refers to hypertension, abnormal edema, or **proteinuria** during pregnancy, whereas eclampsia is the disease's most extreme form, manifested by severe convulsions, coma, and even death. Eclampsia is a leading cause of maternal and fetal mortality and can cause stillbirths and premature labor. Medical experts remain confused about the cause of this disorder and have no effective way to cure the disease other than to terminate pregnancy by delivering the baby. Through careful prenatal care, however, physicians can usually control the problem, and it is now relatively rare in the United States and Europe.

Not only is the disease difficult to define, but also accurate records of its existence are rare, especially in Third World countries where prenatal care by medical attendants is uncommon. Although eclampsia is among the diseases most troubling to obstetricians, research is difficult because it is found only in humans. Its etiology remains unknown but may be multifactorial.

Characteristics

For reasons not understood, eclampsia seems more common among the economically underprivileged. The typical patient is a young woman in her first pregnancy, of low socioeconomic status, and with little or no prenatal care. It is more common among women with **diabetes**, **high blood pressure**, or renal or vascular disease; who suffer from poor nutrition or hydatiform moles; who are at the age extremes of childbearing years; and who bear twins. It occurs more frequently in spring and summer and in certain locations. It also evinces a familial tendency, suggesting a genetic disorder.

Eclampsia is less likely to occur in women who have experienced a previous case. Few conclusive studies indicate that race is a factor, though it has been suggested that black women in the United States are more likely than their white counterparts to suffer eclampsia because of a greater tendency to develop chronic hypertension on the one hand, and less opportunity for maternal care on the other. The disorder occurs in 6–8 percent of pregnancies. Statistics show it to be more common in urban areas, though this association may reflect only the fact that urban women who experience eclampsia or preeclampsia receive more medical assistance in giving birth than rural women, and thus the condition is more frequently noted and reported. Indeed, it is difficult to determine the frequency of eclampsia in rural areas and Third World nations because women there seldom seek, have access to, or can afford regular prenatal care and a hospital delivery.

Symptoms of eclampsia and preeclampsia include excessive and sudden weight gain, edema, hypertension, and proteinuria. Patients may also suffer from headache, dizziness, visual disturbances, **anorexia**, nausea, vomiting, upper abdominal pain, and swelling of face and extremities. In severe cases, women experience visual and neurological disturbances, **oliguria** (a deficiency of urine excretion), and, of course, convulsions. In addition, cardiac output increases and the kidneys (which seem to be the target organ for the disease) are affected. Eclampsia can lead to lethal complications affecting the liver, kidney, uterus, and brain, such as **abruptio placentae**, acute **renal failure**, **cerebral hemorrhage**, disseminated **intravascular coagulation**, and circulatory collapse. Preeclampsia does not occur before the twentieth week of pregnancy, and eclampsia rarely before the thirty-second week.

History

The writings of Egyptian, Chinese, Indian, and Greek scholars note no convincing cases of eclampsia other than occasional remarks describing a pregnant woman's convulsion, fit, or headache. For centuries, eclampsia was commonly mistaken for **epilepsy**. If discussed at all, it was attributed to uterine suffocation. Therapy focused on encouraging a retrograde motion of the uterus to relieve pressure on the upper body and brain. Medieval writings only hint at the disease, but perhaps this paucity of information was because midwives monopolized birth assistance and failed to record problems they encountered.

In the second century, Galen noted that epilepsy could be fatal to pregnant women, and Eucharius Rösslin in the sixteenth century stated that convulsions and unconsciousness were ominous signs in pregnant women. Jacques Guillimeau in 1612 concluded that convulsions occurred because the fetus was striving to come forth or improper positioning extended the womb. François Mauriceau in 1688 was the first systematically to describe eclampsia, indicating a new concern with the disorder as men entered the field of obstetrics. He also was the first to note that primogravids were at greater risk than multigravids. Mauriceau suggested several causes, including excessive hot blood flowing from the uterus and malignant vapors from a dead fetus. In 1694, he recommended that two or three phlebotomies be performed routinely during pregnancy should a woman exhibit eclamptic tendencies. All early medical experts agreed that it was a dangerous disease.

During the nineteenth century, medical speculation about the causes of eclampsia was widespread. These included a woman's rapidly changing emotions, a sanguine or plethoric state, excessive hemorrhaging, blood to the brain, nutritional deficiency, excessive protein in the system, albuminuria, renal deficiency, retention of urinary constituents, nerve irritation, high blood pressure, seasonal changes, lethargy, melancholia, wealth, improper positioning of the womb, corrupt menstrual flow, a bad seed, an unstable personality, passions of the mind, and interrupted circulation.

Therapy was generally "heroic." Solutions included warm baths, doses of opium, extensive bleeding from the jugular vein or a temporal artery, depletion to rid the body of toxins, removal of meat or milk from the diet, mustard poultices, ice or cold water on the head, snuff, clysters, emollients to dilate the cervix, and plasters to the lower body to draw the uterus downward.

In 1768, Thomas Denman wrote one of the earliest English monographs on the disease. John Lever and James Simpson in 1843 simultaneously discovered the consistent occurrence of proteinuria in preeclamptic patients. This major breakthrough meant the disease could be considered a toxemia rather than one caused by mechanical pressure. Until the twentieth century, eclampsia was associated with wealthy women, probably because they used male doctors who wrote about the disorder. Not until the 1930s were poor women viewed as susceptible. Unwed mothers were also seen as vulnerable, perhaps because their infants were more likely to be primogravids. Early in the twentieth century, eclampsia was usually associated with hypertension, though speculation as to its origin was still common.

Today, physicians depend on careful monitoring of blood pressure and proteinuria during pregnancy, while watching for edema and excessive weight gain. Early detection is essential. If a woman should suffer preeclampsia, physicians recommend rest and constant monitoring. If a patient suffers convulsions, attendants take immediate measures to prevent physical injury by suctioning her air passage, providing oxygen, and employing magnesium sulfate to control the seizures. Seizures can cause fetal death because the convulsive woman is not breathing and thus the baby is cut off from its oxygen supply. If the baby is near term, doctors make every effort to deliver it once convulsions have subsided and the patient is conscious.

Sally McMillen

46. Emphysema

Pulmonary **emphysema** is defined in morphological rather than clinical terms. In 1958, emphysema was defined as an "increase beyond the normal of air spaces, distal to the terminal bronchiole, either from dilation or from destruction of their walls." A 1962 statement made anatomic destruction a part of the definition: "Emphysema is an anatomic alteration of the lung characterized by an abnormal enlargement of the air spaces distal to the terminal, nonrespiratory bronchiole, accompanied by destructive changes of the alveolar walls. The definition was further refined in 1985: "Emphysema is defined as a condition of the lung characterized by abnormal, permanent enlargement of airspaces distal to the terminal bronchiole, accompanied by the destruction of their walls, and without obvious fibrosis."

Emphysema can also be subclassified in anatomic terms. If emphysematous changes predominate in the region of respiratory bronchioles, the condition is termed centriacinar or centrilobular emphysema. More uniform involvement constitutes panacinar or panlobular emphysema. Occasionally, emphysema may occur adjacent to a scar or fibrotic process and is called paracicatricial emphysema.

Characteristics

Because emphysema is, by definition, a morphological diagnosis, its presence and prevalence depend on examination and interpretation of the lungs during autopsy. Obvious emphysema is likely to be found in at least 50 percent of an average autopsy population, with a frequency of about 65 percent in men and 15 percent in women. Incidence increases with age, reaching 30 percent by the fourth decade and 60 percent by the seventh decade of life. It has been suggested that at least some emphysema may be a universal finding in elderly adults.

Perhaps because of a younger average age of the population examined and a lower prevalence of cigarette smoking, studies from Africa reveal a lower frequency of emphysema than elsewhere. Yet even when populations are the same age, and lungs examined by the same investigators, national and even regional differences seem prevalent. For example, the frequency of emphysema is greater in parts of Britain than in Sweden or some parts of North America, and lower in some North American cities than in others. These differences may reflect different levels of cigarette smoking or air pollution, or the selection of people autopsied.

Various studies agree that the severity of emphysema increases with advancing age. Cigarette smoking is a primary cause of the dis-

ease, especially of moderate to severe forms, although some forms of mild emphysema are quite common and can occur in nonsmokers. Greater incidence in males may reflect their greater prevalence of smoking; if that is the case, then as more women take up cigarette smoking, this sex preference may change. Although emphysema is remarkably common, it causes – or contributes to – death in only a small percentage of cases.

The patient with clinically significant emphysema is typically an older male smoker with a history of breathing difficulties that increase in severity over time. He is usually thin, with a thoracic configuration (barrel-chested) suggesting hyperinflation, and has markedly diminished breath sounds on auscultation. Airflow obstruction can be demonstrated. However, this "typical" clinical picture is more often the exception than the rule. In several autopsy series, moderate to severe emphysema was found in a significant proportion of individuals who exhibited no clinical evidence of disease. Most often, emphysema occurs in conjunction with chronic **bronchitis** and is accompanied by a chronic productive cough.

The presumptive diagnosis of emphysema cannot be made without pulmonary function tests. Chronic airflow obstruction manifested by slowing of forced expiration is characteristic of moderate to severe emphysema, although even this finding may not be universal. When emphysema increases in severity, hyperinflation is reflected by an increase in total lung capacity and residual volume, and carbon monoxide diffusing capacity is reduced. Loss of lung elastic recoil is commonly associated with emphysema. Such physiological data provide more sensitive indicators of the presence of emphysema than do clinical symptoms or radiological findings.

History

In 1698, John Floyer described bullous emphysema, together with hyperinflation and loss of lung elastic recoil, in a horse he dissected. In 1793, Matthew Baillie described human emphysema with tissue destruction leading to airspace enlargement. Good evidence indicates that the lung illustrated in Baillie's book was that of Samuel Johnson, whose lungs, at autopsy, were permanently distended and failed to collapse on opening the chest. In his classic *Treatise on the Diseases of the Chest* that appeared in 1819, René Laennec provided the first description of pulmonary emphysema, its destructive nature, and its association with chronic bronchitis. James Jackson accumulated a series of emphysema cases and noted that the disease exhibited a familial predisposition. (Though he died in 1834, his work was published in 1837.) But not until 1963 was emphysema's genetic alpha-1-antitrypsin deficiency described. Physiological changes associated with emphysema have attracted the attention of many investigators over the years. The precise mechanisms causing emphysema's characteristic lung destruction are under current investigation.

Ronald J. Knudson

47. Encephalitis Lethargica

Foremost among recorded **encephalitis** epidemics was the global pandemic of **encephalitis lethargica** that spread from Europe during World War I and repeatedly struck throughout the world during the 1920s. This pandemic both accompanied and followed the 1918 **influenza** pandemic.

Characteristics

Encephalitis lethargica was often a sequel to influenza. Patients developed the triad signs of fever, lethargy, and disturbances of eye movement, along with other symptoms including headache, tremor, weakness, depression, delirium, convulsions, and inability to articulate ideas, coordinate movements, or recognize sensory stimuli, as well as psychosis and stupor. **Oculogyric crisis** (fixed eyeballs) and other eye-movement disorders – the most frequent sign

of localized damage to the nervous system – occurred in three-fourths of cases. Lethargy lasted a few days in some patients, but in others it persisted much longer, sometimes until death from comatose respiratory failure. Spasmodic twitching and severe psychic and behavior changes often persisted long after the illness. Approximately one-third of patients died of acute disease, and 80 percent of survivors later developed **parkinsonism**.

The main findings were a diffuse inflammatory reaction in the meninges and blood vessels of the brain and spinal cord, and degenerative changes in the neurons, especially in the brainstem, basal ganglia, and cerebellum, but also including the cortex and subcortical white matter. In the spinal cord, both white and gray matter were involved in the disease process.

Although epidemics of encephalitic disease had occurred in conjunction with many influenza epidemics (1580, 1658, 1673–75, 1711–12, 1729, 1767, 1780–82, 1830-33, 1847–78, and especially 1889–92), the pandemic associated with the 1918 influenza pandemic was unparalleled in virulence and sequelae. Along with its unique time distribution (1917–26), the encephalitis lethargica epidemic had a pronounced seasonal predilection for winter months.

Encephalitis cases were so closely associated with influenza attacks that many initially believed the disease was caused by influenza. Subsequently, however, many epidemics of encephalitis occurred when no influenza activity existed, which generated skepticism that influenza could be the cause. Long latent intervals and slow viruses were not well recognized in 1918; moreover, influenza was contagious and encephalitis was not. All this was misinterpreted as indicating that these were unrelated diseases rather than different manifestations of the same viral agent. Even the name "encephalitis lethargica" generated ongoing diagnostic confusion.

Although early reports of encephalitis preceded the explosive dissemination of influenza in 1918, influenza was active during the winter of 1916–17. Encephalitis was reported in Britain,

Scandinavia, Germany, the United States, and other countries in 1918, but its epidemic peaks occurred in 1919–20 and subsequent winters.

Attack rates for encephalitis lethargica during the pandemic years 1918–26 approached 1 case per 1,000 population in the United States and Europe. Reports indicate that rates may have been similar worldwide, except in some areas, most notably American Samoa, where neither influenza nor encephalitis occurred during the pandemic years. The world total of encephalitis lethargica cases was probably more than 1.5 million, of whom about 500,000 died of acute illness. More died from parkinsonism and other complications in later stages.

Leading researchers of the 1920s judged the relationship between influenza and encephalitis to be inconsistent, and stated the etiology of encephalitis lethargica to be "unknown." But in recent decades, from research undertaken in Seattle and Samoa, the disease's etiology seems clear. Seattle records show a characteristic lag of approximately a year from influenza/**pneumonia** death peaks to onset of encephalitis lethargica clusters, providing strong evidence that encephalitis cases were actually late sequelae of influenza.

In the Samoan Islands, the sharply contrasting experiences of Western and American Samoa provided a unique basis for studying the pandemic. In Western Samoa, nearly 20 percent of the population died of influenza during two months in 1918 alone. Meanwhile, American Samoa, just 70 kilometers away and inhabited by the same racial stock, avoided the infection. Despite the rudimentary nature of Western Samoan records, it is clear that that territory suffered heavily from both influenza/pneumonia and encephalitis lethargica during the years 1918–22. American Samoa was remarkably free of both diseases during those years.

The evidence, then, is compelling that the pandemic of influenza beginning in 1918 and the pandemic of encephalitis lethargica generally beginning the following year had a common etiology. Both pandemics were globally distributed and closely related in time, and only one agent (influenza virus) has been reliably identified. Local, regional, and national influenza/pneumonia epidemics preceded local, regional, and national epidemics of encephalitis lethargica. A large proportion of encephalitis cases had had influenza. Later, when patterns shifted from massive epidemic to sporadic endemic, the relationship between the two diseases became progressively obscured.

History

From among all causes of encephalitis – structural, chemical, and microbiological – it was difficult to identify specific infectious organisms and routes of transmission. But in the late nineteenth and twentieth centuries, many agents and vectors of encephalitis became known, among them the **syphilis** spirochete, the trypanosome of **African sleeping sickness**, the bacterial toxin of **botulism, yellow fever, Japanese B encephalitis, equine encephalitis, rabies**, influenza, **mumps, measles**, the enteroviruses, and most recently the **human immunodeficiency virus**. Adding to diagnostic confusion were many cases of stuporous encephalitic reactions to various toxins and drugs, especially **Reye's syndrome**, caused by aspirin, the etiology of which became known only in the 1980s.

But the main causative agent of epidemic encephalitis during the pandemic years was the influenza virus. Successive peaks of encephalitis occurred in European, Asian, African, and American countries. In the United States, encephalitis lethargica progressed across the country from east to west in 1919, just as influenza had the previous year, reaching peak occurrence in New York during January 1919; in Virginia during February; and in Illinois, Louisiana, and Texas during March. In California it peaked in April, and in Seattle the first cases were reported in October.

Research has tended to disregard the influenza/encephalitis/parkinsonism puzzle, apparently on the assumption that these epidemics are of little importance to current and future health. But failure to identify influenza virus as the cause of encephalitis lethargica and parkinsonism has crippled progress toward the understanding needed to prevent these elusive but exceedingly important diseases. Almost every disease of the central nervous system (CNS) may follow influenza. Thus we should examine CNS damage caused by influenza attacks during earlier life when seeking the keys to serious **CNS disease**, especially **Alzheimer's disease**.

R. T. Ravenholt

48. Enterobiasis

The **pinworm** *Enterobius vermicularis* is a common parasite around the world and is the most prevalent parasitic helminth in developed countries today. **Enterobiasis** has afflicted humans from ancient times; it was known to ancient Chinese, classical, and Islamic writers and was present in pre-Columbian America. Humans are the only hosts. Mature worms of 2–13 millimeters inhabit the cecum and adjacent regions of the intestines. Gravid females migrate out the host's anus and deposit thousands of eggs on the skin of the perianal region. The eggs mature quickly and are infectious within hours. Infection by ingestion of eggs from the hands is common, as the worms induce itching and scratching. Eggs are frequently eaten with contaminated food, and, because they are light, they are easily inhaled in household dust. Eggs hatch in the small intestine and develop into mature adults in as little as 4 weeks. Retroinfection, when eggs hatch on the perianal skin and the larvae crawl back into the rectum, is possible but rare. Pinworms are especially prevalent among small children and often become a family affair.

Enterobiasis is rarely a serious disease. Intestinal disturbances, if any, are minor, but pinworms can cause great discomfort, and scratching can lead to secondary infections. Migrating worms occasionally reach the vagina or appendix, but rarely cause serious harm. Rectal itching and consequent insomnia, especially in children, are suggestive of pinworm infection.

The condition normally is self-limiting in the absence of continuing reinfection. Drug treatment is safe and effective, but often an entire family or living group must be treated simultaneously, and bedding and clothing must be thoroughly cleaned. Even the most fastidious housekeepers may find it difficult to rid a home of airborne eggs. Personal hygiene is the best preventive measure.

K. David Patterson

49. Epilepsy

Epilepsy is characterized by repeated seizures resulting from recurrent, abnormal, excessive, synchronous discharges of cerebral neurons. It has probably been in existence since the dawn of humanity. The condition is chronic but rarely fatal. Modern medications can control seizures, and the limitations imposed by the disorder may be negligible. Unfortunately, epileptics are all too frequently stigmatized and excluded from many activities. Outdated beliefs and misconceptions about epilepsy have only recently shown signs of lessening in the United States and other industrialized societies.

Characteristics

Although epilepsy can begin at any age, most patients have their first seizure before 20. In fact, age of onset is often related to etiology. Perinatal injuries, severe hypoxia, developmental brain defects, and genetic metabolic defects are common causes of epilepsy among infants and the newborn. Brain infections such as **meningitis** and **encephalitis** often damage brain cells, with subsequent development of epilepsy. Many children experience seizures during high fever caused by infection elsewhere than the brain; however, only a tiny percentage of such febrile seizures persist after the age of 4. In urban ghettoes, **lead poisoning** and drug addiction are among the leading causes of epilepsy. Head trauma is a common cause of seizures among adults, although **brain tumor** must also be suspected, as about 40 percent of patients with brain tumors have seizures. Later in life, seizure may result from **cerebrovascular attack**.

Despite medicine's increased ability to determine various causes of epilepsy, many seizures proceed from no definitively known or reasonably presumed cause. That genetic factors are involved, however, is indicated by the fact that people with family histories of epilepsy have a higher incidence of seizures than the general population. Moreover, according to electroencephalograms (EEGs), asymptomatic relatives of epileptic patients exhibit greater abnormal discharge than among the general population.

Epilepsy is characterized by *recurrent* seizures; thus, a single seizure does not of itself indicate an epileptic condition. Nervous system infection, metabolic imbalance, and head injury may all result in a seizure episode without further risk. Among epileptics, however, any number of stimuli may trigger seizure activity. Fatigue, alcohol abuse, and infection, for example, commonly precipitate attacks in people whose epilepsy is otherwise well controlled.

Since the 1960s, epidemiological surveys of epilepsy have reported crude prevalence rates between 3.6 and 5.5 per 1,000 population. Such studies, however, are plagued with problems, most importantly a lack of agreement on the definition of epilepsy itself as well as what constitutes an active or an inactive case. Moreover, some cases are simply not identified by survey procedures.

Epilepsies are classified by localization of the electrical abnormality in the brain. The major division is between generalized (centrencephalic) seizures – with brain activity throughout the cerebral cortex – and partial (focal) seizures occurring in only one part of the brain. Generalized seizures exhibit bilateral motor activity and loss of consciousness, which may or may not occur in partial seizures depending upon the part of the brain initially affected and subsequent involvement of other structures. The clinical manifestation of the seizure approximately corresponds with the brain site where electrical abnormality occurs.

"Epilepsy" was first used to denote the symptoms of major (*grand mal*) seizure, currently termed "tonic-clonic" seizure. Over 60 percent of all epileptics have tonic-clonic seizures. A sudden burst of discharges involving the whole brain occurs without warning. The patient falls to the ground unconscious. Then, in the tonic phase, the patient goes rigid and often gives a short cry because of diaphragm and chest-muscle contraction. The eyes may roll upward or sidewise, and the tongue may be bitten. After this, jerky clonic spasms alternately flex and extend muscles of the head, face, and extremities. During this phase, the patient may become injured as well as incontinent. **Cyanosis** is usually marked. Breathing is deep, with sweating and salivation. Subsequent to the seizure, the patient may awaken in a confused state (the "postictal twilight state") and even display some bizarre behavior. Sometimes patients are difficult to rouse, sleep for hours, and awaken with headache or sore muscles. Although most tonic-clonic seizures last for only a few minutes, some develop into a series of seizures with no letup, or a continuous prolonged seizure. This serious condition (*status epilepticus*) may lead to death without immediate care.

A variety of generalized seizures have been recognized. Sometimes patients exhibit only the tonic or clonic aspects of the seizure. Between ages 4 and 12, "absence" seizures often occur. These have been called *petit mal* because their brief duration – only a few seconds – often renders them unrecognized and untreated. During the brief lapse of consciousness, the child stares vacantly, neither speaking nor hearing. Subsequent activity is resumed with no period of stupor. Equally brief are "atonic" seizures, during which the child simply falls to the ground;

"myoclonic" seizures, which are sudden, brief, and massive, involving the entire body or confined to extremities, face, or trunk; and "infantile spasms," during which the child is jerked into a fetal position with the knees drawn up. Many children with infantile spasms are also mentally retarded.

All partial seizures begin in one part of the brain, and because different parts of the brain control different parts of the body (as well as mental and sensory functions), their signs are varied and often complex. Many patients exhibit behaviors easily mistaken for psychiatric problems, hindering accurate diagnosis. Victims of partial seizures may display bizarre, learned, culturally conditioned behavior.

Simple partial seizures have been variously called "focal," "focal motor," or "focal sensory" seizures. Although symptoms may be motor, autonomic, psychic, sensory, or a combination, they are all linked to the affected area of the brain. The patient remains conscious as a general rule, and the attacks last no more than 30 seconds. One type of simple partial seizure has been called the "Jacksonian" – it characteristically begins with the twitching of one foot or hand.

Complex partial seizures are characterized by complex symptoms and impairment of consciousness. Often the patient appears conscious but later has no recollection of the episode. These seizures are usually associated with the temporal or frontal lobe and often begin with an "aura" warning of the impending attack. Auras include any number of sensations. Some of those most commonly reported are nausea; faintness; dizziness; numbness of the hands, lips, and tongue; choking sensations; and chest pain. Less often, patients report visions, palpitation, or disturbances of smell or hearing. Some patients' sensations may begin hours or even days before the seizure. These symptoms are called the "prodrome" and most often involve irritability or uneasiness. Psychomotor symptoms appearing during a seizure are generally semipurposeful and inappropriate actions such as clumsy attempts to dis-

robe. Patients often stagger about uttering guttural sounds. Such behavior is alarming to onlookers and often confused with psychiatric disorder.

Secondarily generalized partial seizures begin with a focal onset, then spread throughout the brain and produce generalized tonic-clonic seizures. Because the generalized phase is so dramatic, people often overlook the focal onset. The presence of an aura indicates a probable focal onset and the need to observe the initial phase more closely.

Eliciting the type of epileptic seizure is important in confirming diagnosis and choosing antiepileptic medication. An accurate medical history is crucially important. EEGs administered between seizures may or may not reveal patterns suggestive of epilepsy. Nevertheless, because they often do reveal abnormal discharges, routine administration of EEGs is of significant value in evaluating any possibly epileptic patient.

By conservative estimates, some 50 percent of patients can control recurrent seizures without side effects with optimal medical treatment. Another 30 percent can achieve seizure control but experience some side effects of the medication. For some patients whose seizures cannot be controlled by medication, surgery may succeed if a distinct piece of brain tissue causing the seizures can be identified, and if its removal will not cause unacceptable neurological deficits.

History
The antiquity of epilepsy is attested to by an ancient Akkadian text. The Greeks called it the "sacred disease" as well as epilepsy ("seizure"), which may derive from the idea that diseases represented attacks by supernatural beings. The term "sacred disease" is found first in the writings of Heraclitus and Herodotus and is explicitly identified with epilepsy in the Hippocratic collection of medical writings (c. 400 B.C.), which includes the earliest monograph on epilepsy we possess.

Underlying various explanations offered by the ancients was the basic belief that epilepsy is an affliction or possession by a higher power and that its cure must be supernatural. The disease was also believed contagious: Epileptics were unclean, and anyone touching them might become prey to the demon. This supposed contagion was one of the factors that stigmatized epileptics and made their lives a misery. To the ancients, the epileptic was an object of horror and disgust – not a saint or prophet as has sometimes been contended. Physicians of antiquity differentiated the sacred disease from hysterical attacks as well as madness.

In the struggle between supernatural and scientific explanations of disease, science has gradually emerged victorious in the Western world. The fight, however, has been long and eventful, and in it epilepsy held one of the key positions. Showing both physical and psychic symptoms, epilepsy more than any other disease was open to interpretation both as a physiological process and as the effect of supernatural influences. The Hippocratic texts provide the first record we have of the battle in an attack on popular superstition about the "sacred disease." The text maintained that epilepsy was hereditary, that its cause lay in the brain, and that it be treated by diet and drugs as long as it was not yet chronic. It is here we first find the fundamental statement that the seat of the disease is in the brain and that the brain is the organ of all psychic processes both normal and pathological. Moreover, not only epilepsy but all mental diseases were to be explained by disturbances in the brain.

During the Middle Ages, literature on epilepsy propounded two contrasting views. On one hand, the "falling evil" was bound to demoniac beliefs and theological speculations; on the other, physicians clung to the idea of a definite natural disease. Little effort was made to force the issue; physicians rarely discussed the theological aspects and anyway were apparently unable to rid themselves of traditional definitions and explanations. By the end of the sixteenth century, however, this changed: Debate became open, involving the role of the devil, witchcraft, and various magical treatments. Despite many efforts to define epilepsy and classify seizures, little medical progress was made, although gradually the idea of epilepsy as a natural disease gained more credence, especially after the Enlightenment.

By the beginning of the nineteenth century, epileptics were hospitalized, although unlike the insane, they were allowed to go to church on Sundays. Moreover, confined epileptics became subjects of systematic medical attention. It was slow going at first, and only in 1838 were epileptic children in Paris removed from the Hospital of the Incurably Ill and provided some kind of education. In addition, the separation of hospitalized epileptics from the insane was motivated less by solicitude for the epileptics than by a belief that epilepsy was infectious and would affect the insane even more than it did the healthy. The confinement of epileptics in separate wards of lunatic asylums became established procedure in Europe around 1850 and was soon followed by requests for special institutions for epileptics.

Nonetheless, during the early nineteenth century, valuable contributions were made by physicians in hospitals and asylums, and new terminology, increased use of statistics, and interest in the psychiatric side of epilepsy developed. The terms *grand mal, petit mal,* "absence," *status epilepticus,* and "aura," for example, came into common usage and survive to this day. The use of statistics fostered investigation into the heritability of epilepsy and its causes. Despite the increased attention, however, modern medicine's understanding of the disease began around 1880 with the work of John Jackson in England and Jean Charcot in France. Jackson outlined a neurological theory of epilepsy, while Charcot separated epilepsy from **hysteria** more emphatically than any of his predecessors. In 1888, Jackson's principles were vindicated by William Macewen, who demonstrated the connection between physical seizure symptoms and specific brain sites of abnormal discharge.

Jerrold E. Levy

50. Ergotism

Ergotism is a disease condition acquired by eating cereal grains infected with ergot fungus. Known since the time of Galen, it was prevalent in medieval Europe, particularly among the poor who, during famine, consumed bread made from spoiled rye. Ergot (*secale cornutum*, "spur of the corn," "horned rye," "womb grain"), the dried sclerotium of *Claviceps purpurea*, develops on the ovary of common rye, or on corn, where it was previously known as "corn smut." The actual cause of ergot in grasses was hotly debated by early naturalists, some of whom thought it occurred in rainy weather and was attributable to fog or impure atmosphere. Others believed it was the work of worms or butterflies, whereas still others regarded it as the product of improper fecundation or perhaps the cooking of the sexual parts of the plants.

Characteristics

Ergotism has two forms: "convulsive" or "spasmodic" (also known as "creeping"), which affects the central nervous system; and "gangrenous," which affects blood vessels and blood supply to the extremities. Common names for **gangrenous ergotism** are "Saint Anthony's fire" (after the patron saint of the disease), "hidden fire," "saint's fire," "evil fire," "devil's fire," and "holy fire." Early imprecision in disease specificity led physicians to confuse ergotism with **plague** and various other diseases including **leprosy**, **anthrax**, **typhus**, **smallpox**, and **scurvy**.

Convulsive ergotism causes areas of degeneration in the spinal cord. Early German accounts mentioned tingling and mortification in fingers and toes – occasionally extending to the rest of the body – and vomiting, diarrhea, intense hunger, anxiety, unrest, headache, vertigo, noises in the ear, stupor, and insomnia. Often the limbs became stiff, accompanied by convulsive muscle contractions leading to staggering and awkward movements, often aggravated by touch. Although many victims recovered, symptoms sometimes remained for long periods, resulting in permanent stiffness of joints, muscular weakness, optic disorders, and occasional imbecility.

Midwives and empirics discovered that spasmodic ergotism caused abortion or miscarriage in pregnant women, the drying up of milk in lactating mothers, and **amenhorrea** in young girls. This abortifacient or oxytocic effect was later noted by orthodox medicine and led to the widespread use of ergot to accelerate uterine action. Before long, doctors began distinguishing ergot with sobriquets such as *poudre obstetrical*, "forcing powders," or more commonly, "forcing drops." Not surprisingly, it also played a major role among quacks, charlatans, and "private specialists" who promised a quick and painless cure for women desiring to "regulate" their menstrual cycles, a euphemism for terminating a pregnancy. For some, ergot substituted for the more common borax, cinnamon, and turpentine as an abortifacient.

Gangrenous ergotism often began with itching and formications in the feet, or sensations of extreme cold, followed by burning pain, or a crop of blisters. A dark spot usually appeared on the nose or affected extremity, leading to loss of sensibility in the part. Early nineteenth century accounts mentioned headache, dizziness, nausea, vomiting, diarrhea, and spreading erysipelatous redness. The epidermis was raised by serous exudation, and the surface assumed the appearance of **gangrene** with the extremities becoming withered and blackened. Usually the gangrene was dry, but the moist variety was not unknown. The patient suffered from continual low fever and phthisical symptoms and faced eventual death from exhaustion or **septicemia**, but recovery often followed loss of the affected limb. When gangrene attacked the viscera, however, death occurred quickly.

History

First allusions to ergotism are concurrent with French monastic hospices, which cared for the common people and took special note of the disease. Along with these observations came the designation of patron saints for ergotism, including Saints Benedict of Umbria, Martial of Limoges, Geneviève of Paris, Martin of Tours, and Anthony of Egypt, whose remains were carried to France in the eleventh century. From this last saint, the name "Saint Anthony's fire" was derived.

One authority has recorded 132 epidemics of ergotism between 591 and 1789. The *Annals of the Convent at Xanten,* near the Rhine, also describe outbreaks, as did François Eudes de Mézeray in the seventeenth century. French epidemics of the gangrenous type reportedly killed 40,000 in 922 and 14,000 in Paris alone during 1128–29. The spasmodic form occurred in Spain in 1581 and 1590 and in Germany in 1595; epidemics in France, Germany, and Switzerland recurred throughout the seventeenth century. The French districts of Sologne and Dauphiné, frequently subject to flooding, suffered continuously from outbreaks of ergotism, as did Artois, Lorraine, and Limousin. The disease also affected the Netherlands, Sweden, Majorca, Italy, Poland, and central Russia, where outbreaks were reported as late as 1926. Three epidemics were recorded in Britain. During the American Revolutionary War, soldiers in upper New York reportedly sickened on ergotted flour shipped from Ohio. A later American outbreak reportedly occurred at a New York prison in 1825.

Recent research has raised the possibility that ergotism can explain the convulsions and hallucinations that attended religious revivals, including the Salem witchcraft affair, as well as the "Great Fear" (July 20–August 6, 1789) that swept the countryside prior to the French Revolution, and even the seasonability of mortality and conception patterns in Europe.

Research in the 1930s suggested that the distribution of convulsive and gangrenous ergotism was a function of the presence or absence of vitamin A in the diet. Analysis of the 1770 epidemic of gangrenous ergotism in Sologne and convulsive ergotism in Hanover indicated that Sologne, on the left bank of the Rhine, was a dairy district that provided a diet rich in vitamin A, whereas Hanover, on the right bank, was unable to sustain a dairy economy. The striking difference in the effects of ergot on the two communities in close proximity caused researchers to undertake feeding experiments, which confirmed the efficacy of vitamin A in mitigating the effects of ergotism.

Similarly, although some researchers believed that England's relative freedom from ergotism resulted from abundant ingestion of meat and potatoes, others demonstrated that the English diet's richness in milk and butter products was actually responsible. In areas rich in dairy products, phytase and bowel bacteria broke down the poisonous phytates of the grain into comparatively innocuous inorganic phosphates. Thus, the convulsive ergotism common to nondairy areas was virtually absent in England and certain sections of France.

John S. Haller, Jr.

51. Erysipelas

The term **erysipelas** (from Greek meaning "red" and "skin") was often used in Hippocratic times to describe classic **cellulitis**. Since the late nineteenth century, however, erysipelas has commonly referred to infection of the derma with a streptococcal organism, usually *Streptococcus pyogenes.*

Characteristics

Infection with a group A beta-hemolytic streptococcus can produce a painful, red, edematous indurated skin lesion called *peau d'orange* for its resemblance to the texture of an orange skin. Sharp borders of the infection extend rapidly, dissecting the underlying dermis from the epidermis. Erysipelas usually appears on the face, producing a butterfly rash over cheeks and nose. The same streptococci that cause erysipelas also cause **scarlet fever**, giving both diseases a fairly distinctive age pattern: Erysipelas is more common among adults, who generally escape scarlet fever, whereas the latter normally attacks the young. The prognosis for untreated erysipelas is especially serious when this infection is secondary to some other insult such as laryngeal infection, or **puerperal sepsis**. Indeed distinctions are still made among **gangrenous erysipelas**, **erysipelas grave internum** (a form of **puerperal fever**), **surgical erysipelas** (which occurs after a surgical procedure), and **traumatic erysipelas** (which begins in a wound).

History

Early accounts of erysipelas are often confusing because they lumped purulent and gangrenous afflictions under this rubric. Thus, Hippocrates distinguished between "traumatic" erysipelas, which accompanied wounds, and a myriad of other skin lesions that had no known external cause. Galen in turn distinguished between **phlegmon** (including suppurative ulcers and gangrene) and nonnecrotic celluliti – but viewed both as forms of erysipelas. Celsus, in the first century A.D., considered septic ulcers, "canker," erythematous wound infections, and *ignes sacer* ("sacred fire") all to be types of erysipelas.

Such confusion has continued into modern times, with some historians interpreting epidemics of *ignes sacer* or "Saint Anthony's fire" as ergotism, whereas others have viewed these scourges as recurrent erysipelas. Before the modern period, however, physicians tended to embrace the distinctions made by Galen and consequently included a wide variety of ailments among the varieties of erysipelas.

During the nineteenth century, physicians began giving greater attention to the causes and prevalence of erysipelas because, on the one hand, the disease seemed connected to wound infection, and, on the other hand, epidemics of erysipelas were occurring simultaneously with peak years of puerperal sepsis, or "childbed fever." Their investigations eventually led to the discovery of streptococci and the distinctions that have provided us with our current definitions of erysipelas.

In 1795, Alexander Gordon first formally associated erysipelas with puerperal fever. Then, around the middle of the nineteenth century, two seminal studies appeared: In 1842, Oliver Wendell Holmes published an essay on the contagiousness of puerperal fever, and in 1861, Philip Ignaz Semmelweis published his classic study of "childbed fever." Both men blamed physicians for carrying infective particles to the bedsides of parturient women. French clinician Armand Trousseau, writing during the same period, regarded even trivial skin injuries as precursors to erysipelas.

In 1882, following the discovery of streptococci, Friedrich Fehleisen published a study of the etiology of erysipelas, which he associated with *S. pyogenes*. In follow-up studies, another German surgeon, Friedrich Rosenbach, described how the erysipelas-causing streptococci spread through host tissues without causing suppuration. This research was of paramount interest to surgeons trying to control the omnipresent infections – occasionally called "hospitalism" – that killed survivors of otherwise "successful" operations.

Although the use of aseptic and antiseptic techniques led to dramatic reductions in postsurgical mortality rates, maternal mortality still remained high. During the 1920s and 1930s, research permitted identification and typing of streptococci strains. This, in turn, led to irrefutable evidence that puerperal fever was an exogenous infection, usually transmitted from a physician, midwife, or nurse attending a parturient woman. Yet even family and friends could communicate the streptococci that caused puerperal sepsis in women in labor, for these were the same streptococci that caused erysipelas. Consequently, maternal mortality from puerperal fever declined only after effective antibiotics became available. Despite well-known changes in the virulence of streptococcal organisms historically, no sudden, spontaneous decline in virulence can account for the abrupt decline in mortality from erysipelas, scarlet fever, and puerperal fever. Instead, credit for moderating these ancient scourges belongs to the beginning of the antibiotic era and, in particular, to the use of sulfonamides.

Ann G. Carmichael

52. Fascioliasis

The **liver fluke** *Fasciola hepatica* is usually a parasite of sheep and cattle. "Liver rot" in sheep was described in a French work in 1379, and the first human case was described in 1760. The fluke's life cycle was discovered in 1881. **Fascioliasis** is a significant veterinary problem, but human infection is also fairly common. The fluke's life cycle is much like that of *Fasciolopsis buski* (see **Fasciolopsiasis**) with people or herbivores infected by eating raw watercress or other plants contaminated by the cysts of the fluke. Adult worms settle in the bile ducts after a period of wandering in the liver. Mild infestations may cause little damage, but fever, **jaundice**, and right upper quadrant abdominal pain radiating to the shoulder blade are common symptoms. Bile ducts may become partially or totally obstructed, and liver destruction can be severe.

F. hepatica is cosmopolitan in distribution, with important foci of human infection in southern France, Algeria, and South America. Treatment is generally effective.

K. David Patterson

53. Fasciolopsiasis

Fasciolopsiasis is caused by the **giant intestinal fluke**, *Fasciolopsis buski*. Discovered in 1843, the organism occurs in China, Korea, Southeast Asia, and parts of India and Indonesia. The adult worm, with a lifespan of only 6 months, attaches itself to the wall of the human small intestine. Pigs and dogs can also be infected and sometimes are important reservoir hosts. Eggs produced by the hermaphroditic adults pass out in the feces and, if they reach fresh water, produce motile larvae that penetrate into the tissues of certain planorbid snails. After two generations of reproduction, another motile form leaves the snail, finds a plant like the water chestnut, water caltrop, or water bamboo, and encysts on it. Humans become infected with cysts by peeling raw fruits with their teeth or eating them un-

cooked. The disease can become quite prevalent in areas where such plants are cultivated with human feces as fertilizer.

Mild infections are often asymptomatic, but flukes can irritate and even ulcerate the intestinal mucosa. Abdominal pain, **diarrhea**, **anemia**, and fluid accumulation in the abdomen are common symptoms. Extreme cases can be fatal. Drug therapy is usually effective.

K. David Patterson

54. Favism

Favism is an acute hemolytic reaction triggered by exposure either to fava beans (*Vicia faba*) or to certain drugs (e.g., sulfa-based antibiotics or primaquine) in people with an inherited deficiency of the enzyme glucose-6-phosphate dehydrogenase (G6PD). In favism, the patient can suffer destruction of red blood cells, severe **anemia**, and possibly death. The bean is a dietary staple in areas where favism is reported. Only about 20 percent of those who are G6PD deficient are likely to experience episodes of favism. With modern medical conditions, the hemolytic anemia caused by favism is only rarely fatal (about 1–4 percent of reported cases). Strong evidence suggests that both the gene for **G6PD deficiency** and the cultural practice of fava bean consumption are evolutionarily adaptive traits that protect against death from **malaria**. Favism, then, could be described as a negative outcome of the interaction of the positive adaptive qualities of both the gene and the bean.

Characteristics
Favism is found primarily in the Mediterranean and Middle East regions, where fava beans are a staple food and the Mediterranean variant of G6PD-deficiency gene is relatively common. It is frequently encountered in Greece, Sardinia, Italy, Cyprus, Egypt, Lebanon, Israel, Iran, Iraq, Algeria, and Bulgaria and is particularly common among Sephardic Jews. Favism has also been sporadically reported in China, Germany,

France, Poland, Romania, Yugoslavia, Britain, and the United States. The disease is considered a serious public-health problem in Greece.

Favism is generally a pediatric illness. Most victims are between 2 and 5 years old, although cases as young as 6 months and as old as 65 years have been reported. The disease has a marked seasonal cycle corresponding to the fava bean harvest between April and July, although where beans are dried for later consumption, cases can occur all year.

Evidence suggests that the toxic factor inducing the favism crisis has four characteristics: It is in the skin of the bean; it is heat stable; it can enter the breast milk of lactating women; and its toxicity decreases when the beans are dried and their skin changes color. Active biochemical agents in the skin – vicine, isouramil, divicine, and L–dopa – are probably responsible. These same agents are believed to provide some protection against malaria for people of normal genotype when they eat fresh fava beans.

Boys are much more likely to suffer favism than girls, because G6PD deficiency is a sex-linked trait. Only carrier males (hemizygotes) and homozygous females can suffer from favism. Heterozygous females appear to have an evolutionary advantage because they have no risk of favism and also enjoy some protection against malaria. Over 200 varieties of the G6PD-deficiency gene have been identified, and their distribution correlates with the historical distribution of malaria.

The G6PD enzyme, found in all tissues, has important housekeeping functions in red-blood-cell metabolism. The cells of enzyme-deficient individuals tend to become oxidant-sensitive, and any exogenous sources of increased oxidants (malaria parasites, antimalarial drugs, or fava beans) can result in the lysis (explosion) of the cell, resulting in either favism or protection from severe malaria infection, depending on the context.

Favism is characterized by five general symptoms: weakness, fatigue, pallor, **jaundice**, and **hemoglobinuria** (blood in the urine). The anemia caused by hemolysis is severe. In populations at risk, this set of symptoms is recognized as a distinct illness, often referred to as "fava-bean poisoning."

History

The historical puzzle of favism is that peoples of Mediterranean and Middle Eastern societies would continue to eat a food that regularly causes illness and even death. From an evolutionary perspective, both fava bean consumption and G6PD deficiency appear to be retained in populations because they provide some protection from malaria. The correlation between the geographic distribution of these traits and malaria is one line of evidence for this relationship. Fava bean cultivation dates back to the Neolithic period in areas that have favism. Ancient Indo-European culture, and particularly Greek culture, placed remarkable emphasis on the symbolic rather than nutritional qualities of the fava bean.

Fava beans have had three primary symbolic associations: the life principle, the souls of the dead, and the generative powers of male sexuality. They are ritualistically eaten at certain times of the year, a practice that continues in European folk cultures. However, taboos against consumption of fava beans for certain groups, particularly priests, have been reported in ancient Greece, Egypt, India, and Africa. The most famous case of such a taboo was among the Pythagoreans, who had the maxim, "It is an equal crime to eat beans and the heads of one's parents." Although many historical analyses of this taboo have been suggested, a medically informed hypothesis based on the risk of favism appears most reasonable.

In the history of medicine, early clinical descriptions by Italian physician Antonio Gasbarrini were a landmark for diagnosis and treatment of favism attacks. Within the tradition of Galenic medicine, treatment, although not always for favism attacks, emphasized reinforcement of the blood with red wine among other things. Understanding the evolutionary history of favism has been a recent development paralleling the discovery of the malaria connection with other genetic polymorphisms like **thalassemia** and **sickle-cell anemia**. The analytical connection with G6PD deficiency was first suggested in 1956, and development of a genetic screening technique for the trait created a wealth of population genetic data during the 1960s. Such data on genetic markers in populations – for example, the variants of G6PD deficiency – have a potential for historical reconstruction of population movements and culture contact.

Peter J. Brown

55. Filariasis

The term **filariasis** refers to several diseases of both humans and animals caused by infection with a specific group of parasitic nematodes called **filarial worms**. Those that affect humans include *Wuchereria bancrofti* and *Brugia malayi*, common causes of **elephantiasis** (extreme swelling and thickening of legs, scrotum, labia, or arms) and **chyluria** (lymph and emulsified fat globules in the urine); *Loa loa*, the "eye worm"; and *Onchocerca volvulus*, the cause of **onchocerciasis**. Adult filarial worms reside in the lymphatic system, subcutaneous tissues, or peritoneal and pleural cavities. Their embryos (microfilariae) are ingested from blood or skin by an intermediate host (a mosquito, fly, or other arthropod). The microfilariae become larvae in the intermediate host and then reenter a human or animal host through skin bites by the intermediate host. *L. loa* is endemic in West and central Africa, whereas onchocerciasis is found in Mexico, Central America, and West Africa. Discussion of **human lymphatic filariasis** in this chapter is, however, limited to its most prevalent (90 percent of infections) form – that caused by *W. bancrofti*.

Characteristics
Bancroftian filariasis is widely distributed throughout the tropics. Though it no longer exists in areas such as North America, southern Europe, Australia, and some Caribbean islands, and is decreasing in prevalence in the Western Hemisphere generally, *W. bancrofti* is becoming more prevalent in parts of Asia. At some time most regions of the tropics or subtropics as well as temperate parts of China and Japan have experienced this infection.

In 1984, the World Health Organization estimated the number of people infected with *W. bancrofti* at more than 81 million. Prevalence is highest in Asia (especially China, India, and Indonesia) and Africa. The disease affects primarily working-age poor people in areas where mosquitoes abound.

Adult *W. bancrofti* lie coiled in human lymphatic vessels and lymph glands and can live up to 18 years. Within 6 months to 1 year of infection, the microfilariae leave the adult female and enter the host's blood and lymph channels. Microfilariae move freely through the lymph or blood. Nocturnal microfilariae (the most common form) reside in the arterioles of the lungs during the day, whereas the diurnal strain appears in the peripheral blood continuously, although periodically in reduced numbers. Nocturnal microfilariae are generally found west of 140° east longitude, and diurnal microfilariae are present east of 180° east longitude. Both types may be found between these two meridians. The largest concentrations of diurnal microfilariae exist in the Polynesian and New Caledonian regions of the Pacific.

Bancroftian filariasis is transmitted only by mosquito. There is no known animal reservoir of *W. bancrofti*. Microfilariae may be transmitted between humans through blood sharing (as in pregnancy) or transfusion, but such microfilariae never develop into adults.

Microfilariae have adapted their daily cycles to either day- or night-feeding mosquitoes, depending on the species present in a particular geographic area. Once inside a mosquito, microfilariae become infective larvae within 2 weeks, then escape onto the skin of the next human host when the mosquito feeds. The larvae burrow into the skin through the tiny puncture wound and find their way to lymph vessels where they mature and mate, producing more microfilariae.

Filarial disease may not manifest itself for many years despite the presence of micro-filaremia. If reexposure to larvae does not occur, infection usually disappears within 8 years. Repeated exposure over many years generally results in clinical disease during adulthood. Symptoms occur throughout the body because of widespread disruption of the lymphatics.

Once the filarial larva settles in a human lymph channel and begins to mature, it provokes a localized response involving lymph-vessel dilation and slowing of lymph flow. The body responds immunologically, sending eosinophils, plasma cells, and macrophages to the site of infection. **Lymphangitis** (inflammation of lymph channels) usually results in swelling and pain, and varices form when the lymph vessels become hypertrophied. Fibrosis of the vessel occurs, killing the adult worm, which is absorbed or calcified. Obliteration of the vessel forces extravasation of lymph into the tissue, where it accumulates, causing the typical **lymphedema** of filarial elephantiasis. The swelling, consisting of lymph, fat, and fibrotic tissue under stretched and thickened skin, can become quite large.

In highly endemic areas, people are exposed to repeated infections from a young age, and the children show little effect of infection. When the larvae move into lymph vessels, they fail to provoke a strong immunologic response, thus allowing new microfilariae to travel through the now-dilated lymph channels. The worms survive for years, and their offspring are passed on in their larval stage by mosquitoes to other human hosts. As the adult worms eventually die in their tolerant human hosts' lymphatics, fibrosis and calcification occur. As lymph channels become obstructed, elephantoid manifestations develop, especially in the groin and lower extremities. People in highly endemic areas are infected repeatedly over the years and so will manifest various stages of filariasis simultaneously.

Uninfected adults newly arrived in an endemic region generally show an inflammatory response to filarial infection. Their immune systems react strongly, sending a variety of cellular defenders to the affected areas. The worms are surrounded, ultimately causing **stenosis** of the lymphatics as well as painful swellings and fever. Such a powerful response generally kills the worm, preventing the development of microfilariae but also causing disruption of the lymphatic system and the early development of elephantiasis. Chronic obstructive filariasis can result in lymph gland enlargement, chyluria, **lymph scrotum**, **hydrocele**, and elephantiasis of the legs, scrotum, labia, arms, or (rarely) breasts.

Several microfilaricidal drugs exist; the most effective is diethylcarbamazine citrate (DEC), first used in 1947. This drug also kills adult worms. When DEC is used in conjunction with a comprehensive mosquito control plan, the rate of *W. bancrofti* infection in an area declines dramatically. Other measures of prevention and treatment, such as mosquito control or avoidance by itself, or surgical treatment of the elephantiasis, are usually not highly effective.

History

Evidence indicates that bancroftian filariasis existed in the ancient tropical world. Discussions of something called elephantiasis appear in the works of ancient Greek and Roman authors, but many of them were probably describing **leprosy**, which was called *elephantiasis graecorum* to distinguish it from another disease, *elephantiasis arabum* (probably bancroftian filariasis).

Bancroftian filariasis was probably not endemic in the ancient Mediterranean except for certain parts of the Nile Delta. Travelers brought knowledge of the condition to residents of the region, and an occasional newcomer undoubtedly carried the disease there from his or her home country. Ancient descriptions of a condition resembling bancroftian filariasis also exist in records from the Nile Delta, Polynesian islands, and India. Moreover, medieval Arab writers discussed an elephantiasis that was probably filariasis and not leprosy.

It has been argued that bancroftian filariasis originated in Southeast Asia and spread with the migration of peoples to Polynesia and Africa. The filarial worm adapted to the mosquito vectors available in these new areas, thus explaining the existence of both diurnal and nocturnal strains. The continued migration of peoples and the opening of the tropical world to trade over the past few centuries, plus the adaptability of *W. bancrofti*, resulted in the spread of the parasite throughout the tropics, including China and India. Filariasis came to the New World, most likely via the slave trade. A legacy of the slave trade in the United States was the establishment of a focus of bancroftian filariasis in Charleston, South Carolina and its surrounding "Low Country," which survived until the early twentieth century.

European observers described numerous cases of elephantiasis, endemic hydrocele, and lymph scrotum. A few even recognized the development of elephantiasis from fever through lymphangitis, lymphadenitis, and swelling. Though these writers located the disease in the lymphatics, none could identify the cause. That discovery awaited widespread medical application of the microscope in the latter half of the nineteenth century.

The first breakthrough in understanding elephantiasis occurred in 1863 when a French physician, Jean-Nicolas Demarquay, described microfilariae he observed in fluid drawn from a Cuban patient. Demarquay could not explain the worms' presence but hoped that there would be some scientific value for others in publishing the case.

Four years later in Brazil, Otto Wucherer found "some threadlike worms" in a patient's blood clot. Wucherer could not identify the species from books on human parasites, so he published his story "as an incentive for some of my colleagues…to attempt to shed light on a disease, the etiology of which is still enigmatic today."

In 1870 in India, Timothy Lewis found worms like those Wucherer had described. The patient left the hospital before Lewis could study the condition further, but a second patient entered the hospital a few days later. Lewis now went beyond Demarquay and Wucherer, removing blood from the new patient's finger and studying it microscopically. He found what he called filariae in this blood and also in the patient's urine. Lewis's report of these and other patients, published in 1872, documented for the first time both the presence of microfilariae and the presence of any microorganism in human peripheral blood. He also described, but could not explain, the disappearance of microfilariae from the blood.

All three of these researchers knew they had identified an immature form of the filarial worm. Nor were they the only ones; both T. Spencer Cobbold of London and M. Robin of Reunion Island reported similar findings in the early 1870s.

It remained for Patrick Manson to synthesize the various bits of knowledge about human filarial infection and produce a useful theory. Manson spent his early career, beginning in 1866, as a medical officer in the Chinese Customs Service. He treated many elephantiasis patients, recognized and named the condition called "lymph scrotum," and devised an operation to remove scrotal tumors. On leave in England in 1875, he read the literature on the conditions he had been treating, including descriptions of lymph scrotum in India, the relation of lymph scrotum to elephantiasis, and Lewis's papers on filarial worms in the blood and lymph of tropical chyluria patients. In articles published in 1876–77, Manson presented studies to show that the three diseases were all caused by the filarial worm described by Lewis, seated in lymphatics. But Manson apparently knew nothing of Demarquay's and Wucherer's earlier findings.

Manson tried to obtain adult filarial worms from newly deceased patients, but Chinese traditions discouraged human autopsies. He suggested that physicians in India, less hampered by such prejudice, seek out adult worms in patients who had died with similar symptoms. However, the first demonstration of adult filariae in humans occurred not in India but in Australia. Joseph Bancroft in Queensland studied a number of patients with lymphatic conditions, though not elephantiasis. His first adult worm came from a lymphatic abscess of the arm. He obtained another four from a hydrocele of the spermatic cord.

In 1877, he forwarded these specimens to Cobbold, the leading British helminthologist. Cobbold had previously encouraged Bancroft to look for the adults after Bancroft sent him immature filariae obtained from these patients. It was Cobbold who suggested naming the filarial worm for Bancroft, and a colleague of Wucherer suggested that Wucherer deserved credit for discovering it. As a result, the filaria is known as *Wuchereria bancrofti*.

How did the worm find its way into humans? Manson, continuing his work in China, published a key suggestion in 1878. The worms' embryos, he argued, could not mature and enter the bloodstream without overwhelming their human host by sheer numbers. Manson suggested and then demonstrated that the mosquito was the "nurse" of the filarial embryo. The insect ingested filariae in its blood meal, and the young worms developed in the body of this intermediate host. The need for a specific mosquito in addition to the human host, Manson concluded, explained "the limitation of the distribution of elephantoid diseases to certain districts and zones ... where the mosquito flourishes."

Another filarial mystery remained: the disappearance and reappearance of worm embryos in the blood of infected patients. Manson discovered that the number of microfilariae increased and decreased in a regular diurnal pattern, the embryos reaching their peak presence in the hours just before and after midnight. He concluded that the microfilariae were "adapted to the nocturnal habits of the mosquito...another of the many wonderful instances of adaptation so constantly met with in nature."

What happened to the filariae during the rest of the day? Manson asked that question in 1879 but could not answer it for nearly 20 years.

In 1897 in London, he studied the organs of a patient with filariasis who had opportunely committed suicide at 8:30 in the morning, presumably just after the worms left the peripheral blood for the day. Postmortem examination revealed huge numbers of the parasites in the small blood vessels of the lungs and others in the large vessels.

The next few years produced the answer to a question Manson had asked in 1877: How did the filariae pass from mosquitoes to humans? In 1900, the work of Thomas Bancroft, Joseph Bancroft's son, and of Manson's protégé, George C. Low, who studied mosquito specimens Bancroft sent to Manson, suggested that filarial embryos exited from the mosquito's proboscis and entered human skin while the insect was biting – a hypothesis confirmed by B. Grassi and G. Noe later the same year.

Nineteenth century physicians working in various tropical areas had made almost every breakthrough in uncovering the mystery of filarial infection. By 1900, the medical world possessed an understanding of a disease that had puzzled people since ancient times.

Todd L. Savitt

56. Fungus Infections (Mycoses)

Although some 200 fungi are established as pathogenic for humans, through the mid-nineteenth century only two human diseases caused by fungi were generally recognized. These were **ringworm** and **thrush**, known since Roman times. Two important additions came at the end of the century: **mycetoma** of the foot and **aspergillosis**.

Fungi were the first pathogenic microorganisms to be recognized. By the early nineteenth century, they had been shown to cause disease in plants and insects, and during the 1840s both ringworm and thrush were shown to be mycotic in origin. For a short period, fungi were blamed for many diseases (for example, **cholera**). But with recognition of the role played by bacteria (and later, viruses) in the etiology of human disease, fungi were neglected. Only since the 1930s has the character and ecology of pathogenic fungi been clarified. In general, the geographic distribution of **mycoses** has been established, and the relation of mycoses to other human diseases has been determined.

Some fungi causing human disease show clear adaptations for the pathogenic state, whereas others do not. Probably none are dependent on a human or animal host for survival. Most are also pathogenic for animals, both domesticated and wild. Many fungi pathogenic for humans apparently belong to the normal environmental flora. Mycoses have often been termed according to the part of the body affected (e.g., "ringworm of the scalp," "athlete's foot") or the name of the pathogen (e.g., aspergillosis, **dermatophytosis**), and they have been categorized as cutaneous, subcutaneous, systemic, opportunistic, and iatrogenic, although these divisions are not mutually exclusive.

Ringworm (Tinea, Dermatophytosis)

Favus (Latin for "honeycomb"), a distinctive type of ringworm, was described by Celsus in the first century. He called it *porrigo*, a term also used by Pliny in the same century and by dermatologists up to the nineteenth century. It is now, however, obsolete, having been replaced by **tinea**. Celsus also described the inflammatory lesion of some forms of ringworm, which is termed the "kerion of Celsus."

Not until the mid-1840s was the mycotic nature of *favus* recognized by three independent workers: J. L. Schoenlein and Robert Remak in Berlin, and David Gruby in Paris. The latter also differentiated **microsporosis** and the ectothrix and endothrix **trichophytosis**, which he showed to be caused by distinct fungi.

A period of mycologic confusion followed, complicated by the difficulty of determining the life histories of the pathogens and whether there was one ringworm fungus or many. Gruby's findings were forgotten and had to be rediscovered during the 1890s by Parisian

dermatologist Raymond Sabouraud, who published his research in 1910. Many ringworm fungi were classified variously according to mycologic and clinical features. Some thousand different names had been proposed up to 1934 when C. W. Emmons in the United States showed that the many species could be accommodated in three genera: *Microsporum*, *Trichophyton*, and *Epidermophyton*. Today the accepted number of ringworm fungi is around 30. Evidence indicates that dermatophytes are closely related to a group of predominantly soil fungi. Two historical landmarks in the treatment of ringworm were the introduction of X-ray epilation for head ringworm in the opening years of the twentieth century and the development of the antibiotic griseofulvin in 1958.

The geographic distribution of ringworm fungi varies. Some, such as *Trichophyton mentagrophytes* (causing **tinea pedis**, etc.) and *Epidermophyton floccosum* (**tinea cruris**), occur worldwide. *Microsporum audouinii* (**tinea capitis**; the classical ringworm of children), which appears to have originated in Europe, is now endemic in North America. Although frequently introduced into the tropics, it has never established itself there. Likewise *Trichophyton concentricum* (**tinea imbricata**) is endemic in Southwest Asia and the South Sea islands, where it was reported by William Dampier in 1686. It has other minor endemic centers in South America and, although frequently seen in Europe, has never become endemic there. By contrast, *Trichophyton rubrum*, probably introduced into Britain by soldiers returning from the Boer War, is now widespread in north temperate regions.

In similar fashion, *Trichophyton ferrugineum* established itself in western parts of Russia after introduction by troops from the Far East. Classical *favus* in Western Europe is caused by *Trichophyton schoenleinii*, but in North Africa and the Mediterranean by *Trichophyton violaceum*. *Microsporum canis* (**tinea canis** [cat and dog ringworm], tinea capitis, and **tinea corporis**), coextensive with dogs and cats as pets, has become endemic in New Zealand in feral cats. Human infections are also contracted from cattle (*Trichophyton verrucosum*), horses, and other farm animals. *Microsporum gypseum* has a worldwide distribution, but outbreaks in humans are usually short-lived.

Candidiasis (Including Thrush)

Reports of the diverse manifestations of **candidiasis** caused by *Candida albicans* and other *Candida* species have made a major contribution to the literature of medical mycology. As with ringworm, a stable taxonomic base was necessary to underpin research on this mycotic complex. It was mainly a group of yeast specialists working in the Netherlands who clarified the taxonomy; the genus *Candida* was proposed in 1923.

Thrush (**oral candidiasis**), an infection of mucous membranes (especially of the mouth) in infants, was mentioned in the Hippocratic corpus (400 B.C.) and later by Galen and others under the heading *aphthae*. Over the centuries, references to thrush in the young, as a feature of terminal illness, and as a vaginal infection continued. Candidiasis, like ringworm, was proved mycotic by three independent workers in the 1840s: B. Langenbeck in Berlin, F. T. Berg in Stockholm, and Gruby in Paris. In 1844, J. H. Bennett in Edinburgh described what was probably *C. albicans* from the human lung.

A wide range of pathological conditions attributed to *Candida* were subsequently recorded. Numerous surveys have shown that many apparently normal individuals carry *C. albicans* in the mouth, in the vagina, and in the feces and gut. Although *C. albicans* has occasionally been isolated from soil, from hospital bedding, and from animals, it is clear that most human infections have an endogenous origin. Infection seems always to be determined by predisposing factors that may be environmental. Age, debility, dentures, and drugs also can predispose one to infection. The patenting of the antibiotic nystatin in 1956 was a notable contribution to the therapy of candidiasis.

Systemic Mycoses

The first case of **coccidioidomycosis** was described from Argentina by Alejandro Posadas in 1892. A case was also studied in California by E. Rixford and T. C. Gilchrist, who attributed the cause to a protozoan, which in 1896 they named *Coccidioides immitis*. In 1905, however, W. Opuls established its mycotic nature. It was known only as a rare and often fatal disease. In 1938, Myrnie A. Grifford and E. Dickson established that "valley fever," prevalent in the San Joaquin Valley of California, was a mild form of coccidioidomycosis. Further investigations showed subclinical *Coccidioides* infection to be widespread in parts of California and neighboring states and to induce lifelong immunity to subsequent attack. Emmons showed rodents to be infected, and they were thought to constitute an animal reservoir of infection. But it became clear that rodents, like humans, were subject to infection by this soil-inhabiting fungus. The dry, airborne spores of the pathogen are extremely infectious (many laboratory infections have occurred); coccidioidomycosis can be contracted, for example, by servicing automobiles that have been driven through endemic areas. Although light- and dark-skinned peoples appear to be equally susceptible, the disease is more likely to be systemic in those with pigmented skin. Coccidioidomycosis is endemic in warm, dry regions of the United States, Mexico, and parts of Central and South America.

Histoplasmosis (*Histoplasma capsulatum*) shows many parallels with coccidioidomycosis and may be a humid-region equivalent. At first considered a protozoan disease, it has been shown to be mycotic. A mild form affects millions of people in the midwestern United States.

Blastomycosis (North American blastomycosis, caused by *B. dermatitidis*) and **paracoccidioidomycosis** (South American blastomycosis, caused by *Paracoccidioides brasiliensis*) are both diseases of the skin and internal organs, characterized by budding cells of the pathogen in the infected tissues. Blastomycosis was first described by Gilchrist in 1894, and paracoccidioidomycosis by Adolfo Lutz in Brazil during 1908. Neither has a mild form, and the natural habitats of these fungi have not been established with certainty. Paracoccidioidomycosis is confined to Central and South America. Blastomycosis is endemic to the western and southeastern United States, where epidemics occur; there are also records of the disease from tropical African countries.

Sporotrichosis is a cutaneous and subcutaneous infection characterized by nodular lesions, often affecting lymph nodes. Infection is frequently initiated by a lesion of the hand. It is caused by *Sporothrix schenckii* and was first described in the United States by B. R. Schenck in 1898. Subsequently, many cases were reported from Europe, especially France, where the disease was discussed by C. L. de Beurmann and H. Gougerot in 1912. Sporotrichosis is sporadic in north temperate regions and has been recorded in Central and South America. In Uruguay, J. E. Mackinnon attempted to correlate the disease with the weather and determined that infection occurred during moist warm weather. *S. schenckii* is one of the rare fungus pathogens of humans that has been shown to cause disease in plants. The largest outbreak ever recorded occurred in gold mines in South Africa during the 1940s. Approximately 3,000 miners were infected, but the epidemic was brought under control.

Opportunistic and Iatrogenic Infections

Mycetoma is a disease characterized by swelling that affects subcutaneous tissues, with sinuses discharging granules of the pathogen that vary in color. The foot is most frequently involved ("Madura foot"), but other parts may be infected. Its geographic distribution is mainly tropical.

The condition was first recorded in Indian vedic medical treatises (c. 2000–1000 B.C.) as *padaavalmika* ("foot ant-hill") and later described by members of the Indian Medical Service during the mid-nineteenth century. H. Vandyke Carter, who coined the designation "mycetoma," wrote about it in 1874. Carter suspected the disease to be mycotic and submitted material to M. J. Berkeley, the leading British mycologist, who described a fungus he obtained from it. From the turn of the century onward, more than 25 diverse fungi and actinomycetes responsible for the condition were identified by workers in North Africa and elsewhere. The color of the grains often indicates the pathogen's identity.

Carter distinguished "melanoid" and "ochroid" mycetoma. His black-grained form was caused by *Madurella mycetomatis*, the most important cause of mycetoma, taxonomized by E. Brumpt in 1905. In 1894, H. Vincent described the actinomycete that caused yellow-grained mycetoma as *Streptothrix madurae* (now *Actinomadura madurae*). Later, A. J. Chalmers and R. G. Archibald in Sudan introduced the term "madura mycosis" for mycetoma caused by actinomycetes. Today the terms **eumycetoma** and **actinomycetoma** are preferred.

Mycetoma occurs most frequently in a band of the tropics extending from India across Africa to Central and South America. Incidence is particularly high in India, Sudan, Senegal, and Mexico. *Pseudallescheria boydii* seems to favor more humid conditions, with species of *Nocardia* responsible for mycetoma in temperate Europe and North America. *Madurella grisea* is limited to South America, whereas cephalosporium infections are cosmopolitan. Early thought held that infection was initiated by injury, particularly injury from plant thorns. Sometimes the pathogen grows as a saprobe on thorns, or the thorn may provide the point of entry for an organism present in the environment.

Cryptococcosis is a chronic infection of the lungs, skin, or other parts, caused by the yeast *Cryptococcus neoformans*, which is widely distributed in nature. Human cases have frequently been associated with inhalation of the pathogen when clearing pigeon roosts. The most frequent infections are self-limiting. Fatal and more generalized infection occurs mostly in debilitated patients or those "compromised" by drugs.

Identified in Europe in 1894, cryptococcosis has a worldwide distribution. In 1946, L. B. Cox and Jean C. Tolhurst published 13 Australian cases termed "torulosis" caused by *Torula histolytica*. In 1956, a comprehensive study of the disease was published by M. L. Littman and L. E. Zimmerman.

Rhinosporidiosis, an infection of mucous tissue (especially of the nose), forms large polyps. The causal agent, *Rhinosporidium seeberi*, has not been cultured, and its taxonomic position is uncertain. Outbreaks of the disease have been associated with water and soil. Rhinosporidiosis was first reported from Argentina in 1900. It occurs sporadically throughout the tropics, especially in India and Sri Lanka.

Species of *Aspergillus* and mucoraceous fungi are a ubiquitous component of "common mold." They are frequently found as contaminants of cultures. Human infections (aspergillosis and **mucormycosis**) by these and similar molds occur sporadically and have been reported worldwide.

Aspergillus fumigatus, widespread in the environment on decaying vegetation, has spores that are readily airborne. It is favored by high temperature. *A. fumigatus* is able to cause fatal infections, particularly in birds. It was first recorded early in the nineteenth century. J. Fresenius in 1850 proposed the name *Aspergillus fumigatus*, and Rudolf Virchow in Germany in 1856 described human pulmonary aspergillosis. The classical cases of this disease occurred in French squab-feeders in the late 1890s, who chewed the same grain used for fattening the birds.

Other species of *Aspergillus* are also pathogenic. *Aspergillus niger* is associated with infection of the ear, whereas aspergillomas or "fungus balls" are associated with pulmonary disease. Diverse mucoraceous fungi are sporadically recorded in north temperate countries. Human infections of the rhino-facial-cerebral region are often fatal. Debility is a predisposing factor.

Several of the diseases addressed in this chapter might also be termed "dependent mycoses." During World War II, for example, ringworm symptoms disappeared in prisoners held under starvation conditions only to reappear on the restoration of a full diet. Tinea capitis (*M. audouinii*) in children, although persistent, resolves spontaneously at puberty for reasons not fully understood. Tinea pedis has been claimed as an occupational disease of workers who wear heavy boots. Candida infection is affected by pregnancy, and metabolic disorders such as **diabetes** are frequently associated with it. Iatrogenic mycoses have resulted from the use of antibacterials. Moreover, immunosuppressive drugs used in organ transplantation have resulted in *Candida* **endocarditis** and mycotic **septicemia**. Antimycotic therapy is now a routine supplementary practice.

Geoffrey C. Ainsworth

57. Fungus Poisoning

Two categories of fungus poisoning may be distinguished: (1) **mycetism**, caused by eating poisonous fungi mistaken for an edible variety (which has a long history and worldwide incidence); and (2) **mycotoxicosis**, from inadvertent ingestion of food containing fungi-produced toxins. The latter, also of worldwide incidence, was (with the exception of **ergotism**) generally recognized only during the twentieth century.

Mycetism

Calamities tend to impress, and the first reference to fungi in the Greek classics is an epigram by Euripides (c. 450 B.C.) commemorating the deaths of a woman and her two children after eating poisonous fungi. During Roman times, edible fungi were a delicacy, and diverse advice was offered by authors such as Horace, Celsus, Dioscorides, Galen, and Pliny about how to avoid poisonous species, how to render poisonous forms harmless, and how to treat fungus poisoning.

Much of the ancient folklore on precautions to ensure edibility was compiled by the authors of the first printed herbals in the fourteenth and fifteenth centuries, and some has even survived to this day. It is, however, invariably unreliable because the distribution of poisonous and edible species seems to be random. For example, the esteemed esculents *Amanita caesarea* ("Caesar's mushroom," a Roman favorite) and *Amanita rubescens* ("the blusher") are congeneric with *Amanita phalloides* ("death cap") and several related species (*Amanita pantherina, Amanita verna, Amanita virosa*) that have caused – and still do – most fungus-poisoning fatalities in north temperate regions. The only reliable guide is correct identification.

The most frequent effect of fungus poisoning is gastroenteric disturbance of greater or lesser severity. *A. phalloides* toxins, symptoms of which occur 4 or more hours after ingestion, also cause severe damage to the liver and kidneys. Other *Amanita* toxins have a hemolytic effect, and hallucinogenic species cause psychosomatic symptoms. Fever is unusual.

The chemistry of toxic fungi has been under investigation since muscarine was isolated in 1869. That name came from the "fly agaric" (*Amanita muscaria*), which has been equated with the Indian *soma*. *Amanita* toxins include amatoxins, phallotoxins, and virotoxins.

The species of fungi implicated in mycetism depend on the locality, and local variations occur in reported incidence. For example, more reports of mycetism are published in France, where edible fungi are widely collected from the wild for sale, than in Britain, where wild forms are regarded with suspicion. Most poisonous fungi are larger basidiomycetes, but a few ascomycetes with large fruit bodies are poisonous.

In the later twentieth century, increased incidence of fungus poisoning originated from ethnomycological studies drawing attention to the hallucinogenic properties of some larger fungi, particularly species of *Psilocybe* containing psilocin, a compound that induces psychotropic effects similar to lysergic acid and mescalin. Collection of such forms in the wild for self-administration or illegal sale has resulted in misidentifications or overdoses and the need for medical attention.

Mycotoxicosis

Until the 1900s, the only mycotoxicosis of humans generally recognized in the West was ergotism, although serious outbreaks of human mycotoxicoses had occurred in Russia and Japan. **Kaschin-Beck disease** of children is characterized by generalized **osteoarthritis** caused by eating moldy grain. It was prevalent among the Cossacks and endemic in both Asiatic and European Russia and in northern Korea and China in the 1860s. A similar mycotoxicosis – "drunken (or intoxicating) bread syndrome" – was also prevalent in Russia. But the most extensively documented of such ills in Russia is **alimentary toxic aleukia** (or **septic angina**); it was known before World War I and became epidemic in the Russian grain belt during World War II, when some 10 percent of the population was affected and suffered high mortality. In affected districts, it was the practice to allow the ripe cereal crop to winter under the snow. When the snow cover was so heavy that the underlying soil did not freeze deeply, and the spring was mild with frequent thawing and freezing, the grain was molded by *Fusarium* species and other fungi that produced toxins (mostly trichothecines).

Known in Japan from the seventeenth century, a form of **cardiac beriberi** was shown in 1891 to be caused by eating moldy rice. In 1940, the toxin involved was identified as citreoviridin, produced by *Penicillium citreoviride*. After World War II, a severe outbreak was recorded in Japan of a similar but different mycotoxicosis from eating rice that had deteriorated in storage ("yellowed rice").

Several major mycotoxicoses of farm animals have been documented in Russia, and a few more have been reported elsewhere. Significant attention was focused on mycotoxicoses after the summer of 1960, when more than 100,000 turkeys and other poultry died in Britain after eating a ration containing ground peanut (*Arachis hypogea*) meal imported from Brazil.

Cattle and pigs were also affected, and feeding experiments induced liver cancer in rats. The toxin, produced by strains of *Aspergillus flavus*, was designated aflatoxin. At first, testing for aflatoxin was limited to using 1-day-old ducklings, which are particularly sensitive to it, but a reliable chemical test was soon developed.

Aflatoxin was shown to be widespread in foods containing peanuts, and in parts of Africa and Asia the incidence of human **liver cancer** has been correlated with aflatoxin intake. The U.S. Food and Drug Administration has set an aflatoxin tolerance of 20 parts per billion for peanut products. Interest in **aflatoxicosis**, because of its carcinogenic potential, is still intense.

Geoffrey C. Ainsworth

58. Gallstones (Cholelithiasis)

Gallstones are common in modern populations, occurring in nearly 20 percent of autopsies. Though often asymptomatic, they can produce significant morbidity, leading to **cholecystitis**, **cholangitis**, **biliary cirrhosis**, and **pancreatitis**.

Characteristics
Descriptively, there are four major types of gallstones: pure cholesterol stones, mixed stones (cholesterol, bilirubin, and calcium), combined stones (with a cholesterol center and laminated exterior of cholesterol, bilirubin, and calcium), and pigmented stones (calcium bilirubinate). The first three types comprise the vast majority of gallstones and are grouped together as cholesterol-based stones, related to abnormal cholesterol and bile salt metabolism. Black pigmented stones are associated with chronic hemolysis, particularly **sickle-cell disease**. Brown pigmented stones are associated with infection and were historically more common in China and Japan.

Though incompletely understood, the three major factors in gallstone formation are abnormal bile composition, **biliary stasis**, and gallbladder infection. These factors are interrelated, but current thinking ascribes the primary role to abnormal bile composition, related to cholesterol and bile acid metabolism. This in turn is affected by dietary, genetic, and hormonal factors.

A common medical maxim describes a typical gallstone patient as "fat, fair, female, and forty." Obesity is associated with increased cholesterol secretion, producing supersaturated or lithogenic bile. Overconsumption of calories, particularly through refined sugar and flour, appears to be the major factor causing high incidence in Western countries. It also explains the increasing prevalence of cholesterol and mixed gallstones among Japanese, Eskimo, and African populations adopting a more Western diet. A diet high in cholesterol-rich foods may have a secondary role.

Gallstones are two to four times more common in females than in males. Estrogen increases secretion of cholesterol and decreases production of bile salts that form soluble micelles with cholesterol. Moreover, childbearing elevates estrogen in the third trimester and also promotes biliary stasis; thus multiparity is a risk factor.

Gallstone prevalence increases steadily with advancing age. Clinically, symptoms of gallbladder disease related to gallstones most commonly present between ages 40 and 60.

Conclusions regarding geographic distribution of gallstones are based on autopsy, hospital-admission, and population-survey data. The large Framingham, Massachusetts, study showed prevalence of gallbladder disease among adult (ages 30–62) males as 1.3 percent and among adult females as 5.9 percent. Many studies have shown a higher prevalence among American Indians, particularly in the Southwest. For example, a study of the Pima Indians using identical criteria and age groups as the Framingham study showed a prevalence of 5.9 percent among adult males and 36 percent among females.

Gallstones are usually asymptomatic, which along with increased prevalence with age explains the much higher incidence of gall-stones at autopsy. A large autopsy series spanning the years 1920–49 demonstrated gall-stones in 7.8 percent of males and 16.8 percent of females. The incidence among blacks was less than half that among whites. Another series of adult whites found gallstones in 16.0 percent of males and 32.5 percent of females.

Gallstones are relatively uncommon in oriental countries; prevalence rates as low as 1.8 percent among adult men and 3.9 percent of adult women are found. Prevalence remains low in Japan; however, there has been a shift from the infection-related pigmented stones to the Western diet-related cholesterol stones. Most African populations demonstrate an extremely low prevalence of gallstones. A review of records shows an increasing prevalence in Europe, North America, Japan, Chile, and Australia.

A genetic tendency to develop gallstones under certain dietary conditions may account for the high rates of gallstones noted in various American Indian groups, including Pima, Navajo, and Chippewa, as well as in groups with significant Indian admixture from Mexico, Bolivia, Chile, and Peru. It has been postulated that a genetic defect in conversion of cholesterol to bile acid results in lithogenic bile.

The geographic epidemiology of gallstones indicates a susceptibility in New World populations that is not shared by their Asian ancestral relatives. The Americas were settled by crossing the Bering land bridge formed during glacial epochs. Survival under the harsh climatic conditions depended on hunting and gathering strategies with unpredictable periods of near starvation. Individuals who could rapidly store excess calories as fat would have had a pronounced survival advantage over individuals lacking this trait. This is the "thrifty gene" theory postulated to explain the prevalence of **diabetes** among American Indians and possibly accounting for the association of **obesity**, parity, and puberty with the formation of gallstones in Indians now exposed to a perpetual "feast" of calories and sedentary living. Indeed, the worldwide distribution of other populations with high gall-stone risk corresponds closely to the area covered by the last glacial epoch.

History

Hippocrates and Aristotle were familiar with the clinical findings of **jaundice** and **biliary disease**, but their writings do not specifically mention gallstones. Hippocrates differentiated four types of jaundice but did not describe any cause related to obstruction. Diocles of Carystus referred to possible mechanical obstruction of the flow of bile. Accounts of Alexander the Great's illness prior to his death in 323 B.C. are suggestive of gallstones and cholecystitis.

Galen described various types of jaundice, including obstructive jaundice. He stated that small foreign bodies such as grain or fig and pomegranate seeds could obstruct the common bile duct. Given the close similarity of small gall-stones to certain seeds, Galen may in fact be referring to gallstones. Gallstones in lower animals had been recognized for centuries, and crushed gallstones constituted an important ingredient in yellow pigment. The codified Talmudic law of the fourth century A.D. considered animals with sharp-edged gallstones unfit to eat (*terefah*), but kosher if the gallstones were smooth.

Sixth century Byzantine physician Alexander of Tralles described both gallstones and renal calculi. Tenth century Persian physician Haly Abbas (often quoted in early Renaissance medicine) recorded the presence of calculi in the gallbladder and liver.

Mundinus was professor of anatomy and surgery at the University of Bologna from 1295 to 1326. His manuscript on anatomy was based on Hippocrates, Galen, and Arabic authors and was widely used for nearly 250 years. He also mentions stones formed within the gallbladder and kidneys. Gentile da Foligno was a graduate of Bologna and professor at Padua, who died of **plague** in 1348. In 1341, he performed one of the earliest autopsies on record, an account of which mentions a gallstone found embedded in the cystic duct of the gallbladder.

Antonio Benivieni wrote the first book devoted to pathological anatomy, published posthumously in 1507. It contains 111 observations based on 20 autopsies, including two descriptions of gallstones found within the gallbladder and liver. Numerous other Renaissance physicians were familiar with gallstones encountered in clinical practice or more often at autopsy.

In 1761, Giovanni Battista Morgagni provided a vast array of pathological findings related to the clinical picture for a large number of diseases, including gallstones. Morgagni noted their increased frequency with age, the greater preponderance of women sufferers, variation by locale, and association with a sedentary life. Bile stasis again figured as a prominent factor in gallstone formation. He also considered irritation or inflammation of the glands within the gallbladder wall as a cause of stones.

Gallstones have been recovered in excavations, which greatly extends the known antiquity of the disease. Given their frequency, more such examples should be expected. The earliest case comes from Mycenae, Greece, dating from 1600–1500 B.C. Other early Old World examples are associated with tenth century B.C. (and later) Egypt, China in the Han Dynasty (206 B.C. to 220 A.D.), and early medieval Europe.

In the New World, gallstones were found at the Libben site in Ohio, a Late Woodland site dating from 1000 to 1200 A.D., and in northern Chile at a site dating from 100 to 300 A.D. A variable frequency in ancient human populations is to be expected, and because of dietary factors, gallstones may have been quite rare in many instances.

R. Ted Steinbock

59. Gangrene

The term **gangrene** describes local death of tissue (**necrosis**) in the living body. Gangrene implies a fairly rapid process extending over a visible area, with an obvious inability of the tissues to repair or replace the gangrenous part. Although gangrene can occur in internal organs, it generally means a process on the body's surface, involving only skin or possibly deeper tissues as well.

Gangrene is either dry or moist. **Dry gangrene** is necrosis of tissues resulting from vascular occlusion, as in severe **arteriosclerosis** of the legs. **Moist gangrene** occurs when bacteria invade dead tissue, producing putrefaction. When gasforming bacteria are involved, **gas gangrene** occurs. An originally dry gangrene may be converted to moist by invading bacteria.

General Characteristics

In dry gangrene, arterial supply is gradually cut off, and drying of the tissues results. Inflammation is frequently absent, but pain may precede the color changes. Soft tissues progressively shrink, and the color deepens until the area is coal black. Constitutional symptoms may occur but are less severe than in moist gangrene.

Moist gangrene may be preceded by inflammation or trauma. The part is initially swollen and painful. The color is red, then blue, and finally green black. There is boggy swelling and putrid odor. If the gangrene is extensive, constitutional symptoms such as fever may occur.

Gangrene has many causes. Some are now quite rare but once were common. Some have been of major consequence throughout history.

Vascular Causes

Historically, **ergotism** resulted from ingesting rye bread contaminated by the fungus *Claviceps purpurea*. It caused a permanent decrease in the caliber of arterioles, eventually leading to dry gangrene of fingers and toes and, less commonly, of the ears and nose. Ergotism caused many gangrene epidemics in medieval Europe. Along with **erysipelas**, it was called "Saint Anthony's fire." Although rare, ergotism still occurs today.

Raynaud's syndrome is characterized by vascular spasms of the extremities. During an attack (often triggered by cold or stress), one or more digits turn white. Some minutes later, the color changes to bluish red. Normal color returns slowly. In severe cases, gangrene may ensue in fingers or toes. Once known as "relapsing gangrene," Raynaud's syndrome may occur alone (**Raynaud's disease**) or with another condition such as **scleroderma**, **lupus**, or **rheumatoid arthritis**. It may be an occupational hazard for people who operate vibratory machinery such as jackhammers.

Embolism is the sudden occlusion of an artery by blood-borne particles. These may be dislodged atheromatous material, vegetations from infected heart valves, fat particles, gas, abnormal proteins, or blood clots. Acute vascular compromise can lead to gangrene, usually dry.

Arteriosclerosis may cause embolisms and can also induce local vascular occlusion (**thrombosis**) of large and medium-sized arteries. It is common in the elderly and therefore called **senile gangrene**. It occurs mainly in the foot and was previously called "Pott's disease of the toe." A special form of arteriosclerosis is **thromboangiitis obliterans** or **Buerger's disease**, occurring in men who smoke heavily. **Diabetes** can predispose to arteriosclerosis with eventual gangrene of the feet. Other factors that may predispose to arteriosclerosis include heredity, fat consumption, lack of exercise, and smoking.

Physical Causes

Various injuries – such as frostbite, compound fractures, contusions, gunshot wounds, and burns – may trigger gangrene. However, this complication was more prevalent before effective medical care became widely available.

Chemical Causes

Tissue can also be destroyed by chemicals of either exogenous or endogenous origin. Caustics such as carbolic acid can cause gangrene. Venoms of certain snakes, spiders, and jellyfish can cause local necrosis at the site of attack. Chemotherapeutic agents may inadvertently lead to local tissue destruction. Some systemically administered drugs may cause gangrene.

Microbiological Causes

Many organisms produce toxins that directly cause cell death. Other toxins cause **vascular spasm** or **vasculitis**. Some organisms produce enzymes that destroy tissue locally. Other organisms – in particular, viruses – destroy cells by invasion.

Streptococci (including *Streptococcus pyogenes*) have caused certain varieties of gangrene. Of historical importance is **hospital gangrene**, also known as **necrotizing fasciitis** and *pourriture des hôpitaux*. This gangrene was the scourge of hospitals in the preantiseptic era but today is almost never seen. Trauma is usually the initiating factor. Within days, gangrene rapidly set into a wound and characteristically was deeply destructive. Patients became febrile and eventually succumbed.

Organisms other than *S. pyogenes* (alone or in combination) may give a similar clinical picture. Another acute streptococcal disease is **Fournier's gangrene**, localized to the scrotum. Finally, anaerobic streptococci in combination with other bacteria such as *Staphylococcus aureus* are the cause of **postoperative synergistic gangrene**.

History

Ergotism has long been a major cause of gangrene epidemics. Gangrene of the limbs has been recognized since ancient times, and a description of gangrene following trauma appears in Hippocrates. Probably gangrene in ancient Greece and Rome resulted mainly from trauma infections.

In temperate and arctic zones, cold injuries causing frostbite and gangrene have always occurred. Explorers of cold regions were often affected, and gangrene produced by cold injury has also been a problem in military activities. For example, gangrene was quite prevalent during Napoleon Bonaparte's invasion of Russia. Yet frostbite was only one of the military causes of gangrene. Penetrating wounds, contusions, and compound fractures were often the initial insult. In the sixteenth century, the introduction of gunpowder in Europe produced tremendous loss of life and limbs from gangrene. Poor hygiene and overcrowding in hospitals led to epidemic wound infections. Because hospital gangrene was rapidly progressive and lethal, many lives were lost, particularly during the Napoleonic Wars, the Crimean War, and the American Civil War. In many cases, gangrenous wounds killed almost as many soldiers as were killed in action.

By World War I, hospital gangrene was much less prevalent. The art of amputation and setting of fractures was advanced by surgeons such as Ambroise Paré in the sixteenth century, Pierre-Joseph Desault in the eighteenth, and John Bell at the turn of the nineteenth, among others. Their work significantly contributed to decreased gangrene mortality. In the late nineteenth century, Louis Pasteur introduced the concept of antisepsis and asepsis. This concept, applied to management of wounds, is known as "Listerism" in honor of Joseph Lister, who first recognized the clinical value of Pasteur's discovery. Finally, the introduction of penicillin in the early 1940s totally eradicated hospital gangrene.

Arteriosclerosis is probably as old as humankind. In the fifteenth century, Leonardo da Vinci illustrated senile arteriosclerosis in one of his anatomic sketches. In the early nineteenth century, it gradually became clear that arterial occlusion could cause dry gangrene. In 1862, Maurice Raynaud suggested that an arterial disease might produce gangrene without arterial obliteration being present. Only recently were diabetes, **hypertension**, and lifestyle recognized as contributing factors in arteriosclerosis. Fortunately, widespread education is contributing to the decline of vascular disease and associated gangrene.

In advanced countries, gangrene is much less common. Infectious gangrenes are easily treated or avoided. But a growing number of individuals are immunosuppressed from chemotherapeutic agents and corticosteroids.

In such a state, these patients are at increased risk of developing infectious gangrenes whose agents may not be easily recognized or readily treatable.

Diane Quintal and Robert Jackson

60. **Genetic Disease**

The idea of physical heredity is probably as old as our species. Clearly, the concept of "like begets like" found expression in the domestication of animals; breeding stock was chosen for favorable traits. The first tangible evidence of the notion of heredity lies in the domestication of dogs some 10,000 years ago. Yet only in recent times have we begun to understand the workings of heredity.

The term "hereditary" refers only to passage from generation to generation. We may regard a hereditary trait as "genetic" only when its passage from generation to generation is determined at least partly by genes. In much the same way, the term "congenital" signifies only that a trait is present at birth. A congenital trait is not necessarily genetic or even hereditary. Thus, the purview of medical genetics includes those traits, both congenital and otherwise, whose origins lie in single genes, in groups of genes, or in the size or number of the chromosomes.

In recent years, medical geneticists have utilized a battery of advanced analytic tools and laboratory techniques to determine the transmission of various traits. These methods are derived from what is called the multifactorial model, according to which the observed variation in a trait (such as clinical presentation of a **genetic disease**, or liability to a complex disorder like **heart disease**) is determined by the joint effects of major gene loci plus multiple minor loci (a polygenic effect) and a nongenetic component (an environmental effect). This model has provided a theoretical underpinning for the field of genetic epidemiology and has become a heuristic device through which clinical presentation of a disease can be assessed.

It is suggested that a network of effects leads from the gene to the final outward manifestation, the phenotype. From this perspective, no gene underlying a human disease exists in a vacuum. It exists in a milieu of its own locus, its chromosomal position and close neighbors, the various effects of other genes elsewhere in the genome, the intercellular and intracellular environment, and the external environment in which it ultimately finds expression. However, the mechanisms governing this multitude of effects are only just being discovered.

History

As already stated, the idea that parents' features were transmitted to offspring was applied early in history to animal domestication. Some knowledge of "good inheritance" (transmission of favorable features) undoubtedly came from observations of "bad inheritance." Thus, for some 10,000 years we have known, in some degree, that certain diseases are hereditary, if not genetic.

By the time of the ancient Greeks, people were clearly cognizant of heredity. Vertical transmission was widely accepted, although its workings were unknown. Amid scholarly speculation, the Hippocratic theory of its mechanism emerged to survive until the Renaissance. In the fourth century B.C., Hippocrates postulated that each organ and tissue produced its own specific component of semen. The composite semen, transmitted to a woman through coitus, then incubated to become a human baby. Hippocrates's theory accounted for inheritance of both desirable traits and abnormal or undesirable ones, and by the same mechanism.

In discussing hereditary traits, the Greeks usually mentioned abstract qualities such as good and evil, or characteristics such as eye color, strength, speed, and beauty. They also noted the shocking and fantastic, gross malformations, and severe illness. Empedocles suggested in the fifth century B.C. that "monsters" (grossly malformed infants) resulted from an excess or deficit of semen. Other writers held similar views, which presumably became part of the Hippocratic heredity theory. Abnormal infants received roughly the same treatment everywhere in the ancient world: abandonment or outright slaughter. Often, mothers suffered the same fate as offspring. The destruction of abnormal infants was advocated by Hippocrates, Plato, Aristotle, and virtually all others. Yet the practice was not universal, as evidenced by the mummy of an anencephalic infant at Hermopolis. It seems that this baby, who was stillborn or nearly so, was an object of worship.

The mechanistic interpretation of **birth defects** was modified by the somewhat mystical Roman attitude. In the first century A.D., Pliny wrote that mental impressions formed during pregnancy were sufficient to produce monsters: Such children were warnings from the gods transmitted to pregnant women. Thus, a black queen of ancient Ethiopia presented her husband, the black king, with a white child. It was concluded that the queen had gazed on a statue of the goddess Andromeda during her pregnancy. The description of the infant, however, is reminiscent of an albino, particularly given that royalty often married close relatives.

The decline of reason that marked the Middle Ages was reflected in interpretations of malformed infants. Such children were called "devil's brats," conceived in a union with Satan. As with any perceived deviation from piety, the fate of both infant and mother was ruthlessly determined. Later, however, astrological beliefs sometimes produced surprising outcomes. For example, in the thirteenth century, a deformed calf said to appear half human was born. The cowherd was immediately accused of an unnatural act and was in danger of burning at the stake. Fortunately for him, it was noted that a particular conjunction of the planets – often the cause of oddities of nature – had recently occurred. The cowherd's life was spared.

As the Renaissance dawned, reason returned to discourses on heredity. Classical works were rediscovered, and development of a science of heredity was once again under way. The writings of Hippocrates and Aristotle were translated and amplified by medical scholars such as

Fabricius and his pupil William Harvey. In addition, there was a growing interest in rare and unusual medical cases. For Harvey and many others, rare pathology was not a source of revulsion or the workings of Satan but, rather, a subject demanding study and understanding. The debt owed to scholars such as Harvey would be acknowledged in the twentieth century, when medical genetics came into full bloom.

With the Enlightenment, the floodgates were opened, and medical science progressed on many fronts. However, despite eloquent writings on heredity in general and on rare cases in particular, few references to specific genetic diseases were made before the twentieth century. Yet among those few instances were some brilliant insights.

Between 1745 and 1757, French natural philosopher Pierre Louis Moreau de Maupertuis conducted studies on the heredity of **polydactyly** (an abnormal number of fingers and/or toes) and published the pedigree of a family with polydactyly in four successive generations. He formulated a theory of heredity, suggesting that particles of inheritance were paired in the "semens" of the father and the mother and that hereditary pathologies were accidental products of the semen. He correctly predicted genes, dominance, and mutation. Moreover, estimating the probability of polydactyly at 1 per 20,000 by his own survey, he noted that if the disorder was not hereditary, the chance of a joint occurrence of an affected parent and an affected offspring was 1 per 400,000,000 and that of an affected grandparent, parent, and offspring in sequence was 1 per 8,000,000,000,000. Obviously, the probability of his four-generation family being the product of chance was so small as to be immediately dismissed. Here, then, was also the first use of statistics in a study of heredity.

Various sex-linked (or X-linked) disorders such as **color blindness** and **hemophilia** were accurately described in the late eighteenth and early nineteenth centuries. In 1820, German physician Christian Nasse presented a detailed pedigree of X-linked recessive hemophilia and noted that although "bleeders" were always male, the trait was transmitted by females.

Perhaps the most remarkable instance before the work of Gregor Mendel was an 1814 publication by British physician Joseph Adams. In this study, he distinguished between "familial" diseases (confined to a single generation) and "hereditary" diseases (passed from generation to generation). Moreover, Adams defined **congenital disorders** as appearing at birth and regarded them as more likely familial than hereditary. He observed that familial diseases were often so severe that subsequent transmission from the affected individual was ruled out by early death. Such conditions increased among offspring and were often found in isolated districts where inbreeding was common. Clearly, Adams's familial diseases were what we term recessive and his hereditary diseases were what we term dominant.

Adams concluded that hereditary diseases (in the modern sense) were not always apparent at birth but might have later ages of onset, that correlations existed among family members with regard to clinical features, and that hereditary diseases might be treatable. Adams hinted at mutation in remarking that a severe disease would last only a single generation except that normal parents occasionally produced offspring in whom the disease originated. Finally, he called for establishment of hereditary-disease registers to assist the study of these diseases.

The basic hereditary laws of segregation and independent assortment were discovered by Austrian monk Gregor Mendel and subsequently rediscovered by Carl Correns, Hugo de Vries, and Erich von Tschermak some decades later. Mendel, conducting hybridization experiments with pea plants in his monastery garden at Brno, Czechoslovakia, demonstrated that alternative hereditary "characters" for a single trait segregated from one another each generation, and that the characters for multiple traits assorted independently in each generation. Moreover, the observed distribution of characters for multiple traits followed a precise mathematical formulation – a binomial series.

Mendel reported his results to the Natural Science Association of Brno in 1865 and published them the following year, but his work was virtually ignored until 1899. By then, numerous researchers were investigating heredity. Dutch botanist Hugo de Vries discovered Mendel's report, which contained the solution to the problems he was studying. De Vries had already formulated his own law of segregation but in 1900 published Mendel's results as well, stressing their importance. At the same time, both German botanist Correns and Austrian botanist von Tschermak independently discovered the Mendelian laws and recognized their significance. All three published translations of Mendel's paper. English biologist and evolutionist William Bateson was also interested in plant hybridization. In 1900, he read de Vries's account of Mendel's experiments, and soon thereafter, as we shall see, made an almost offhand comment that became a fundamental contribution to the study of human genetic diseases.

In 1897, London physician Sir Archibald Garrod began studying **alkaptonuria**, a nonfatal congenital disorder characterized by excretion of homogentisic acid in the urine – turning the urine dark – and often accompanied in later years by **arthritis** and black pigmentation of cartilage and collagenous tissues. At the time, the disease was considered infectious, and the excretion of homogentisic acid was thought to result from bacterial action in the intestine. Garrod believed instead that the condition was a congenital error of **abnormal metabolism**. He published this theory in 1899.

Soon, however, Garrod made a crucial observation. He noted that among four families with alkaptonuric offspring and two unaffected parents, three of the parental pairs were first cousins. (This circumstance would hardly have surprised Joseph Adams, who had commented on inbreeding nearly 90 years earlier.) Garrod discussed his findings with Bateson, who recognized that the pathology was "all or none," affected or normal. Moreover, the high incidence of consanguinity and the characteristic pattern of normal parents having affected off-

spring was precisely what would be expected were the abnormality determined by a rare, recessive Mendelian character.

In Bateson's interpretation of the situation, Garrod saw the solution. In 1902, Garrod published a landmark paper on nine families of alkaptonurics, adding further clinical data, incorporating the hereditary mechanism proposed by Bateson, and suggesting that the laws of heredity discovered by Mendel and relayed by Bateson offered an explanation of the disorder as an example of a Mendelian recessive character. Indeed, Garrod went beyond alkaptonuria to include the possibility of other disorders sharing the same hereditary mechanism. Later, he studied **cystinuria**, **albinism**, and **pentosuria** and classed them all with alkaptonuria.

By 1908, the impact of Mendelism was fully felt. Few doubted that these and other diseases were caused by Mendelian characters, and that the study of families – particularly inbred ones – was crucial to obtaining new insights into old disease entities. Garrod suggested that the pathology of inborn errors of metabolism consisted of a blockade in the normal pathway and that this blockade was caused by congenital deficiency of a specific enzyme. By the mid-twentieth century, the truth of his insight – that transmitted enzymic defects cause disease – led to the "one gene, one enzyme" hypothesis and to the theory of gene action. Garrod has since been called the "father of chemical genetics."

From our contemporary perspective, the work and insights of Garrod are landmarks. The incorporation of Mendelian laws of heredity into the study of human diseases was the turning point for medical genetics. Surprisingly, however, Garrod's theories went largely unnoticed for several decades. One reason for this slow recognition was that it was impossible in Garrod's time for most geneticists to reduce Mendel's laws to purely chemical phenomena. Indeed, in the earliest days of the rediscovery of Mendel, much effort was devoted to dealing with a growing list of exceptions to those laws.

Nevertheless, progress in understanding the hereditary nature of numerous human diseases was made, although it failed fully to coalesce until the middle of the twentieth century. Two disorders that contributed greatly to this progress were **sickle-cell anemia** and **Down syndrome**.

Molecular Medicine

The first case of sickle-cell anemia was reported in 1910 by Chicago physician J. B. Herrick. On examining a young black man from Grenada, he found, among other features, an anemia in which many red blood cells had a "sickle-like shape." Soon after, a similar case was reported, and in 1917 the phenomenon was described by V. E. Emmel. Emmel showed that the sickling was developmental, with seemingly normal red cells undergoing the change as they matured. He further showed that no red cells from controls or from any other type of **anemia** or **leukemia** could be induced to sickle. However, Emmel noted that a small proportion of red cells from the patient's father, who was not anemic, did undergo sickling.

Even though the father showed traces of the sickling trait and three of the patient's siblings had died early of severe anemia, Emmel failed to infer a possible hereditary factor. The first such suggestion was offered six years later by J. G. Huck, who – in addition to reporting the first large clinical sample (17 patients) – displayed the pedigrees of two sickle-cell families. In one, *both* parents were affected but had produced one normal offspring along with two affected children. The significance of these families was noted: "Apparently the 'sickle cell' condition in man is inherited according to the Mendelian law for the inheritance of a single factor." Moreover, "one interesting feature of this inheritance is the fact that the sickle cell condition is dominant over the normal condition." In 13 years, reports of a unique pathological finding had led to recognition of a hereditary disease – sickle-cell anemia.

After this good start, study of the disease slowed dramatically – partly because most investigators failed to differentiate between sickle-cell anemia and the nonanemic

sickle-cell trait, believing that the latter was merely the dormant stage of the former. In 1933, L. W. Diggs and colleagues suggested this to be incorrect, showing that hemoglobin determinations among black schoolchildren with sickle-cell trait were similar to those of controls. Moreover, no pathology was significantly associated with the sickle-cell trait.

As the distinction between the trait and the anemia became accepted, the pace of research on sickle-cell anemia quickened, and in 1949 two milestones were reached. First, two investigators independently discovered that the sickle-cell trait appears as a heterozygote with the normal allele, whereas sickle-cell anemia is the homozygous state of the gene, meaning that it must be inherited from both parents. These findings led to recognition that most dominant genetic diseases are heterozygous.

Then, L. Pauling and colleagues showed that the hemoglobin molecules in individuals with sickle-cell anemia and those in normal controls were fundamentally different. They predicted that the abnormality would be found in the globin part of the molecule and not in the heme groups, that the sickling process involved abnormal interactions of altered molecules, and that the alteration resulted in two to four more net positive charges per molecule. Their predictions were all correct, as was shown by V. M. Ingram in 1956. Abnormal (sickle-cell) hemoglobin differed in only one "spot," which had a net positive charge. Within three years it was demonstrated that the charge was caused by alteration of a single amino acid through mutation.

Since the moment the puzzle of sickle-cell anemia was solved, the study of mutant globins and associated disorders has signaled nearly every major advance in molecular biology. In 1978, R. M. Lawn and colleagues and Y. W. Kan and A.M.Dozy independently demonstrated the first human restriction fragment length polymorphisms (RFLPs) in the hemoglobin molecule. This led to recombinant-DNA-based studies on genetic diseases as well as human gene mapping. The discovery of repetitive DNA sequences in globin genes resulted in the development of DNA probes. Moreover, other recombinant DNA techniques for molecular diagnosis of genetic diseases were pioneered by Kan and Dozy and are now applied to a wide range of disorders, including **cancer** and infectious diseases.

Cytogenetics

The chromosome theory of heredity, that the Mendelian characters were contained in the chromosomes, developed soon after the rediscovery of Mendel's laws and was largely a result of Mendel's own observations. W. S. Sutton concluded that parallels between the organization and behavior of chromosomes and the laws of segregation and independent assortment could not be mere chance. He proposed that multiple characters would be found on a single chromosome.

Spurred by the work of Sutton and others, T. H. Morgan began studying inheritance of unit characters, the individual factors of Mendelian transmission. Using the fruit fly *Drosophila*, by 1914 Morgan concluded that the Mendelian factors, or genes, were physical entities present in the chromosomes in a linear manner. In 1923, T. S. Painter suggested that the number of human chromosomes was 48, and this was accepted for 23 years. Improved cytological techniques eventually led to establishment of the correct number as 46. So strong was the belief in Painter's estimate of 48 that a previous study had been abandoned because researchers could count only 46.

Not long afterward, the solution to an old medical puzzle became apparent. A syndrome called **furfuraceous idiocy**, described in 1846 by French physician E. Séguin, included characteristic facial features, incomplete growth, and mental retardation. In 1867, J. Langdon Down ascribed these traits to the Mongol type. From his publication the term "Mongolian idiot" replaced the previous name, and later "Down syndrome" became an interchangeable term. But repeated studies of Down syndrome failed to produce a viable etiologic hypothesis. In 1939, L. S. Penrose noted that the disorder had failed to meet Mendelian expectations – though some favored "irregular dominance" as an explanation – and that the only clear correlate was late maternal age. Two decades later, the improvements in cytological techniques that allowed determination of the correct number of human chromosomes also provided the solution to Down syndrome. In 1959, three French cytologists announced that patients with Down syndrome had an extra chromosome.

This first example of a disorder caused by at least one triploid chromosome in an otherwise diploid set (now called **trisomy**) led to a spate of similar findings, including **Turner's syndrome** (lack of one X-chromosome – XO), **Kleinfelter's syndrome** (XXY), **trisomy 13**, and **trisomy 18**. The discovery of chromosome banding techniques enabled chromosomes to be identified individually, and these techniques have been refined to the point that regions within them can be identified.

Finally, the advent of recombinant DNA techniques and analytic tools for estimating genetic linkage enabled one group to focus on the cause of the trisomy. A. C. Warren and colleagues demonstrated that recombination among DNA markers that have undergone **nondisjunction** (the event leading to a trisomy) occurs to a significantly lesser extent in Down-syndrome patients than it does in controls. Reduced recombination is indicative of **asynapsis**, or a failure of normal chromosome pairing. This result will likely lead to the discovery of the molecular mechanism of chromosome pairing.

In sum, the history of the study of human genetic diseases has been marked by periods of superstition and pseudoscience as well as by flashes of brilliant insight such as those of Maupertuis, Adams, and Garrod. It has also been characterized by an exponential increase in fundamental understanding coupled with technological and methodological breakthroughs, as clearly exemplified by sickle-cell anemia and Down syndrome. The development of recombinant DNA technology has inaugurated a revolution in the study of genetic disease matched only by the revelation of Mendel's laws in 1900.

The future of medical genetics is bright indeed. Systematic screening of the human genome has revealed hundreds of DNA sequence variants, exploitation of which has made it possible to establish genetic linkage and chromosome map locations for a large number of hereditary human illnesses. Moreover, the disease genes themselves have been cloned. These successes have made a genetic map of the entire human genome a feasible imperative. Clearly, the day of an exact science of molecular medical genetics has dawned, and with it has come the potential for treating and even curing genetic diseases.

Eric J. Devor

61. Giardiasis

Infection with the small flagellate *Giardia lamblia* is found around the world. This protozoan inhabits the small intestine of humans and is especially common in children. Other mammals, including beavers and muskrats, also harbor *Giardia* and are important reservoir hosts. The parasite was first seen by Anton van Leeuwenhoek in 1681 and described scientifically in 1859.

Adult parasites (trophozoites) attach to the intestinal wall with sucking disks. As trophozoites detach and pass down the intestinal tract, they transform themselves into cysts that are able to resist many environmental pressures, including water filtration and chlorination. Humans almost always acquire infection by swallowing fecally contaminated food or water. In developed countries, many cases of **giardiasis** have been traced to campers who drank from streams that appeared to be pure but had been contaminated by animals. Because of the cysts' resistance to normal water-purification methods, public water supplies can become infected, as happened in two Colorado ski resorts in 1964 and 1978.

Giardiasis is a frequent cause of "traveler's diarrhea," and tourist groups in Leningrad have suffered well-publicized outbreaks. In 1983, 22 of New York City's 55 police and fire department scuba divers had *Giardia*, presumably from the harbor's heavily polluted water. Prevalence rates in developing countries are 8–20 percent and higher. In poor countries such as Bangladesh, most children and many adults repeatedly acquire infection.

There has been considerable dispute about the clinical importance of *Giardia* infection. Although many cases are asymptomatic, it is now clear that the flagellates damage the intestinal wall and heavy infestations can cause nutritionally significant malabsorption of food. Symptoms include diarrhea, flatulence, abdominal discomfort, and light-colored, fatty stools. Repeated examinations and use of serologic techniques developed in the 1980s yield more reliable diagnoses for either individual patients or an entire population. Most infections are self-limiting, and treatment is effective, but reinfestation must be avoided. Some evidence indicates that mothers' milk helps protect infants against infection.

K. David Patterson

62. Glomerulonephritis (Bright's Disease)

Glomerulonephritis, an immunologic disease of the kidneys, affects the glomerulus, a cluster of capillaries that is the filter in the functioning unit of the kidney, the nephron. Inflammation, initiated by immune complexes, injures the glomerulus. Often the disease is acute, but it may be completely undetected until signs of kidney failure appear. This silent disease may prove fatal.

The urine-secreting structure (nephron) consists of the glomerulus and its tubular system. Each glomerulus consists of a tangle of capillaries branching between two tiny arteries (arterioles). The glomerulus is a blood filter that controls passage of molecules through the basement membrane. Normally red blood cells and albumin are not permitted to pass. The tubules reabsorb, secrete, synthesize, and excrete solutes and metabolites, thereby maintaining physiological equilibrium.

Poststreptococcal glomerulonephritis, studied by Richard Bright during the nineteenth century, still bears his name (**Bright's disease**). Related diseases include the **glomerulopathies**, seen in **diabetes** and **amyloidosis**.

Characteristics

Glomerulonephritis occurs worldwide and was seen frequently in Europe during the eighteenth and nineteenth centuries as a complication of **scarlet fever**. Today glomerulonephritis occurs sporadically. Since the 1950s, epidemics have struck Trinidad, the United States, and Venezuela. The disease appears more prevalent in the Western world, probably because modern diagnostic aids are available. Children contract it more commonly than adults. Because it is often silent, the incidence of glomerulonephritis remains unknown.

Physicians have long known that swelling (**dropsy**) occurred in some individuals 10–14 days after bouts of scarlet fever (**scarlatina**). Early physicians believed that toxins released during fever caused the dropsy, and long after Bright associated post-scarlatina dropsy with kidney changes, the role of scarlet fever remained unknown. In the latter nineteenth century, physicians learned that the scarlatina rash resulted from streptococcal toxins.

Only in the mid-twentieth century did researchers find that rabbits developed glomerulonephritis when injected with foreign proteins. Following injections, the glomerulus sustained injury from immune complexes. An immune complex consists of an antigen (the protein), an antibody (produced by the rabbit), and a complement. Immune complexes localize in the glomerulus and damage the basement membrane, which leaks protein and red blood cells into the urine. Swollen cells block the glomerular capillaries.

In humans, events mimicking this model follow certain **streptococcal infections**. Before antibiotics, glomerulonephritis usually followed attacks of scarlet fever. Today, it often follows streptococcal infections, as scarlet fever is uncommon.

History

About 100 A.D., Rufus of Ephesus noted hardened kidneys in patients who produced little urine, suffered no pain, and sometimes developed dropsy. This description could certainly be chronic glomerulonephritis. Around 1000 A.D., Avicenna, an Arab who authored perhaps the most famous medical text ever, mentioned patients with "chronic nephritis." Gulielmus de Saliceto's treatise, written in the mid-thirteenth century but not published until 1476, discusses dropsy, scanty urine, and hardened kidneys. This is **chronic kidney disease** – very likely glomerulonephritis.

Scientific urinalysis, representing a major step forward from the "looking and tasting" of the "Pisse Prophets," commenced with Frederick Dekkers, who discovered in 1695 that some urine samples, like serum, coagulated when heated or combined with acetic acid. In the next century, Neapolitan anatomist Domenico Cotugno attended a soldier with a febrile illness, who "had a wonderful eruption of intercutaneous water." This fluid and the urine "contained a coagulable matter." Whether Cotugno knew of Dekkers' observation is unknown, but Cotugno may have been first to note albumin in the urine associated with dropsy. About the same time, Swedish physician Nils Rosén von Rosenstein wrote an early, accurate account of poststreptococcal glomerulonephritis he observed during the scarlatina epidemic in Upsala in 1741.

The relationship between scarlet fever and dropsy was well recognized over the next 50 years. Thomas Bateman described post-scarlatina dropsy patients seen between 1804 and 1816 in London. In 1811, William Wells observed that the urine of such patients frequently contained blood constituents. Unaware of Cotugno's writings, he credited another with first noting "serum" in the urine of dropsy patients. Wells found serum in the urine of 78 of 130 such patients and also noted increased urine volumes. He observed altered kidneys in one dropsical patient at autopsy but thought this limited observation did not justify associating the urine anomalies with the kidney abnormalities.

In 1818, John Blackall also observed dropsy, **albuminuria**, and bloody urine after scarlatina. He also noted hardened kidneys. Soon afterward, Bright, a giant of medicine, was studying patients with post-scarlatina dropsy and albuminuria. In 1827, he first reported his findings. Bright's meticulous account of the disease and illustrations of the renal changes remain a model report today, but he did not explain how albumin enters the urine. This question could not be answered until nephron structure was further defined.

Marcello Malpighi had tried to answer the question in 1666 at Bologna. He knew of the glomeruli but was frustrated in attempting to establish their function. In the nineteenth century, Johannes Peter Mueller knew of Malpighi's study of the glomeruli, but he considered them as simply receptacles of blood. He believed that urine was secreted by the epithelium of the proximal tubules. In 1842, however, William Bowman wondered, as Malpighi had, why the glomerulus ended blindly in a space opening into the tubules. Bowman suggested that protein and red cells might pass through the glomerulus under abnormal circumstances!

A few years later, German physiologist Carl Ludwig supplemented Bowman's observations with the view that the glomerulus was a semipermeable filter. In 1861, Thomas Graham showed that membranes could block colloids but permit passage of crystalloids. The glomerulus was established as the source of urine, but albuminuria was still attributed to tubular epithelium. Even as microscopic studies advanced, pathologists adhered to this view. The source of dropsical urinary albumin was not determined for another century.

Rudolph Virchow established the cellular basis for pathology in 1858, and classified Bright's disease into three categories – involving the tubules, the connective tissue, and the blood vessels. In later writings, he referred to glomerular changes, but he believed the main changes were in the tubules. The first pathologist to use the word "glomerulonephritis" was Edwin Klebs in 1879. The term became synonymous with Bright's disease after its incorporation in a 1914 classification, which remained in use with little modification for nearly a half century.

The use of biopsy to evaluate kidney disorders was also an important contribution. As biopsy experience accumulated in the 1950s, 1960s, and 1970s, many classifications of Bright's disease appeared. Understanding of the role of the immune system in glomerulonephritis was achieved, and the glomerular basement membrane was established as the site of albuminuric leakage. The tubule is not the source of the urine protein, but altered tubular reabsorption possibly plays a role in albuminuria. The major contributions of the twentieth century were the use of thin sections, immunofluorescent techniques, and electron microscopy in biopsy interpretation.

Today, Bright's disease consists of many disorders, all of which can be considered glomerulonephritis. Their diagnosis and management will continue to challenge medical science as the twenty-first century progresses.

Donald M. Larson

63. Goiter

Goiter is an ancient disease that has always been more common in some places than in others. It was known in China at least by the third century B.C. and possibly earlier. The Romans knew the disease well by the second century A.D.; indeed, a major focus of **endemic goiter** was in the European Alps. The word "goiter" (*goitre* in Europe) derives from the Latin *gutter*, but the meaning has shifted from "throat" to mean specifically an **enlarged thyroid**. An ancient Greek synonym was *bronchocele*. Modern synonyms are the Spanish *bocio*, the Italian *gozzo*, and the German *Kropf.* The ancient

Latin word *struma*, probably used originally to describe inflamed lymph nodes in the neck, was later used to indicate goiter.

This semantical confusion is understandable because the thyroid gland was unknown until the sixteenth century. Leonardo da Vinci may have drawn it about the year 1500, but the drawing was not published until much later. Andreas Vesalius noted "laryngeal glands" in 1543, but not in humans. By the end of the century, however, anatomists had identified the human thyroid as a discrete structure: Bartolomeo Eustachi in 1552, Realdo Colombo in 1558, and Giulio Casserio in 1600. In 1619, Hieronymus Fabricius realized that goiter arises from an enlargement of this gland, and in 1656 Thomas Wharfton named the gland by virtue of its proximity to the thyroid cartilage.

Characteristics

Other diseases of the neck confounded the connection between goiter and the thyroid gland. The main confounder was **scrofula**, which in medieval Latin meant "swelling of the glands" and is still used to connote tuberculous lymph glands in the neck. In regions where goiter was endemic, affecting large portions of the population, its connection with the thyroid was fairly clear. But where only a few individuals exhibited the disease, it was called **sporadic goiter**. If the swelling was small and moved with swallowing, it was called an enlarged thyroid. But if the mass was immovable, then it was considered to arise from tuberculous nodes. This confusion persisted until the mid-nineteenth century. Jean Louis Alibert, for example, in 1835 classified endemic goiter as a type of scrofula found in rural areas. Today goiter is (arbitrarily) defined as endemic if more than 10 percent of a population is goitrous.

Large and disfiguring goiters were cosmetically distressing and sometimes blocked breathing. Moreover, endemic goiter areas produced a number of people who were retarded from birth, with disfigured faces, and sometimes deaf and mute. Most but not all had goiter, which was also common in their mothers. They were called "cretins," and their disease **endemic cretinism**. The word "cretin" probably derives from the French *cretien*, and thence from the Latin *christianus* ("christian") and was likely used to make clear that these persons were truly human. Travelers' observations of cretinism in the Alps date from the thirteenth century, but clinical allusions begin with Paracelsus, who around 1527 connected cretinism with goiter. Good descriptions begin with Felix Platter, who probably observed it in 1562 and who also associated the two maladies.

By the seventeenth century, the concept of goiter as an abnormally enlarged thyroid gland was reasonably well established, as was its association with cretinism and with the alpine areas of Europe. Yet, cretinism in particular was rare, and most physicians never saw it. Just as goiter could be confounded with other neck diseases, so could cretinism with any sort of **mental retardation**. Thus a certain amount of diagnostic "fuzziness" persisted.

Today goiter means only an enlarged thyroid. The thyroid may be uniformly enlarged (**simple goiter**) or have several lumps (**multinodular goiter**). The World Health Organization assigns gradations to the disorder:

Grade 0 = no goiter
Grade 1 = palpable but invisible goiter
Grade 2 = easily visible goiter
Grade 3 = goiter visible at 30 meters.

Some goiters are malignant (e.g., **thyroid cancer** or **lymphoma**), but most are benign. Some are associated with specific thyroid diseases such as **hyperthyroidism, hypothyroidism**, and **thyroiditis**. These and other conditions overlap considerably and continue to cause confusion in diagnosis and treatment.

Goiter is not particularly harmful unless it compresses the trachea or causes emotional upset. For a large goiter requiring treatment, however, the only solution until the twentieth century was surgery. But the operation commonly killed the patient, and some surgeons objected to it in principle. Others, such as E. Theodor Kocher in Berne and the cousins

Jacques-Louis and Auguste Reverdin in Geneva persisted, and by the 1880s were able to remove all or most of a goitrous thyroid with death rates under 1 percent.

It became clear, however, that removing the entire thyroid caused symptoms resembling cretinism. In 1883, Felix Semon in London suggested that cretins, thyroidectomy patients, and adults with a mysterious disorder called **myxedema** all suffered because they lacked thyroid glands; in 1888, he was found to be correct. **Thyroid deficiency**, myxedema, and hypothyroidism are now synonyms for decreased or lacking thyroid function.

History

Many theories have attempted to explain goiter. One ancient idea was that goiter comes from an excess of phlegm descending from the head into the throat. Many saw excessive flexing of the head as the cause – including Michelangelo, who suggested it in 1509. Geographic peculiarities and climatic factors were frequently blamed as well. Finally, some thought hereditary or constitutional factors important.

During the nineteenth century, major theories of goiter focused at least in part on some peculiarity of drinking water, lack of iodine, an infection of some sort, or some combination of these. Climatic factors had been dismissed. High altitude had been rejected as well, for the disease was not limited to mountainous regions.

The long process of linking goiter and cretinism to **iodine deficiency** began in 1811, when Bernard Courtois discovered iodine while making saltpeter for gunpowder during the Napoleonic Wars. He noticed it as a violet vapor released from the residue of burnt seaweed. It was subsequently named iodine from the Greek word for "violet." The key was the seaweed. For centuries, dating from the 1100s in Europe and from considerably earlier in China, seaweed had been among the many remedies for goiter. Within a few years, iodine was detected in various seaweeds.

In 1818, J.-F. Coindet, a Geneva physician, suggested that iodine might be the active principle in treating goiter. Chemist Jean-Baptiste Dumas looked for iodine in marine sponge and found it. Coindet then gave iodine to goitrous patients, with good results that were soon confirmed by other physicians. As early as 1825, another chemist, Jean Baptiste Boussingault, suggested that iodine deficiency might be the cause of goiter and recommended the addition of iodine to table salt to prevent it, but little came of this suggestion.

A generation later, Jean-Louis Prévost, another Geneva physician, made the same suggestion as Boussingault. But iodine had fallen into disfavor as therapy for goiter because of toxic side effects, including hyperthyroidism. Coindet himself had seen this and had cautioned against too high a dose, but to no avail.

In the 1850s, Adolphe Chatin, a French pharmacist and botanist, found iodine in *freshwater* plants and suggested that these be used to prevent goiter. He measured iodine in water samples from all over France, and in some foods as well, and concluded that in certain areas a lack of iodine in drinking water appeared to be the principal cause of goiter. But in 1852, a French Academy of Sciences committee – although congratulating Chatin on his work – viewed his association between lack of iodine and goiter as unproven.

Meanwhile, in South America in 1835 and in Savoy in the 1840s there had been successful trials of iodine against endemic goiter. Yet the success of iodine as a goiter preventive was not pursued. The reluctance to accept iodine deficiency as a cause of goiter is understandable: There was then no good example of a disease caused by a deficiency. Further, the theory did not explain why only some people in low-iodine areas got goiter while others did not. This problem remains unresolved today.

After the discovery of the bacterial cause of many diseases, it was postulated that goiter was caused by either a bacterium or a bacterial toxin, perhaps in water. Edwin Klebs believed he had found such an agent in 1877, and August Hirsch around 1885 stated flatly that "endemic goitre and cretinism have to be reckoned among the infective diseases." Indeed, the notion that goiter has an infectious cause persisted into the early twentieth century despite unconvincing evidence. But the parallel notion of a toxin in the water, possibly of bacterial origin, is still alive and warrants serious consideration, particularly where there is much goiter despite adequate iodine intake.

Until the 1890s, there was no resolution of the cause of endemic goiter or cretinism. No clear choice was possible among the drinking-water, iodine-deficiency, or toxic-infective hypotheses. Fear of serious side effects if everyone took iodine in salt or food was widespread: After all, iodine was a known poison. Nonetheless, substantial advances began to be made in goiter research. George R. Murray discovered in 1891 that a glycerin extract of sheep thyroid cured myxedema, and investigators began to look for iodine in the thyroid itself. For example, while looking for the active compound in the thyroid, Eugen Baumann produced an extract. When analyzing it, he routinely looked for iodine, not expecting to find it; to his surprise it was there.

From this point research diverged. One path led to the 1914 isolation of a specific thyroid hormone, thyroxine, by Edward C. Kendall. Researchers also began to study goiter in relation to the iodine content of the thyroid rather than that of the environment. By 1910, David Marine in Cleveland, Ohio, had demonstrated that iodine prevented goiter in brook trout. He gave iodine to hospital patients and to children of friends to prevent goiter. In fact, he tried to give it to all schoolchildren in Cleveland, but the school board, led by a goiter surgeon, said it would poison the children. Several years later, Marine conducted a large-scale study of iodine prophylaxis for goiter. The results were clear-cut: Sixty-five percent of goiters became smaller, and new goiter was largely prevented. This study provided the impetus for the use of iodized salt in the United States.

Marine had shown iodine to be both treatment and preventive for goiter but had not proven that his patients were iodine deficient. It remained for J. F. McClendon, an army nutrition officer during World War I, to measure iodine in water and food. He showed that there was a correlation between lower iodine and the presence of human goiter and also that rats on a low-iodine diet got goiter. He later gathered worldwide data to support his thesis that low iodine in drinking water causes goiter.

By 1924, Michigan offered iodized salt to the public after an education campaign; within 12 years, goiter prevalence fell from 37 percent to 8 percent – and by 1951 to 2 percent. Since Marine's study, iodine intake in the United States has increased several times, not only because of iodized salt but because of widespread use of foods that contain iodine, such as bread and milk. Thus, in the United States, few can develop iodine deficiency, and goiter is mostly sporadic, occurring either spontaneously or as a result of factors other than iodine deficiency. Yet, some areas of endemic goiter persist in the United States, especially in parts of Appalachia, and may be caused by a "goitrogen" (a substance that causes goiter). Goitrogens certainly exist, but how much they contribute to human goiter is unclear.

In many other parts of the world, goiter remains endemic. Persons in an endemic area could have any of the diseases that cause sporadic goiter, which is one reason why goiter prevalence never falls to zero even with iodine repletion. For some areas, goiter is a major public-health problem, and millions of people remain at risk. The disease is almost always associated with low iodine intake and iodine deficiency, and while there remains no good explanation of why some do not develop goiter in areas of low dietary iodine, iodine does prevent the disease. The issue then becomes a social and political one of providing iodine to those in deficient areas and then getting them to take it. Iodine is not, however, the answer to all endemic goiter, and we now face the challenge of teasing out several probable factors in addition to iodine deficiency, as well as the political challenge involved in iodine prophylaxis on a worldwide basis.

Clark T. Sawin

64. Gonorrhea

The name **gonorrhea** ("flow of seed") and its vernacular counterparts ("clap," "dose," "strain") reflect a hazy comprehension of the disease. The only accurate term in common use is "drip," which acknowledges the white-to-yellowish milky discharge from the male penis. But even this more realistic designation indicates only the male urethral aspect of a broader syndrome.

Gonorrhea is an infection of mucosal surfaces caused by a bacterium, the gonococcus *Neisseria gonorrhoeae*, whose only natural reservoir is humans. Its presence in the genital tract defines the condition gonorrhea; otherwise, the adjective "gonococcal" is used (as in **gonococcal endocarditis**). Though gonorrhea is transmitted primarily (through sexual contact) to genital mucosa, it may disseminate elsewhere, with infection of the skin, heart valves, joints, and central nervous system. It is rarely the cause of death but can produce serious sequelae. The gonococcus occupies an ecological niche requiring a surprisingly complex assortment of attributes necessary for survival, not least among which is a propitious set of social and sexual mores among its hosts. As history demonstrates, the seemingly delicate balance among such factors has been universally available.

Characteristics

In male genital infections, pus issuing from the penile opening, accompanied by discomfort on urination, is the most frequent symptom of gonorrhea. The gonococcus adheres to cells lining the urethra, establishing an inflammatory reaction. This primary pathological process is basically the same at all mucosal sites of infection. The majority of men will become symptomatic in 3–5 days. In perhaps one-quarter of cases, symptoms are insufficient to cause the patient to seek medical care. A substantial proportion of men with gonorrhea will be asymptomatic.

Though women have long been known to harbor the organism, only recently have distinct syndromes been identified. This is because asymptomatic infection probably occurs more frequently in women. Infection of the urethra occurs in 70–90 percent of women with gonorrhea, but the more important manifestation of the disease is infection of the uterine cervix.

The major concern about gonorrhea is its potential for destruction of female reproductive organs. The gonococcus may spread from the cervix to inflame the uterine lining and ultimately cause **peritonitis**. Once established, **pelvic inflammatory disease** (PID) becomes chronic, with serious consequences. About 20 percent of women will have a recurrence after treatment. Studies in Sweden indicate that the risk of **sterility** is 12–16 percent after a single episode and rises to 60 percent after three episodes.

A distinctive picture appears when the gonococcus is spread via the bloodstream, including infection of various sites along with characteristic skin lesions and **arthritis**. This is **disseminated gonococcal infection** (DGI). The lesions are small and generally number fewer than 20. Infected joints usually exhibit the classic features of arthritis. Patients with DGI usually respond well to routine treatment.

Another major mode of transmission of the gonococcus is from mother to child. The most common manifestation is **gonococcal ophthalmia**. The typical syndrome includes relatively rapid progression to generalized involvement, scarring, and blindness. Children may develop gonorrhea in sexual sites as well. It is apparent that the majority of infected children have suffered sexual abuse.

The importance of gonorrhea is measured not only by its considerable burden of acute disease and long-term consequences, but also by some of its extraordinary biological characteristics. The virulence of the gonococcus rests in its ability to adhere to muscosal surfaces, to resist immunological defenses, to cause asymptomatic infection, and to resist antibiotic killing. These qualities have been important in the development of four major classification schemes based upon the following:

1. The presence or absence of *pili* (long, filamentous projections on the surface of the gonococcus), which determine adherence to mucosal cells. Their presence is, in turn, reflected in the size, shape, and opacity of gonococcal bacterial colonies and formed the basis of the earliest classification scheme used.
2. The nutritional requirements of the gonococci. Typing of organisms based on their need for certain amino acids (auxotyping) has identified special strains that are more or less sensitive to antibiotics and have a greater propensity to cause disseminated infection.
3. The antigenic structure of the gonococcal cell envelope, which provides a mechanism for classification (serovars). Serovars have been used in conjunction with auxotyping to indicate distribution patterns and link cases epidemiologically.
4. Susceptibility to antibiotics. Four transferable pieces of genetic material (plasmids) help in geographic localization of cases.

These systems for classification reflect the considerable pathogenetic repertoire available to the gonococcus. In contrast, the immunologic armamentarium of the host seems inadequate. Genital secretions may have some inhibitory effect but are not protective. Local immunoglobulin production may be counteracted by the gonococcus. Serum antibody is usually demonstrable, but resistance to serum killing is a typical feature of gonococci. Studies to date simply reflect the time-honored observation that people may contract gonorrhea again and again. There is no apparent protective immunity.

Gonorrhea is found worldwide, but its true extent is unknown. Direct comparisons of incidence among nations are difficult to make. The disease is widespread in both industrialized and developing countries, but the burden on developing nations is likely greater. Incidence in some African cities may be as high as 10,000 per 100,000 population. Surveys of women attending clinics in Africa disclose prevalence as high as 17 percent. Among prostitutes in Latin America, Asia, and Africa, the prevalence of gonorrhea may be 30–50 percent. These data provide some sense of the potential magnitude of the problem.

Some industrialized nations practice systematic reporting of gonorrhea. Statistics have documented the major event in the history of gonorrhea: a worldwide pandemic that began in the late 1950s and peaked in the mid-1970s. A comparison of disease rates in the United States, Britain, Sweden, and Canada indicates a rise in gonorrhea after World War II, with a subsequent fall to a nadir in the mid-1950s. Then each nation experienced an increase throughout the 1960s, peaking by the mid-1970s. At the peak, rates among industrialized nations differed as much as tenfold. Rates among developing nations differed even more wildly, but inconsistent reporting clearly plays an important role.

The impact of the pandemic is demonstrated by the history of the disease in the United States during this period. Between 1956 and 1985, rates of gonorrhea increased in all age groups of both sexes. Rates for females were higher at younger ages and peaked at ages 15–19. Rates for males peaked at ages 20–24. The origin of this increase, and of the pandemic in general, is often attributed to changes in sexual mores during the 1960s and 1970s. Major increases were reported in the frequency of premarital sexual experiences; availability of contraceptive technology was considerably greater; and there was an unusual increase (the "baby-boom" generation) in the number of people reaching the age of sexual activity. It is likely that the pandemic has not yet had its full impact on the developing world, though the peak in industrialized nations seems to have passed.

History

Gonorrhea is the oldest as well as the most common of the **venereal diseases**. An Egyptian papyrus from approximately 3500 B.C. prescribes plant extracts to soothe painful urination. The Hebrew Bible mentions treatment of genital exudates. In the fourth century B.C., Hippocrates recognized the venereal nature of transmission, and Galen, in the second century A.D., is believed to have coined the name. In the fourteenth century, a description of the ailment stressed a major symptom, *chaude pisse* ("hot piss"), the disease's appellation in French.

By 1500 or so, interest centered on the distinction between **syphilis** and gonorrhea. Majority opinion held that they were different manifestations of the same disease. But in the middle of the sixteenth century, French physician Jean Fernel described gonorrhea as a disease separate from syphilis, and British physician Francis Balfour (some two centuries later) also receives credit for distinguishing between the two.

In the late eighteenth century, however, John Hunter argued that the cause of both diseases was the same. He infected himself with discharge from a patient he thought had gonorrhea, but he developed syphilis instead. This was an unfortunate instance of a brilliant and heroic use of scientific method gone wrong, and it postponed understanding of the two diseases for decades.

During the same period, the most lucid literary account of gonorrhea appeared. James Boswell, the biographer of Samuel Johnson, kept a diary of his own encounters with gonorrhea. The diary details 19 episodes. There is little question of the impact of gonorrhea on his life and on the lives of countless others in the era. He is believed to have died of gonorrheal complications.

In the 1790s, Benjamin Bell of Edinburgh, who disagreed with Hunter, published several tracts exploring evidence that gonorrhea and syphilis were separate entities. He posed several simple questions: Why is gonorrhea more common when the skin of the penis is at greater risk of exposure than the urethra? Why are there geographic differences in the distribution of the two diseases? Why have their manifestations appeared in the same populations at different points in time?

It remained, however, for Philippe Ricord, in a series of experiments in the mid-1800s, to provide a definitive distinction between the diseases. He inoculated 17 prisoners with gonorrheal pus, producing occasional ulcers with prompt healing but no evidence of syphilis.

In 1879, Albert Neisser in Breslau, Germany, published findings that confirmed Ricord's conclusions. Neisser described the organism that now bears his name. In 1882, the organism was grown in vitro by Ernst von Bumm, and the first major preventive action was taken in 1883, when Karl Siegmund Credé in Leipsig instilled a silver nitrate solution in the eyes of newborns. The occurrence of gonococcal ophthalmia diminished rapidly with the widespread adoption of this procedure.

After this, however, there were no major improvements in the understanding of gonorrhea until sulfonamides were introduced in 1937. This success was short-lived, and true antibiosis for gonorrhea appeared only in the 1950s with the general availability of penicillin. It is only in recent times that gonorrhea's effect on us and our ability to alter its course have dramatically changed.

In the late 1970s, analysis of thousands of geocoded cases – based on the routine reporting of gonorrhea morbidity data – revealed a general geographic pattern. Intense concentrations of gonorrhea exist in a small number of core areas in inner cities. In a concentric circle surrounding the core are a group of adjacent areas with somewhat lessened gonorrhea rates. The rest of the city constitutes a peripheral area with a markedly diminished gonorrhea burden. This pattern was repeated in all cities studied, and all the core areas are similarly characterized by high population density and low socioeconomic status. Such a pattern has been documented in Buffalo, New York; Colorado Springs and Denver, Colorado; Liverpool, England; Miami, Florida; and Seville, Spain; among other localities.

It cannot be assumed that these geographic characteristics are universal. Differences in human ecology and sexuality in developing countries may dictate a different pattern, and data are not yet available. It might be concluded, however, that a concentric pattern of gonorrhea risk, which diminishes outward from the central inner city, exists in many major urban areas. The potential for use of geographic patterns in the development of disease control strategies, and in the understanding of other sexually transmitted syndromes, is an area for further development.

Richard B. Rothenberg

65. Gout

Gout is a chronic, intermittently symptomatic disease. It is manifested primarily by small numbers of acutely painful, swollen joints that result from an inflammatory reaction to the precipitation of crystals of monosodium urate.

Characteristics

The predisposing metabolic factor for **primary gout** is an abnormally high or rapidly changing concentration of uric acid in the blood. **Hyperuricemia** may result from an accelerated synthesis of uric acid, or decreased excretory capacity for uric acid in otherwise normal kidneys as a result of unidentified but probably heritable causes. Hyperuricemia leading to **secondary gout** occurs particularly (1) in diseases of the blood-forming tissues that increase the availability of precursors of uric acid; (2) in kidney failure, which limits the excretion of uric acid; or (3) as a result of medications that either accelerate the breakdown of purine-rich cells (e.g., antineoplastic drugs) or interfere with the renal excretory mechanism (e.g., some diuretics). Dissolved in the serum, uric acid is harmless. However, because of unidentified local circumstances it may leak from capillaries and crystallize. The crystals of monosodium urate elicit the inflammatory reaction, which is the **gouty attack**, and the microscopic identification of the crystals in synovial fluid confirms the diagnosis. Why this inflammation occurs predominantly in joints, and why much more commonly in some joints (such as those of the feet or in the knee) than in others (such as the hip or those of the vertebral column) are unexplained characteristics. Unexplained as well is the question why "tophi," which are urate deposits that form beneath the skin, are usually painless and the antiuricemic effect of estrogens.

Ninety to 95 percent of gout patients are male. Gout rarely develops in women before menopause. The first attack usually occurs in the fifth decade in men and the sixth decade in women. The rate of production of uric acid thereafter diminishes. The normal uric acid content in men is about 1.2 grams, and in women 0.6 gram.

Uric acid accumulates in part as the subcutaneous deposits called tophi. About 50 percent of untreated patients have tophi 10 years after their first attack of gout. After tophi, the most common uratic manifestation of gout is **kidney stones (nephrolithiasis)**. This association has been noted since at least the sixteenth century. Uric acid stones constitute no more than 5 percent of all kidney stones, but about 80 percent in cases of gout. How close the relationship between gout and urate nephrolithiasis may be is uncertain. Allopurinol therapy, which reduces the uric acid pool, decreases the incidence of uratic kidney stones and has the same effect in nongouty urate hyperexcretors who have a history of calcium stone formation.

History

For many centuries, "gout" was a nonspecific term. The differentiation of the disease was begun in the late seventeenth century by Thomas Sydenham; his contemporary, Anton van Leeuwenhoek, described crystals from a tophus. In 1776, Swedish pharmacist Karl W. Scheele discovered an organic acid in urinary concretions – he called it "lithic acid." In 1797 at Cambridge, William H. Wollaston found that tophi contained lithic acid. In 1798, lithic acid was renamed *acide ourique* ("uric acid") by French chemist Antoine F. de Fourcroy because he found it was present in urine.

A half century passed. In 1847 and in 1854, London physician Alfred B. Garrod devised two tests whereby uric acid could be detected in hyperuricemic states such as gout. He demonstrated urate in subcutaneous tissue and cartilage in cases of gout. Garrod hypothesized that gout resulted from either loss of excretory capacity or increased formation of uric acid. A century after his 1859 monograph on gout, both concepts were proved correct. In 1876 Garrod postulated that gout results from precipitation of sodium urate in or near a joint, and this was proven in 1962.

Beginning in 1871 numerous assays of uric acid were devised, but none was sensitive enough. Lack of understanding of uric acid metabolism cast doubt on the relationship of uric acid to gout, and two effects resulted. One was that the old belief in a "gouty poison" – that caused a wide variety of symptoms or diseases – gained new adherents. The other was that clinicians virtually ceased diagnosing gout.

The first practical technique sensitive enough to detect normal concentrations of uric acid was devised by Otto Folin at Harvard in 1912. Its sensitivity was improved so that in 1938, uric acid content was shown to be greater in men than in women, thereby correlating with the rarity of gout in women. However, physicians continued to be poorly aware of true gout. Specificity in uric acid determination was achieved in 1953 with a technique employing the enzyme uricase. Nevertheless, most laboratories use less specific methods that give somewhat higher than "true" values.

Therapy of gout has two components: treatment of the acute attack and prophylaxis to decrease uric acid content. Colchicum in various alcoholic or aqueous extracts from the meadow saffron came into use in the nineteenth century in France and England. It was included in an American "Dispensatory" in 1836, although its use was advocated somewhat earlier. Colchicum was toxic, however, causing severe **diarrhea**, which was believed to constitute its therapeutic effect. Its active component, colchicine, was isolated in 1820 and available in pill form by 1900, but crude tinctures were still in use in the 1950s.

Until about 1910, when cinchophen was introduced, colchicine was the only remedy for gout. Cinchophen not only was effective against gouty attacks but also was an analgesic. However, by the 1930s it became evident that cinchophen may cause severe, even fatal, liver damage. Its use faded, and colchicine again became the standard treatment.

Two pharmaceutical breakthroughs occurred in 1951. Probenecid, a drug developed to retard excretion of penicillin, was found to accelerate the excretion of uric acid and was well tolerated and convenient to take. The other discovery was phenylbutazone, which proved to have effects similar to cinchophen. Like probenecid, it increased excretion of uric acid, and like colchicine, it counteracted attacks. However, it proved to be toxic and has fallen into disfavor.

Another pair of pharmaceutical products was introduced in 1963. Indomethacin counteracts gouty attacks, and it gradually superseded phenylbutazone. Allopurinol lowers uric acid like probenecid but by a different mechanism. Like probenecid, allopurinol lacks value against gouty attack, but it is effective during **renal failure** and is convenient.

Dietetic attempts to treat gout are ancient and based on belief in the virtue of moderation. Gout was thought to be caused largely by excessive consumption of food and alcohol, but in 1924 it was shown that starvation results in increased uric acid concentration. Since the 1960s, it has been found that certain circumstances may operate to block excretion of uric acid and thereby increase the possibility of gouty attack. Starvation, alcohol ingestion (especially without eating), and uncontrolled **diabetes mellitus** are among such conditions.

Uric acid is synthesized from foodstuffs, particularly those rich in nucleoproteins. A low-fat, largely vegetarian diet reduces uric acid concentration, but the effect such diets have on reducing gouty attacks is equivocal. Since the advent of urate-depleting drugs, dietetic therapy has become irrelevant except for the advantages of weight reduction for obese patients.

Gout is rarely a direct cause of death, although it is commonly associated with **hypertension** or **arteriosclerosis**, and untreated hypertension with normal renal function is frequently associated with hyperuricemia. **Hyperlipidemia** appears not to correlate with hyperuricemia; rather, both are associated with hypertension and **obesity**. **Angina pectoris** is twice as frequent among gouty men, and one study found that causes of death among 427 gout patients were cardiovascular in 66 percent of cases.

Although a rough correlation does exist between hyperuricemia and the likelihood of a gouty attack, its predictive value is poor. The most important measurable factors affecting uric acid concentration are the protein content of the diet and overweight. Weight and rate of uric acid metabolism are to some extent genetically predetermined. However, the immediate cause of a gouty attack remains unknown.

Worldwide, the prevalence of gout has changed since the 1940s. In developed countries, the disease is now rarely disabling. Elsewhere, however, it has become more prevalent, predominantly because of "improved" diets. Hypotheses about whether ethnic differences are genetic or the result of environmental changes are weakened by a lack of data.

Several American surveys have compared the uric acid levels of executives and either lower-level employees or age-matched population samples. The executives have consistently been found to have higher urate concentrations and a larger proportion of cases of hyperuricemia. This finding, which has been inconsistently confirmed in Europe, has not been explained by differences in physiognomy, blood pressure, or medications.

Most reports of gout in non-Caucasian populations are relatively recent. The first case was a 31-year-old African servant who died in 1807 in Edinburgh, where he had often suffered severe pains that occurred in his great toes. A medical missionary in Hawaii in the early 1830s reported that **rheumatism** frequently occurred there, and although gout might also be expected to be common, the mild quality of the food suggested otherwise. Similarly, a military surgeon in New Zealand in the 1850s found that although "rheumatic affections" were much more frequent among New Zealanders than among the English, gout was unknown. A leading expert wrote in 1948 that gout "is common in England and France, less common but increasing in North America. Hebrews are affected, prosperous American Negroes occasionally." Another specialist stated in 1952 that gout "is unknown in China, Japan, and the tropics [and] is rare in Negroes."

Such statements may have reflected either ignorance or changing circumstances but clearly are incorrect now. Probably the most ubiquitous factor underlying an increased prevalence of gout is the increased proportion of proteins in many diets, which increases the amount of uric acid. Comparisons of uric acid values of most adequately nourished populations give similar values. The exceptions remind us that there are unidentified (presumably genetic) factors that result in differences among groups that would be assumed not to differ empirically.

Generally, the ability of gouty individuals to excrete uric acid is normal, but differences in excretory capacity can be identified. One hypothesis suggests that some ethnic groups may include a large proportion of persons who have a (genetically determined) relatively low limit to their renal excretory capacity. As long as such individuals consume a low-protein diet, such as the Asian rice-based diets, or diets based on yams, their excretory mechanism is not saturated, urate remains in the normal range, and gout rarely occurs. When the protein consumption of such persons increases – as their diet becomes "Westernized" – the excretory capacity is overwhelmed, urate accumulates, and gout becomes more frequent.

There is a marked difference in the prevalence of hyperuricemia between Caucasian and various Pacific island populations. Less than 10 percent of most unselected Caucasian populations, but more than 40 percent of many Pacific populations, exceed "normal upper limits." Many surveys have been conducted since the 1960s. The hyperuricemia cannot be attributed entirely to dietary changes, nor is alcohol consumption necessarily a factor. The highest prevalence of hyperuricemia has been found on the Micronesian island of Nauru. The diet there had largely become Westernized by the time these surveys were conducted. However, some groups were hyperuricemic on their traditional diets. The complexity of the uricemia – gout relationship is illustrated by the unexplained observation that although the New Zealand Maoris, Tokelauans, and Rarotongans have the same high prevalence of hyperuricemia, a fourfold difference exists in the prevalence of gout.

Surveys in the early 1960s in the Osaka district of Japan showed an extremely low prevalence of hyperuricemia. With continued Westernization of the diet, however, an anticipated increase in the prevalence of gout is occurring. The clinical characteristics of gout are the same and occur in similar frequencies as in Caucasian populations.

A Chinese author claimed that the first case of gout to be described in China occurred in 1948, and that by 1959 he could collect only 12 cases, 10 with tophi. This almost certainly reflects socioeconomic rather than biological circumstances. The prevalence of gout may indeed have been low because of the widespread, inadequately low protein diet, but this would have pertained particularly to the large segment of the population that lacked medical care. In regard to the well-nourished upper classes, a lack of diagnostic acumen may have been at least partially responsible.

Aside from South Africa, there is little relevant information from the African continent. The effect on uricemia of the urbanization of primitive people has been well illustrated by studies in South Africa that showed the lowest values in a tribal population, higher values in a village, and the highest levels, equal to those of urban whites, in urban blacks. The combined three black populations contained no cases of gout. A survey in Ethiopia similarly showed the lowest values among rural Ethiopians, intermediate values among urban Ethiopians, and the normal, highest value among Caucasian and Indian urban professionals.

Data from Israel are analogous. Desert Bedouins were found to have lower uric acid values than villagers of the same Arabic stock, and the latter results were the same as those that were obtained from a nearby Jewish population in Haifa. These variations are presumed to be related to changes in nutrition associated with changes in life style.

Thomas G. Benedek

66. Heart-Related Diseases

In many ways, the year 1628 marks the beginning of modern Western conceptions of **heart disease**. In that year, London physician William Harvey showed that the blood must circulate, rather than being continuously regenerated as earlier theories suggested. He also showed that the heart drives the blood on its circuit around the body. Harvey's revolutionary achievement failed to bring about any immediate changes in medicine's approach to heart disease, but over the next few centuries many people tried to discover what was going on within the chests of patients who showed the debilitating signs of **cardiac disease**.

During the mid-eighteenth century, Leopold Auenbrugger, working in Vienna, described a new diagnostic technique. By percussing the chest – that is, by striking the chest and both listening to and feeling the reverberation – he could tell, to some extent, what lay within. His method enabled him to ascertain the size of the heart and to determine the presence of fluid in the chest, a common manifestation of **heart**

failure. However, Auenbrugger's technique attracted little attention until after the French Revolution.

That revolution radically changed French hospitals and medical schools, and physicians working in these institutions changed their perception of disease, emphasizing the location and nature of specific lesions in the body. In the early nineteenth century, Parisian physicians daily went from bedside to bedside, examining patients with all manner of diseases. All too often they had the opportunity to correlate their findings with autopsy results. In this milieu, René Laennec invented the stethoscope for listening to chest sounds, and Auenbrugger's percussion technique became widely used. Although both were used primarily to diagnose lung disease, they also helped investigate heart problems.

Auscultation with the stethoscope was a skill requiring experience and could yield misleading results. Moreover, it was useless in discovering cardiac diseases, such as **coronary heart disease**, that produced no outward signs. (Coronary heart disease, encompassing **angina pectoris** and **myocardial infarction** or "heart attack," was manifested by chest pain and is now understood to be caused by occlusion of coronary arteries.) So, in addition to anatomic studies, practitioners published descriptions of patients' reported symptoms. In 1768, William Heberden of London coined the term "angina pectoris" and differentiated it from other chest pains.

Heberden focused on the symptoms of the disease, not its cause. However, others had described disease of the coronary arteries. English surgeon John Hunter, after performing an autopsy on a person who had died in a fit of anger, declared: "My life is in the hands of any rascal who chooses to annoy me." Hunter's words proved true. In 1793, he collapsed and died soon after leaving an acrimonious meeting.

Different manifestations of coronary heart disease were noted over the next century. Although the first diagnosis before death probably occurred in 1878, recognition of the condition remained limited until technological means of diagnosis became common in the twentieth century. The new technology owed something to an ancient diagnostic technique – feeling the pulse, practiced at least since antiquity. The rate and pattern of the pulse were analyzed, with rhythmic abnormalities of particular concern. John Floyer, who in 1709 constructed a portable clock to time patients' pulses, noted that rates varied according to geographic location, age, and sex.

An extremely slow pulse – among the most striking abnormalities – was often associated with **syncope**. This condition has come to be known as **Stokes–Adams disease** after Dublin physicians Robert Adams and William Stokes, who described it in the first half of the nineteenth century. Today the condition is treated with pacemakers. In 1859, French physiologist Etienne-Jules Marey devised an instrument that produced a record of cardiac pulsations on a drum of paper. With this device, Marey recorded the pressure within a horse's heart, and also made pressure tracings from human surface arteries. In the 1890s, English physician James Mackenzie developed the polygraph, which recorded blood-vessel pulsations onto a continuous strip of paper, and he subsequently described many pulse abnormalities, identifying the cardiac causes of several. London physician Thomas Lewis analyzed cardiac rhythms with the electrocardiogram (EKG), a new instrument that recorded electrical signals generated by the heart. Invented in 1902 by Willem Einthoven, the EKG earned its inventor a 1924 Nobel Prize.

James Herrick of Chicago saw that the EKG could help diagnose diseases undetectable by the unaided senses – such as coronary artery disease. Herrick's 1912 description of this condition received little attention; however, after collaborating in 1918–19 with Fred Smith to describe the characteristic EKG changes, Herrick's definition of coronary artery disease became widely recognized. This was an early example of a pattern repeated throughout the twentieth century: A disease first described clinically would become more widely accepted as a disease once it was defined in terms of a laboratory technique.

In 1628, Harvey was unable to measure the pressures and volumes in human hearts. Physicians' regular use of such measurements today largely results from a self-experiment. In 1929, Werner Forssmann, working in a small German hospital, became fascinated by a nineteenth century diagram showing Marey's recorded pressures from a horse's heart. Forssmann decided to perform a similar procedure on himself, passing a catheter from the main vein in his arm up into his heart. However, he needed cooperation from the surgical nurse, who controlled access to the instruments. Forssmann was so successful in convincing the nurse that she insisted he perform the experiment on her. He persuaded her to lie on a cart, where he strapped her down. With the nurse immobilized, Forssmann inserted the catheter into his own arm, pushed it through the veins into his heart, and then released the nurse. She helped him walk downstairs, and X-rays confirmed the catheter's placement within his heart. The experiment earned Forssmann some praise but more hostility, and he abandoned working on cardiac catheterization.

Others, however, went forward with Forssmann's method. In 1932, Dickinson Richards and André Cournand at New York Hospital needed blood samples from the right atrium, the cardiac chamber that collects blood from the body before pumping it to the lungs to receive oxygen. They practiced Forssmann's technique on animals and determined that it did not significantly interfere with cardiac functioning. Although their first attempt on a patient was unsuccessful, Cournand eventually showed that it was safe to insert a catheter routinely into the right side of the heart.

During the next few years, Richards, Cournand, and colleagues designed a new catheter and constructed a device that recorded four different pressure tracings along with the EKG. In 1942, they advanced the catheter into the right ventricle, and in 1944 into the pulmonary artery, making it possible to measure hemodynamic pressure and the oxygen content of the blood at each stage of passage through the right side of the heart. They outlined the profound effects of reduced blood volume on cardiac output and described how to reverse the condition by blood replacement. Later, they used the same technique to diagnose congenital and acquired cardiac defects, particularly diseases of the heart valves. Richards and Cournand shared a 1956 Nobel Prize with Forssmann.

Soon, the technique was extended to measure pressures on the left side of the heart, which greatly aided understanding of various forms of **congestive heart failure**. Other investigators have shown how injecting dye into the heart can aid diagnosis. Today, passing diagnostic catheters into the heart is so routine that patients may not even spend a night in the hospital.

Western ideas about heart disease are based increasingly on technological diagnosis and the ability to invade the thorax for purposes of diagnosis and intervention. Along with increased use of technology has come the pervasive assumption that diagnosis has finally become objective, transcultural, and reflective of some inevitable underlying system. The validity of this assumption is doubtful. Historical analysis shows that definitions of heart disease are products of both biology and culture.

Anatomic linkage of the heart and vessels as a single unit was common in the nineteenth century. Around the end of that century, however, the conceptualization of heart disease changed fundamentally. British physicians started to consider the heart in terms of functional capacity rather than anatomy. This led them to regard **cardiac murmurs**, such as are detected by a stethoscope, as less important than physiological measurements of function.

This conceptual change was particularly apparent regarding a military ailment once called **DaCosta's syndrome** and later – at the start of World War I – "soldier's heart." Afflicted by breathlessness and a feeling of impending doom, soldiers with this syndrome were initially treated with extended bedrest. The presence of a cardiac murmur was taken as ipso facto evidence of heart disease. However, as the war continued, heart disease became a serious military, economic, and political problem. It was the third most common reason for military discharge. Yet heart disease offered far more hope of return to service than did the most common cause of discharge, "wounds and injuries." Nonetheless, the long convalescence strained both military hospitals and the political fortunes of England's leaders, who instituted a military draft in 1916. Given the political exigencies, physicians reconceptualized the disease as **effort syndrome**. They decided that heart murmurs were important only insofar as they impaired working ability and prescribed regulated exercise rather than hospitalization. Thus, many soldiers previously declared unfit for service were reclassified as "fit." All of this demonstrates that some notions about what constitutes heart disease are informed by social needs.

Physicians' ideas continue to be shaped by social context. For example, studies of incidence of heart disease in black Americans in the early twentieth century led many to conclude that **coronary disease** was rare in blacks, largely because they were considered less likely to experience stress and less intellectually alert.

In another example from the late twentieth century, it was suggested that failure to appreciate differences between the German and American concepts of heart disease could lead to the erroneous conclusion that death rates from **ischemic heart disease** are lower in Germany than in the United States. In fact, the rates are similar, but that condition is more likely to be called "ischemic heart disease" in the United States and **cardiac insufficiency** in Germany.

Changes in disease classification reflect both social and biological events. There has been a significant change in the types of disease from which people die. During the twentieth century, classification methods helped make heart disease an increasingly important cause of death and disability. The predominant causes of sickness and death were once infectious diseases. In the mid-nineteenth century, for example, **tuberculosis** caused possibly one-seventh of all deaths in Western Europe. Yet infectious diseases have subsequently decreased in many parts of the world.

Two major forms of heart disease related to infection have undergone a dramatic shift. **Rheumatic fever**, caused by a **streptococcal infection**, was once a major agent of heart disease in the West. In industrialized countries, it has now become relatively minor, but in other parts of the world, **rheumatic heart disease** remains a serious problem.

Endocarditis, an infection of the heart valves, carried an almost certain death sentence before the advent of antibiotics. At one time, it primarily afflicted people with **valvular damage** caused by rheumatic heart disease. Now endocarditis is most often a disease of intravenous drug abusers.

There has also been an increase in average life expectancy. People now live long enough to succumb to diseases that develop slowly, such as many cardiac diseases, particularly coronary heart disease. Lifestyles, too, have changed. Lack of physical activity and changes in diet may contribute to increased coronary heart disease.

Coronary disease has become the major form of heart disease in industrialized countries and is a major object of attention, much of which is focused on explaining geographic and historical changes in the pattern of disease. Accounting for 47 percent of all deaths in the United States in 1986, heart disease is by far the leading cause of death, with myocardial infarction the most common diagnosis. Many more people suffer from heart disease than die from it. The physical activity of one-quarter of heart-disease patients is limited, making the condition an important cause of disability as well as death.

As a cause of death in the United States, heart disease was once behind **pneumonia, influenza,** tuberculosis, **diarrhea, enteritis,** and **intestinal ulceration.** A sharp upward trend in coronary disease became apparent around 1920, and it was recognized with increasing frequency throughout the first half of the twentieth century. By 1940, only two disease categories with death rates of more than 100 per 100,000 remained: **cancer** and diseases of the heart.

The death rate from heart diseases then began a dramatic series of changes, peaking in 1963 and declining continuously since then. However, that decline has been unevenly distributed. Heart-disease mortality in California, for example, peaked relatively early, around 1955, and the subsequent decline there was repeated in other parts of the United States throughout the 1960s and 1970s. By 1986, the death rate for coronary heart disease was 55 percent of the 1966 rate.

Countries such as Australia, New Zealand, and Canada have experienced similar declines in coronary-disease mortality among men. Other countries, however, have seen significant increases, from Scotland and Northern Ireland (initially comparable to the United States) to Poland and Switzerland (initially having death rates much lower than the United States).

Studies of changing patterns of cardiac disease have contributed to the invention of "risk factor," a notion receiving widespread attention as a way of conceptualizing the causes of many diseases. Current explanations for historical and geographic differences in coronary-disease mortality derive much from the concept of risk factor. Studies have identified several factors contributing to the likelihood of coronary heart disease. Some of these cannot be modified. For example, men are more likely to suffer heart disease than women; older people are more likely to develop it than younger ones; and those having a family history of early cardiac disease are at greater risk than those without such history.

However, other factors can be modified. Cigarette smoking dramatically increases the likelihood of a coronary event and constitutes the greatest and most preventable cause of heart disease. Once a person stops smoking, the risk rapidly declines to approximately the same level as if the person had never smoked. **High blood pressure** and **diabetes** are also important risk factors.

Studies have clearly demonstrated a consistently positive relationship between increased serum cholesterol level in the form of low density lipoprotein and the rate of heart disease. At high levels the association is particularly strong. Good evidence exists that lowering cholesterol levels with drug therapy will lower death rates from coronary disease. Exercise, too, has a beneficial effect on the types of lipids circulating in the bloodstream.

Alcohol intake in small quantities – two or fewer drinks per day – may diminish the risk of coronary disease. However, alcohol in greater amounts is clearly associated with greater morbidity and mortality from both cardiac and noncardiac disease.

In many parts of the world, other types of heart disease are more common than coronary disease. **Endomyocardial fibrosis**, for example, is common in the tropical belts of Africa and South America. The disease characteristically leads to heart failure, accounting for up to 20 percent of such patients in Uganda, Sudan, and Nigeria. It affects indigenous people as well as foreign visitors. Its precise cause is yet unknown.

In much of South America, the parasite *Schistosoma mansoni* is a common cause of heart disease. Also common in South America is **Chagas' disease**. Other heart diseases having characteristic geographic patterns include forms of **congenital heart disease** that are significant for people living at high altitudes, where the concentration of oxygen is reduced. **Peripartum cardiac failure** develops in up to 1 percent of women in Nigeria and appears to result largely from cultural patterns. In this respect it resembles coronary heart disease, which is linked to Western culture in ways that we identify as risk factors and in ways that we do not fully understand.

The heart continues to have a central place in Western medicine. In the past few decades, many new approaches have been directed at heart disease. Concepts of heart disease are drawn from general cultural concepts of what it means to be human, and studies of how and when they change will increase our understanding not only of the history of medicine but of history in general.

Joel D. Howell

67. Herpes Simplex

Herpes simplex is caused by the herpes virus *hominis*, of which there are two types, HSV-1 and HSV-2. In general, the first causes disease above the waist, such as **cold sores**; the second causes disease below the waist, especially **genital herpes**. The active phase is followed by prolonged latency, but the virus can be reactivated by infection, stress, exposure, or any number of other circumstances.

Characteristics

Herpes viruses are visible by electron microscopy and may be grown in the laboratory. Some animals react differently to HSV-1 and HSV-2. Infection with herpes simplex results from person-to-person contact.

HSV-1 is commonly transmitted through kissing or sharing eating utensils, and thus infection can easily spread within a family. Normally, **HSV-1 infection** is bothersome but has no serious consequences, except when the virus invades the cornea. **Corneal herpes** may produce scars that impair vision.

HSV-2 infection is generally the result of sexual transmission. Lesions appear on the penis, vulva, buttocks, and adjacent areas. The prevalence of HSV-2 infection during pregnancy and its incidence in neonates are related to the socioeconomic level, age, and sexual activity of a population. Infants are safe from infection if the mother's condition clears 3–4 weeks before delivery. But women who suffer from genital herpes during pregnancy may be three times more likely to abort during the first 20 weeks

than other women. Neonatal infection is usually HSV-2 from an infected birth canal. In addition, some evidence links HSV-2 to **cervical cancer**.

Unknown factors cause reactivation of the virus (**recurrent herpes**). Studies of reccurent herpes show inexplicable differences in recurrence: 45 percent in Britain, 40 percent in North America, 30 percent in Europe and Africa, 17 percent in Asia, and 16 percent in South America.

HSV-2 has been studied more intensively in recent years than HSV-1. Most observers agree that **herpes genitalis** has been on the increase. In 1983 there were an estimated 20 million cases in the United States, with 300,000–500,000 new cases developing annually. Publicity and wider use of diagnostic tests may account for some of the apparent increase. Certainly, publicity has alerted the public and the medical profession to the disease.

The initial lesion is a small, reddened area that develops into a small, thin-walled, blisterlike vesicle filled with clear fluid. **Labial herpes** only occasionally represents the initial HSV-1 lesion, but the "cold sore" or "fever blister" of the lip is the most common lesion of recurrent disease. Here a cluster of vesicles appears, to last up to 10 days. These usually appear at the line of the skin of the lower lip or on the skin of the upper lip, at times extending to or into the nostril. **Conjunctivitis** may also be the primary lesion of the infection. **Cutaneous herpes** (HSV-1) may involve the skin of the body, anywhere above the waist and including the feet.

Herpes genitalis has an incubation period of several days. It may be subclinical, especially in women. Infection is more obvious in men with localized pain and development of vesicles on the penis. Urethral involvement in both sexes is manifested by **dysuria** (painful urination), and a discharge may be noted in male patients. Pelvic pain accompanying dysuria is common in women. Infection with HSV-2 often is accompanied by systemic symptoms during the first several days.

Some studies show recurrences within the first year in 80 percent of HSV-2 infections. Recurrent cases commonly show milder symptoms, are of shorter duration, and rarely exhibit overt systemic symptoms. The lesions appear on the genitalia and adjacent areas. In some patients, recurrences cease some years following the onset of disease. In others, however, recurrences last many years. Febrile illness may be a provoking factor in HSV-1 recurrences, but what triggers recurrent genital herpes is unclear. Stress, fever, heat, trauma, and coitus have all been suggested.

History

"Herpes" derives from the Greek "to creep." The oldest record of disease of the genitalia appears in the *Ebers Papyrus* (c. 1550 B.C.), with nonspecific commentary on a patient's inflamed vulva and thighs. The same papyrus, however, describes "herpes of the face." Hippocrates mentioned "herpetic sores," "ulcerations of the mouth, [and] frequent fluxations of the genital organs." Herodotus described eruptions "which appear about the mouth at the crisis of simple fevers," and both Hebrew and Byzantine texts contain references to what was probably herpes.

The first definitive description of herpes was published by Jean Astruc in 1736. His description of vesicles strongly suggests those of herpes genitalis. Toward the end of the eighteenth century, English physician Robert Willan developed a classification of the many skin diseases, including a category of vesiculae.

In 1818, Thomas Bateman described **herpes labialis**. He emphasized the hazard of interpreting a cluster of vesicles as a **syphilitic chancre**. He discussed the development of the vesicles and their course to healing and noted that the disease was "liable to recur in the same individual."

Later, in 1832, Jean Louis Alibert not only described **herpes praeputialis** but stated that the lesion may occur at the introitus of the vagina. In 1853, F. L. Legendre described **herpes of the vulva**, with the observation that it may recur some days before menstruation.

Herpes progenitalis was discussed in 1881 by Boston physician F. B. Greenough. He made the important observation that one of the "three" venereal diseases had existed before the appearance of herpes genitalis. In addition, Greenough made the surprising observation that he had never seen an instance of genital herpes in a woman. This prompted an investigation into the incidence of the disease among women, and in 1883 Paul Unna of Hamburg not only concluded that women did contract herpes, but suggested that women who were prostitutes contracted it at a greater rate than men.

In 1890, R. Bergh of Copenhagen confirmed a high incidence of herpes genitalis among prostitutes, but he rejected any relationship between herpes genitalis and venereal disease and concluded the lesions were of a nervous origin, resulting from congestion of the parts.

In 1921, B. Lipschütz successfully inoculated material from genital vesicles into the skin of human subjects. Four years later, S. Flexner and H. L. Amos demonstrated the herpes virus, and in 1934 Albert Sabin isolated it. In 1962, K. E. Schneweiss identified two strains of herpes, a finding confirmed by W. R. Dowdle and A. I. Nahmias in 1967. Research in subsequent years has contributed to knowledge concerning epidemiology and immunology.

R. H. Kampmeier

68. Herpesviruses

The family of **herpesviruses** (Herpetoviridae) includes **herpes simplex** 1 and 2, **varicella zoster, Epstein–Barr virus,** and **cytomegalovirus.** All are double-stranded DNA viruses of icosahedral form, enclosed in a lipid-containing envelope, and ranging in size from 120 to 180 nanometers. See: **Cytomegalovirus Infection, Herpes Simplex, Infectious Mononucleosis, Varicella-Zoster Virus Disease (Chickenpox).**

R. H. Kampmeier

69. Histoplasmosis

Histoplasmosis is an infection caused by inhaling *Histoplasma capsulatum,* a soil fungus; the primary infection is in the lung. The disease is usually benign and self-limited, despite a strong tendency to invade the bloodstream during primary infection. This **fungemia** seeds reticuloendothelial organs throughout the body. Under favorable conditions, the organism can cause progressive disease at multiple sites, resulting in a wide variety of clinical manifestations.

Characteristics

H. capsulatum is most common in temperate climates along river valleys and has been found in North, Central, and South America; India; Southeast Asia; and Europe. By far the most heavily endemic region in the world is the east central United States, particularly the Mississippi and Ohio river valleys. It is most prevalent in the states of Ohio, Kentucky, Indiana, Illinois, Kentucky, Tennessee, and Arkansas. Surrounding states also have many infections.

Infection is almost universal in heavily endemic areas. Skin-test surveys reveal that over 90 percent of persons in some central U.S. counties have had histoplasmosis before age 20. Probably 40–50 million people in the central United States have had histoplasmosis, and several hundred thousand new cases occur each year. However, the number of serious infections requiring diagnosis and treatment is negligible, perhaps 1 or 2 percent of the total.

H. capsulatum grows as a fluffy white mycelium, which bears microconidia; the organism is free-living in nature in this form. In warmer temperatures, it grows as a yeast – and takes this form in infected tissue.

A minor disturbance of fungus-laden soil may scatter spores into the air. The microconidia are inhaled, causing infection. Within the lung, the organism converts to the yeast phase, which is not infectious. Person-to-person transmission does not occur. So-called epidemics of histoplasmosis are more accurately point-source outbreaks. Most cases, however, are sporadic, resulting from casual exposure to environmental spores. Patients with sporadic illness probably inhale fewer spores and are more likely to be asymptomatic or minimally symptomatic. Most infections are never recognized and are known to exist only as a result of skin-test surveys.

Primary pulmonary histoplasmosis is asymptomatic at least half the time. Symptomatic patients become ill about 2 weeks after exposure, with influenza-like fever, chills, myalgias, headache, and a nonproductive cough. Rare manifestations include **arthralgias, arthritis,** and **erythema nodosum**. With or without symptoms, the chest roentgenogram may show patchy areas of **pneumonitis** and prominent **hilar adenopathy**. Following exposure to an unusually heavy inoculum, more diffuse pulmonary involvement may occur, with extensive nodular infiltrate on the chest roentgenogram. **Dyspnea** may appear alongside other symptoms, and symptoms are more severe and last longer. Most patients recover without treatment, but extreme cases may progress to respiratory failure.

Chronic cavitary histoplasmosis may occur anywhere in the lung but usually involves both upper lobes and closely resembles reinfection **tuberculosis**. The mechanism of infection, however, is not endogenous reactivation. Rather, the infection is the result of a primary infection in abnormal lungs, typically the lungs of middle-aged or older male smokers who have centrilobular **emphysema**. **Acute pulmonary histoplasmosis** in this setting usually resolves uneventfully although very slowly. In about a third of cases, infected air spaces persist. A progressive fibrosing and cavitary process gradually destroys adjacent areas of the lung. Chronic cough is the most common symptom. Constitutional symptoms, including low-grade fever, night sweats, and weight loss, increase as the illness progresses.

Disseminated histoplasmosis is any progressive extrapulmonary infection. There is a range of infection with different tissue responses. At one extreme there are massive numbers of organisms in all reticuloendothelial organs with little tendency to granuloma formation. This type of disseminated histoplasmosis has been called the "infantile" form and may lead to death within days or weeks. Other patients, often older adults, have a more indolent illness, many months in duration, characterized by low or moderate fever, weight loss, and skin and mucous membrane lesions. The condition can also occur as an opportunistic infection.

Disseminated histoplasmosis often presents as a nonspecific systemic febrile illness rather than as a pulmonary infection. There is usually no cough. The chest roentgenogram may be normal. The disease may also present as a more localized infection, such as histoplasmosis of the central nervous system; **meningeal histoplasmosis**; and isolated **gastrointestinal histoplasmosis**, which often involves the terminal ileum. All are extremely rare.

The histoplasmin skin test is a valuable epidemiological tool that has permitted mapping of the endemic area. However, it is worthless in individual case diagnosis. A positive skin test means only that the person is one of many millions who have had histoplasmosis, probably remotely and without sequelae. It does not mean that a current illness under investigation is being caused by the fungus.

Primary histoplasmosis is usually not diagnosed at all. Serologic tests are most useful for diagnosing patients who have already recovered. Patients with rapidly progressive **pneumonia** not responding to antibacterial antibiotics need urgent diagnosis, especially if respiratory failure is impending or actually develops. Some patients are diagnosed by serology. Others require lung biopsy for histopathological diagnosis.

Chronic cavitary histoplasmosis is easier to diagnose. The pace is slower. Tuberculosis is suspected first, but the tuberculin skin test is negative and the sputum is negative for tuberculosis. Sputum cultures for *H. capsulatum* are usually positive, as are serologic tests. Disseminated histoplasmosis is difficult to diagnose because it is so nonspecific. Serologic tests are positive in over half of cases and may provide an important clue. Histopathological examination of tissue biopsies is the method of diagnosis in most cases. Bone marrow biopsy is particularly valuable in febrile illnesses without localizing features. Cultures of blood, bone marrow, and other tissues and of body fluids may also give the diagnosis.

History

In 1906, Samuel Darling described an infection of the reticuloendothelial system caused by an organism that he believed was protozoan. Macrophages were filled with small organisms. Within a few years, he reported two other cases. In 1913, H. da Rocha-Lima speculated that the organism might be a fungus rather than a protozoan.

In 1926, W. Riley and C. Watson credited Darling with being first to describe the infection in 1906. Later, however, some confusion arose as to whether a 1906 report by R. Strong had described histoplasmosis first. But in a personal letter many years later, Strong stated that the case he had described was not histoplasmosis but rather a rare human infection with *Cryptococcus farciminosus*, the cause of **farcy** in horses. Thus credit for the first case description remains with Darling, who recognized the disease as previously undescribed and named the organism and the illness.

Scattered reports of similar cases followed, mostly from the central United States. Then in 1934, the first premortem diagnosis of such a patient was made. The infectious agent was isolated and proved to be a fungus, and its thermal dimorphism was demonstrated.

In 1945, a review of 78 cases concluded that histoplasmosis was a rare systemic infection that was nearly always fatal. However, in the same year, A. Christie and J. Peterson and also C. Palmer demonstrated that great numbers of asymptomatic persons in the central United States had been infected with the fungus. Furthermore, they showed that almost all tuberculin-negative persons with chest calcifications had positive histoplasmin skin tests. The endemic area was mapped, and fungus was isolated from the soil. The new conclusion was that histoplasmosis is very common and almost invariably benign and self-limited. Fatal cases were rare and exceptional.

Most skin-test reactors in early surveys had had asymptomatic or minimally symptomatic nonspecific infections. The retrospective discovery of a highly symptomatic but also self-limited form of primary histoplasmosis soon followed. Small groups of patients exposed to high concentrations of organisms, often in closed spaces, had been verified as victims of epidemics of an unknown but relatively severe pulmonary illness. An epidemiological investigation of one such outbreak, which occurred in 1944 and was reported 3 years later, demonstrated convincingly that *H. capsulatum* had been the offending agent. Upper-lobe cavitary histoplasmosis resembling tuberculosis was first described in 1956 among sanitorium patients being treated for tuberculosis.

In 1955 came the isolation of amphotericin B, and within a few years the drug was available for treatment of a wide variety of fungal infections. This drug, despite some toxicity, proved highly effective for histoplasmosis and remains the agent to which newer alternatives must be compared. Ketoconazole, a nontoxic oral imidazole, arrived in the 1980s. It is not as effective as amphotericin B but is reasonable therapy for mild to moderately ill patients with chronic cavitary disease and indolent forms of disseminated disease.

With the increase in the use of glucocorticoids and cytotoxic drugs for malignant and nonmalignant diseases, disseminated histoplasmosis assumed increasing importance. Endogenous reactivation was suspected as a mechanism in some cases because the illness presented as a nonspecific febrile illness. Treatment with amphotericin B was very effective if the diagnosis was made quickly and if the patient had some degree of cell-mediated immune response.

Finally, **AIDS** brought a new level of suppression of the cell-mediated immune system. The concept of endogenous reactivation

received further support: Unlike other immunosuppressed patients, even those AIDS patients who respond to treatment are not cured but require long-term suppressive therapy to prevent relapse of infection.

Scott F. Davies

70. Hookworm Infection

Ancylostomiasis, or **hookworm disease**, is caused by **hookworm infection** and is characterized by progressive **anemia**. Perhaps one billion people, mostly in tropical and subtropical regions, are afflicted to some extent with hookworm infection, although it is not known how many thus infected can be said to be victims of hookworm disease. A host whose diet contains adequate amounts of iron may sustain a worm burden without debilitating consequences that would render a malnourished person anemic. A person exhibiting signs of the anemia, therefore, may be said to have hookworm disease regardless of the number of parasites present. Hookworm disease is an important contributing factor in millions of deaths annually and a source in its own right of widespread human suffering.

Characteristics

Two species of intestinal **nematode**, *Ancylostoma duodenale* and *Necator americanus*, are the parasites that cause ancylostomiasis. *A. duodenale* can be ingested in contaminated food, water, or possibly breast milk, but the more common route of infection, and the only one for *N. americanus*, is through penetration of the skin. Larvae in the soil typically enter through the skin of the feet, frequently causing **dermatitis**, once called "ground itch" or "dew poison" in the southern United States, and "water itch" or "coolie itch" in India. The parasites travel through the bloodstream to the alveoli of the lungs, climb the respiratory tree, and make their way into the esophagus. During their migration through the airways, the host sometimes develops a cough, wheeziness, or temporary hoarseness.

The hookworms are swallowed and pass into the gut, where some successfully attach themselves to the small intestinal mucosa and begin nourishing themselves on their host's blood. In the small intestine, hookworms grow to about 1 centimeter, maturing in 6–8 weeks. Depending on the species, hookworms generally live from 1–5 years, although a few apparently live longer. The adult female may produce thousands of ova per day, which pass out of the body with the host's feces. If deposited on warm, moist soil, the eggs produce larvae that can survive in a free-living state for over a month before finding a host.

Hookworms thrive on human ignorance and poverty. If the billions of people living in areas of hookworm infestation were able to eat moderately well, wear good shoes, and defecate in latrines, hookworm disease would soon no longer pose a serious threat to human health. Understood as an index of socioeconomic status, hookworm infection will likely remain a daunting public-health problem as long as there are poor people, inadequately educated, living in warm climates.

The earliest global survey of hookworm distribution, in 1910, led to a preliminary description of a "hookworm belt" girdling the Earth between 30° south latitude and 36° north. Another survey conducted at the same time estimated that 40 percent of the inhabitants of the southern United States suffered in varying degrees from hookworm infection. Although infection has not been eliminated in the United States, the public-health menace of hookworm disease has disappeared, largely as an incidental consequence of the concentration of the population in cities and towns with sewer systems, and the general improvement in sanitary conditions and the standard of living for those remaining on the farms. Likewise in Europe, where the disease was sometimes found in mines, hookworm infection is no longer a problem. In Japan as well, rising living standards and antihookworm campaigns have eradicated the disease.

It is still, however, a chronic fact of life in most of the rest of the regions within the old "hookworm belt." In the Caribbean, Central and South America, Africa, China, India, Southeast Asia, and Oceania, endemic hookworm infection remains widespread and largely untreated. After a flurry of activity in the first three decades of the twentieth century, hookworm prevention and treatment programs have been sporadic and uncoordinated. This recent history of neglect has made it difficult even to estimate the incidence of hookworm disease in areas of the world where hookworm infection is known to be prevalent.

Hookworm disease shares many of the clinical symptoms accompanying other kinds of anemia. Severely infected persons have a pale and wan appearance, a telltale yellow-green pallor that explains why the disease was sometimes called "Egyptian chlorosis" or "tropical chlorosis." In children, growth may be significantly retarded. A distended abdomen and pronounced, sharply pointed shoulder blades ("pot belly" and "angel wings" in the American South) were once thought to identify children with hookworm disease, although the same features often accompany malnutrition as well.

In pregnant women, hookworm infection increases the likelihood of fetal morbidity. Victims of hookworm anemia may be chronically sluggish, listless, and easily tired, symptoms that prompted a facetious journalist early in the twentieth century to dub hookworm the "germ of laziness." **Dropsy**, dizziness or giddiness, **indigestion**, shortness of breath, **tachycardia**, and in extreme cases **congestive heart failure** have also all been associated with advanced hookworm disease. Hookworm sufferers sometimes eat dirt, chalk, or clay as well.

Since the nineteenth century, dozens of anthelmintic drugs have been tried, including thymol, oil of chenopodium, carbon tetrachloride, and tetrachloroethylene. More recently developed hookworm vermifuges include bephenium, mebendazole, pyrantel, and thiabendazole. A regimen combining chemotherapy with simultaneous administration of iron tablets now seems to be the most effective way to eliminate the parasites and at the same time to restore the hemoglobin to a normal level quickly. The probability of reinfection is high, however, if a person thus treated continues to walk barefooted on ground contaminated with hookworm larvae. This discouraging realization has bedeviled public-health workers since the days of the massive control programs.

History

The *Ebers Papyrus* (c. 1550 B.C.) describes a mysterious affliction, "a-a-a disease," thought by some to be **hookworm anemia**, but by others, **schistosomiasis**. In the fifth century B.C., Hippocrates described a pathological condition marked by dirt eating, intestinal distress, and a yellowish complexion. A handful of other sketchy descriptions from the Mediterranean basin in the ancient and early medieval periods appear to be reports of hookworm disease. From the Western Hemisphere in the centuries after European colonization came scattered accounts from English, French, Spanish, and Portuguese settlers of epidemics among their slaves, called by a rich variety of colloquial names and now thought to be widespread hookworm infestation.

Italian physician Angelo Dubini was first to report hookworms in a human, detecting them during autopsy in 1838. Dubini examined 100 cadavers for hookworms and found them in more than 20. He provided a detailed description of the parasite, which he named "*Agchylostoma*" (a faulty transliteration of the Greek words for "hook" and "mouth") *duodenale*. By 1846, Dubini's parasites had been found in Egypt and, by 1865, in Brazil. In 1878, Italian scientists announced their detection of hookworm ova in feces of anemic patients, making it possible for anyone with a microscope to diagnose hookworm infection. In the 1880s, Edoardo Perroncito argued that the presence of hookworms in large numbers was causally related to a major epidemic of anemia. In 1881, Camillo Bozzolo reported his success using thymol to treat the infection. For the next 35 years, thymol remained the most widely used drug in the treatment of hookworm disease.

In 1898, Arthur Looss first suggested that hookworm larvae could penetrate the skin. He had accidentally infected himself by spilling water contaminated with hookworm larvae on his hand. Shortly afterward, the spot on his hand where the water had spilled began to burn and turned red. Although Looss's announcement was initially greeted with considerable skepticism, further experimentation had by 1901 confirmed beyond doubt the percutaneous route of infection. Looss would later describe the migratory path of the hookworm within the host.

While Looss was developing his theory of skin penetration in Egypt, a U.S. Army physician stationed in Puerto Rico, Bailey K. Ashford, discovered in 1899 that hookworm infection was rampant among agricultural workers in the cane fields. In 1903, Ashford persuaded the governor to budget funds for the creation of the Anemia Commission of Puerto Rico, the first large antihookworm program of its kind.

Ashford believed that the hookworms he found in Puerto Rico were *A. duodenale*. At the time of his discovery, no other species was known to infect humans. Charles Stiles examined Ashford's hookworms and others from different parts of the United States. He compared them with samples of *A. duodenale* and concluded in 1902 that the former were a different species indigenous to the Western Hemisphere, which he named *Necator americanus*. In 1905, Looss found *N. americanus* in Central African pygmies and speculated that it originated in the Eastern Hemisphere and was brought to the Americas by African slaves. Within 2 years, *N. americanus* had been found extensively not only in Africa but also in India and Australia. Whether *A. duodenale* might also have been introduced into the Americas at about the same time via early European contact has been disputed. The theory that *A. duodenale* existed in pre-Columbian America was bolstered by the 1974 discovery of what appears to be *A. duodenale* in the intestine of a Peruvian mummy dating from about 900 A.D. Both species are widespread in both hemispheres, although their origins remain murky.

In 1909, John D. Rockefeller created an organization to eradicate hookworm disease in the southern United States, although Stiles maintained that eradication was an unrealistic goal. With $1 million, the Rockefeller Sanitary Commission established operations in 11 American states. Over its 5-year existence, it awakened the public to the nature and extent of the threat, stimulated widespread concern for improved sanitation, treated almost 700,000 people, and invigorated long-moribund state boards of health. It failed, however, to eradicate hookworm infection anywhere.

In 1914, the Rockefeller Foundation undertook a worldwide campaign modeled on the experience of the Rockefeller Sanitary Commission, opening operations in the British West Indies before extending into British Guiana, Egypt, Ceylon, and Malaya. By the end of World War I, Rockefeller programs were under way or planned in Central America, Brazil, and China, and soon thereafter were in place in most tropical countries. The earlier experience in the southern United States led administrators to employ a dual approach. The dispensary method attracted people from the surrounding area to a day-long demonstration conducted by a Rockefeller physician assisted by microscopists, during which examinations were carried out and treatments dispensed, while the crowd heard lectures on prevention and improved sanitation. The intensive method involved selection of a clearly delimited area for a saturation campaign of aggressive hookworm treatment and latrine construction.

Beginning in the early 1920s, the Rockefeller Foundation began to rethink its basic approach. The extensive, protracted campaigns had produced negligible results. The incidence of hookworm infection in Puerto Rico, for example, was as high in 1920 as it had been in 1903, just before Ashford's Anemia Commission began its work. Not yet prepared to abandon hookworm work altogether, the Rockefeller Foundation gradually withdrew from massive treatment campaigns and redirected its efforts toward laboratory research, with fieldwork restricted to data gathering and testing hypotheses and drugs.

By the mid-1920s, disillusionment had set in and the days of the antihookworm crusades were over. Since then, although laboratory work has revealed much more about the relationship between humans and hookworms, little has been done in a practical way to rid the former of the latter, except where living conditions have improved.

John Ettling

71. Huntington's Disease (Chorea)

Huntington's disease (HD) is a rare progressive neurological disorder, in which normal central nervous system development is succeeded in early adulthood by premature and selective neuronal death. First-rank symptoms consist of rapid, involuntary jerking movements, or **chorea**, caused by lesions in the putamen and the caudate nucleus, and a progressive **dementia** from loss of cells in the cerebral cortex. Onset of symptoms is typically in the third or fourth decade, and the clinical course is progressive and relentless over a period of 10–30 years. At autopsy, gross examination of HD brains reveals severe, symmetrical atrophy of frontal and temporal lobes as well as, to a lesser degree, the parietal and occipital lobes. The caudate nucleus is profoundly involved, and diffuse neuronal loss extends into the cerebral cortex, basal ganglia, thalamus, and spinal motor neurons. Various neurotransmitter systems are also progressively affected.

References to the disorder as early as 1841 have been found, but the first full description was by George Huntington in 1872. Discussing a large family on Long Island, Huntington distinguished the condition from other known choreiform movement disorders such as **Sydenham's chorea** ("Saint Vitus's dance"). The remarkable history of HD in the New World was recounted in 1932. Carriers of the mutant gene responsible for nearly all known cases of the disease sailed for Massachusetts from Suffolk in 1630. Upon arrival, these individuals founded family lines that included not only the Long Island cases but also the celebrated "Groton witch," whose violent and uncontrollable movements were recorded in 1671 as evidence of possession. Pedigrees encompassing the various branches of the families demonstrate a clear pattern of autosomal dominant transmission, meaning the disease will appear in one-half the offspring of an affected parent.

Since the first description of HD, numerous biochemical and histological studies have been undertaken, but the primary defect remains unknown. A major breakthrough occurred in 1983, when researchers announced discovery of an anonymous DNA sequence closely linked to the putative HD gene. This molecular probe, which has been refined by subcloning, is now a tool for presymptomatic diagnosis of HD.

Eric J. Devor

72. Hypertension

Hypertension is a condition of abnormally high blood pressure. Blood pressure is measured by the force exerted against artery walls during each heartbeat or pulse. The peak of the pressure wave occurs when the heart contracts (systole) and is called systolic pressure. The valley of the pressure wave occurs when the heart relaxes (diastole) and is termed diastolic pressure. Blood pressure is recorded as systolic over diastolic.

Although even slight blood-pressure elevations are associated with increased risk of premature death, the World Health Organization has recommended the following categories for classifying adults:

Hypertensive: Greater than or equal to 160
    millimeters of mercury (mmHg) systolic

and/or greater than or equal to 95 mmHg
    diastolic.
Normotensive: Less than or equal to 140
    mmHg systolic and less than or equal to 90
    mmHg diastolic.
Borderline hypertensive: Between hypertensive
    and normotensive.

The condition is also divided etiologically into two types. **Secondary hypertension**, resulting from some known cause (such as **kidney disease**), represents less than 10 percent of total hypertension incidence. **Primary hypertension** (also called **essential hypertension**), representing more than 90 percent of total incidence, arises from unknown causes.

Characteristics

In most societies, average blood-pressure levels and diseases associated with hypertension increase as people age; however, this is not the case in all populations. Indeed, hypertension seems virtually nonexistent in "Stone Age" societies. But surveys indicate that hypertension in developing countries is increasing.

Many have hypothesized that environmental factors cause hypertension, principally because when members of unacculturated populations – normally free of hypertension – migrate to urban areas, their blood pressures rise. Some postulate that dietary changes (especially salt intake) and/or weight gain occasion this phenomenon. Others suggest that increased psychosocial stress is to blame. Still others surmise that those with the greatest rise in blood pressure have a genetic predisposition to the disease that is sparked by environmental phenomena such as salt or stress.

Dietary factors that may affect blood pressure include salt (sodium chloride), potassium, magnesium, calcium, fat, and even licorice. Most interest has centered around salt – specifically its sodium component. The most compelling evidence for the influence of salt on blood pressure is that every low-salt-intake population ever studied has manifested low blood pressure without age-linked increases. Some surveys have suggested that stressful societies have higher mean blood-pressure levels than less stressful ones. Unfortunately, stress is difficult to measure, and any association between stress and blood pressure has been difficult to demonstrate in humans. Heredity is an important contributor to blood-pressure regulation, and hence to hypertension. Like many genetic traits, high blood pressure tends to run in families. Genetic influence is also revealed by the concordance of hypertension in siblings, especially identical twins.

Some humans are "salt sensitive" and others are not, which may represent an interactive relationship between genes and environment. In former times, isolated populations migrated into different ecological systems and perhaps experienced different "selection pressures" related to salt metabolism. These included different temperatures, salt intake, and mortality from salt-depletive diseases such as **diarrhea**, possibly resulting in a new genotype that enhanced survival in new environments by protecting against salt-depletive conditions. If this genotype included enhanced sodium-conserving ability, then such adaptations may predispose to **salt-sensitive hypertension** today. This may have occurred when many sub-Saharan Africans were forced to migrate to the Western Hemisphere. Mortality from salt-depletive diseases was high, and those with superior salt-retaining ability may have survived to pass their genes on to present-day African Americans. This enhanced salt-conserving ability may, therefore, be found more among Western Hemisphere blacks than among West African blacks and may help explain why the former group has a higher prevalence of hypertension than the latter.

History

For centuries, the only way to assess blood pressure was to feel the pulse and interpret its force and rhythm. About 2500 B.C., a Chinese physician remarked: "When the pulse is abundant but tense and hard like a cord, there are dropsical swellings."

Over 4,000 years later, in 1827, British physician Richard Bright suggested that certain dropsical swellings resulted from obstruction in the kidney's circulatory system. Bright's argument was so persuasive that throughout the nineteenth century most physicians considered a strong or tense pulse a symptom of kidney disease.

By the late nineteenth century, discoveries relating to systolic blood pressure led to invention of the sphygmomanometer (blood-pressure cuff). With the 1905 description of diastolic blood pressure, this device effectively replaced diagnosis by "pulse," and its widespread use led observers to realize that most hypertension patients did not have kidney disorders. The newly discovered condition was given various names: **angiosclerosis, presclerosis, hyperpiesis, primary hypertensive cardiovascular disease**, and essential hypertension. It was soon recognized as among the most common cardiovascular disorders.

During the 1930s and 1940s, researchers studied the influence of the sympathetic nervous system, the endocrine system, and the renal system on arterial pressure, noting several types of secondary hypertension. **Pheochromocytoma** was first reported in 1929, **Cushing's syndrome** in 1932, **pyelonephritis** in 1937, **renal artery stenosis** in 1938, and **Conn's syndrome** in 1955. In some cases, these "secondary" causes of hypertension were cured through surgery, but in most cases – those with essential hypertension – the cause remained unknown. One important breakthrough occurred among researchers in animal physiology.

In the 1920s, Harry Goldblatt progressively constricted blood flow to a dog's kidney, producing rapidly developing hypertension that resulted in death from heart failure. The experiment sparked a worldwide search for a renal-based pressor substance that produced hypertension. By the end of the 1930s, two teams, one in the United States and one in Argentina, simultaneously discovered that blood from "Goldblatt kidneys" contained a substance that caused vasoconstriction. The

North American group called the substance "angiotonin," while the Argentine group christened the compound "hypertensin." The two teams decided they were working on the same substance and combined the names for it; the substance became "angiotensin." These discoveries led to extensive research into the neural, cellular, and hemodynamic systems that control blood pressure, and eventually to the development of today's antihypertensive medications. These discoveries were extremely important, but researchers were still a long way from finding the cause of the disease.

In the 1950s and 1960s, two British physicians debated the influence of heredity on hypertension. Robert Platt argued that it was a "qualitative" disease, controlled by a single gene, with a bimodal population distribution. George Pickering reasoned that "hypertension" was only the upper end of a continuous unimodal distribution of blood-pressure levels. He thought that hypertension was a "quantitative" disease and was controlled by multiple genes in combination with environmental influences. The debate was never resolved. Research since then has tended to favor Pickering's quantitative definition, but not entirely.

Today, both environmental and genetic factors are under examination at the individual and population levels, but the cause of hypertension remains unknown. Fortunately, blood pressure is successfully being lowered through diet, stress reduction, exercise, weight control, and medication, in the hope that premature deaths from hypertension will be reduced.

Thomas W. Wilson and Clarence E. Grim

73. Infectious Hepatitis

The term **hepatitis** literally means any inflammation of the liver. Even when restricted by the term "infectious," it has many causes, including **malaria**, **yellow fever**, and numerous viruses. By convention, however, **infectious hepatitis** usually refers to a small group of diseases caused by several unrelated viruses, whose most obvious and consistent symptoms result from liver damage.

History

Until the mid-1900s, hepatitis was frequently equated with **jaundice**, although jaundice is only a sign of failure to clear normal breakdown products from the blood. Under this terminology, hepatitis and other liver diseases played an important role in early medical writings, but it is difficult to determine which references relate to hepatitis as we now know it, and which refer to various other causes of jaundice. It is even more difficult to distinguish one type of hepatitis from another in the early references. Hippocrates identified at least four kinds of jaundice, one of which he considered epidemic and thus, by implication, infectious. Another was "autumnal hepatitis"; this condition could have been **hepatitis A**. An emphasis on the liver has persisted into modern times in French popular medicine, where the liver is commonly blamed for ill-defined ailments.

Postclassical writers continued to have difficulty in distinguishing infectious forms from noninfectious forms of jaundice because of the variable incubation periods of infectious diseases. Clear recognition of the infectivity of hepatitis is usually ascribed to Pope Zacharias, who in the eighth century advocated quarantine of cases. This had little effect on general thinking, however, because of the variety of circumstances associated with different outbreaks. Many cases seemed to be sporadic, but epidemics of what must have been hepatitis A (or **enterically transmitted non-A, non-B hepatitis**, known as ET-NANBH) were known from the early seventeenth century to be common in troops under campaign conditions. An epidemic of **hepatitis B**, associated with a single lot of **smallpox** vaccine, was described in 1885. In spite of this, as late as 1908, the dominant medical opinion held that all hepatitis was due to obstruction of the bile duct. The picture did not begin to clear until the mid-twentieth century.

Hepatitis A

Hepatitis A is caused by an RNA virus 27 nanometers in diameter. It is very similar to **poliovirus** in general structure and also in its ability to spread through fecal contamination of food and water. The virus is fastidious in its host range. It is known to infect only humans, apes, and marmosets.

The virus of hepatitis A is essentially worldwide in distribution but is much commoner where drinking water is unsafe and sanitation inadequate. The prevalence of disease is often inversely related to the prevalence of virus. In less-developed countries, most people become immune through infection in childhood, often with no apparent illness. Persons from developed countries, however, especially when traveling in less-developed areas, are likely to become infected as adults with serious consequences.

Hepatitis A is manifested by general malaise, loss of appetite, and often jaundice. Specific diagnosis can be confirmed only by electron-microscopic examination of feces or, more practically, by demonstration of specific antibodies. The disease is seldom fatal when uncomplicated and rarely leaves sequelae. Recovery normally occurs in 4–8 weeks.

Specific identification of hepatitis A was not accomplished until the 1960s and afterward. Then, the development of methods for recognizing hepatitis B, and the demonstration of two distinct agents in studies of children, made its existence apparent. The agent of this disease remained enigmatic because it could not be propagated, except in humans. The virus was identified in 1973. An attenuated vaccine has been produced and successfully tested but not marketed because of continuing production problems.

Hepatitis B

The cause of hepatitis B is a very unusual virus. Most important, it is unusually stable and can withstand boiling temperatures and drying without inactivation. Although the virus is of moderate size, 45 nanometer in diameter, it has the smallest DNA genome known. The protein forming the external surface of the virus is produced in such excess that the host immune system cannot cope and becomes paralyzed. The virus DNA can be integrated into human genetic material, to provide a secure resting place for the virus and, perhaps, to interfere with the host's growth-control mechanism and cause **cancer**.

The stability of hepatitis B virus means that it can persist on any article that is contaminated with blood, most significantly used needles and surgical instruments. In developed countries, it has usually been transmitted in this way. Precautions have reduced the incidence of this disease in most of the population, but it continues to be a serious problem among intravenous drug abusers.

Hepatitis B can also be sexually transmitted. It is excreted in the semen and transmitted from male to female and from male to male in this way. Because the heterosexual transmission does not form a complete cycle, this has been less of a problem among heterosexuals than in the male homosexual communities of Europe and North America.

The ability of the virus to remain infectious when dried means that it can persist on sharp stones and thorns along paths and, perhaps, also on the proboscises of mosquitoes. This provides a particularly important mode of spread in primitive societies.

The most serious pattern of hepatitis B infection is seen in South Asia and sub-Saharan Africa, where transmission from mother to child is common. Infection may occur during birth or via mother's milk. The significance of this pattern of transmission is that persistent infection is particularly likely to follow infection in early life, and **liver cancer** is a common sequela to persistent infection. In these parts of the world, cancer of the liver is the most common of all cancers and a major cause of death in middle age. The situation is self-perpetuating, in that persons infected in infancy are most likely to become carriers and, hence, most likely to transmit to the next generation.

Infection with hepatitis B can have a variety of outcomes. It may be inapparent, or it may cause a disease indistinguishable from that caused by hepatitis A. It may also, however, cause **chronic active hepatitis** with or without **cirrhosis**. Any of these forms may lead to a chronic carrier state, which may damage the kidneys or lead to cancer. Thus, although uncomplicated hepatitis B is not often fatal in the acute phase, the total mortality it causes can be great.

A good vaccine is available. It was proven effective in an extraordinary trial carried out with the help of the New York male homosexual community. Thousands participated, either as vaccine recipients or as part of a placebo group. Because of the high homosexual transmission rate, the incidence of disease in the unvaccinated group was high enough to provide a good level of significance in the results. Bacterial clones have now been developed that carry the gene for the virus antigen, and the product of these clones has now replaced blood as a source of antigen in the United States. This technology has been expensive, however, and blood-derived vaccine is still used elsewhere.

It must be remembered that the vaccine only prevents infection. There is as yet no way to cure the disease or abort the carrier state. A person who becomes a carrier is likely to remain so for many years. This means that many people already infected are still doomed to liver cancer.

Although it had been clear for many years that blood products could transmit hepatitis, the full import of this fact did not register on the medical profession. In 1942, a new yellow fever vaccine, mixed with human serum, was administered to U.S. troops headed overseas: Of those vaccinated, 28,000 developed hepatitis, and many died.

The discovery of hepatitis B virus followed an unusual course. In the early 1960s, an antigen was found in the blood of Australian aborigines. Later, a researcher who worked with the blood samples was discovered to have acquired the "Australia antigen," and it was recognized as infectious. Ultimately, it turned out that this antigen was the surface protein of the hepatitis B virus.

Hepatitis C

The virus of **hepatitis C** has been neither seen nor cultured. However, in 1989, a strand of RNA from the blood of an infected chimpanzee was transcribed into DNA. Propagated into a bacterial clone, this DNA codes for an antigen that crossreacts with the agent of an important transfusion-transmitted hepatitis virus. The discoverers suggested that this "hepatitis C virus" might be structurally similar to the virus of yellow fever or **equine encephalitis**. This implies that the virus genetic material was the original RNA strand, not DNA. Hepatitis C is inactivated by chloroform, showing that, unlike the viruses of hepatitis A and B, it has a lipid-containing envelope. The agent of some other transfusion-transmitted non-A, non-B hepatitis is resistant to chloroform, indicating the existence of at least one more unidentified agent of this disease.

Wherever hepatitis A and B have been distinguished, a residuum of non-A, non-B cases has remained. Some of these cases are associated with blood transfusions, whereas others are not. Hepatitis C is the most common transfusion-transmitted non-A, non-B in the United States, but its role in the rest of the world is unknown. Although it is important as a cause of posttransfusion hepatitis, this is not its main mode of transmission, and it is seen sporadically in untransfused persons. Transmission by intravenous drug use is more frequent, and sexual transmission seems also to occur.

Hepatitis C is a serious disease in that a high proportion of cases develop permanent liver damage. In spite of the paucity of our knowledge about this disease, it is almost unique among viral infections in being treatable. Alpha interferon results in dramatic improvement of hepatitis C liver disease. Unfortunately, the disease often recurs when treatment stops, and the treatment is both expensive and accompanied by unpleasant side effects.

Delta Agent

A fourth hepatitis virus, the **delta agent**, is unable to grow independently; it grows only in cells that are also infected with hepatitis B. Its defect is an inability to make coat protein, and it must, therefore, wrap itself in the surface protein of another virus to become infectious. Envelopment in the other's coat also gives delta the advantage of hepatitis B virus's freedom from immune attack, and the fact that hepatitis B is commonly persistent in infected persons gives delta a reasonably large field in which to forage. Infection with delta virus has the highest acute fatality rate of all the hepatitides. Outbreaks of unusually severe hepatitis have often proven to be caused by it. No vaccine is available as yet.

ET-NANBH

Enterically transmitted non-A, non-B hepatitis (ET-NANBH) is a virus structurally similar to but immunologically distinct from hepatitis A. It has recently been associated with a number of previously inexplicable hepatitis epidemics. The virus has been identified by electron microscopy. Most ET-NANBH epidemics have occurred in less-developed countries at times when even normally limited sanitation procedures have broken down. All ages are commonly affected, but there may actually be a preponderance of adult cases. These circumstances suggest that ET-NANBH virus is less infectious than hepatitis A and that, even in conditions of generally poor sanitation, most people remain only minimally susceptible. ET-NANBH is usually indistinguishable from hepatitis A or B. However, infected pregnant women have an unusually high mortality rate, which may reach 20 percent.

Francis L. Black

74. Infectious Mononucleosis

Infectious mononucleosis is an acute infectious disease of children, adolescents, and young adults. It is caused by the **Epstein-Barr virus** (EBV) and is followed by lifelong immunity.

Characteristics

Based on populations investigated, it seems that infectious mononucleosis occurs worldwide but attacks only people with no EBV antibodies. The virus replicates in the salivary glands, is present in the oropharyngeal secretions of patients ill with the disease, and continues to be shed for months following convalescence. As a lifelong inhabitant of the lymphoid tissues, it is excreted intermittently into the oropharynx.

In underdeveloped countries, it is a disease of childhood, and as it spreads via oral secretions, crowding and unhygienic surroundings favor its transmission. In developed countries, it strikes especially among the 15- to 25-year age group. In the United States, on college campuses, it is commonly known as the "kissing disease."

Children of low socioeconomic status almost universally show antibodies to the virus. In Ghana, for example, 84 percent of infants have such antibodies. In a worldwide study of 5,000 children and young adults without EBV antibodies, 29 percent developed antibodies within 4–8 years. Among susceptible college students, annual incidence is about 15 percent.

Although pathological findings may be multivisceral, **follicular hyperplasia** of the lymph nodes predominates. Lymphoid tissues show diffuse proliferation of atypical lymphocytes in the spleen, blood-vessel walls, liver, and peripheral bloodstream. These monocytoid lymphocytes (Downey cells) may constitute 10 percent or more of white cells and are of diagnostic significance.

In childhood, the disease is subclinical or masquerades as one of many episodes of upper respiratory infection. In the typical youthful adult, after incubating 5–6 weeks, clinical disease presents with prodromes of malaise, fatigue, headache, and chilliness followed by high fever, sore throat, tender swollen cervical lymph nodes, and a transient **maculopapular rash**. **Palpebral edema** and/or **periorbital**

edema may develop. Mild **jaundice** appears in some 10 percent of patients. Rarely are symptoms related to the central nervous system.

In most patients the disease is mild, and recovery occurs within several weeks. College students are generally up and about within a week or so. Complications in the nervous system may occasionally occur in adults, but death from the disease is extremely rare, splenic rupture being the most serious complication.

History

This disease was described in 1885 by Russian pediatrician Nil Filatov as **idiopathic adenitis**. Four years later, German physician Emil Pfeiffer also described a disease that was epidemic in children and characterized by glandular enlargement. He gave it the name *Drüsenfieber* ("glandular fever"). In 1896, J. West wrote of a similar epidemic in the United States, but only in 1920 did Thomas Sprunt give it the name infectious mononucleosis. The characteristic mononuclear leucocytes were described in 1923. EBV was identified in 1968.

R. H. Kampmeier

75. Inflammatory Bowel Disease (Crohn's Disease, Ulcerative Colitis)

The **inflammatory bowel diseases** (IBD) are disorders of the intestines that remain obscure. Their course is acute and chronic, with unpredictable remissions and exacerbations and numerous complications. The economic and emotional impact of these diseases is enormous. In these contexts, IBD is one of the major contemporary challenges in medicine.

Ulcerative Colitis

Symptoms of **ulcerative colitis** are rectal bleeding, constipation, **diarrhea**, cramping, pain, fever, **anorexia**, fatigue, and weight loss. Examinations demonstrate inflammation and ulceration of the rectum and colon and the adjoining terminal ileum. Ulcerative colitis begins in the inner bowel surface of the colon; in severe colitis the entire bowel wall may be involved. The white blood cell count is usually normal except with complications. The hemoglobin and red cell count are decreased in proportion to blood loss. Blood proteins including albumin are often diminished. The stools contain blood. Complications are numerous. In the colon, they include perforation, **peritonitis**, hemorrhage, obstruction, polyps, and **carcinoma**. Systemic complications include **anemia**, protein loss, **malnutrition**, **arthritis**, skin problems, **nephrolithiasis**, and **liver disease**.

The therapeutic emphasis in ulcerative colitis involves a general program of nutritional restoration, emotional support, medications, and various surgical alternatives in selected patients. The prognosis of ulcerative colitis has improved considerably, and mortality is less than 1 percent because of medical and surgical advances.

Ulcerative colitis is common among young people, especially below the age of 40, but the number of older patients is increasing. The circumstances of onset are not known; patients usually appear to be in good health. Occasionally, symptoms appear after visits to foreign countries, implicating an **enteric infection**. Initial thoughts emphasized a microbial infection, and this possibility continues today. Many organisms have been implicated and discarded. Immunologic mechanisms have been implicated and may involve defective immunoregulation.

Various circumstances may act as "trigger mechanisms," precipitating the disease in vulnerable persons. Genetic influences may be expressed through the immune response genes and the mucosal immune system of the bowel. Emotional disturbances are common in ulcerative colitis patients but probably do not initiate the disease. Investigation of interactions among the nervous system, the gut, and the endocrine and immune systems is ongoing.

Crohn's Disease

Crohn's disease is an acute and chronic inflammatory disease of the small intestine, especially the terminal ileum, but actually involving the entire gastrointestinal tract. It occurs frequently among children and young adults but is increasing in people over the age of 60. There is a slight female-to-male predominance. Clinical manifestations include fever, diarrhea, cramping, pain, anemia, and weight loss. Symptoms may include arthritis, gynecological difficulties, urinary symptoms, or a combination of severe appetite loss, weight loss, and depression. Occasionally, the initial presentation is indistinguishable from an acute **appendicitis**.

Findings include a normal or elevated white blood cell count, anemia, decreased total proteins and serum albumin, and evidence of undernutrition. The intestinal lumen is ulcerated and narrowed, and fistulas are not uncommon. Complications of Crohn's disease include most of the problems enumerated for ulcerative colitis along with abscesses, **fistulas**, and intestinal obstruction and carcinoma.

As in ulcerative colitis, medical treatment is symptomatic and individualized, with emphasis upon medication and restoration of nutrition. Surgery is necessary for complications, especially abscesses and fistulas, unrelenting intestinal obstruction, and uncontrollable hemorrhage. The recurrence rate is high.

Etiologic hypotheses vary widely, from excessive eating of cornflakes, sugars, or margarine to bottle-feeding, pollutants, antibiotics, and oral contraceptives. A variety of bacteria and viruses have been implicated, and the "new" pathogens have renewed interest in microbial possibilities. Other suggested but unproven etiologies have included blunt trauma to the abdominal wall, ingestion of foreign material, and nutritional deficiencies.

General Characteristics

Ulcerative colitis and Crohn's disease share similar demographic features. Ulcerative colitis apparently has stabilized or diminished in many areas of the world, with several exceptions. It appears to be more prevalent in Britain, New Zealand, Australia, the United States, and northern Europe. It is less frequent in central and southern Europe, infrequent in the Middle East, uncommon in South America and Africa, but increasing in Japan.

Similarly, Crohn's disease is common in Britain, the United States, and Scandinavia, on the rise in Japan, but less frequent in central and southern Europe and uncommon in Africa and South America. It has been increasing throughout much of the world but appears to have stabilized in some localities. The worldwide prevalence of Crohn's disease, especially in industrialized areas, and the similarity of its features regardless of geographic and sociocultural differences, are noteworthy.

The IBD are more frequent among whites than blacks, but Crohn's disease is increasing among black populations of the United States and Britain. Ulcerative colitis and especially Crohn's disease are much more common among Jews of the United States, Britain, and Sweden than among other groups. Ulcerative colitis and Crohn's disease occur among all ethnic groups, including Maoris, Arabs, and probably the Chinese, albeit infrequently. There is a scarcity of cigarette smokers among ulcerative colitis patients, and ex-smokers apparently have an increased vulnerability to it. By contrast, there is an excess of smokers in Crohn's disease populations. This intriguing observation, however, has yet to be explained.

Ulcerative colitis and Crohn's disease are not "classic" genetic disorders. However, genetic influences are important in both, as reflected in their familial clustering (20 percent for ulcerative colitis and up to 40 percent for Crohn's disease). In addition to the initial patient, one more member of the family is usually affected, but up to 8 patients have been observed in a family. IBD occurs with a high degree of concordance among monozygotic twins. The nature of the genetic influence in IBD is not known. The occasional occurrence of IBD in the adopted child or mate of an IBD patient supports an environmental mechanism. Current studies focus upon an abnormality in immune response genes among other possibilities.

Both disorders have significant familial associations. Approximately 25 percent of families with multiple instances of IBD show both ulcerative colitis and Crohn's disease. Both share epidemiological and demographic features. They also share many symptoms, local complications, and systemic complications. However, ulcerative colitis is a continuous mucosal disease, at least initially, with diffuse involvement of the colon. Crohn's disease is a transmural process, focal in distribution, penetrating through the bowel wall, and producing abscesses and fistulas. **Granulomas** and prominent **lymphoid aggregates** are much more common in Crohn's disease than in ulcerative colitis.

Ulcerative colitis is limited to the colon and occasionally a short segment of terminal ileum; Crohn's disease may involve any segment of the alimentary tract. Ulcerative colitis is a continuous inflammatory reaction; Crohn's disease, wherever located, is a discontinuous, focal process. Perianal suppuration and fistula formation characterize Crohn's disease, but not ulcerative colitis. Immune-modulating drugs are more helpful in Crohn's disease than in ulcerative colitis. Surgery is often curative in ulcerative colitis, but the same operations in Crohn's disease carry a recurrence rate of 15–20 percent.

History of Ulcerative Colitis

Hippocrates recognized that diarrhea was not a single disease entity, whereas Aretaeus described many types, including one with "foul evacuations," chiefly in older children and adults. An apparent "ulcerative colitis" was described by Roman physicians, including Ephesus in the eleventh century. "Noncontagious diarrhea" flourished for centuries under many labels, such as Thomas Sydenham's "bloody flux" in 1666. In 1865, U.S. Army physicians described the features of an "ulcerative colitis-like" process. (Several of these cases actually suggest Crohn's disease more than ulcerative colitis.)

During the 1880s and 1890s, an ulcerative colitis was described by numerous physicians from England, France, Germany, Italy, and other European countries. In 1895 W. Hale-White reported the association of liver disease and ulcerative colitis, and in 1920 R. F. Weir performed appendicostomy to facilitate "colonic drainage" in ulcerative colitis. J. P. Lockhart-Mummery in 1907 described **colon carcinoma** in patients with ulcerative colitis, and emphasized the diagnostic value of sigmoidoscopy. In 1909 W. H. Allchin recorded perhaps the first "familial" ulcerative colitis. Additional instances were noted at the Paris Congress of Medicine in 1913, and in the same year, J. Y. Brown may have been the first to suggest ileostomy in the surgical management of ulcerative colitis.

During the 1920s, the number of reports increased steadily and included those by H. Rolleston, C. E. Smith, J. M. Lynch and J. Felsen, A. F. Hurst, and E. Spriggs. Hermann Strauss may have been the first to recommend blood transfusions in the treatment of ulcerative colitis. In 1924, J. A. Bargen published his studies implicating the diplostreptococcus in ulcerative colitis – a notion later discarded. More important was his 1946 study of the course, complications, and management of "thrombo-ulcerative colitis." C. D. Murray in 1930 drew attention to the psychogenic aspects, and this initiated a period (1930s–60s) of intense psychiatric interest in ulcerative colitis.

Worldwide attention was directed to the disease at the 1935 International Congress of Gastroenterology, and the amount of literature increased rapidly after this. By the 1940s, ulcerative colitis was recognized more often than Crohn's disease. However, by the end of World War II, Crohn's disease had become more frequent. Concurrently with an apparent stabilization of ulcerative colitis in the United States, Crohn's disease has been the more prominent.

History of Crohn's Disease

The initial description of Crohn's disease may date back to Giovanni Morgagni, who in 1761 described **ileal ulceration** and enlarged mesenteric lymph nodes in a young man who died of an ileal perforation. More suggestive early instances of Crohn's disease include an 1806 report by H. Saunders and one in 1813 by C. Combe and Saunders. Nineteenth century descriptions of disease consistent with today's concept of Crohn's disease were authored by J. deGroote, J. Abercrombie, J. S. Bristowe, N. Moore, and S. Wilks.

In 1913, T. Kennedy Dalziel described a group of patients with findings closely resembling those recorded in 1932 by B. B. Crohn, L. Ginzburg, and G. D. Oppenheimer. Many reports of a chronic inflammation of the last portion of the small bowel appeared subsequently. F. J. Nuboer in 1932 described two patients manifesting the same findings that Crohn described. Soon after Crohn's 1932 paper, A. D. Bissell reported on two patients. The first had symptoms including cramps, diarrhea, and weight loss and required resection of an ileocecal mass. The second required resection of the terminal ileum and cecum. These early case reports depicted Crohn's disease as a mass-producing, bowel-narrowing process, virtually always requiring surgical intervention. The principal clinical differentiation in the early part of the twentieth century included intestinal **tuberculosis** and granuloma formation simulating tumor in the bowel.

In other notable articles, H. Mock in 1931 and R. Colp in 1933 chronicled involvement of the colon. C. Gotlieb and S. Alpert in 1937 described regional **jejunitis**, and J. R. Ross in 1949 identified "regional gastritis." W. A. Jackman and J. L. Kantor in 1934 and R. Marshak in 1951 described the roentgenographic appearance of Crohn's disease, and in 1936 Harold Edwards described a resected terminal ileum with "the consistency of a hosepipe."

Authoritative descriptions of Crohn's disease have been provided by S. Warren and S. C. Sommers, G. Hadfield, and H. Rappaport. In 1952, Charles Wells distinguished between ulcerative colitis and what he termed "segmental colitis" and suggested that this latter form was a variant of Crohn's disease. In 1955 Bryan Brooke and W. Trevor Cooke recognized "right-sided colitis" as Crohn's disease, but it was not

until reports in 1959 and 1960 by Lockhart-Mummery and B. C. Morson that Crohn's disease of the colon was accepted as a valid entity. It is to the credit of Crohn, Ginzburg, and Oppenheimer that their description stimulated worldwide interest in this disease. Certainly much credit belongs to Crohn for his long interest in the illness, his many publications on the subject, and his encouragement of others in its further investigation.

Joseph B. Kirsner

76. Influenza

Influenza, also known as "flu," "grip," and "grippe," is a disease of humans, pigs, horses, and other mammals, as well as of a number of species of birds. Among humans it is a contagious respiratory disease characterized by sudden onset and symptoms of sore throat, cough, often a runny nose, fever, chills, headache, weakness, generalized muscle and joint pain, and prostration. It is difficult to differentiate between single cases of influenza and feverish **colds**, but when a sudden outbreak of symptoms occurs among a number of people, the correct diagnosis is almost always influenza.

There is at present no specific cure effective against this viral disease. In mild cases, symptoms disappear in 7–10 days, although physical or mental depression may occasionally persist. Influenzal **pneumonia** is rare but often fatal. **Bronchitis, sinusitis**, and bacterial pneumonia are among the more common complications, and the last can be fatal if untreated. Influenza is generally benign, and even in pandemic years, mortality is usually low – 1 percent or less – the disease being truly life-threatening for only the very young, the immunosuppressed, and the elderly. However, this infection is so contagious that in most years multitudes contract it, and thus the number of deaths in absolute terms is usually quite high. The sequelae of influenza are often difficult to define, but evidence indicates that the 1920s global pandemic of

encephalitis lethargica had its origin in the great pandemic of 1918–19.

Characteristics

In seemingly every year, there are at least some cases of influenza on every populated continent and most large islands. During epidemics, which occur somewhere almost annually, the malady sweeps large regions, even entire continents. During pandemics, a number of which have occurred every century for several hundred years, the disease infects a large percentage of the world's population and, ever since the 1889–90 pandemic, in all probability a majority of that population. Not everyone so infected becomes clinically sick; nonetheless, influenza pandemics are among the most awesome of earthly phenomena. The disease strikes so many so quickly and over such vast areas that eighteenth century Italians blamed it on the influence of heavenly bodies and called it *influenza*.

The causative agents of influenza are three myxoviruses: influenza viruses A, B, and C. The B and C viruses are associated with sporadic epidemics among children and young adults, and do not cause pandemics. The A virus is the cause of most cases during and between pandemics. It exists in a number of subtypes, which usually do not induce cross-immunity. In most instances, influenza viruses pass from person to person by breath-borne droplets, and from animal to animal by this and other routes. Its epidemics in temperate zones usually appear in winter, when people gather together indoors under conditions of poor ventilation. Geographically, the malady spreads as fast as its victims travel, which in our time can mean circumnavigation of the globe in a few months, with the pandemic veering to the north and south of the tropics with the changing seasons.

Influenza A virus is distinctive in its genetic instability, which probably makes permanent immunity to the disease impossible, no matter how many times it is contracted. This genetic instability is the likeliest explanation of why even during pandemics the virus seems to change sufficiently to produce repeating waves of infection in a given locale. Several times a century, the virus has changed radically, rendering obsolete the immunologic defenses of most humans. In the mildest of these pandemics, millions fall ill and thousands die.

The cause of the major changes in the virus that set off the pandemics is still a matter of mystery. The three most plausible theories are that the influenza A virus itself mutates into a new version of infection-producing organism; that an animal influenza virus abruptly gains the ability to cause disease in humans; or that a human virus and an animal virus "cross-breed," producing a new infectious organism unfamiliar to human immune systems. The first of these seems least likely and the last most likely. Nothing, however, is certain yet, and the cause of influenza pandemics remains unknown.

History

Influenza's origins, too, are unknown. It does not afflict our primate relatives and so is probably not a very old human disease. It is unlikely to have been common among our Paleolithic ancestors or their herd animals before the advent of agriculture, cities, and concentrated populations. In small populations, it would have burnt itself out by killing or immunizing all available victims quickly.

Although influenza could have been acquired from pigs or ducks or other animals thousands of years ago, no clear evidence exists of its spread among humans until Europe's Middle Ages, and no undeniable evidence until the fifteenth and sixteenth centuries. Since that time, however, the malady has been our unfailing companion, never absent for more than a few decades, if that. Its associations and characteristics suggest that it was restricted to the Old World until the end of the fifteenth century, after which it spread overseas with Europeans and their livestock – and may account for much of the clinically undefined morbidity and mortality among the indigenes of Europe's empires. Large-scale epidemics rolled over Europe in 1510, 1557, and 1580. The latter – the first unambiguous pandemic of influenza – extended into Africa and Asia as well. Further European epidemics occurred in the seventeenth century, but seemingly of only a regional nature.

At least three pandemics of influenza occurred in Europe during the eighteenth century (1729–30, 1732–33, and 1781–82), and several epidemics, two of which (1761–62 and 1788–89) may have been extensive enough to be termed pandemics. The pandemic of 1781–82 was, in geographic spread and number of people infected, among the greatest manifestations of disease of all history.

By the end of the eighteenth century, population growth, urbanization, and improving transportation were changing the world in ways that enhanced the transmission of microbes across long distances. There were at least three influenza pandemics in the nineteenth century (1830–31, 1833, and 1889–90) and several major epidemics as well. Even so, one of the most intriguing aspects of the history of influenza in this century was the long hiatus between the second and third pandemics. In fact, in Europe, after the epidemic of 1847–48, only a few minor upsurges occurred until 1889.

When influenza rose up again in 1889, medical science was making rapid advances, and public health had become a matter of governmental concern. The 1889–90 pandemic was the first for which we have detailed records. It reached Europe from the east (hence its nickname, the "Russian flu"), and such was the efficiency of transatlantic shipping that it swept over western Europe and appeared in North America in the same month, December of 1889. It struck Nebraska, Saskatchewan, Rio de Janeiro, Buenos Aires, Montevideo, and Singapore in February, 1890, and Australia and New Zealand in March. By spring the pandemic was firmly established and widespread in Asia and Africa. Waves of the infection continued to roll across large regions of the world for the rest of the century, and although mortality in this pandemic was quite low, the total of deaths was high. By conservative estimate, 250,000 died in Europe, and the world total must have been at

the very least two or three times greater. Influenza killed many more than **cholera** did in the nineteenth century, but much of the mortality was restricted to the elderly, and thus its reputation as an unpleasant but not dangerous infection was preserved.

Its history for the first 17 years of the next century reinforced this view. Although rarely absent for long, influenza attracted little attention until the appearance of the unprecedentedly virulent pandemic of 1918–19. What was probably its first wave rose in the spring of 1918, perhaps first in the United States, attracting little attention because its death rate was low. Its most ominous characteristic was that many of the dead were young adults, in contradistinction to the malady's previous record. That spring and summer, this new influenza circumnavigated the globe, infecting millions, killing hundreds of thousands, and hindering the waging of war in Europe and the Middle East. The name given this new disease was the "Spanish flu," not because Spain's morbidity and mortality were higher than elsewhere but because Spain was not a belligerent and thus the ravages of the malady in that country were not screened from world attention by censorship. As in previous pandemics, morbidity was vastly greater than mortality, and the latter, as a percentage of the former, was not impressive.

In August, that changed, as death rates doubled, tripled, and more. A second wave arose, sending hundreds of millions to sickbeds and killing millions. This wave tended to subside toward the end of the year but returned again in a third wave in the winter and spring. In both the fall and winter waves, about half the deaths were in the 20–40 age group. Fully 550,000 died in the United States, about 10 times the number of battle deaths of Americans in World War I. In remote parts of the world, where influenza had never or rarely reached before, the death rate was often extremely high. The total of deaths in the world was in excess of 21 million, a figure estimated in the 1920s before historians and demographers sifted through the records of Latin

America, Africa, and Asia, adding many more – millions, certainly – to the world total.

It is possible that the 1918–19 pandemic was, in terms of absolute numbers, the greatest single demographic shock that the human species has ever received. The Black Death and World Wars I and II killed higher percentages of the populations at risk, but took years to do so and were not universal in their destruction. The so-called Spanish flu did most of its killing in a 6-month period and reached almost every human population on Earth. Moreover, its impact was even greater than these numbers indicate because so many young adults died. To this day, we do not know what made the 1918–19 influenza such a killer. Perhaps as has been suggested, a chance synergy of viral and bacterial infection produced an exceptionally deadly pneumonia, or perhaps the 1918 virus was so distinctive antigenically that it provoked a massive immune response, choking the victims with inflammation and **edema**. We have no way of proving or disproving such theories.

In 1920, another wave of the disease rolled over the world, but morbidity and mortality soon shrank back to normal, and the disease lost most of its power to kill young adults. The medical profession, however, has subsequently worried about a resurgence of the killer virus and has devoted great energy to identifying it, learning its secrets, and studying how to disarm it.

It is possible that more is now known about the influenza virus than about any other, but its changing nature has defeated all efforts thus far to make a vaccine against the disease that will be effective for more than a few years at most. Vaccines were produced in the 1940s to protect the soldiers of World War II from a repetition of the pandemic that had killed so many of them in World War I, and influenza vaccines developed since have enabled millions, particularly the elderly, to live through epidemics without illness or with only minor illness. But the ability of the A virus to change – sometimes radically – and to race around the globe faster than suitable vaccines can be produced and delivered has so far frustrated all efforts to abort pandemics.

At present, a worldwide network of 100 or so centers, most of them national laboratories, cooperate under the direction of the World Health Organization to identify new strains of influenza virus as quickly as they appear in order to minimize the time between the beginning of epidemics and the production and distribution of relevant vaccines. The efficiency of this organization has been impressive, and certainly has saved many lives, but influenza is not yet under control.

Alfred W. Crosby

77. Japanese B Encephalitis

Japanese B encephalitis is a relatively uncommon disease even in areas where the infection is endemic. The disease is one of several caused by arthropod-borne viruses (arboviruses) and is carried by mosquitoes of the genus *Culex*. The virus belongs to the genus *Flavivirus* and is an RNA virus. The most common insect vector for the virus is *Culex tritaeniorhyncus*.

The disease was recognized and described in 1871, and the virus was isolated in 1935. The infection may appear in epidemic or sporadic outbreaks and is carried particularly in swine but also has been isolated from a variety of birds and equine animals. The virus is distributed principally in East and Southeast Asia.

Epidemic outbreaks of Japanese B encephalitis tend to occur in regions that are usually dry and arid and therefore relatively free of viral activity; such areas may accumulate many individuals who are relatively susceptible. Then, with rain and conditions favorable to the insect vector, epidemic outbreaks may occur, particularly among relatively dense populations of human and animal hosts. In some arboviruses, a change occurs in the relative virulence of the infecting strain, which may also account for an epidemic outbreak.

Why, given the presence of Japanese B encephalitis in birds with wide-ranging migratory patterns, the disease remains localized to certain geographic areas is unclear but presumably has to do with the specificity of the insect vector in carrying the infectious agent. The mosquito vector, *C. tritaeniorhyncus*, is found in rice fields and feeds on pigs and birds as well as human and other hosts. However, the Japanese custom of raising pigs in the fall, after the flooding of rice paddies is over, and of taking the pigs to market early the following year may help account for the general lack of large outbreaks as well as for the usual pattern of sporadic cases.

Most information on the early stages of the disease has been gained from studies in the mouse. Pathological features of fatal human cases have generally been consistent with experimental findings. Early in the disease, focal hemorrhages, congestion, and **edema** are found in the brain. Microscopically widespread damage to Purkinje cells of the cerebellum is noted, with perivascular inflammation and multiple foci of degeneration and **necrosis**. Extraneural evidence of spread of the virus is found in the form of **hyperplasia** of the germinal centers of the lymph nodes and of the spleen; multiple foci of round-cell infiltration in many organs, including the heart, kidneys, and lungs; and, in pregnancy, infiltration of the placenta with corresponding abortion and stillbirth. Multiple lesions in the offspring indicate cross-placental passage of the virus.

The clinical disease consists of the usual signs and symptoms of encephalitis, and no syndrome has been elicited that is specific for Japanese B encephalitis. Within a few days to several weeks after an infective mosquito bite, the susceptible patient manifests fever and evidence of damage to the central nervous system, which may include **meningism**, delirium, drowsiness, confusion, stupor, **paralysis** (especially of facial muscles), and – in the most severe cases – coma and death within a few days. Definitive diagnosis is made only from studies of the antibody status of the affected individual.

The disease is among the most fatal arboviruses, with case-fatality rates of 50–70 percent in outbreaks. Recovery may be complete, or there may be residual damage to the central nervous system; Japanese B encephalitis, in contrast to other arboviral encephalitides, has relatively high rates of complete recovery despite high case-fatality rates.

There is no specific treatment, and supportive care is the major intervention that can be offered. The protective effect of antibody suggests that convalescent serum or other sources of antibody might have some therapeutic value, but this has not been systematically investigated on a suitable scale.

Vaccines have been available for many years for immunization of humans and livestock. Live attenuated vaccines have been available in Japan since 1972, and in China more recently, and their effectiveness is shown by seroconversion rates of up to 96 percent. Widespread immunization campaigns have been successful in Japan, Taiwan, and China. At present, vaccines are composed principally of the prototype Nakayama strain, and reasonable control of the disease has been achieved.

Vector control has been investigated in some detail. Larvicides and adulticides aimed at the chief mosquito vector have reduced attack rates in test areas. Insect-control programs, clearing irrigation channels, and spraying insecticides in livestock pens have had some success in China. Under epidemic conditions, spraying with appropriate insecticides has sometimes been necessary.

Edward H. Kass

78. Lactose Intolerance and Malabsorption

The inability to digest lactose (sometimes called "milk sugar") is related to the enzyme lactase in the intestine. **Lactose intolerance** means that the individual is unable to tolerate the lactose in milk and other foods because of insufficient lactase activity. Such intolerance has been recognized for some time. Early in the twentieth century, physicians began to realize that much infantile **diarrhea** resulted from a lack of "ferments" necessary for carbohydrate digestion. By the 1950s, attention was focused on **lactose malabsorption**.

Characteristics

Lactose is found in the milk of most mammals in concentrations ranging up to 7 percent. It is digested in the small intestine by lactase, which is anchored to the membrane by amino acids. In most mammals, lactase activity is high during the perinatal period but declines by about 90 percent after weaning. In certain human groups, however, lactase activity remains elevated throughout the lifetime of most individuals. Examples of such groups include northern Europeans, people of Magyar-Finnish extraction, and two African tribes, the Fulani and the Tussi.

Clinical manifestations of lactose intolerance include abdominal discomfort, **borborygmus**, flatulence, and fermentative diarrhea. These symptoms primarily result from the level of lactase activity relative to the quantity of dietary lactose. The lower the activity, the less the capacity for hydrolysis of lactose, although other factors – such as intestinal motility and the presence of other nutrients – also play a role in this phenomenon. When the capacity of the lactase is exceeded, the nonhydrolyzed lactose passes into the large bowel, where it is fermented by myriad bacteria. This action yields propionic acid, hydrogen, methane, and alcohols, resulting in a watery diarrhea.

Lactose malabsorption can be classified into three categories: congenital, documented only in rare cases; primary, encountered in most humans after 5–7 years of age and in other animals after weaning; and acquired malabsorption from illness and other causes.

History

The ability to digest lactose is clearly associated with evolutionary pressures. During the Neolithic period, human adults began drinking milk, probably in association with animal domestication. The ancient pastoralists who originated in the Euphrates Valley were nomadic, constantly in search of new pastures. Presumably they migrated in two main directions: northwest toward Europe and southwest toward Central Africa. When this occurred is unknown, but the nomadic pastoralists of Africa and Europe may have their origins in these migrations.

By contrast, in the Americas, no pastoral groups existed, and no post-weaning ingestion of milk occurred until the Europeans arrived. This was also the case in Australia, the Pacific islands, Japan, and the rest of Asia. In these regions, the weaned individual obtained calcium from bones, limestone, vegetables, and fermented or pressed dairy products (much reduced in lactose).

Thus the present-day geographic distribution of lactose-tolerant and lactose-intolerant peoples matches historical knowledge of the distribution of ancient pastoral groups and the milking of animals. Data support the cultural hypothesis of Frederick Simoons – first promulgated in 1970 – that ability to digest lactose is associated only with populations that have a history of pastoralism. The hereditary pattern for this ability appears to follow straightforward Mendelian genetics. Individuals who can digest lactose carry the mutated gene, which is dominant; lactose nonabsorbers carry a recessive gene. Consequently, crosses between lactose malabsorbers always yield progeny who are malabsorbers, thus perpetuating the lactose-intolerant population.

Today, lactose malabsorbers who desire to drink milk can purchase "lactase" preparations that "digest" lactose before ingestion. Others can overcome potential dietary calcium deficiency by consuming various calcium-rich foods. The worldwide distribution of lactose intolerance among human adults and all other mammals argues that this condition is the normal physiological state. It is only the bias of the milk-oriented societies of Europe and North America that casts lactose malabsorption as abnormal.

Norman Kretchmer

79. Lassa Fever

Recognition of Africa's major human diseases was apparently well advanced by 1900. **Malaria, trypanosomiasis, yellow fever, schistosomiasis, typhoid, brucellosis,** and many others had been characterized. But in 1969, a new member of the coterie was discovered: **Lassa fever**.

Events leading to the discovery were dramatic. A nurse at a mission hospital in Lassa, Nigeria, became ill, progressed unfavorably, and died, despite thorough modern treatment. This death, as a statistic, would probably have been labeled "malaria" in national and international disease records. But another nurse, who attended the first, also became ill. She was moved to the Evangel Hospital in Jos, Nigeria, where she too died. Again, there was no firm diagnosis, and then *her* nurse got sick. Doctors were thoroughly alarmed; this third patient was evacuated to America and admitted at the medical college of Columbia University.

The Yale Arbovirus Research Unit in New Haven, Connecticut, secured specimens from the patient (who ultimately recovered), and a previously unknown virus was isolated and named "Lassa" after the locale of the first outbreak. Two laboratory-acquired cases occurred in Yale personnel working on the virus: One died; the other was given plasma from the recovered nurse and was cured. In due course, Lassa virus was designated an *Arenavirus* in the family Arenaviridae, a grouping of nearly worldwide distribution, including other entities such as **lymphocytic choriomeningitis, Tacaribe virus, Junin virus**, and **Machupo virus**. Several other outbreaks of Lassa fever are known to have occurred in Africa since 1969.

High fever associated with malaise, muscle and joint pains, sore throat, retrosternal pain, nausea, liver involvement, bleeding, **proteinuria**, and **erythematous maculopapular rash** with petechiae are features of the illness but not of themselves particularly diagnostic. Some consider an **enanthem** in the oropharynx to have specific diagnostic importance.

In early stages, the disease simulates many African illnesses, prominent among them malaria. Sporadically occurring Lassa cases are infrequently diagnosed. When epidemics arise, the clumping of cases of mysterious illness has attracted attention, leading to diagnosis. It has become recognized that there are many mild Lassa cases. Mortality is directly associated with level of **viremia**, although it must be noted that by the time viremia figures are received from the overseas laboratory, the patient is either recovered or dead. Generally, fatalities in infections are estimated at 1–2 percent, a rate lower than estimates based on hospitalized patients. How widely such findings can be extrapolated in West Africa is unknown. However, it is clear that prognosis is highly unfavorable for seriously ill patients, even when the best therapeutic regimes are applied.

Diagnostic tests have been developed. Viremia is a constant feature, and the virus can be identified in cell culture. Progress has been made in survey methodology. Serum specimens taken in samplings can be examined for the presence of antibody to Lassa, using a special test plate developed in U.S. Army laboratories. This method has led to greater knowledge of several deadly African diseases and is a major step toward understanding their geographic distribution. All work with Lassa virus must be conducted under conditions of highest security, because it can pass from human to human via blood, urine, feces, and saliva – which, of course, slows down laboratory work. Several deaths have occurred among laboratory workers, nonetheless.

The association with the Arenavirus group helped determine the transmission cycle of Lassa virus. Predictably, like its congeners, it is an infection of small rodents, usually house-frequenting. *Praomys* (*Mastomys*) *natalensis* in sub-Saharan Africa is the most common house-frequenting rodent and has been found infected in several African regions afflicted with Lassa. The infection in the rodent is persistent, with virus in the urine a common feature. As epidemics occurred in Nigeria, Liberia, and Sierra

Leone over several years, it became apparent that Lassa virus is widespread in West Africa and may also be found in East Africa. At present, it is especially prevalent in eastern Sierra Leone and is also found in Senegal, Gambia, Guinea, Ghana, Mali, and Cote d'Ivoire.

Wilbur G. Downs

80. Lead Poisoning

Lead poisoning or **plumbism** simply means the undesirable health effects induced by lead. Many are "nonspecific" and are similar to effects produced by other causes, and some are so subtle they require laboratory identification. This chapter deals primarily with overt effects apparent upon even casual observation. Principal among these are **abdominal colic**, muscle **paralysis** resulting from lead-damaged nerves, and **convulsions**.

Characteristics
Lead enters the body mainly through inhalation and ingestion. Residents of industrialized nations acquire half of their "body burden" of lead from polluted air. Healthy adults absorb 10 percent of ingested lead, but children may absorb half the lead they ingest. Lead is also absorbed through the skin: Lead-containing cosmetics, for example, may cause health-threatening effects. The body's ability to excrete lead is extremely limited, and 95 percent of unexcretable lead is stored in bone, where it will remain for decades in an adult. If absorption ceases, such lead is leached from the skeleton over many years and excreted. Lead may be transferred to the fetus via the placenta.

Lead interferes with almost every body function. At low blood concentration, it may impair intellectual development in children, an effect of potentially greater significance than more overt symptoms. Intense exposure may cause temporary arrest of long bone growth. Lead produces moderate **anemia** by poisoning enzymes necessary for the formation of hemoglobin. It can poison kidney cells, eventually causing fatal **renal failure**.

The symptom of lead poisoning most commonly encountered in historical literature is abdominal pain. It is usually attributed to intestinal spasm, though the abdominal muscles may undergo the painful, uncontrolled contractions called "colic." Similar pain is seen in **diarrhea**, but lead poisoning is instead accompanied by constipation; hence the abdominal pain of lead intoxication is termed "dry bellyache."

Lead also has a destructive effect on the nerves that transmit electrical impulses to muscles, producing muscle paralysis. Muscles raising the wrist or foot are especially affected, causing "wrist drop" (often termed "the dangles") and "foot drop." Behavioral disturbances leading to convulsions, coma, and death are the most severe of lead's effects. Children are notoriously susceptible to such brain toxicity, and even a single episode of convulsions, when not fatal, often causes permanent cerebral damage. Finally, plumbism may cause **gout** because of the reduced ability of lead-poisoned kidneys to excrete uric acid. The full etiology of gout is obscure, but when the kidney injury is caused by lead, the condition is called **saturnine gout**.

History
The prevalence of plumbism correlates with practices and traditions of lead use. Because galena is the most abundant lead ore in Europe and Asia, and because it produces little toxicity for its miners, lead poisoning probably was not common before the popularization of smelting about 3500 B.C. The cupellation process, discovered about 3000 B.C., permitted separation of the small amounts of silver from the much larger quantities of lead. A substantial increase in lead production was a byproduct of the pursuit of silver, and during this period, many involved in lead production in the Middle East and Mediterranean regions must have been exposed to a toxigenic degree. Introduction of coinage resulted in increased silver (and lead) production, which eventually Rome exaggerated to the point of ore exhaustion and a marked reduction

in that form of mining. Not until the late Middle Ages did lead production rise again in Europe. But it was the Industrial Revolution, with its enormous surge in lead production, that created the recurrent endemics of plumbism in France, Italy, Spain, Germany, and especially Britain, and later their colonies. Since Roman times, productivity has expanded from 80,000 to more than 3 million tons worldwide today. With this rise has come a staggering degree of lead exposure in Western nations.

The use of lead in prehistoric times is evidenced by various artifacts dating from the fifth through the second millennia B.C. in the Near and Middle East, South and Southeast Asia, and China. By 2000 B.C., not only had lead smelting become common, but cupellation was also widely practiced. Lead had broad utilitarian applications and was widely traded. Such widespread use of the metal must have been accompanied by **lead intoxication**, at least among industrial workers and those using lead products including foodware, but there is no evidence of severe or widespread lead poisoning in this era.

Much of our knowledge about lead use in the Greco-Roman period is related to mines such as the one at Lavrion near Athens. The Athenians called Lavrion a "silver mine" even though they had to separate 100 to 200 ounces of lead for each ounce of silver. Similar mines were operated in the Mediterranean islands, Asia Minor, Spain, France, Italy, and Britain. With the generation of huge quantities of lead as a byproduct of silver, the obvious utilitarian value of lead was also exploited. Applications included tableware, storage containers for oil and other fluids, construction materials, sheathing for ships' hulls, coins, toys, statues, various alloys, coffins, tablets, solder, and many others. The most intensive Roman use of lead related to their water systems: Lead sheets not only lined aqueducts and cisterns but also were rolled and soldered to make water pipes.

Another dangerous application of lead was its use in food and beverage containers and, even worse, as a food additive. The Romans used con-centrated fruit juice as a sweetening agent. Such juice was concentrated by boiling in lead-lined containers, and lead was leached from the containers by the juice's acids. Replications of original Roman juice recipes contain lead concentrations up to 800 milligrams per liter, 16,000 times the upper limit for potable water defined by the U.S. Environmental Protection Agency! Eventually Romans became so addicted to the sweet flavor of lead acetate that it was employed as a seasoning in wine.

Clearly, then, the majority of urban Romans were exposed to lead. Roman customs, however, probably resulted in unequal exposure. Poor and middle-class citizens shared ingestion of lead-contaminated water from public water systems. But wealthier people additionally contaminated their wine and food through the use of lead-lined containers, expensive pewter tableware, and food additives.

By this time, contemporary writers were aware of health problems associated with excessive lead exposure. The Greek physician-poet Nicander is credited with the first unequivocal description of plumbism in the second century B.C., and other early warnings came from Lucretius and Vitruvius in the first century B.C. and Pliny and Celsus in the first century A.D. Moreover, the emperor Augustus prohibited the use of lead for water pipes, though there is little evidence of the edict's enforcement.

Well-known historical arguments suggest that the lead poisoning endemic in Roman society may have helped cause the decline of the Roman aristocracy during the first and second centuries. It may also explain the bizarre behavior of many Roman emperors and their alleged afflictions of gout, and may even have been a major factor in the decline of the Roman Empire.

As already mentioned, only in the late medieval and early modern periods did lead production return to levels approaching those of Rome. Then the rapid production increase during the Industrial Revolution and its subsequent explosive growth (including the modern era of lead fuel additives) shifted the scene of lead poisoning. From the sixteenth to the eighteenth centuries and even into the nineteenth, recurrent epidemics of tardily recognized lead poisoning swept over Europe. Most of these were traced to either industrial exposure or ingestion of lead-contaminated substances. The concept of industrial exposure as a cause of disease was crystallized in 1700 by Bernardino Ramazzini. His studies established clear relationships between certain diseases and occupations – among them, lead poisoning in miners, potters, and painters.

Epidemics of lead poisoning were even more difficult to pin down. A French epidemic, called the "colic of Poitou," had begun in the late sixteenth century, but over 100 years passed before lead-contaminated wine was identified as its cause. Similarly, a half-century-long colic endemic, which began in Madrid about 1730, was not associated until 1797 with badly glazed lead food containers. In the mid-eighteenth century, the "colica pictonum" in Holland was traced to lead water pipes.

Interestingly, the eighteenth and nineteenth centuries were characterized by British importation of port wine in prodigious quantities. The brandy used to fortify such wines was often prepared in stills containing lead parts, and fortified wines may have been responsible for an epidemic of gout so widespread that the period is called "the golden age of gout" in England. In the same vein, "the colic of Devonshire" raged for decades in mid-eighteenth century England, but in 1767 George Baker published a milestone report in the history of plumbism, establishing that the epidemic was caused by cider contaminated with lead during the manufacturing process. Subsequent preventive practices led to a gradual subsidence of the epidemic.

Similarly, for many decades in the eighteenth and early nineteenth centuries, Paris's Charity Hospital had become famous for its treatment of patients with various "dry colic" syndromes. In 1839, L. Tanquerel des Planches demonstrated that most were engaged in occupations involving lead exposure. His detailed observations included such a thorough description of the symptoms comprising plumbism that it can be used as a medical teaching exercise even today.

Colics also appeared in the American colonies. There, settlers had arrived with limited tools and machinery; malleable lead was employed to create many items normally manufactured out of steel, with consequent opportunities for lead exposure. One source of exposure was lead-contaminated liquor. By 1685, epidemics of "dry bellyache" or "dry gripes" were common in North Carolina and Virginia. Complaints of lead-contaminated New England rum led to the enactment of the Massachusetts Bay Law of 1723, prohibiting the use of lead parts in stills.

Although the law is often hailed as the first public-health law in the colonies, it appears the legislators were motivated more by trade than by health concerns. Similar afflictions occurred at Caribbean island plantations. Barbados was especially affected, with literature from the latter seventeenth and much of the eighteenth centuries replete with references to "dry bellyache." Sufficient lead has been found in archaeologically excavated bones to suggest that at least one-third of Barbadian slaves had lead-poisoning symptoms of moderate or greater severity.

In 1745, Benjamin Franklin published Thomas Cadawaler's treatise that defined the role of lead in dry gripes. Franklin may have carried this knowledge to Europe, because Baker of Devonshire quoted Franklin in his 1767 article. In 1788 John Hunter detailed dry gripes symptoms in Jamaica and specifically attributed them to lead. The condition subsided in the West Indies toward the end of the century.

Another source of lead poisoning in colonial America was pewter houseware. Plates and goblets were commonly of pewter in wealthier colonial homes, and perishables and beverages were stored in lead-lined containers. Indeed, in such a wealthy home almost everything the family ate or drank contained some lead. Colonists were also exposed through their use of lead bottles, funnels, nipple shields, dram cups, candlesticks, lamps, pipes, roof gutters, and other items.

Mining also claimed its New World victims. Eastern American mines were largely of poorly soluble galena ore and generated little morbidity. But in western mines, with predominantly lead carbonate ore, lead poisoning reached epidemic proportions. Thousands of miners suffered from plumbism between 1870 and 1900.

Even in modern times, the ongoing use of lead provides new opportunities for exposure. **Lead encephalopathy** acquired by infants nursing at the breasts of mothers using lead-containing cosmetics constituted the fourth most common, fatal, pediatric malady in Manchuria in 1925. Poisoning from lead fumes occurred in a Baltimore neighborhood in 1933 when poor families burned battery casings as cheap fuel. Even in the early 1980s, lead solder was still used to seal food cans. The common practice among children of **pica** (dirt eating) has become especially dangerous for those playing in yards whose soils are badly contaminated by factory- and vehicle-exhausted lead and from the chips of old, lead-laden paint peeling from aging inner-city houses. Many surviving victims of childhood lead poisoning in Australia suffered failure of lead-poisoned kidneys several decades later. And in recent times plumbism has been rampant among "moonshiners" using lead-containing distillation units (automobile radiators soldered with lead) in the United States.

American lead production peaked about 1975, with at least half converted into automobile-fuel additive. Recent partial control of exhaust fumes has been accompanied by a 37 percent reduction in average lead levels in Americans.

Humanity's flirtation with lead frequently has been its undoing. No other metal is so easily extracted from the soil and so readily fashioned into needed items. In every age, however, writers sounding the warning of its toxic hazards were ignored. It may be that the nonspecificity of the lead intoxication syndrome confused earlier diagnosticians because other conditions can simulate some of lead's toxic effects. Perhaps even more relevant is the fact that during most of history the cause-and-effect relationship between specific agents (like lead) and specific symptoms was only vaguely appreciated by physicians whose theoretical concepts did not readily embrace such an association. Such physicians were apt to attribute a broad range of symptoms to general environmental (often climatic) disturbances. Even nineteenth century French naval surgeons, while accepting lead as the cause of the lead poisoning syndrome, rejected it as the cause of an identical symptom complex in tropical sailors. They attributed it instead to the effect of high tropical temperatures, thus delaying recognition of its true origin in their custom of shipboard food storage in lead containers.

Lack of a system for regular publication and wide dissemination of medical knowledge also contributed to delay in grasping the etiology of lead poisoning. As early as 1656, Samuel Stockhausen, a physician to the lead miners of northern Germany, published his realization that their affliction was the toxic effect of the lead ore they mined. Forty years later, that observation led his southern German colleague, Eberhard Gockel, to recognize lead contamination of wine as the cause of an identical problem in his clerical patients, and it was to be more than another century (and many more "colicdemics") before the translation of Stockhausen's report into French enabled Tanquerel to identify the same problem.

Serious and major efforts to reduce lead exposure, such as the 1971 Lead-Based Poisoning Prevention Act in the United States and more recent legislation involving lead air pollution by automobiles, are phenomena primarily since the 1970s. The history of the past two millennia, however, suggests that our knowledge of lead's potential hazards will not prevent at least some continuing problems with its health effects.

Arthur C. Aufderheide

81. Legionnaires' Disease (Legionellosis, Pontiac Fever, *Legionella* Pneumonia)

Legionnaires' disease is an acute infection principally manifested by **pneumonia** and caused by bacteria of the genus *Legionella*. Typically, the attack rate – the proportion of people exposed to the bacterium who become ill – is less than 5 percent. Without specific antibiotic treatment, 15 percent or more of cases are fatal, although that percentage rises sharply in immunosuppressed patients.

Legionnaires' disease is one form of presentation of *Legionella* infections, which are generally termed **legionellosis**. Another version of legionellosis, **Pontiac fever**, affects 45–100 percent of those exposed; no pneumonia occurs, and all patients recover. More than 20 species of *Legionella* have been identified, 10 of which are proven causes of legionellosis in humans.

Characteristics

The weak staining of *Legionella* and its failure to grow on common bacterial media allowed it to be missed for many years in evaluation of pneumonia patients. Once the right diagnostic procedures were identified, *Legionella* was found to cause 1–2 percent of the pneumonia in the United States, perhaps 25,000–50,000 cases annually.

Legionellae live in unsalty warm water and are widely distributed. They thrive particularly well at or slightly above human-body temperature, and may be commonly found in various hot-water systems, including heat-exchange devices. The various ways in which legionellae can go from their watery environment to infect humans are not all worked out, but one method is clear. Aerosols created by some disturbance of contaminated water, such as in a cooling tower, can on occasion infect people downwind. It is likely that, after the aerosol is generated, the water droplets evaporate, leaving the bacteria airborne to travel a considerable distance and be inhaled. Potable-water systems also originate legionellosis outbreaks, but whether this occurs via aerosols, inhalation succeeding throat colonization, direct inoculation, or ingestion is unknown.

Many outbreaks have been recognized, but most cases occur individually or sporadically. The risk of **Legionella pneumonia** (including Legionnaires' disease) increases with age and is two to four times higher in men than in women. Nosocomial (hospital-acquired) legionellosis is an important problem, probably because particularly susceptible people are gathered in a building with water systems that *Legionella* can contaminate.

Legionellosis occurs throughout the year but is most common in summer. This pattern prevails even in outbreaks unrelated to air-conditioning systems, but whether or not warmer weather causes the bacteria to flourish is unknown. Most bacterial and viral pneumonias are more prevalent in winter, making the seasonality of legionellosis one clue in diagnosis. Legionellosis does not seem to spread from one person to another.

Legionnaires' disease is multisystemic, characterized by pneumonia, high fever, chills, muscle aches, chest pain, headache, **diarrhea**, and confusion. Pneumonia usually worsens over the first week of illness and resolves gradually thereafter. In the lungs, air sacs are filled with macrophages, other inflammatory cells, and fibrin. With the proper stain, large numbers of legionellae can be seen, mostly in macrophages. The larger airways are generally spared, which may explain the relative lack of sputum and of contagiousness. Pontiac fever is characterized by fever, chills, muscle aches, and headache. Cough and chest pain are much less common than in Legionnaires' disease.

History

In July 1976, the Pennsylvania American Legion held its annual meeting in Philadelphia, with headquarters in the Bellevue Stratford Hotel. Within days of the convention, many conventioneers sickened. A massive investigation uncovered 221 cases among legionnaires who had attended the convention and others who had been in or near the hotel. Ninety percent of those who became ill developed pneumonia, and 16 percent died. Diagnostic tests for known agents of pneumonia were negative. The epidemiological investigation suggested airborne spread of the agent, because risk of "Legionnaires' disease," as the press dubbed it, increased with the amount of time spent in the hotel's lobby and on the nearby sidewalk but was unrelated to contact with other people or animals, eating, or participation in specific convention events. Those who drank water at the Bellevue Stratford had higher risk than others, suggesting a waterborne agent, but 49 of the cases had only been on the sidewalk outside and had drunk no water there. The outbreak received considerable notoriety and prompted a congressional investigation. Failure to identify the agent immediately led to much public speculation about toxic chemicals and sabotage.

In August, Joseph McDade of the U.S. Public Health Service tested specimens from legionnaires for evidence of **rickettsiae**. The experiments were complicated by an apparent bacterial contamination but overall yielded negative results. In November, McDade noted that the liver was involved in many experimental guinea pigs, a sign reminiscent of **Q fever**, the rickettsial infection most commonly associated with pneumonia. Within a month, he discovered a cluster of what seemed to be large rickettsiae or small bacteria in the liver section of a guinea pig that had been inoculated with a deceased legionnaire's lung tissue. McDade was able to grow these organisms (which have since become known as *Legionella pneumophila*) and showed them convincingly to be the causative agent.

In previous years, the Centers for Disease Control and Prevention (CDC) had investigated other epidemics of mysterious respiratory disease. One, in 1965, involved 81 patients at St. Elizabeth's Hospital in Washington, D.C. In autumn 1976, it was suggested that the same agent had caused both outbreaks. Fortunately, specimens from the St. Elizabeth's outbreak had been stored at the Centers, and tests in January 1977 unequivocally proved the suggestion correct.

In 1968, a remarkable outbreak of a severe, self-limited illness involved 95 of 100 employees in a health-department building in Pontiac, Michigan. Some investigators from the CDC succumbed also, but only those who entered the building when the air-conditioning was on. Inspection of the system showed that the exhaust from the evaporative condenser discharged on the roof just a few feet from the fresh air intake. In addition, the exhaust duct and an adjacent chilled-air duct had defects allowing droplets from the former to puddle in the latter.

When materials from the 1968 investigation of the "Pontiac fever" were used in the tests that succeeded for Legionnaires' disease, scientists were intrigued to find positive results. Not only did Pontiac-fever convalescents show specific antibody to *L. pneumophila*, but also *L. pneumophila* was recovered from stored lung tissue of exposed guinea pigs. Thus a very different disease – both epidemiologically and clinically – was shown to result from a bacterium indistinguishable from that causing Legionnaires' disease.

Investigations of legionellosis proceeded both forward and backward in time. In the summer of 1977, outbreaks of Legionnaires' disease were quickly recognized in Vermont, Ohio, and Tennessee. In 1978 an outbreak at a Memphis hospital started shortly after a flood knocked out the primary cooling tower, requiring operation of an auxiliary that had been out of use for 2 years. Cases clustered downwind from the auxiliary cooling tower but stopped occurring 10 days after it was shut off. *L. pneumophila* was isolated from both patients and the cooling-tower water, confirming the epidemiological evidence that Legionnaires' disease, like Pontiac fever, could be caused by *L. pneumophila* contamination of cooling systems.

Other previously unsolved outbreaks were found to have been legionellosis. In 1973, 10 men cleaning a steam-turbine condenser at a power plant in Virginia had developed what in retrospect seemed to have been Pontiac fever. Testing of stored serum specimens confirmed this. An outbreak of hospitalized cases of pneumonia in Austin, Minnesota, in the summer of 1957 was further investigated in 1979, confirming a diagnosis of Legionnaires' disease in this earliest proven epidemic of legionellosis.

As further studies were reported, the picture emerged of *Legionella* as a group of freshwater-associated bacteria causing pneumonia in humans when particularly susceptible people are exposed by aerosols, or perhaps otherwise, to contaminated water. The presence of running hot water and other thermal pollution, often from industrial processes, favors its growth, suggesting that legionellosis may be particularly common in developed countries. However, the disease appears to be worldwide in its distribution.

David W. Fraser

82. Leishmaniasis

Leishmaniasis is primarily a skin disease produced by **protozoa** of the genus *Leishmania*. The disease takes three basic forms, within which are variants caused by different species, subspecies, or strains of the pathogen. The intermediate host is the sandfly.

Characteristics
Cutaneous leishmaniasis ("oriental sore") is found in Armenia, Azerbaijan, Turkmenistan, Uzbekistan, Afghanistan, India, Iran, much of the Middle East and North Africa, the savanna states from Sudan to Senegal, Kenya, and Ethiopia. In the New World, variants occur in Central America, the Amazon Basin, the Guyanas, and the Andes, especially Venezuela and Peru. In eastern South America, a variant mainly afflicting children extends from Argentina to Venezuela and north to Mexico.

Mucocutaneous leishmaniasis is restricted to the New World. It occurs in Brazil, Peru, Paraguay, Ecuador, Colombia, and Venezuela.

Visceral leishmaniasis (*kala-azar*) is found in India, Burma, Bangladesh, China, Thailand, Somalia, Chad, Kenya, Gabon, Sudan, and Niger. A variant mainly afflicting children inhabits southern Europe, North Africa, the Middle East, Romania, and southern central Asia.

In endemic areas, high levels of disease in rodent and dog populations make leishmaniasis so common that it marks every inhabitant. Some 12 million individuals are estimated to suffer from this infection. Thus, leishmaniasis is second only to **malaria** among the protozoal diseases. Although mortality is low for the skin disease, the organ variant is almost always fatal.

All forms of leishmaniasis are zoonoses transmitted to humans via the sandfly (usually *Phlebotomus*). The leishmanial form of the parasite lives in reticuloendothelial cells of a mammalian host, where it divides by binary fission to destroy the host cell. The parasites are ingested by the sandfly while feeding on the host's skin and develop into leptomonad forms in the insect's intestine. These reproduce enormously, moving to the pharynx and buccal cavity. Individual leishmaniae are restricted to specific sandflies, even though many species may be available.

Cutaneous leishmaniasis is caused by members of *Leishmania tropica*, producing chronic skin lesions that mostly ulcerate. Some forms tend to be "urban" and closely linked to dogs. Others are "rural," with reservoirs including rodents, marsupials, and foxes. In the Americas, sandflies of the genus *Lutzomyia* are often vectors. The initial lesion usually heals spontaneously but leaves a disfiguring scar.

Mucocutaneous leishmaniasis is caused by *Leishmania braziliensis*. In the form called *espundia* in Brazil, the initial lesion becomes an infection of nasal and oral mucosal tissues, resulting in gross deformities and sometimes death from secondary infections. *Lutzomyia* flies are the major vectors.

Visceral leishmaniasis, or *kala-azar*, is caused by members of *Leishmania donovani*. In visceral leishmaniasis, unlike other forms, the organisms parasitize cells beyond subcutaneous and mucosal tissues. Internal organs may be involved. Symptoms include liver and spleen swelling, fever, **diarrhea**, emaciation, **anemia**, skin darkening, and gross abdominal enlargement. Mortality in untreated cases has reached 95 percent.

History

Leishmaniasis is an ancient disease of both the Old and the New Worlds. Old World cutaneous leishmaniasis was first described in English in the mid-eighteenth century. New World pottery clearly depicts the disfiguring disease. Pre-Columbian Incas knew the dangers of leishmaniasis in the lowlands, where coca grew, and used captives to cultivate it. The Spaniards, who later took over the coca trade, were less aware of the problem; their labor policies resulted in much disfigurement and death.

Nineteenth-century British physicians in India knew visceral leishmaniasis as *kala-azar* or "Dumdum fever," its symptoms attributed variously to malaria, **Malta fever**, and other diseases. In 1900, W. B. Leishman noticed the similarity of the parasite to that of **trypanosomiasis**, and soon it was revealed as the cause of *kala-azar*. Leishman published his findings in 1903, yet Charles Donovan independently duplicated his work. Leishman's name was given to the genus, but the agent of *kala-azar* got its specific name from Donovan.

"Oriental sore" had long afflicted Africa and India, where it was known locally as "Delhi boil," "Aleppo boil," and so forth. The first description of *L. tropica* was published in 1898 by Peter Borovsky in a Russian military journal; however, his paper was unknown in the West, and discovery of the organism is often credited to James Wright, who in 1903 found it in an Armenian child's ulcer.

Cutaneous disease in the Americas was described by A. Carini and V. Paranhos in Brazil in 1909 – the same year that mucocutaneous leishmaniasis was described, also in Brazil. Gasper Oliveira de Vianna named the agent *Leishmania braziliensis* in 1911. The American visceral form was first seen in Paraguay in 1913.

Phlebotomus was suspected of being the vector as early as 1911, but this was not proven until 1941.

Marvin J. Allison

83. Leprosy (Hansen's Disease)

Leprosy occurs only in humans and is caused by *Mycobacterium leprae.* Known since the nineteenth century as **Hansen's disease** after Norwegian microbiologist A. G. H. Hansen, who first isolated the microorganism in 1873, true leprosy is a chronic, debilitating, and disfiguring infection. The history of conditions attributed to leprosy undoubtedly includes many afflictions that only resembled leprosy symptoms.

Characteristics

The leprosy bacillus multiplies slowly, usually in the sheaths of peripheral nerves. Losing sensation in discrete, patchy areas of skin is often the earliest symptom of infection. Lacking adequate innervation, the affected dermis can be damaged without evoking a pain response. Tissue repair is then hindered by poor regulation of local blood supply. Hence, secondary infection and inflammation are common, leading to scarring and callusing of surviving tissues. This process can result in loss of fingers, toes, nasal tissue, or other body parts frequently exposed. A "bear-claw" foot or hand is among the characteristic features of leprosy. Involvement of nasal cartilage and vocal cords – common sites for the organism's growth – leads to profound facial disfiguration and also to the raspy, honking voice described in historical accounts.

Earlier physiological signs of leprosy have been noted consistently only since the nineteenth century. The heavily innervated face loses "free play" of expression and affect. Eyelashes and part of the eyebrows disappear long before grosser signs betray infection.

Leprosy occurs commonly only in tropical and subtropical regions. At least 15 million lepers reside mostly in Africa, South and

Southeast Asia, and South America. However, this geographic distribution more likely reflects poverty than it does the possibility that elevated temperatures and humidity facilitate infection. Despite cheap, effective medication (dapsone), leprosy continues to spread in rural regions of Africa and South and Southeast Asia. Because lepers are stigmatized socially, leading to loss of employment, alienation from family and community, and ultimately confinement in a leprosarium, they often deny infection or evade treatment as long as possible, thus ensuring transmission of the disease to others. Leprosy passes between individuals only with sustained exposure, but the disease continues to spread even in areas with Western medicine, because of the high social costs of early identification and treatment.

In the past, leprosy probably extended north to the Arctic Circle. Extensive investigations of medieval gravesites have produced evidence of leprosy among thirteenth century Danes and Norwegians. Interestingly, the distribution of leprosy in medieval Europe, like that of today, appears to have been rural, and evidence of leprosy disappears with urbanization. The disappearance of leprosy in Europe historically progressed northward from the urban Mediterranean areas of Italy and Spain. Cases of leprosy were still reported in Britain during the fourteenth and fifteenth centuries, and it persisted in Scandinavia until the late nineteenth century, when Hansen discovered the leprosy bacillus.

One odd feature of leprotic distribution is increased prevalence on islands or near seacoasts. Early theorists attributed the cause of the disease to a fish diet, an explanation now discredited. Undoubtedly leprosy's low infectivity and association with poverty contribute to the slow spread inland.

It is possible that *Mycobacterium tuberculosis*, a related organism that also conveys limited cross-immunity to *M. leprae*, has affected the long-term distribution and incidence of leprosy. Other atypical mycobacterial infections, such as **scrofula**, may be involved as well. Increased population density facilitates the spread of **tu-berculosis**, which may have contributed to a decline in leprosy as large towns appeared. In West Africa today, leprosy in rural villages increases with distance from a city, whereas tuberculosis increases dramatically with population density. There is little evidence that leprosy existed in the Western Hemisphere, Australia, or Oceania before it was introduced from the Old World.

This epidemiological relationship between tuberculosis and leprosy, however, is obscured in individual patients. For despite cross-immunity, the most common associated cause of death among lepers is tuberculosis, illustrating how long-suffering victims lose the ability to combat other infections. Moreover, geographic determinants alone cannot explain the high prevalence of leprosy in densely settled eastern India. It could be that successful control of tuberculosis in the region permitted the persistence of leprosy and that stigmatization of lepers effectively delayed treatment of the illness.

Members of the family Mycobacteriaceae can infect mammalian and avian hosts, and, as exemplified by **bovine tuberculosis** and **avian tu-berculosis**, a pathogen dominant in one host species can successfully infect another. Thus humans have suffered from bovine tuberculosis transmitted through contaminated milk and from atypical mycobacterial infections. But among these, only leprosy and tuberculosis can be transmitted from one human to another, and *M. leprae* is the only one that cannot be transmitted naturally to nonhuman species. The organism usually enters a new host via respiration or the skin. Because the incubation period is lengthy, the microorganism's growth and dissemination through the body is poorly understood. Early symptoms usually appear 3–5 years after infection, but clinical evidence may appear in as few as 6 months or as long as 20 years.

As with other chronic infections, clinical features of leprosy can vary. Indeed, leprosy is called a **bipolar disease** because of two different forms of the illness, with "mixed" or "intermediate" reactions possible but infrequent. In **tuberculoid leprosy**, one polar type, skin areas of "patchy anesthesia" heal relatively quickly after injury, but new areas appear, more extensive and severe, involving peripheral nerves to the extent that desensitized skin cannot be protected from burns, exposure, or other insults. Even though tuberculoid leprosy is considered milder than **lepromatous leprosy** – possibly because of a stronger immune response – infections secondary to skin injury make it a serious disease.

In the "leonine facies" of lepromatous leprosy, the other polar type, the skin reaction is severely disfiguring: Intermediate healing produces thick, corrugated scar tissue. Lesions often teem with infective bacilli. Lepromatous leprosy and tuberculoid leprosy arise from morphologically indistinguishable *M. leprae* bacilli. Thus, both strong and weak immunologic responses (if this difference is the "cause" of the two forms) produce crippling and disfigurement.

The leonine form is more distinctive and thus more frequent in historical accounts. However, grossly disfiguring ulceration of face and limbs is not necessarily caused by leprosy. **Syphilis, frostbite**, or **diabetes** could also explain the descriptions in some reports. Moreover, other illnesses such as **psoriasis, pellagra, eczema**, and **lupus erythematosus** could easily lend themselves to the historical "diagnosis" of leprosy. Thus the more subtle changes of early leprosy provide more assurance of a correct diagnosis than simply loathsome appearance.

History

The history of leprosy has been dominated by three problems. One concerns stigmatization. Most ancient societies identified some individuals as "lepers," who were stigmatized, although surely "lepers" included many suffering from something besides Hansen's disease. Stigmatization of lepers has persisted into the present despite advances in diagnosis and treatment. The second problem focuses on medical evidence for leprosy's changing prevalence over time, particularly in Western Europe between the years 500 and 1500. Finally, the world distribution of leprosy and failure to impede its spread has emerged as a historical problem of recent centuries.

In the biblical book of *Leviticus*, the disease **zara'ath** or **tsara'ath** was identified by priests, and its victims cast "outside the camp" as unclean and uncleansable. They were viewed as both chosen and rejected by God and, consequently, not exiled altogether from the community – as were criminals – but rather made to live apart. Thus, central problems posed by the disease involved on one hand the spiritual identity of diseased individuals, who though probably morally "tainted" were not apparently responsible for their disease; and on the other hand the delegation of diagnosis to religious, not medical, authorities.

The opprobrium attached to leprosy was handled dramatically by Old Testament writers, and this Judaeo-Christian tradition was of central importance in European history for the next 2,000 years. Stigmatization of the leper was derived from religious, medical, and social responses to individuals carrying the diagnosis. Thus, during the High Middle Ages (1100–1300 A.D.), lepers were identified by spiritual authorities and then separated from the general community, often ritualistically. Considered "dead to society," last rites might be said in the leper's presence, sometimes as the victim stood symbolically in a grave. Thereafter access to his or her city or village was severely limited. Italian cities, for example, posted guards to identify lepers and deny them entrance except under carefully controlled circumstances. Leprosaria (hospitals to isolate and house lepers) were constructed at church or communal expense, although medical services were limited. Where public services were lacking, lepers depended upon begging or alms.

Laws in Western Europe illustrated the exaggerated fear of contagion lepers generated. Lepers had to be identifiable at a distance, leading to the creation of legendary symbols of leprosy: a yellow cross sewn to cape or vestment, a clapper or bell to warn passersby, and a long pole for indicating wanted items or for retrieving an alms cup placed closer to the road than lepers were allowed to go.

The stigmatization of lepers, however, was not limited to Western tradition. Most past societies denied lepers legal rights as well as socially ostracizing them. In both East and South Asia, marriage to a leper or a leper's offspring was prohibited. As in Western tradition, the disease was often attributed to sin as well as contagion. The stereotype of the leper as filthy, rotten, nauseating, and repulsive is so strong that most hansenologists today advocate rejection of "leprosy" in favor of "Hansen's disease." The only exception to the pattern of stigmatization seems to be in Islamic society, where lepers are neither exiled nor considered morally repulsive.

In contrast to ancient Chinese texts that describe in detail leprosy's destruction of the face, evidence for leprosy in the ancient Mediterranean is meager. Nowhere in the Biblical tradition is there more than a general description of the disease. Hippocratic texts provide no evidence that true leprosy existed in ancient Greece, but the Greek word *lepra*, probably describing psoriasis, gave origin to the disease's name. Thus a coherent and powerful Western tradition stigmatizing lepers apparently began in the absence of any organized, accurate medical description of the condition. Indeed, the earliest Western clinical description of leprosy appears in the writings of tenth century Persian physician Avicenna; his is the description upon which medieval Europeans relied.

The decline of leprosy in Europe coincided with increasing sophistication in diagnosis. This decline may have resulted from several factors: an increase in another disease, such as tuberculosis; improvement of living standards; high catastrophic mortality from **plague** and other epidemics, reducing the number of lepers in the population; or the simple fact that medical authorities began to participate in diagnosis of leprosy. Surely other skin afflictions were better recognized in the late Middle Ages. Nonetheless, true leprosy certainly existed in Europe, as exhumations of medieval remains have illustrated.

Knowledge of leprosy in modern terms evolved during the nineteenth century, coincident with the germ theory of disease. During this period, the description of lepromatous leprosy by Danish physician Daniel Danielssen in the 1840s, the discovery of the microorganism by Hansen in 1873, and widespread attention to leprosy in European colonies identified it as a contagious tropical infection. As such it was believed eradicable by Western medicine and public-health intervention.

In the same year that Hansen found the causal organism of leprosy, Catholic priest Damien de Veuster drew worldwide attention in attempting to humanize the treatment of leprosy by going to live among lepers in Hawaii. But he may have underscored the fear of contagion, because he eventually contracted the disease. Thus in modern times, increasing medical knowledge of *M. leprae* may have increased alarm as leprosy was "discovered" to be the resilient global problem it remains.

Ann G. Carmichael

84. Leptospirosis

Leptospirosis manifested by severe **jaundice** was first described in 1886 by A. Weil. Named "Weil's disease," it designated an infectious jaundice. Not until later was it known that leptospirosis was caused by leptospires triggering various syndromes. The first pathogens were discovered in 1915 among Japanese mineworkers and German soldiers. *Leptospira*, a genus of family Treponemataceae, order Spirochaetales, is a fine threadlike organism with hooked ends that is pathogenic for humans and other mammals, producing **meningitis**, **hepatitis**, and **nephritis**. Leptospirosis once killed up to 40 percent of those infected; modern treatment has reduced mortality to about 5 percent. Rodents are the natural reservoir.

Characteristics

Leptospires are obligate aerobes and are classified serologically as bacteria, subdivided into two species. *Leptospira biflexa* includes various water spirochetes; *Leptospira interrogans* embraces parasitic strains. The species *interrogans* (so named because it appears like a question mark) is subdivided into 187 serotypes. Human leptospirosis generally results from exposure to infected animal urine, although it is also transmitted via contact, animal bites, and ingestion of contaminated food and water. Leptospires enter the body through breaks in the skin as well as through mouth, nose, and eye linings.

Leptospirosis is mostly seen during warmer weather and heavy rainfall, and the presence of the disease in mud and swamps has often placed soldiers at special risk. Usually, it causes isolated cases, but small clusters and even large outbreaks have occurred.

Leptospirosis is frequently an occupational disease. Fieldworkers and husbandmen are at risk, as are employees of slaughterhouses and poultry and fish processors, and workers in sewers, mines, and other wet places infested with rodents. Infected wild rodents are the source of infection in domesticated animals, especially dogs, pigs, and cattle.

Localized leptospirosis infections produced by one or another strain occur worldwide. Pig-raising areas of Europe, Australia, and Argentina see one form called "swineherd's disease." Similarly, sugarcane plantation regions of East Asia and rice-growing regions of Spain and Italy harbor other forms. Local names for various leptospiroses often reflect the circumstances of contraction, as in "harvest" or "swamp" fever. In Germany, agricultural workers contracted "field fever"; in Silesia, "mud fever"; in Russia, "water fever"; and in Germany and Switzerland, "pea-pickers' disease." Leptospirosis can also be an urban disease carried by rats as well as by dogs.

The first phase of leptospirosis involves acute onset of high fever, headache, malaise, conjunctival reddening, muscle pain, **meningism**, renal irritation, **hypotonia**, and **bradycardia**. In the second stage, danger of organ involvement is accompanied by the appearance of specific antibodies. Frequently, the liver becomes enlarged and painful, and life-threatening complications arise when renal damage is severe. **Icterus** can be intense and lasting. The most common second-stage symptom is **serosal meningitis**, and less frequently **encephalomyelitis** or **neuritis**. Other damage is rare. When death occurs, renal and hepatic failure is usually the cause. Hemorrhages can be found in almost any organ and in muscles and subcutaneous tissue. Antibiotics are effective against leptospires but only if employed within the first few days. After this, efforts are directed at avoiding complications.

History

Much of the history of leptospirosis appears as efforts to separate leptospiral jaundice and meningitis from other infections. Clinical history began with Weil's 1886 description, followed by isolation of the germs in 1915. In 1918, the newly discovered bacteria were named *Leptospira*. About the same time, researchers found cases without jaundice – the 7-day **Nanukayami fever**, carried by field mice. In subsequent decades, numerous serotypes were found throughout the world. After 1950, a new classification grouped the serotypes into malignant and benign human leptospires as well as animal ones.

After over a century of leptospirosis research, it seems remarkable that widespread epidemics have been infrequent. Today, incidence of leptospirosis has been reduced in developed countries, probably because of decreased rodent populations and improved human hygiene in the presence of domestic animals.

Otto R. Gsell

85. Leukemia

Leukemia, commonly known as **cancer of the blood**, denotes a group of malignant disorders in the blood-forming cells. The bone marrow (where blood cells are made) malfunctions, producing abnormal white (leukemic) cells to the detriment of other essential blood cells.

Blood consists of plasma, the fluid component; red blood cells (erythrocytes), which transport oxygen; white blood cells (leukocytes, categorized as monocytes, granulocytes, or lymphocytes), which help defend the body against infection; and platelets, which control bleeding. Blood-cell formation (hematopoiesis) starts in bone marrow, the spongy interior of the large bones, with undifferentiated "pluripotent stem cells," which contain characteristics of all blood cells. These cells divide, producing specialized cells. The production process is continual, with cell characteristics becoming increasingly defined. Eventually, the cells are "committed" to evolution into one specific cell type (red, white, or platelet) and are released into the bloodstream at a rate consistent with the body's needs and the death of old cells. In normal health, immature stem cells ("blasts") are present in the blood only in small numbers.

Every day at least 200 billion red cells, 10 billion white cells, and over 400 billion platelets are produced in the marrow. In normal circulating blood there are approximately 1,000 red cells to each white cell. But in leukemia, normal production of blood cells fails. White blood cells reproduce abnormally and create immature blasts or poorly developed cells. These leukemic cells overpopulate the bone marrow, enter the bloodstream and lymph system, and infiltrate organs and glands, causing them to enlarge and malfunction. The bone marrow becomes unable to produce sufficient levels of red cells and platelets; consequently, the balance of the blood cell population is seriously disturbed, and the body's defenses based on white blood cells and platelets are rendered ineffective.

Characteristics

Leukemia is classified according to the type of white cell affected. The two main types of the disease are **myeloid** (affecting monocytes and granulocytes) and **lymphatic** (affecting lymphocytes). These are further subdivided into **acute** and **chronic**. In **acute leukemias**, there is abnormal growth of immature blast cells, whereas in **chronic leukemias**, more mature cells proliferate, although immature cells may be present. The following are the diseases that mainly arise:

1. **Acute myeloid leukemia** (AML) – also called **acute myelogenous leukemia**, **acute myelocytic leukemia**, **acute myeloblastic leukemia**, and **acute granulocytic leukemia** – is synonymous with the group known as **acute nonlymphocytic leukemia** (ANLL), which includes some of the rarer subtypes of the disease (e.g., **monocytic leukemia**). AML involves the neutrophils (one of the granulocytes) that stem from the myeloid progenitor cell line.

2. **Chronic myeloid leukemia** (CML) – also called **chronic myelogenous leukemia**, **chronic myelocytic leukemia**, and **chronic granulocytic leukemia** (CGL) – produces excessive numbers of granulocytes that accumulate in the bone marrow and bloodstream.

3. **Acute lymphoblastic leukemia** (ALL) – also called **acute lymphocytic leukemia** and **acute lymphatic leukemia** – arises as a result of abnormal immature lymphocytes, which proliferate in the bone marrow and bloodstream and affect the lymphocytes (B cells and T cells) stemming from the lymphoid cell line.

4. **Chronic lymphocytic leukemia** (CLL) – also called **chronic lymphatic leukemia** and **chronic lymphogenous leukemia** – produces an abnormal increase in lymphocytes that lack infection-fighting ability. It is the major type of a group of diseases known as **lymphoproliferative disorders**, which includes rarer forms of leukemia such as **hairy-cell leukemia** and **adult T-cell leukemia**.

Leukemia occurs worldwide and represents about 5 percent of all cancers. The disease has no regular pattern. Its comparative rarity helps explain its irregularity. Leukemia can strike anyone, at any time, at any age. Because of variable medical standards, comparing the worldwide incidence of leukemia and other cancers can present problems. The estimated incidence of leukemia in the developed world is 10 per 100,000 population, the most common being AML and its subgroups, followed by CLL including its rarer forms, then CML, and lastly ALL. Rates vary in some countries and among some ethnic groups, but no variation is significant. The male/female ratio is about 1.7:1.

What causes a healthy cell to become malignant and to proliferate in that state? The consensus of opinion is that leukemia results from the interaction of several factors, and investigations are being pursued into genetic factors (some studies indicate that certain individuals are more susceptible than others), disorders of the immune system, radiation, chemicals that suppress bone marrow function, and viral infection (retroviruses are known to cause leukemia in certain animal species).

Because of the occasional occurrence of "clusters" of the disease, investigations are often launched to find a cause, and identification of possible contributory factors within the environment is one approach. The most established cause of human leukemias is ionizing radiation. The atom bombs dropped on Hiroshima and Nagasaki in 1945, for example, increased the incidence of leukemia beginning about 3 years after the attack, peaking at 6 years, and then slowly declining to normal incidence at 20 years. The greatest incidence was among those closest to the explosions, whereas from 2,000 meters the risk of leukemia was no greater than among the general population. Increased numbers of clusters of leukemia have been reported in areas surrounding nuclear power stations, and childhood cases appear to be more prominent than usual in these clusters. But if nuclear power stations are emitting radiation, relatively few people are affected – again raising the question of individual susceptibility.

Early symptoms of leukemia are similar to those of infectious illness. The leukemias share common signs arising from the infiltration of the bone marrow. Lack of red cells causes fatigue and **anemia**, lack of normal white cells results in infections, and lack of platelets produces bleeding and bruising. Lymph nodes, spleen, and liver may become enlarged with infiltrating leukemic cells. Bone or joint pains are associated symptoms. Marked differences, however, exist between acute and chronic leukemias in their presentation. In acute leukemias, **influenza**-like symptoms signal the sudden and rapid progress of the disease. By contrast, symptoms of chronic leukemias are subtler. Often, the disease is discovered accidentally during a routine blood test. Common symptoms are weakness, tiredness, fever, night sweats, and loss of appetite.

Remedies for leukemia in the nineteenth century were few, and none helped control the disease for any length of time. Quinine was used for combating fever; morphine and opium, for **diarrhea**; iron, for anemia; iodine, for external use as an antibacterial; and arsenic. In 1865, a German physician prescribed arsenic trioxide for a woman with CML. The patient was temporarily restored to health, and arsenic became the first beneficial agent against certain forms of leukemia.

The 1895 discovery of X-rays by Wilhelm Röntgen soon led to X-ray therapy of leukemia with results similar to those of arsenic. X-rays seemed more advantageous because they could prevent cell division and inhibit cell growth, but patients could become resistant to X-rays. Nowadays, irradiation is used to attack leukemic cells that accumulate in certain areas of the body where chemotherapy is less effective.

As late as 1938, one researcher wrote that although chronic leukemia patients could be made more comfortable, acute leukemia did not respond to any form of therapy. During the 1940s, however, some X-ray-resistant leukemia patients responded to treatment with chemical analogues of poisonous mustard gas. This triggered intensive efforts to find less toxic and more specific agents. The result was the beginning of chemotherapy, in which various drugs, often given in combination, are used to attack the leukemic cells. As these drugs can affect both leukemic and normal cells, their use must be controlled with great care.

In nearly all cases, modern therapy can effect remission. The next stage is to keep the patient in remission through "consolidation therapy," followed by "maintenance therapy," which aims to destroy any remaining or undetected leukemic cells. Complete remission, however, does not always mean cure. A further form of treatment in suitable cases is bone marrow transplantation, although graft-versus-host disease may cause a major complication. This therapy, however, has controlled the disease in cases when other means would not have been successful.

History

Leukemia was identified as a disease entity in 1845 by independent researchers John Hughes Bennett and Rudolph Virchow. Virchow named the disease leukemia, Greek for "white blood," and Bennett called it **leucocythemia**, Greek for "white cell blood." During the previous decade, there had already been reports of peculiar conditions of the blood, pus in the blood, and "milky" blood, with some symptoms compatible with leukemia.

Microscopes were crude, and there was no satisfactory means of illuminating specimens being observed. In fact, it is remarkable that the disease was recognized at all. But after recognition, reports of suspected or actual cases of leukemia began to appear, slowly revealing its worldwide distribution. Case reports also indicated the ineffectual nature of known therapies.

The first breakthrough was the discovery by Ernst Neumann in 1868 of the importance of the bone marrow in blood formation; he also investigated changes in the bone marrow in leukemia. Another breakthrough occurred in 1877, when Paul Ehrlich developed a stain that permitted cells to be clearly defined. By then, microscopes were improved, and the new technique of staining enabled features of the blood to be studied with unprecedented clarity.

Thus began a new era in hematology, but nearly 70 years passed before any progress was made in the treatment of leukemia. Experiments indicated that folic acid might stimulate the growth of leukemic cells. This led to the development for trial of new drugs antagonistic to folic acid. Aminopterin was one of these and was used successfully against acute leukemia in the late 1940s. Much research followed, with the result that by the late 1980s there was an established armamentarium of drugs used mostly to achieve a remission and maintain it.

Leukemia is a disease of major interest in both hematology and cancer research. Much progress has been made in terms of patient survival. Moreover, the outstanding "problem areas" of research are now more clearly defined, and research efforts within the fields of cell and molecular biology, immunology, cytogenetics, and virology are ongoing.

Gordon J. Piller

86. Lupus Erythematosus

Lupus erythematosus (LE) is a clinical syndrome with multiple but largely unknown causes. It exhibits a broad spectrum of symptoms ranging in severity from potentially fatal to virtually undiagnosable. When limited to the skin, it is called **discoid lupus erythematosus** (DLE); when viscera are affected, it is **systemic lupus erythematosus** (SLE). The inciting causes activate immunologic mechanisms that mediate the pathological, predominantly inflammatory, tissue responses.

History

Medical use of the term "lupus" has been traced to the fifteenth century, when it designated a **cancer**. The term was reintroduced in England in 1808 to designate **cutaneous tuberculosis**, particularly when it affected the face. Cutaneous tuberculosis was eventually designated **lupus vulgaris**. In 1851, a French physician used the term *lupus erythemateaux* to describe a condition later named discoid lupus erythematosus (DLE) by Moriz Kaposi in 1872. Kaposi concluded that DLE was more common and more severe in women and further believed that it was not related to **tuberculosis**. Such a causal relationship, however, was advocated by other researchers (particularly French dermatologists), and the question was debated until the 1930s.

Kaposi used the term **disseminated lupus erythematosus** for cases with widespread skin lesions rather than visceral involvement. Nevertheless, he described some cases having fever, **pleuropneumonia**, **arthralgia**, and **arthritis**. Slowly, recognition developed that various visceral manifestations are attributes of the systemic disease rather than coincidences. From 1894 to 1903, William Osler saw 29 patients presenting an "erythema with visceral lesions"; he provided the first clear descriptions of SLE. Osler added kidney and central nervous system involvement to Kaposi's description, and it was soon recognized that **pneumonia** also belongs to the syndrome.

Before the 1940s, most publication on lupus erythematosus was by dermatologists; consequently, skin lesions were considered essential to diagnosis. In 1923, a report described four cases of noninfectious **endocarditis** (heart inflammation) of which three had the skin lesions. A 1932 review of 11 such cases found that 5 lacked the skin eruption. In 1936, a study concluded that this form of **heart disease** is a manifestation of SLE. **Leukopenia** and sensitivity to sunlight were convincingly related to SLE in 1939, but only in the 1940s was it accepted that skin eruption is not a necessary component of SLE. Data indicate that only about 40 percent of patients ever have the "butterfly" facial rash and that eruptions on the body occur in about 75 percent of cases. That DLE and SLE are manifestations of the same disease was first proposed in 1937, but two decades passed before the concept achieved general acceptance.

SLE was perceived to be rare and uniformly fatal because only the most severe cases – identified by the rash – were diagnosed. For example,

at University Hospital in Prague, there were just 8 cases from 1897 to 1908. At Johns Hopkins Hospital, only 3 cases were diagnosed between 1919 and 1923. In fact, among 7,500 autopsies of cases above 13 years of age reviewed at the same hospital in 1936, there were just 5 instances of SLE. Five cases were diagnosed at the Mayo Clinic between 1918 and 1921, but as the disease became more familiar, 132 cases were recognized during the decade 1938–47.

In 1948, however, "LE cells" were reported in bone marrow, initiating numerous efforts to demonstrate these new entities more easily and reliably. In 1954, researchers discovered that LE cells result from reactions between a serum factor and leukocyte nuclei, and in 1957, a quantifiable test for this reaction was developed. Such tests have greatly increased case findings and brought about recognition that SLE exhibits a broad range of severity.

The next advance was standardization of the criteria for diagnosis. In 1971, American rheumatologists published a battery of clinical and laboratory findings of which a specified number were required for acceptable diagnosis. This schema was well received, and a 1982 modification was adopted in many countries.

In the 1940s, it was generally acknowledged that no effective treatment existed for LE. The initial breakthrough occurred in 1949 with the discovery that corticosteroids exert a dramatic suppression of most SLE symptoms. Prednisone, a synthetic derivative of cortisone introduced in 1955, has become the most commonly used oral corticosteroid. Only cutaneous and renal manifestations are frequently refractory. In 1951, quinacrine, an antimalarial drug, was found effective against DLE. Soon, other antimalarials were found similarly useful, and hydroxychloroquine is now principally employed. In SLE, antimalarials are most effective against the rash but may also ameliorate some visceral symptoms. The third major therapeutic category is immunosuppressive drugs: The first was nitrogen mustard, in 1950; now the most common are azathioprine and cyclophosphamide.

Modern therapy and the recognition of milder cases have not only improved the quality of life for SLE patients but also greatly prolonged their survival. Before corticosteroids, one-half of patients died within 3 years of diagnosis. Later, the mean survival of 15 years beyond diagnosis reached 75 percent.

Characteristics

SLE mortality is influenced by race and sex. According to U.S. data, annual mortality – relative to 1.0 for white males – is 1.6 for black males, 3.7 for white females, and 10.5 for black females.

The proportion of DLE cases in dermatology clinics has been reported since the early twentieth century; incidence between 0.25 and 0.75 percent has consistently been found in various parts of the world. The early belief that the disease is rare in the tropics and among black populations has been disproved.

The only epidemiological conclusion about SLE until the 1950s was that it occurred predominantly in young women. In 1952, an ethnic predisposition was postulated, based on the frequently deleterious effect of sun exposure: Redheaded, freckled persons – unable to tan – were deemed most susceptible. This was contradicted, however, by a 1964 study indicating that SLE is actually more common among blacks. More recent studies have substantiated an increased susceptibility of blacks, particularly black women.

Unlike diseases such as **rheumatic fever** or tuberculosis, SLE appears unrelated to socioeconomic factors. Annual incidence in the United States has been estimated at about 5 per 100,000, with black females about three times more susceptible and black males two times more susceptible than their white counterparts. The mean age of onset is 28–30 years, but the preponderance of female patients varies with age. About twice as many females as males are afflicted during the first decade of life and from the seventh decade on. But between ages 20 and 40, there are 8 female patients for every male.

Studies also indicate greater susceptibility of Chinese than other ethnic groups, and the SLE death rate for Oriental women in the United States (nearly three times that of white women) is similar to that of black women. Prevalence of SLE among Polynesians also exceeds that of Caucasians. In the predominantly black population of Jamaica, SLE constitutes a remarkably large proportion of treated **rheumatic diseases**. In view of the prevalence of SLE among nonwhite populations elsewhere, the apparent rarity of the disease among African blacks has been perplexing. The possibility of differences in susceptibility of various African ethnic groups must be considered. The data from much of the world remain inadequate to draw firm conclusions about ethnic and other possible variables related to SLE.

Thomas G. Benedek

87. Lyme Borreliosis (Lyme Disease)

Lyme borreliosis is a tick-borne spirochetal disease caused by *Borrelia burgdorferi*. This systemic illness potentially involves the dermatologic, neurological, cardiac, and articular systems. It can mimic various other diseases such as juvenile **rheumatoid arthritis, multiple sclerosis**, and **syphilis**.

Characteristics
Lyme disease is the most frequently diagnosed tick-transmitted illness in the United States, where its three major geographic loci are the northeastern and Middle Atlantic coastal regions, the upper Midwest, and the Pacific Northwest. The disease is also found in Europe, Australia, the former U.S.S.R., China, Japan, and Africa. The vector of Lyme disease is a tick, *Ixodes dammini* (or related *Ixodes* species such as *pacificus, scapularis,* and *ricinus*).

B. burgdorferi has also been found in other ticks, horseflies, deerflies, and mosquitoes, but whether these insects are possible secondary vectors has not been established. Reservoirs of *B. burgdorferi* occur in animals parasitized by infected ticks. *Ixodes* is a three-host tick with a life cycle of 2 years. Adult ticks mate and feed primarily on deer in late fall; the female deposits eggs on the ground, which produce larvae that are active late the following summer. The tiny larvae obtain blood meals from infected rodents such as white-footed mice, shrews, chipmunks, and squirrels, which are primary reservoirs for *B. burgdorferi*. Ground-foraging birds are also important hosts for the larvae and nymphs. After a blood meal, the larva molts to a nymphal form, which is active the following spring and into midsummer. It seeks an animal host, obtains a blood meal, and molts to the adult stage to complete the 2-year life cycle. Animal hosts include humans, dogs, deer, cattle, horses, raccoons, cats, skunks, bears, and opossums.

Each developmental stage of the tick requires feeding once and may take several days. *B. burgdorferi* is transmitted to the host during the blood meal. The longer the time the infected tick is attached to the host, the greater probability of transmission.

Lyme borreliosis is arbitrarily categorized in three stages: Stage I involves the dermatologic system and is diagnosed by the classic rash, **erythema chronicum migrans** (ECM); Stage II involves the neurological or cardiac system months to years after infection; Stage III involves the joints, also months to years after infection. These three stages may overlap and occasionally present simultaneously. Moreover, any of these stages may occur in the absence of the others.

The ECM rash is pathognomonic for Stage I Lyme borreliosis and begins as a small flat (macule) or swollen (papule) spot at the site of the tick bite. It then expands to a large oval or round lesion with a red-to-pink outer border and a clear central area. Viable *B. burgdorferi* occasionally can be cultured in the advancing margins. Blood-borne spread of the spirochetes may produce multiple secondary lesions days to weeks later. The rash persists a few days or weeks, usually unaccompanied by systemic symptoms, although occasional fever, chills, and fatigue may occur. Because the rash can be asymptomatic or unobserved, many people

may go undiagnosed. More than 20 percent of adults with Lyme borreliosis fail to remember the rash, and the percentage is much higher in children.

Stage II of Lyme borreliosis may involve the neurological system. Of patients, 10–15 percent may present a **meningitis**-like picture or have **cranial nerve palsies**. The most commonly involved cranial nerve is the seventh, interfering with proper control of facial musculature. In individuals with meningeal irritation, episodic headaches, neck pain, and stiffness may occur. Occasionally, patients with **stroke** syndromes including **hemiparesis** as well as cases mimicking multiple sclerosis or **encephalitis** have been reported. Individuals may have associated confusion, agitation, disorientation, and memory loss. The symptoms and signs may wax and wane over weeks and months. Heart involvement in Stage II is rare. Cardiac manifestations are commonly detected only as first-degree **heart block** on electrocardiographic tracings, although some patients can have a more serious second- or third-degree heart block and present with episodic fainting spells.

The most common late manifestation of Lyme borreliosis is **arthritis**, usually occurring several months after the tick bite – but the range is 1 week to over 10 years. It is usually **oligoarticular arthritis** (fewer than four joints) involving large joints such as the knee or ankle. Attacks may last from a few days to several months. Some individuals experience recurrence with variable periods of remission. The intensity of articular involvement is variable: Some patients complain only of aches (**arthralgias**), whereas others demonstrate joint swelling (arthritis).

B. burgdorferi infection can be spread transplacentally in humans. Infections during pregnancy can result in spontaneous abortion, premature delivery, low birth weight, and congenital malformation – complications similar to those caused by the spirochete *Treponema pallidum*, the causative agent of syphilis.

Lyme borreliosis is treated with antibiotics. The best results are achieved with prompt administration of oral antibiotics at the time of initial infection (Stage I). The duration of the rash and associated symptoms is abbreviated by a 3-week course of oral tetracycline, penicillin, or erythromycin therapy. In Stage III Lyme borreliosis, 3 weeks of parenteral medicine or ceftriaxone are the drugs of choice. The earlier antibiotics are instituted, the more likely a cure may be achieved. A delay in starting antibiotics may result in lifelong residual symptoms – intermittent or even chronic – from the disease.

History
In 1909, Swedish dermatologist Arvid Afzelius described a rash (which he labeled **erythema migrans**) that succeeded an *Ixodes* tick bite. In 1913, an Austrian physician described a similar lesion and labeled it erythema chronicum migrans. Recognition of ECM's association with systemic symptoms occurred in France in 1922. Investigators described tick-bite patients with subsequent erythema migrans and nervous-system involvement. In 1934, a German dentist described erythema migrans with associated joint symptoms. And in 1951, the beneficial effects of penicillin in treating a patient with ECM and meningitis suggested a bacterial etiology.

In the United States, the first documented case of ECM occurred in Wisconsin in 1969. In 1975, state health officials learned that several children living close together in Lyme, Connecticut, had developed arthritis. An investigation by Allen Steere revealed ECM in 25 percent of patients. He named the syndrome "Lyme disease" after the town.

In 1977, it was observed that an *I. dammini* tick bite preceded the ECM rash. Willy Burgdorfer and colleagues isolated a spirochete from the midgut of the tick; this spirochete was subsequently named *B. burgdorferi*. The following year, Steere isolated the spirochete from blood, skin, and spinal fluid of Lyme disease patients and concluded that it was the causative agent. Also, in 1983 in West Germany, H. Pfister and colleagues concluded that *B. burgdorferi* isolated in spinal fluid from a **lymphocytic meningoradiculitis** ("Bannwarth's syndrome") patient was causative, and they im-

plied that the original 1941 description of 13 patients provided by A. Bannwarth may have resulted from the same organism. In 1984, Klaus Weber and colleagues, also in West Germany, noted an elevation of IgG antibodies in the blood of patients with the skin lesion **acrodermatitis chronica atrophicans** (ACA). ACA is an uncommon late dermatologic manifestation of Lyme borreliosis. German physician Alfred Buchwald first described ACA in 1883, which may have been the first reported case of Lyme borreliosis.

Robert D. Leff

88. Malaria

Malaria results from infection by protozoans of the genus *Plasmodium*. These parasites are transmitted from one human host to the next by infected mosquitoes of the genus *Anopheles*. Although malaria receded from many temperate regions in the twentieth century, it continues to be a major cause of morbidity and mortality in tropical and subtropical countries. Three of the species – *Plasmodium vivax*, *Plasmodium falciparum*, and *Plasmodium malariae* – are widely distributed; the fourth, *Plasmodium ovale*, is principally found in tropical Africa. *P. vivax* (causing **benign tertian malaria**) and *P. falciparum* (causing **malignant tertian malaria**) are responsible for the great majority of malaria cases throughout the world.

Characteristics
Malaria is characteristically paroxysmal and periodic. The classical episode begins with chills, extends through a bout of fever, and ends with sweating, subsiding fever, a sense of relief, and sleep. Between early paroxysms, infected persons may feel quite well; as the disease progresses, however, patients are increasingly burdened by symptoms. *P. falciparum* infection is particularly dangerous because of associated complications.

The term "malaria," from the Italian *mala* and *aria* ("bad air"), was in use by the seventeenth century and referred to the cause of **intermittent fevers** (thought to result from exposure to marsh air). However, past writers used the term for the presumed cause rather than the disease. Only after the pathogenic agents were identified did usage shift so that "malaria" came to mean the disease rather than the agent.

Protozoa of the genus *Plasmodium* are parasitic in many vertebrate animals. Most primate species are hosts for plasmodia. It is generally accepted that malaria parasites evolved in association with early humans, perhaps differentiating into the four recognized species during the mid-Pleistocene.

All mammalian plasmodia have similar two-phase life cycles: an asexual (schizogonic) phase in the vertebrate host and a sexual (sporogonic) phase in female *Anopheles* mosquitoes. These cycles reflect ancient relationships that seem to date from at least the Oligocene.

The sexual phase is initiated as the mosquito takes a blood meal. Parasites in ingested red blood cells are released as male and female gametes in the stomach of the mosquito. Fusion of the gametes produces a zygote, which encysts in the stomach wall. After 10–20 days, this oocyst releases thousands of sporozoites that migrate to the salivary glands. When the now infective mosquito probes for blood, these sporozoites are injected into the new host in saliva.

The sporozoites follow the bloodstream to the liver and there reproduce by nuclear division into large numbers (10,000–20,000) of merozoites. These enter the bloodstream, invade red blood cells (erythrocytes), and break down the hemoglobin contained therein. The parasite again divides, producing 8–24 merozoites. When it reaches maturity, the erythrocyte bursts and the merozoites are released. Again some invade uninfected red cells. The process may continue through repeated cycles, destroying more and more red cells. Immune responses or intervention can check the process short of profound anemia, complications, and death. Some red-cell merozoites differentiate as

male and female gametocytes. These circulate in erythrocytes and may eventually be ingested by a female *Anopheles* mosquito to begin a new sexual phase of the life cycle.

Following recovery, *P. vivax* and *P. ovale* can cause relapse even after several years, and recrudescence of **quartan malaria** (*P. malariae*) may occur 30 or more years after infection. *P. falciparum*, however, has a much more limited survival time; if it remains untreated and is not fatal, the infection will terminate spontaneously without relapse, usually in under a year.

Reported cases of malaria are increasing from year to year, especially in areas of Asia and the Americas undergoing agricultural colonization with forest clearing and pioneering of unexploited lands. Eradication campaigns have given way to long-term control programs in most areas where the disease remains endemic, and in some countries control is now being linked to or integrated with systems of primary health care.

The United States, Canada, and most Caribbean islands are essentially free of malaria transmission and report only small numbers of imported cases. Costa Rica, Panama, and several southern South American countries are also nearly free of local transmission. Haiti and the Dominican Republic report only *P. falciparum* cases, although in substantial numbers. *P. vivax* is the prevailing species in Mexico, Central America, and northern South America, although many *P. falciparum* cases are also reported, especially from Brazil, Colombia, and Ecuador.

Malaria is no longer endemic in Europe and the former Soviet Union, but Turkey still reports some autochthonous cases. Only a few small foci of autochthonous transmission persist in North Africa and western Asia. About 90 percent of the population in sub-Saharan Africa is still at risk, and transmission is high in many areas, especially in rural West Africa. *P. falciparum* is the predominant species.

Malaria remains endemic in most countries of central and South Asia. *P. vivax* is predominant, but *P. falciparum* is also important and appears to be increasing in relative prevalence.

The northeastern area of Asia, including Japan, is free of transmission, as are many of the smaller islands and groups in Oceania. Endemic foci persist in some of the larger islands (e.g., Philippines, Solomons, New Guinea, Indonesia) and in Southeast Asia and China. *P. vivax* prevails in China, where incidence is steadily declining. In Thailand (also experiencing a decline), *P. falciparum* is somewhat more prevalent.

Malaria transmission in any locale depends upon the complex interactions of parasites; vector mosquitoes; physical, socioeconomic, and environmental factors; and human biology, demography, and behavior. In 1957, George Macdonald attempted to fit many of these variables into an epidemiological model, and his ideas continue to be influential. Macdonald's definitions of **stable malaria** and **unstable malaria**, for example, are still helpful in studies of epidemiological patterns. Stable malaria is characteristically endemic: There is little seasonal change; transmission continues through most or all of the year; epidemics of malaria are very unlikely to occur; and most individuals have some immunity. Control under these circumstances is likely to be difficult. Malaria in much of tropical Africa corresponds to Macdonald's stable extreme. Unstable malaria may be endemic, but transmission varies from year to year and may be strictly seasonal. Seasonal epidemics may occur; collective immunity varies and may be low; and children as well as infants may be nonimmune. Control is relatively easy; indeed, many countries only recently freed from **endemic malaria** were in the unstable category.

Acquired and innate immunity are important factors in the epidemiology of malaria. Innate resistance has been recognized in some human populations. In parts of Central and West Africa, for example, many individuals are genetically resistant to *P. vivax* infection. Generally, in these areas, *P. ovale* replaces *P. vivax* as the prevailing cause of benign tertian malaria. In endemic *P. falciparum* areas of Africa, individuals heterozygous for hemoglobin AS (**sickle-cell trait**) are more likely to survive malignant tertian malaria. The unfortunate consequences of **sickle-cell disease** (hemoglobin SS) are balanced by the substantial antimalarial advantage conferred by the heterozygous condition, but only as long as *P. falciparum* remains endemic in the area. Another genetic condition, **G6PD deficiency**, also provides some protection against **falciparum malaria**.

Acquired immunity in malaria is species-specific and also specific to stage, that is, to the sporozoite, to the asexual forms in the blood, or to the sexual stages. In endemic areas, newborns may be protected for a few months by maternal antibodies that have crossed the placenta. After this phase, however, infants and toddlers are especially vulnerable; most deaths from malaria in endemic regions occur in these early years. Older children and adults gradually acquire immunity with repeated exposure.

History

Since at least the mid-Pleistocene, thousands of generations of humans have been parasitized by the plasmodia. It is certain that human malaria originated in the Old World, but there has been some debate about the timing of its appearance in the Western Hemisphere. Some have suggested that malaria was present in the New World long before European contact, but a strong case exists that the hemisphere was malaria-free until the end of the fifteenth century.

Malaria could have reached the New World before 1492 only by traveling overland from northeast Asia or via seaborne introductions. The possibility that humans brought malaria into North America from Siberia can almost certainly be discounted; conditions in the far north for malaria transmission were and are unsuitable. It is equally unlikely that the Vikings could have introduced malaria in the centuries before Columbus. They came from northern regions presumably free of malaria at the time and seem to have visited only coasts that were north of any possible anopheline mosquito populations. Similarly, voyagers from the central or eastern Pacific could not have transported the parasites because that region is free of anopheline vectors and thus of locally transmitted malaria. Voyagers reaching American coasts from eastern Asia could conceivably have introduced malaria, but this possibility too is remote.

Moreover, colonial records strongly indicate that malaria was unknown to indigenous Americans, and some areas that had supported large populations soon became dangerously malarious after European contact. The absence in aboriginal American populations of any blood-genetic polymorphisms associated with malaria is another kind of evidence that the Western Hemisphere remained free of the disease until contact.

After 1492, malaria parasites must have been introduced many times from Europe and Africa. Native American anopheline vectors were at hand, and together with **smallpox**, **measles**, and other infectious diseases from the Old World, malaria soon began to contribute to the depopulation of the indigenous peoples. From its early, usually coastal, sites of introduction, malaria spread widely in North, Central, and South America, limited principally by altitude and latitude – factors controlling the distribution of vector mosquitoes. By the nineteenth century in North America, the disease was prevalent in much of the Mississippi Valley, even in the northernmost areas. Malaria transmission extended into the northeastern United States, well north in California, and far to the south in South America. By the eighteenth and nineteenth centuries, malaria had also become established in the American subtropics and tropics.

The Old World gave malaria to the New; the New World, however, provided the first effective remedy for the disease. Cuttings of cinchona bark, taken from a Peruvian tree, were carried to Europe in 1632. The bark was soon discovered to provide relief from certain intermittent fevers. This therapeutic action allowed Richard Morton and Thomas Sydenham in England in 1666, and Francesco Torti in Italy in 1712, to begin to define malaria as a clinical entity separable from other fevers. By the end of the seventeenth

century, cinchona bark was an important medicinal export product from Peru.

In the Old World, malaria was probably endemic in Greece by the fourth century B.C.; Hippocrates described types of the intermittent fevers and noted the enlarged spleens of people who lived in low, marshy districts. In Italy, too, intermittent fevers were well known, for example, to Cicero, and well described by Celsus, Pliny, and Galen.

Malaria was of some importance in the centuries of Roman domination of Europe and the Mediterranean basin. However, it was probably much less destructive than it has been more recently, primarily because *P. falciparum* was absent or rare and the other species were less intensely transmitted. It is suggested that *Anopheles atroparvus*, basically a zoophilic species, was a poor vector for the human parasites. By late classical times, however, two other species, *Anopheles labranchiae* and *Anopheles sacharovi*, were introduced and dispersed along the coasts of southern Europe. These anthropophilic species were much more effective vectors for the plasmodia. By the final centuries of the empire, malaria was a more lethal force and may have contributed to Rome's decline.

After the fall of the Roman Empire, the history of malaria in Europe and the Mediterranean is obscure for many centuries. With few exceptions, medieval writers provide only sketchy accounts of outbreaks that may have been malarial. During the Renaissance, malaria appears not to have represented a major problem. Not until the seventeenth and eighteenth centuries did malaria become resurgent in Europe, not only in the south but periodically as far north as the Netherlands, Germany, Scandinavia, Poland, and Russia.

Through all of these centuries the record of malaria's impact in Asia and Africa is fragmentary. With European colonization, however, it soon became obvious that endemic malaria was a threat almost everywhere in the Old World tropics, especially to the colonizers.

The modern era in malariology began in the last decades of the nineteenth century with the identification of the causal parasites and the recognition of the role of anopheline mosquitoes as vectors. These discoveries provided the rationale for new strategies in malaria control. Malaria control itself was not a new concept; nor was the control of mosquitoes a new idea. Humankind had sought from ancient times to control mosquitoes. The new rationale, however, provided for more specific control directed principally at the anophelines that were important in transmission. Malaria control was further strengthened in the 1930s with the introduction of synthetic antimalarials. The 1940s brought further advances in chemotherapy together with the first of the residual insecticides.

By the late 1940s and early 1950s, attempts at national eradication in a few countries (e.g., Venezuela, Italy, United States) seemed justified. Early successes in local eradication, together with concerns about the emergence of anopheline resistance to insecticides, led to a 1955 decision to commit the World Health Organization (WHO) to malaria eradication. This commitment pushed many countries into supposedly time-limited eradication campaigns, often with considerable financial and advisory support. Some of these campaigns were successful, but others faltered after dramatic initial results. By the end of the eradication era in the early 1970s, some hundreds of millions of people were living in areas where campaigns had eliminated endemic malaria, but in other areas it continued to prevail, forcing a return to long-term control strategies.

In 1980 the WHO began to recommend that malaria control be coordinated with primary health care. Malaria control and therapy continue to be complicated by mosquito resistance to insecticides and parasite resistance to drugs. Vaccine development proceeds, although slowly. The problems posed by malaria persist, but they are not insoluble. Malaria remains endemic in many countries in the twenty-first century, but steady improvement in control is expected.

Frederick L. Dunn

89. Marburg Virus Disease

The so-called **Marburg virus**, presumed to be African in origin, remains among the more mysterious of disease-causing organisms.

History

In 1967, a disease outbreak occurred at a laboratory in Marburg, Germany, where monkey kidneys were being prepared for cell cultures. Twenty-seven laboratory workers (including one in Yugoslavia) fell gravely ill; seven died. Four secondary cases occurred (including a laboratory worker's wife), but none were fatal. Early suspicion focused on **yellow fever**, but subsequently investigators isolated an unknown virus. Electron micrographs revealed a bizarre morphology of a type never seen before: Photographs resembled a mass of spaghetti. The agent was named Marburg virus. Strict monkey quarantines were initiated. No further cases were seen in laboratory workers.

Field studies were initiated in East Africa, the monkeys' homeland. No virus was recovered from any monkeys examined. Later, serologic studies involving humans, primates, and rodents were undertaken in many regions.

The first Marburg cases seen in Africa occurred in 1975. A young Australian couple touring Rhodesia (now Zimbabwe) became ill by the time they reached South Africa. They were admitted to a Johannesburg hospital, where the man died and the woman recovered. A nurse also sickened and recovered. After the disease was determined to be Marburg, a thorough epidemiological inquest investigated the victims' travel route, concentrating particularly on every locale where they spent a night. Animal, insect, and human populations were sampled. No evidence of endemic disease was found.

In 1980, a man from western Kenya entered a Nairobi hospital. He died 6 hours after admission, and a physician attending him also became ill but recovered. Marburg virus was isolated from his blood. Subsequent epidemiological investigations produced a positive finding:

antibodies against Marburg virus in two vervet monkeys among many examined.

Another episode, in 1987, involved a boy who became infected while visiting a park in western Kenya. The boy died. No secondary cases were reported. Since that time, there have been many isolated cases as well as outbreaks – such as that of 1998–99 in civil-war-torn eastern Congo – suspected of being **Marburg virus disease**. In the latter case, this was confirmed by the World Health Organization only after **Ebola virus** was ruled out as the cause of some 50 deaths. Marburg virus disease, however, continues to elude easy diagnosis.

Characteristics

Marburg virus is unrelated to many arboviruses against which it was tested. It most closely resembles Ebola virus. Both Marburg and Ebola have been placed in a new family, Filoviridae, which includes but the two members thus far. A cytopathic effect was observed in *Cercopithecus* kidney cells and human amnion cells.

Incubation following exposure varied from 5–7 days. In six cases with available data, death occurred between days 7 and 16. Onset involved malaise, **myalgia**, and often prostration. Vomiting frequently occurred by the third day, and **conjunctivitis** by the fourth, by which time the temperature had reached 40°C. Rash, beginning on the fifth day, progressed to a **maculopapular rash** that later became more diffuse. In severe cases, a diffuse dark livid **erythema** developed on face, trunk, and extremities. An **enanthem** of the soft palate developed along with the rash. Lymph node enlargement was noted. A **diarrhea** appeared, often with blood. The South African cases differed only in having no enanthem and no lymph node enlargement.

Diagnosis may be easy with a clustering of cases and when epidemiologists are alerted; however, the occurrence of single cases is not likely to arouse suspicion. Moreover, during the first several days, the symptoms could be mistaken for many other diseases. None of the methods of laboratory diagnosis is readily accessible in the usual field situation; yet early di-

agnosis is imperative to abort possible developing epidemics.

Ebola virus is considerably more fatal in humans than is Marburg virus. In secondary Marburg cases studied, the clinical course was less severe than in primary cases, with no mortality. No effective therapy has been found. In one case, therapy employed interferon in conjunction with immune plasma. The patient (a secondary case) recovered. Further clinical trials await further cases.

Basic methods of managing patients with suspected viral hemorrhagic fever include strict isolation and precaution in examination, in taking specimens, and in handling material in the laboratory. Such procedures are not readily applicable in African bush clinics. Medicine awaits further epidemiological information on animal reservoirs, modes of transmission, and the persistence of the virus in nature. For like Ebola, Marburg is the only other disease-causing human virus for which the host and the natural transmission cycle remain unknown.

Wilbur G. Downs

90. Mastoiditis

Infections of the middle ear and mastoid encompass a spectrum of potentially serious medical conditions. Decreased hearing from ear infections may have a lifelong impact and is a major health concern. Because of the anatomic relationship of the middle ear and mastoid to the middle and posterior cranial compartments, life-threatening complications may occur.

Characteristics

Acute suppurative otitis media (AOM) is characterized by obstruction of the eustachian tube, allowing retention and suppuration of secretions. AOM is the term associated with the acute ear infection of childhood. Generally the course of this infection is self-limited, and infected secretions are discharged through either the eustachian tube or a ruptured tympanic membrane.

Acute coalescent mastoiditis can result from failure of these processes to evacuate the abscess. Coalescence of disease within the mastoid leads to pus under pressure and ultimately dissolution of surrounding bone. This condition may require urgent surgical evacuation because the infection is capable of spreading to other structures.

Otitis media with effusion (OME) is an inflammatory condition of the middle ear in which fluid accumulates. Both AOM and OME are precursor conditions to tympanic membrane retractions and perforations. Ongoing **eustachian tube dysfunction** predisposes to persistent secretions in the ear and recurrent attacks of otitis media. Some patients develop a chronic tympanic membrane perforation that may allow eventual aeration of the middle ear and mastoid air-cell spaces and resolution of the underlying disease.

Chronic suppurative otitis media (CSOM) is defined as an ear with a tympanic membrane perforation. **Benign CSOM** is characterized by a dry tympanic membrane perforation unassociated with infection. **Active CSOM** results from intermittent infection often associated with ingrown skin (**cholesteatoma**) in the middle ear and mastoid cavities. **Primary acquired cholesteatoma** occurs through tympanic membrane retraction into the attic of the middle-ear space with subsequent potential for extension into the middle ear and mastoid air-cell systems. **Secondary acquired cholesteatoma** is defined as skin growth through a tympanic membrane perforation into the ear.

Some 80 percent of all children experience one or more episodes of AOM by the age of 6. Together AOM, OME, and CSOM comprise one of the most common disease entities affecting humans. Indeed, AOM may be the most common disease treated with antibiotics.

Complicated infections producing **mastoiditis** have dramatically declined since the advent of antibiotics in the 1930s and 1940s. Prior to that time, acute coalescent mastoiditis complicated AOM in approximately 20 percent of cases. By the 1950s, acute mastoiditis resulting from AOM had declined to 3 percent.

AOM occurs most commonly between 6 and 24 months of age. Subsequently, incidence declines with age except between 5 and 6 years, the age of entrance into school. The incidence of uncomplicated AOM in boys is not significantly different from that in girls. Mastoiditis, however, appears to be more common among males.

The severity of otitic infections is related to factors such as extremes of climate and poverty. During winter months, outpatient visits for AOM are approximately fourfold higher than in summer months. Intake of mother's milk and avoidance of cigarette smoke appear to confer some protection against OME, but no effect on complications is known.

Eustachian tube dysfunction is the most important factor engendering middle ear infections. It commonly occurs in young children; adolescent growth improves the eustachian tube opening. However, poor tubal function may persist for many reasons and induces a relative negative pressure in the middle-ear space. Lack of aeration and accumulation of effusions conduce to the development of OME or AOM.

When AOM continues beyond 2 weeks, progressive thickening of middle-ear mucosa obstructs free drainage of purulent secretions, permitting bone destruction and extension of infection. This process may eventuate in mastoiditis and possibly other extensions of suppuration.

The onset of AOM in childhood is often associated with fever, lethargy, and irritability. Older children may experience earaches and decreased hearing. However, there is considerable variability in the symptoms. OME is often characterized by hearing loss and a history of recurrent episodes of AOM. CSOM in its active form often presents with foul-smelling drainage and longstanding hearing loss. Development of pain in such an ear is a foreboding sign, as it often represents obstruction of drainage and pus under pressure. Local complications of CSOM include bone erosion, facial nerve dysfunction, hearing loss, and "ringing" in the ear. Infection may extend into the bony skull or the soft tissues of the neck and scalp.

History

Studies of 2,600-year-old Egyptian mummies reveal perforations of the tympanic membrane and destruction of mastoid air cells. Suppurative destruction of the mastoid is also evident in skeletons from Persian populations of the second and first millennia B.C.

Hippocrates appreciated the potential seriousness of otitic complications and noted that delirium and death could result; later, Roman physician Celsus agreed. Later still, the Persian Avicenna reasoned incorrectly that ear discharge was caused by **brain disease**. For centuries, infections producing discharges from the ear were considered virtually normal conditions because they occurred so frequently.

Although the seriousness of ear suppuration was appreciated much earlier, the idea of opening the mastoid to relieve infection awaited the sixteenth century. Medieval surgeon Ambroise Paré was summoned to treat Francis II of France. Paré found the boy-king febrile and delirious with a discharging ear. He proposed to drain the infection through an opening in the skull. Francis's wife, Mary "Queen of Scots," consented, but the king's mother, Catherine de Médici, refused to permit the operation, and Francis died.

Notable advances were made in the seventeenth century. In 1683, Joseph DuVerney published an account of the structure, function, and diseases of the ear, including infectious aural pathology and the mechanisms producing earache, **otorrhea**, and hearing loss. He was the first to describe extension of tympanic cavity infection to the mastoid air cells as a cause of mastoiditis.

In 1704, Antonio Valsalva suggested a method of removing purulence from the ear, consisting of exhaling strongly with mouth and nose firmly closed, forcing air to pass into the middle ear through the eustachian tube. (In 1761, Valsalva's student Giovanni Morgagni would demonstrate that aural suppuration was the pri-

mary source of lethal, intracranial abscesses.) Also in the early eighteenth century, Jean Petit of Paris performed probably the first successful operation on the mastoid for the evacuation of pus. He stressed the need for early drainage of mastoid abscesses because of the potential for further damage.

Unfortunately, the advancement of otological surgery suffered a setback when a mastoidectomy was performed on Baron von Berger (personal physician to the King of Denmark), who had heard of Petit's achievement. He persuaded a surgeon to operate upon his mastoid to relieve **tinnitus** and hearing loss. The operation took place but resulted in a wound infection. The baron died of **meningitis** 12 days later, and the mastoidectomy operation fell into disrepute until the middle of the nineteenth century.

One of the first to specialize in otology was Jean Marie Gaspard Itard, a military surgeon in Paris. In 1821, he exposed many errors of his predecessors, particularly the opening of the mastoid cavity as a cure for deafness. Like Itard, Jean Antoine Saissy, another Parisian surgeon, was opposed to puncturing the tympanic membrane for aural suppuration. Instead, he treated suppuration by rinsing through a eustachian catheter, describing the technique in 1829.

In 1853, William Wilde of Dublin (Oscar Wilde's father) recommended incision of the mastoid for mastoiditis when symptoms were life-threatening. The mid-century also saw the beginning of advances in anesthesiology, bacteriology, surgical practice, and other fields that mean so much to modern medicine.

London surgeon James Hinton and Hermann Schwartze of Halle are credited with establishing the specific method of simple mastoidectomy. This operation involved removal of the bony cortex overlying the mastoid air cells. Schwartze's work led to the first account of the operation as a systematic procedure performed according to a definite plan to correct a specific condition. By the end of the nineteenth century, the operation had attained widespread acceptance, overcoming more than a century of prejudice.

In 1861, German surgeon Anton von Troltsch reported successful treatment of mastoiditis with a postauricular incision and wound exploration. He recognized that failure to address disease deeper within the middle ear and mastoid invariably resulted in disease recurrence, and in 1873 proposed extensions of Schwartze's procedure to treat these areas. In 1889, Ernst von Küster and Ernst von Bergmann recommended extending Schwartze's mastoidectomy to include removal of the posterior wall of the external canal and middle ear structures. This extended procedure became known as the radical mastoidectomy. Properly performed, mastoidectomy for well-localized infections proved to be extremely effective in removing the risk of serious complication within the mastoid. The addition of new techniques, as well as earlier diagnosis of mastoiditis, capped this important phase of otologic surgery.

In many cases of radical mastoidectomy, previous infection had destroyed the middle-ear sound-conducting system. Removal of the tympanic membrane and ossicular remnants was necessary in order to extirpate the infection. In 1899, however, Otto Körner demonstrated that the majority of the tympanic membrane and ossicular chain could be left intact, thus maintaining the preoperative hearing level.

In 1910 Gustav Bondy devised the modified radical mastoidectomy. He demonstrated that removal of the superior bone overlying infected tissue adequately exteriorized and exposed disease while preserving hearing. Despite the success of this less radical approach, otologic surgeons were slow to accept it, but it finally gained widespread acceptance by the 1930s.

A marked decline in the need for mastoid operations followed the use of sulfanilamide and penicillin. The favorable results achieved with these antibiotics encouraged their application at earlier stages of severe infections. At first, otologic surgeons were hesitant to abandon established surgical procedures, fearing that antibiotics would mask the clinical picture and lead to late complications. It became evident, however, that if antibiotics were given before coalescences were established, fewer complications requiring surgical intervention would result. Nonetheless, modern-day physicians have recognized that too low a dose given for too little time may indeed mask a developing mastoiditis.

Interest in hearing preservation in surgical treatment of chronic ear infections continued. German surgeons F. Zöllner and H. Wullstein share credit for performing the first successful repair of the tympanic membrane using skin-grafting techniques in 1951. Since the 1950s, emphasis on preservation and restoration of hearing has fostered the development of methods of ossicular reconstruction designed to simulate the middle-ear sound-conducting mechanism. Prostheses made of polyethylene, Teflon, and bioceramic materials have produced mixed results with respect to long-term hearing, stability, and acceptance.

In 1954, B. W. Armstrong reintroduced a procedure (first suggested by Adam Politzer in 1869) to reverse the effects of eustachian tube dysfunction, entailing a limited incision of the tympanic membrane and insertion of a tympanostomy tube. Tympanostomy tubes appear to be beneficial in restoring hearing and preventing middle-ear infections and structural deterioration.

The historical development of otology constituted an evolution in the management of aural infections. The lessons learned by otologists underscore the importance of adequate surgical exposure, removal of irreversibly infected tissue, and regular postoperative follow-up in order to maintain a safe, dry ear.

John L. Kemink, John K. Niparko,
and Steven A. Telian

91. Measles

Measles (*rubeola,* "hard measles," "red measles," "9-day measles," *morbilli*) is a common infectious disease, principally of children, with worldwide distribution, and characterized by fever and a red, blotchy rash. Measles is a vaccine-preventable disease, and its vaccine is among those included in the Expanded Programme on Immunization of the World Health Organization. The disease is known by many local names throughout the world.

Characteristics

Measles is caused by a species of *Morbillivirus* (family Paramyxoviridae). Although this virus does not survive drying on a surface, it can survive drying in microdroplets in the air.

Measles is one of the most communicable diseases, transmitted via contact of susceptible individuals with nose and throat secretions from infected persons, primarily by droplet spread. Measles has no reservoir other than humans, meaning that a continuous chain of susceptible contacts is necessary to sustain transmission. The period of communicability lasts up to 4 days after the start of the rash. There is no carrier state. The incubation period from exposure to rash onset is about 14 days.

In populated areas with no or low vaccination coverage, measles is primarily an endemic disease, with epidemics occurring every few years. In such areas, the greatest incidence is in children under 2 years of age. In more remote and isolated populations, measles is not endemic, and disease is dependent upon introduction from the outside, at which time an epidemic may occur, affecting all persons born since the last epidemic. No evidence indicates any gender difference with respect to incidence or severity, or any racial difference with respect to incidence. Differences in severity among certain populations are most likely the result of nutritional and environmental factors.

Measles mortality is highest in the very young and the very old. In malnourished children in the developing world, the case-fatality rate may be as high as 10 percent or more. Some studies have indicated that multiple cases within a family group may lead to higher mortality rates.

The Expanded Programme on Immunization of the World Health Organization maintains information on reported measles cases and vaccination coverage in member countries.

Because of underreporting, worldwide reported incidence represents only a small fraction of the estimated annual 50 million cases and 1.5 million deaths caused by measles in developing countries. Vaccination – with global coverage estimated at 55 percent for children under 1 year old – currently averts over 40 million cases and 1 million deaths each year in developing countries. A single dose of live attenuated measles virus vaccine confers long-term, probably lifelong, immunity in over 95 percent of susceptible individuals.

The prodromal phase of measles typically presents fever, cough, **coryza**, and **conjunctivitis**. During this stage, small whitish specks on reddened areas of the mucosal lining of the mouth (**Koplik's spots**) are diagnostic. Symptoms continue 3–7 days until the characteristic blotchy reddish rash appears, usually first on the head and then spreading down the body over 4–7 days. After its peak, in uncomplicated cases, all symptoms recede and the rash fades in the same order it appeared.

Complications from secondary infection may occur, however, possibly resulting in **otitis, encephalitis**, or **pneumonia**. **Diarrhea** may also complicate measles and is one of the most important causes of measles-associated mortality in developing countries. Measles is uncommon during pregnancy, and limited available data fail to demonstrate clearly any increased risk of fetal mortality or congenital malformations.

History

The origin of measles is unknown. Francis Black notes that populations of sufficient size to sustain measles transmission would not have developed until sometime after 2500 B.C. He suggests that measles may be an adaptation of another virus of the same genus (which includes **rinderpest** and **canine distemper**). Hippocrates, writing in the fourth century B.C., described no rash illness consistent with measles, even though his case histories document many other infections in ancient Greece.

The history of measles is confused with that of **smallpox** in much early literature.

Although records are scanty, major unidentified epidemics with high mortality spread through the Roman Empire in 165–80 A.D. and again in 251–66 – epidemics that may have signaled the arrival of measles and smallpox. In China, two major epidemics with high mortality were recorded in 161–2 and 310–12 A.D., but again we cannot be certain about the identity of the diseases.

Persian physician Rhazes is generally credited with the first written record of measles by differentiating it from smallpox in approximately 910. Rhazes, however, quoted previous writers, including Hebrew physician El Yahudi, who lived 300 years earlier. Around the year 1000, Avicenna also wrote about measles, and translators of his writings may have introduced the term *rubeola* for the disease.

During medieval times, measles was designated by the Latin *morbilli* ("little disease"). Measles was also called *rossalia* and *rosagia*, as well as *fersa* or *sofersa* (Milanese), *mesles* (English), *maal* and *masern* (German), and *masura* (Sanskrit). The derivation of the English "measles" is in some doubt. One suggestion is that it arose from the Latin *miscellus* or *misella*, a diminutive of the Latin *miser*, meaning "miserable" – a term given to those suffering from **leprosy**. Leprotic sores were called *mesles*, and John of Gaddesden in the early fourteenth century unjustifiably coupled these *mesles* with the disease *morbilli*. Eventually the term "measles" lost its connection with leprosy.

Measles, smallpox, and other rash illnesses continued to be confused in medieval Europe. Physician and epidemiologist Thomas Sydenham studied measles epidemics in 1670 and 1674 and discussed clinical features of the illness and its complications. He is generally credited with differentiating and describing measles in northern Europe. The first clear demonstration that measles was infectious is attributed to Francis Home, who in 1758 attempted to create immunity by placing blood from measles patients beneath the skin or into the noses of susceptible persons. Numerous measles epi-

demics were reported in the seventeenth and eighteenth centuries.

The most famous epidemiological study of measles was conducted by Peter Panum in 1846. Measles attacked about 6,100 Faroe islanders during that year and was associated with the deaths of 102 of the 7,864 inhabitants, who had been completely free of the disease for 65 years. Panum confirmed the respiratory route of transmission, the incubation period, and the lifelong immunity acquired from previous infection. August Hirsch built on Panum's work, recording the universal geographic distribution of measles and noting epidemics from most parts of the world. He noted too that measles reached the Western Hemisphere soon after the arrival of Europeans and followed the westward movement of settlers. He suggested that introduction of the disease into Australia occurred in 1854, after it first appeared in Hawaii in 1848.

Measles was especially dramatic when it struck "virgin-soil" populations with no prior or recent exposure, and thus the outbreak affected most individuals. The disease played an important role in thinning the ranks of Native Americans after 1492, and later high mortality also occurred in epidemics among several Pacific virgin-soil populations during the nineteenth century: 40,000 deaths (out of a population of 150,000) in Hawaii in 1848; 20,000 deaths, comprising 20–25 percent of the Fijian population in 1874; and 645 deaths out of 8,845 cases in Samoa in 1911. Such high case-fatality rates in these settings likely resulted from some of the same factors that cause high mortality among unvaccinated individuals in developing countries today, including lack of supportive care, lack of treatment for complications, and **malnutrition**. In virgin-soil settings where populations were well nourished and had better medical care, mortality was much lower, as seen in the measles outbreak in southern Greenland in 1951. In one district, 4,257 persons out of a population of about 4,400 contracted measles, but only 77 deaths occurred.

Not until 1896 did Henry Koplik publish a description of Koplik's spots, although apparently their significance was independently recognized about a century earlier by John Quier in Jamaica and Richard Hazeltine in Maine.

Research leading to current measles vaccines began about the early twentieth century. In 1911, investigators demonstrated that the illness was caused by a virus. By the 1940s, the virus had been cultured, and in 1954 it was isolated. Subsequent research resulted in an attenuated strain of measles vaccine, which was produced in 1958. In 1963, after field trials, the attenuated ("live") vaccine was licensed for use in the United States. An inactivated ("killed") measles vaccine was also developed, but was shown to be inferior and is no longer available.

With the 1974 establishment of the World Health Organization Expanded Programme on Immunization, measles vaccine has been introduced into the national immunization programs of most countries, and geographic occurrence in endemic regions is related to the immunization coverage with measles vaccine. In countries with sustained, large-scale immunization programs and reliable disease surveillance, the impact of control efforts has been documented through decreasing numbers of reported cases. Global measles eradication is considered technically possible, but experts increasingly recognize that extremely high immunization-coverage levels are necessary to achieve such a goal.

Robert J. Kim-Farley

92. Meningitis

Meningitis means inflammation of the meninges, the membranes covering the brain and spinal cord. It usually results from bacterial infection but can also be caused by other microbial agents and noninfectious conditions. **Meningococcal meningitis**, caused by a bacterium, *Neisseria meningitidis*, is the form occurring in major epidemics. Also called **cerebrospinal meningitis** (CSM), it has been known

in the past as "spotted fever," "cerebrospinal fever," *typhus cerebralis*, and *meningitis epidemica*. **Aseptic meningitis** means inflammation of the meninges without detectable bacterial involvement. The most common causes are any of a number of viruses.

Characteristics

Many bacteria can cause meningitis, but in developed countries over 80 percent of cases in recent years have resulted from only three species: *N. meningitidis, Hemophilus influenzae,* and *Streptococcus (Diplococcus) pneumoniae*. Other common members of the human bacterial flora such as *Escherichia coli* and various streptococci and staphylococci can also produce meningitis under special circumstances, as can members of genera *Listeria, Pseudomonas,* and *Proteus*. Meningitis sometimes develops as a complication of **tuberculosis**.

Aseptic meningitis is usually the result of viral infection. Among the many types of viruses that can be involved are **mumps, echovirus, polio, coxsackievirus, herpes simplex, herpes zoster, hepatitis, measles, rubella,** and several mosquito-borne agents of **encephalitis**. Fungi, most commonly *Cryptococcus*, are other possible agents.

Laboratory study is necessary to determine the cause of any particular case of meningitis, so it is generally difficult to be certain of the exact etiology of past meningitis cases or epidemics. However, despite the current relative significance of *Hemophilus* and *Streptococcus, Neisseria* is the most important pathogen for meningococcal meningitis; it is the only type that commonly occurs in major epidemics and is the most likely to attack adults.

N. meningitidis is closely related to the organism that causes **gonorrhea**. Humans are its only natural host. It is a common inhabitant of the mucosal membranes of the nose and throat, where it normally causes no harm. Up to 50 percent of a population may be asymptomatic carriers without any cases of meningitis developing, but such carriers are crucial to the spread of the disease. The organism is transmitted via droplets sneezed or coughed from the nose and throat. It is very susceptible to desiccation and sunlight.

The majority of victims, especially in sporadic cases and small outbreaks, are children under age 5. Among adults, military recruits crowded into barracks have traditionally been prime targets. Throughout the nineteenth and twentieth centuries, wartime mobilization was always accompanied by sharp increases in meningitis cases.

Meningitis is highly seasonal. In temperate regions, a large preponderance of cases develop in the winter and early spring. The reasons for this are unclear, but indoor crowding, cold temperature, and low humidity may all play a role. Epidemics in sub-Saharan Africa develop during the cool, dry season – when people travel more and sleep indoors to keep warm – and tend to end abruptly when the rains come.

In most cases, bacteria are carried in the nose and pharynx without any symptoms or perhaps a sore throat. Serious disease develops only if the bacteria reach the bloodstream. This can produce **fulminating blood infection**, characterized by sudden prostration, high fever, skin blotches, and collapse. Most cases are fatal unless promptly treated, and death may ensue in only hours, before the meninges become involved.

Meningitis, however, is the more common result, occurring when bacteria travel through the blood to infect the meninges. Fever, headache, stiffness, and vomiting are typical symptoms, and many victims show a rash from blockage of small blood vessels. A thick, purulent exudate covers the brain, and **arthritis**, cardiac damage, and **shock** may develop. Coma, convulsions, and **delirium** are frequent, and death rates for untreated cases range up to 90 percent. Even in epidemic conditions, however, only a small minority of carriers develop clinical disease. It is unknown why most people remain healthy whereas others become desperately ill. Individual susceptibility, damage to mucous membranes, and concomitant infections may all play a role.

History

Meningitis was not described definitively until after 1800, so the antiquity of the disease is unknown, but it is unlikely that it is a "new" infection in humans. Mention of "epidemic convulsion" in tenth century China and a description by T. Willis in England in 1684 could indicate earlier recognition. From the sixteenth century onward, many possible references occur in European literature.

In 1805, an epidemic of CSM occurred in Geneva. Most victims were infants and children. Clinical accounts by Gaspard Vieusseux and autopsy studies by A. Matthey identified the disease. In 1806, a cluster of cases developed in Massachusetts. As in Switzerland, the victims were infants and children; most died despite frantic application of an array of therapies. Case descriptions and autopsies confirmed a diagnosis of CSM. An epidemic of apparent meningitis afflicted British troops in Sicily in 1808, and garrisons in France were struck in 1814. In North America, meningitis epidemics were reported in Canada in 1807; in Virginia, Kentucky, and Ohio in 1808; in New York and Pennsylvania in 1809; and among U.S. troops during the War of 1812. They were described as "sinking typhus" or "spotted fever" in New England from 1814 to 1816.

Little more was heard about the apparently new disease until the years 1837–42, when a series of outbreaks occurred in French garrisons and among nearby civilians. Epidemics in Algeria (1840–47) began among French troops but killed many among the indigenous Moslem population as well. Meningitis was also widespread in Italy in 1839–45 and was reported in Corfu, Ireland, and especially Denmark from 1845 to 1848. There was also a series of small epidemics in the United States in the 1840s, primarily in the South.

The first recorded major epidemic of CSM began in Sweden in 1854, starting in late winter and slowly spreading during the next 5 years. It died out in the summers and resumed a slow, irregular progress during winters. The epidemic declined in 1859, with scattered cases reported in the next several years and a small flare-up in 1865–67. Government returns showed a total of 4,158 meningitis deaths in 1854–60 and 419 in 1865–67.

During the 1860s, small but deadly epidemics occurred in Germany, the Netherlands, England, France, Italy, Portugal, Austria, Hungary, Greece, Turkey, Poland, and Russia. There were numerous outbreaks in the United States during the same decade, with both sides suffering during the Civil War. Everywhere, troops and small children were the most common victims. Scattered cases and sporadic outbreaks continued for the rest of the century, with flurries of activity in the mid-1880s and at the end of the century.

A new burst of meningitis occurred in the first decade of the twentieth century. The first cases from Australia were recorded in 1900–01. Portugal had more than 5,000 cases from 1901 to 1905; a series of North American epidemics in 1904–47 involved much of the United States and Canada, with 2,755 patients in New York alone in 1905. A severe epidemic in Silesia caused almost 10,000 cases from 1905 to 1908.

For most of the twentieth century, meningitis in the developed countries followed a pattern of small, local epidemics and scattered cases, mostly among children. The two world wars caused major spurts as military authorities crammed recruits into crowded barracks. For example, there were 5,839 cases and 2,279 deaths among U.S. soldiers during World War I. In 1942 and 1943, however, although there were 13,922 military cases, thanks to new therapy there were only 559 deaths. Moreover, except for a spurt to about 14 cases per 100,000 people in 1942, civilian case rates in the United States have remained under 4 per 100,000 since the late 1930s. Total meningococcal infections have rarely exceeded 3,000 a year, but reported cases of aseptic meningitis have risen steadily.

The situation in non-Western countries is quite different. Incidence rates tend to be much higher, and there are still major epidemics like those that afflicted Sweden and Silesia in

the past. For example, China has experienced three major epidemics of serogroup-A meningitis since 1949, with rates of 50–400 per 100,000. During the 1963-69 epidemic, there were more than 3 million cases and 166,000 deaths.

Africa has had two kinds of experience with the disease. In most of the continent, meningitis is a sporadic disease, behaving much as it does in the West, although often with higher incidence and fatality rates. However, one terrible epidemic occurred in 1913 in Kenya and Tanganyika, lingering in Tanganyika until 1919. Both territories, as well as neighboring Uganda, had dramatic surges during World War II. In North Africa, Algeria and Egypt experienced epidemics in the nineteenth century, and Morocco had over 6,000 cases in 1967.

The classic area for epidemic CSM, however, has been the savanna zone south of the Sahara from Sudan to Senegal. This "CSM belt" was swept by a series of epidemics during the twentieth century. Indeed, there the disease has behaved differently, advancing on regular fronts and killing tens of thousands each season. Only the Swedish epidemic of the 1850s seems to have displayed a similar broad geographic pattern. In both places, the disease advanced regularly from season to season, but cases were scattered widely and unpredictably within the afflicted zone. The epidemics hopped about, skipping some communities and striking hard at others. Areas struck in one CSM season were usually spared the next.

The antiquity of meningitis in the savanna is unknown, but evidence exists that it had occurred in Sudan and Nigeria by the 1880s. Small outbreaks struck in Senegal in the 1890s and in Ghana in 1900. The first of the great West African epidemics began in Nigeria in 1905. It spread westward to Mali and Ghana in 1906, lingering there until 1908. British authorities guessed the death toll in Ghana at some 34,000; case mortality was estimated at 80 percent. Total deaths in the epidemic are unknown but were clearly disastrous.

The second CSM cycle began in Ghana in 1919, spread to Upper Volta in 1920, and swept

Nigeria and Niger from 1921 to 1924. The death toll in one Nigerian province was put at over 45,000 in 1921 alone, and French officials assumed at least 15,000 deaths in Niger over the 4-year period.

The third cycle began in 1935, when Chad was attacked by an epidemic that had raged the previous year in Sudan – the first and only time that an east-west spread pattern from Sudan was demonstrated. Infection moved westward into Chad, Nigeria, and Niger, with epidemics developing in 1937. CSM hit Upper Volta in 1938 and Mali and Ghana in 1939. Local outbreaks continued through 1941. Even with sulfa drugs, tens of thousands died. CSM was again epidemic in the years 1943–47, with outbreaks reported from Chad to Senegal.

Another cycle developed in 1949 from foci in northern Ghana, northern Nigeria, and Upper Volta, spreading eastward to Sudan by 1952. By this time, meningitis had become well established, and geographic patterns were less distinct. At least 250,000 and perhaps a million or more people died of CSM in West Africa between 1905 and 1960. The disease remains a serious public-health problem in the entire CSM belt.

The late identification of meningitis did not delay study of its etiology. By 1860, researchers widely assumed that a specific poison or agent was involved. In 1887, Austrian pathologist Anton Weichselbaum described the meningococcus. This organism was suspected of being the meningitis pathogen, but its role was not proven until the early twentieth century. By 1910, researchers recognized that the meningococcus was responsible for epidemics and that other bacteria could cause sporadic cases. Lumbar puncture, introduced in 1891 by Heinrich Quincke, made cerebrospinal fluid available for study and sometimes relieved the headaches caused by CSM. The crucial epidemiological role of asymptomatic carriers was appreciated by the turn of the twentieth century.

After 1905, attempts were made to develop a therapeutic serum. Some early successes were reported, but by 1909 it was clear that serologic differences existed among strains. Four serogroups were identified by the end of World War I. Vaccine therapy remained of limited value but – in the absence of anything else – was frequently tried. In the 1930s, French efforts to protect Africans against serogroup A by vaccination had inconclusive results, and similar British trials in Sudan were unsuccessful.

The development of sulfa drugs in the 1930s revolutionized meningitis therapy. Clinical trials showed the almost miraculous impact of sulfanilamide on meningococcal infections in 1937. This drug reduced case-fatality rates to 20 percent and less and saved thousands of lives during the epidemics of World War II. Sulfa drugs were successfully used for prophylaxis by the U.S. Army beginning in 1943, and the technique was widely adopted.

The "wonder drugs" had an especially dramatic impact in the CSM belt of Africa, where they were introduced in 1938. Africans had been well aware that prior European therapies were useless. Preventive measures seemed futile, arbitrary, and even harsh. Victims were quarantined, and cordons thrown around entire districts. Such efforts disrupted trade and other activities but did nothing to impede the spread of the disease. Annoying procedures like "nasopharyngeal disinfection" of travelers or destruction of houses discouraged African cooperation with medical authorities. Sulfa drugs were, however, extremely effective. Africans responded pragmatically and eagerly began to report cases and seek treatment.

In 1963, sulfa-resistant strains of *N. meningitidis* were detected, and their spread has halted sulfa prophylaxis. Penicillin therapy is still effective but has no preventive value. Vaccines against serogroups C and A were introduced in the early 1970s, and improved vaccines have been developed since, although protection against serogroup B is still unavailable. Meningitis remains a public-health problem, especially in underdeveloped countries. Death occurs in about 5 percent of all cases, even with prompt treatment.

K. David Patterson

93. Milk Sickness (Tremetol Poisoning)

Milk sickness, usually called "milksick" by early nineteenth-century American pioneers, denotes what we now know to be poisoning by milk from cows that have eaten either the white snakeroot or the rayless goldenrod plants. The white snakeroot (*Eupatorium urticaefolium*) is common in the Midwest and upper South and also known as "white sanicle," "squaw weed," "snakeweed," "pool wort," and "deer wort." The rayless goldenrod (*Haplopappus heterophyllus*) is found in southwestern states such as Arizona and New Mexico.

Milk sickness has been called variously "alkali poisoning," "puking disease," "sick stomach," the "slows" or "sloes," "stiff joints," "swamp sickness," the "tires," and (in animals) the **trembles**. It is now known as **tremetol poisoning** after a toxic ingredient of white snakeroot and rayless goldenrod. Tremetol is an unsaturated alcohol that in consistency and odor resembles turpentine.

Characteristics

Milk sickness was unknown in Europe or any other region of the world except North America. It appeared in North Carolina as early as the American Revolution near a mountain ridge named Milk Sick. Its highest incidence was in dry years when cows wandered from their brown pastures into the woods in search of forage. As more forests were cleared so that cattle had more adequate pasture, and as fences were built, the incidence of milk sickness decreased rapidly.

The disease wrought havoc in the Midwest, especially in Illinois, Indiana, and Ohio, and in the upper southern states of Kentucky, North Carolina, Tennessee, and Virginia. Milk sickness was, in some years and some localities, the most important obstacle to settlement by the pioneers. Beginning about 1815, a flood of pioneers moved west. As they penetrated the forest wilderness of the Midwest, epidemics of the disease all too frequently caused villages to be abandoned. Physicians in Kentucky and Tennessee described milk sickness as being so widespread that the Kentucky legislature appointed a committee in 1827 to investigate its cause. A few years later, the state medical society of Indiana also attempted a similar investigation. It is said that Evansville, Indiana, became a prominent city only because an early rival, Darlington, was abandoned as a result of milk sickness.

In 1811, an anonymous author wrote that milk sickness was a true poisoning because it involved no fever. He also believed that it was caused by poisonous milk that had a peculiar taste and smell. The source of the poison, he wrote, was vegetation eaten by the cows. He further advised that finding the offending plant would remove a major stumbling block to emigration westward.

In subsequent years, theories as to the cause of milk sickness were numerous. One suggested that the cause was arsenic; another claimed it was a soil organism, whereas another attributed the disease to a mysterious exhalation from soil. Still others incriminated various poisonous minerals and springs. However, no specific toxic plant was identified during the nineteenth century. In the 1880s, the medical revolution following the discoveries of Louis Pasteur and Robert Koch led to the expectation that many obscure diseases such as milk sickness would prove to be of bacterial etiology. This expectation was apparently realized when researchers reported in 1909 that *Bacillus lactimorbi* was the cause of milk sickness in humans and trembles in cattle. Needless to say, they were wrong.

Beginning in 1905, Edwin Moseley of what is now Bowling Green State University in Ohio began a study of the white snakeroot that lasted more than three decades. He established the toxic dose for animals at 6–10 percent body weight. He also found that the stems were less poisonous than the leaves and that neither freezing nor drying destroyed the poison. His book, published in 1941, is the definitive work on milk sickness.

Finally, in 1928 James Couch reported the isolation of three poisonous substances from the white snakeroot: a volatile oil and a resin acid that did not produce trembles, and an oily liquid that did. The last had the characteristics of a secondary alcohol and was identified as $C_{16}H_{22}O_3$. Drawing on the Latin (*tremere*) for "tremble," Couch named it "tremetol."

Heating reduces somewhat the toxicity of poisoned milk, and oxidation destroys the toxic properties of tremetol. Because only a small number of cows are likely to be secreting toxic milk at one time, human illness is seen chiefly when milk from a single animal or herd is consumed. It is now thought that dilution (from collection and distribution at a large milk source) rather than pasteurization is the reason that milk sickness has failed to develop in urban areas and has become extremely rare. Moreover, in rural areas, farmers are now well aware that to avoid trembles or milk sickness, they need only abandon woodland grazing, for the white snakeroot is a woodland plant and almost never found in bright and open pastures.

Animal trembles (occurring chiefly in cattle) causes **anorexia**, weakness, falling, stiffness, and trembling. In humans, symptoms of milk sickness include anorexia, listlessness, severe constipation, and – most important of all, and underlying most other symptoms – profound **acidosis**. The latter, if untreated, leads to coma and death. Because of the acidosis, the breath smells of acetone, described in the past as overpowering. The weakness is thought to arise chiefly from **hypoglycemia**, and death from **ketoacidosis** and marked **fatty degeneration** of liver, kidneys, and muscles. The disease can be chronic or latent and is likely to recur if the patient is subjected to fatigue, starvation, intercurrent infection, or vigorous exercise.

The lethargy that characterizes a milk-sickness convalescent helped give it the name of slows (or sloes). Abraham Lincoln knew it by that name, and, annoyed by the desultory progress of the army early in the Civil War, he once tartly remarked that General McClellan "seemed to have the slows."

History

Milk sickness has vanished from the list of major concerns of modern Americans. Although endemic in the Midwest and upper South, it had never been seen elsewhere in the United States, Europe, or any other continent. The settlers along the Atlantic seaboard knew nothing of it, and if the Indians or their cattle suffered from the disease, they did not inform the early settlers. Not until the pioneers began to push westward beyond the Alleghenies did the disease attract attention.

The first sporadic cases of milk sickness were recognized in North Carolina in the years preceding the Revolution. It was generally known that on the western side of the Allegheny Mountains from Georgia to the Great Lakes a disorder called trembles prevailed among cattle, and that wherever it appeared, the settlers were likely to get a disease, which from its most prominent symptom received at first the name "sick stomach" and from a theory concerning its cause that of "milk sickness."

In 1811, the *Medical Repository* of New York contained an anonymous report entitled "Disease in Ohio, Ascribed to Some Deleterious Quality in the Milk of Cows." This appears to be the earliest surviving reference to a disease that became a frequent cause of death and a major source of misery and mystification in the rural South and Midwest through a large part of the nineteenth century.

In 1834, Anna Pierce Hobbs, a pioneer doctor in Illinois, learned from a Shawnee medicine woman that white snakeroot caused trembles and milk sickness. Hobbs fed a calf several bunches of the root. The calf developed typical trembles, enforcing her conviction that she had found the cause of milk sickness. John Rowe, a farmer of Fayette County, Ohio, wrote in 1838 that he had discovered through similar experimentation that trembles was caused by ingestion of white snakeroot.

During the second half of the nineteenth century, milk sickness occurred sporadically, which made sequential observations difficult, and its cause was lost in the widely held medical belief in miasmas and exhalations from the ground. Moreover, because milk sickness was limited to the Midwest, upper South, and Southwest, influential eastern physicians tended to ignore it or even discount its existence as a disease *sui generis*.

Nonetheless, the solution was eventually found when attention returned to the poisonous plant theory. Although many plants were suspected, such as poison ivy, water hemlock, Virginia creeper, coralberry, spurge, mushrooms, and march marigold, scrutiny finally centered once again on white snakeroot. Yet not until 1928 was white snakeroot established with certainty as the cause of milk sickness – over a century after the anonymous 1811 article appeared. In 1956, an article in the *Journal of the American Medical Association* by William Snively and Louanna Furbee asked the question: "How could a disease, perhaps the leading cause of death and disability in the Midwest and Upper South for over two centuries, go unrecognized by the medical profession at large until 1928?"

Thomas E. Cone, Jr.

94. Multiple Sclerosis

Multiple sclerosis (MS) is a disease of the central nervous system characterized by recurring episodes of neurological disturbance. The course of the disease is quite variable, at one extreme lasting 50 years without significant disability and at the other terminating fatally in a matter of months. Overall, about one-quarter of patients remain able to work up to 15 years after the first recognized manifestation, and mean duration of life is approximately 25 years from that time. Nevertheless, because MS commonly affects young adults, producing disability in the prime of life, the economic burden is heavy, in the United States averaging $15,000 per annum per affected family.

History

Multiple sclerosis is a remarkable disease. It was first clearly described more than 130 years ago in a way that we would recognize as a modern, pathologically based account that discusses the clinical features of the illness and their possible pathophysiology. But only since the 1970s has real progress been made in understanding its nature, course, and pathogenesis. It was discussed in pathological treatises of the 1830s and 1840s, and more knowledge was added in 1873. The "French school" did most to delineate the disease. Good descriptions appeared in neurology textbooks before the end of the nineteenth century, and an exhaustive 1916 account of the pathology of MS remains a standard reference.

The geography of multiple sclerosis is interesting because it is strange and because understanding it may provide a crucial clue to the nature of the disease. Geographic peculiarities were first noted around a century ago when Byron Bramwell argued that the higher incidence of multiple sclerosis in his practice in Edinburgh than that of neurologists in New York reflected a real difference in frequency between the two cities.

Fifty years ago, the notion of the relevance of genetic background as well as latitude was pointed out by Geoffrey Dean on the basis of the lower prevalence of multiple sclerosis among Boers than among British descendants in South Africa; in both groups, the prevalence of the disease in Africa was the same as in their countries of origin. The idea that genetic background was important also received support from the discovery of the rarity of multiple sclerosis among the Japanese. In recent decades, strenuous efforts have been made to determine the consequences of migration at different ages from areas of high to low prevalence, and vice versa. These studies support the general idea of an interaction between latitude and genetic factors determining the geographic distribution of the disease.

Characteristics

The characteristic lesion of multiple sclerosis is the **plaque of demyelination** – patches of varying size in which the myelin sheathing of nerve fibers is destroyed, leaving the axons relatively intact. Small plaques are oriented around small veins (venules), though this orientation is often obscured in large lesions. Venules in areas of active demyelination are surrounded by cells derived from the immune system. Such cells are also present in the substance of the brain – in the lesions, especially at the edges, where they may help limit the spread of damage. The plaques are distributed asymmetrically throughout the brain and spinal cord, but certain sites of predilection determine the characteristic pattern of the disease. The important functional consequence of demyelination is block of electrical conduction in the nerve fibers, which causes many of the symptoms.

In at least 80 percent of patients, the disease follows a relapsing and remitting course, often in the later stages entering a steadily progressive phase. Fully 10–20 percent experience a steadily progressive course from onset. The typical episode of neurological disturbance develops in up to 2 weeks, persists for a few weeks, then resolves over a month or two. Common manifestations include reversible episodes of visual loss (optic **neuritis**), sensory disturbance or weakness in trunk or limbs, vertigo, and bladder disturbance. Obvious disturbance of intellectual function is uncommon – except in severe cases – although subtle defects have been demonstrated early in the course of the disease.

Multiple sclerosis principally affects individuals of northern European Caucasoid origin living in temperate zones, though it does occur infrequently in the tropics and in other racial groups. Females are affected about twice as commonly as men. The average age of onset is 30 years, and it rarely starts over the age of 60 or before puberty. In Caucasoid populations, approximately 10 percent of patients have an affected relative. The concordance rate in twins is about 30 percent for identical twins and 2 percent for nonidentical twins, the latter similar to

the frequency in siblings. The difference in concordance rates between identical and nonidentical twins strongly implicates a genetic factor; however, the rather low concordance of identical twins suggests that an environmental factor is also involved.

Among Caucasoids, the prevalence of MS generally increases with latitude. MS is more common in the northern United States and Canada than in the southern United States, and in southern New Zealand and Australia than in the north. The influence of migration on risk has been studied in several populations. Migration from high-prevalence (e.g., northern Europe and the northern United States) to low-prevalence areas (e.g., Israel, South Africa, or the southern United States) before puberty appears to decrease risk of developing MS, whereas such migration after puberty does not. These and related studies provide further – albeit rather weak – evidence for the operation of an environmental factor in MS.

On the face of it, stronger evidence comes from apparent clusters of cases in the Faroe Islands. No cases were identified in the Faroes before World War II. But between 1943 and 1973, 32 cases occurred, with no new cases since. Some investigators have suggested that the pattern of presentation suggests a point-source epidemic. Noting that patients' residences were close to the location of 1940s army camps, analysts further proposed that an infection was introduced by British troops occupying the islands during that period. Other researchers have challenged these conclusions. Nonetheless, the overall clustering of cases is striking and probably a phenomenon of biological significance, indicating exposure to a newly introduced environmental agent in the early 1940s. Other examples of clustering have been reported but are less convincing.

MS is much less frequent in non-Caucasoid populations. No proven case has yet been described in African blacks, and prevalence is lower in American blacks than in whites in the same areas. The disease is similarly rare among American Indians, New Zealand Maoris,

Hungarian gypsies, and Orientals on the U.S. west coast, but not in the larger populations they live among. MS is also rare among the Japanese, Chinese, and (Asian) Indians in their homelands. It is unreported in Eskimos. Real differences in the frequency of MS in different ethnic groups again suggest the operation of a genetic factor in determining susceptibility.

The most intensively studied genetic associations of multiple sclerosis are those within the human leukocyte antigen (HLA) region of the sixth chromosome. The most frequent association in Caucasoid populations is with HLA-DR2, though others have been reported. There are fewer data for non-Caucasoid populations, although it should be noted that MS is rare in two populations in which DR2 is common: the Hungarian gypsies (of whom 56 percent of controls are DR2 positive) and the Maoris – raising the possibility of an overriding genetic protective effect. The frequency of association with the HLA system suggests that the observations are significant, yet no identified factor alone seems to confer susceptibility to the disease. The simplest explanation is that DR2 acts as a marker for another gene (or genes) conferring susceptibility, and that other genetic factors are involved as well. What is common to all the genetic associations so far identified is that they are concerned in one way or another with control of the immune response.

Much evidence suggests an immunologic basis for MS: abnormal synthesis of antibodies, both inside and outside the brain; changes in the number and activity of peripheral-blood lymphocyte subsets; and the presence of immune-competent cells around the venules in the lesions and in the brain itself. The occurrence of such changes in the retina (where there is no myelin) is evidence that the vascular events are not secondary to myelin breakdown, indicating that vascular change is a critical early event in development of the new lesion.

These processes provide a plausible though incomplete explanation for the development of the lesions in established MS. But what of its initiation? Good evidence from family studies and epidemiology indicates that an environmental trigger, probably infective, is required in the genetically susceptible individual. The most likely infective agent is a virus, though interest in spirochetes has revived as well.

In conclusion, knowledge of the nature and cause of MS seems to be within sight. When we understand the reasons for the peculiar distribution of the disease, we are also likely to understand its etiology and pathogenesis.

W. I. McDonald

95. Mumps

Mumps (also **infectious parotitis** or **epidemic parotitis**) is a common viral infectious disease, principally of children, with worldwide distribution. It is frequently characterized by fever and painful enlargement of one or more salivary glands. Inapparent infection is common, occurring in about one-third of cases. Sometimes, postpubertal males with mumps may develop painful swelling of the testicles, usually only on one side, with sterility an extremely rare complication. Mumps is a vaccine-preventable disease, but the vaccine is not yet widely used on a global basis.

Characteristics

Mumps is caused by the mumps virus, of the genus *Paramyxovirus*. Mumps virus has an irregular spherical shape and contains a single-stranded RNA genome.

Mumps is a contagious disease, only slightly less contagious than **rubella** and **measles**, transmitted from infected persons to susceptible individuals by droplet spread and by direct saliva contact. Mumps virus can also be transmitted across the placenta to the fetus. There is no natural reservoir for mumps other than humans, which means that a continuous chain of susceptible contacts is necessary to sustain transmission. Although the duration of communicability may be as much as 15 days, the period of greatest infectivity is about 48 hours before salivary-gland involvement. There is no carrier state. Mumps incubates about 18 days with a range of 2–3 weeks.

In populated areas with no or low vaccination coverage, mumps is primarily an endemic disease of children, with epidemics occurring in closely associated groups such as schools. Its peak incidence is found in the 6–10 age group, and mumps is rare before 2 years of age. Outbreaks may occur at intervals ranging from 2 to 7 years. Cases concentrate in the cooler seasons in temperate climates, but no apparent seasonality prevails in tropical areas. In remote isolated populations, mumps is not endemic, and disease depends upon introduction from outside, at which time epidemics may occur, affecting all persons born since the previous epidemic. No evidence exists for a sex or racial difference in mumps incidence, although clinically apparent mumps may be more common in males than in females.

Mumps is not a reportable disease in most countries and is underreported even where it is notifiable. In populated areas where mumps is both endemic and epidemic, more than 80 percent of the adult population evidences prior infection. In remote or island populations where mumps is not endemic, a significant proportion of the population can be susceptible, which may lead to large outbreaks when the virus is introduced from outside. In some countries, such as the United States, where mumps is a reportable disease and mumps vaccine has been extensively used (often in combination with measles and rubella vaccine), impressive declines in reported cases have occurred.

Infants usually have a passive immunity to mumps because of maternal antibodies acquired transplacentally from immune mothers. This passive immunity protects an infant from infection for about 6 months, depending on the amount of maternal antibody acquired. Mumps infection in both clinically apparent and inapparent cases induces lifelong immunity. Because a significant percentage of infections are inapparent, persons may develop immunity without realizing they have been infected.

A single dose of live attenuated mumps virus vaccine confers long-term, probably lifelong, immunity in more than 90 percent of susceptible individuals.

The prodromal phase of mumps disease may be absent or include symptoms of low-grade fever, loss of appetite, malaise, and headache. Salivary-gland swelling often follows the prodromal period within a day, although sometimes not for a week or more. The salivary-gland swelling progresses to a maximum in 1–3 days. The gland is painful and tender to the touch. Typically, both parotid salivary glands are affected, usually with one enlarging a few days after the other; hence the name "parotitis." One-sided parotid-gland involvement occurs in approximately one-fourth of patients who have such swelling. The fever lasts for a variable period (1–6 days), and parotid gland enlargement for 6–10 days.

A common manifestation of mumps in 20–30 percent of postpubertal males is painful testicular swelling (**orchitis**), usually one-sided. Sterility is an extremely rare outcome of testicular involvement on both sides, occurring in approximately 2 percent of cases. The next most common manifestation of mumps is central nervous system involvement in the form of **meningitis** – usually benign – occurring in about 10 percent of infections. Uncommon manifestations of mumps include involvement and sometimes painful swelling of other glands such as ovaries, breasts, thyroid, and pancreas. Mumps-associated complications are rare but include **encephalitis, neuritis, arthritis, nephritis, hepatitis, pericarditis**, and hematologic complications. Deafness, usually one-sided and often permanent, is reported to occur once per 20,000 cases. Although increased fetal mortality has been reported in women who contracted mumps during the first trimester, there is no evidence that mumps in pregnancy increases the risk of fetal malformations.

History

Hippocrates (fifth century B.C.) is believed to have first recognized mumps as a distinct clinical entity. He described an outbreak on the island of Thasus. Other ancient Greek and Roman medical writers as well as medieval practitioners at various times recorded cases of mumps-like illnesses, but the disease was relatively little studied. In the sixteenth century, Guillaume de Baillou recorded outbreaks of mumps in Paris. In 1755, Richard Russell described mumps and opined that the disease was communicable.

Mumps is called *Ziegenpeter* or *Bauerwetzel* in German and *oreillons* in French. The origin of the term "mumps" is unclear although it may come from the English noun *mump*, meaning a "lump," or the English verb *mump*, meaning "to be sulky," or even perhaps from the pattern of mumbling speech in individuals with significant salivary gland swelling.

In 1790, Robert Hamilton presented a full description of mumps, emphasizing that orchitis was a manifestation of mumps and suggesting that some mumps patients had symptoms of central nervous system involvement. Study of epidemics helped establish the communicability and wide distribution of the disease. Some 150 epidemics occurred between 1714 and 1859 in temperate, cold, subtropical, and equatorial regions in both hemispheres.

Data have demonstrated the occurrence of epidemic mumps in the closely associated populations of prisons, orphanages, boarding schools, armies, and ships. Indeed, mumps was the most important disease in terms of days lost from active duty in the American Expeditionary Force in France during World War I, and in 1940 the disease was one of the most disabling acute infections among U.S. armed forces recruits, exceeded only by **venereal diseases**.

Despite earlier animal experiments suggesting that salivary-gland fluid was infective, the viral etiology of mumps was not conclusively proved until 1934. In 1945, mumps virus was successfully cultivated in chick embryos. In 1948, the significant percentage of clinically inapparent infections was confirmed. In 1951, an experimental killed-virus vaccine was used in humans. A live mumps virus vaccine has been used in the former U.S.S.R. since the early 1960s. In 1966, researchers reported development of a live attenuated mumps virus vaccine, and successful trials led to its licensure in 1967 in the United States.

Robert J. Kim-Farley

96. Muscular Dystrophy

The **muscular dystrophies** are genetically determined, almost exclusively pediatric diseases. Generally, the earlier the age at which symptoms begin, the poorer the prognosis. Because of a considerable overlap of manifestations and rates of progression and, until recently, the lack of any biochemical test, their classification is still unsettled. As a group, the principal differential diagnosis of muscular dystrophies is from **muscular atrophies**. In the former, the primary defect is in voluntary muscle fibers; in the latter, it is in the innervation of muscles.

The most common of the dystrophies and the first to be described was that delineated by French neurologist Guillaume Duchenne in 1868. **Duchenne muscular dystrophy** (DMD) is a sex-linked recessive disorder. Consequently, it affects only males and is inherited through female carriers of the gene. Affected boys have abnormally elevated concentrations of muscle-cell enzymes such as creatine phosphokinase in their blood; this abnormality is also found in about three-fourths of female carriers. DMD appears to have a rather uniform incidence worldwide of 15–33 cases per 100,000. A family history of DMD is identified in only about one-third of cases. Others are attributed to either a previously unexpressed carrier state or a new mutation.

Cases can be identified during the first week of life by excessive concentration of creatine phosphokinase in the blood, although the infant appears normal. The boy learns to walk somewhat late, falls easily, and has difficulty getting up again. The gait gradually becomes broad-based and waddling. Nevertheless, diagnosis usually is not made before age 5. Without intervention, the parents' risk of producing additional dystrophic children remains high.

The child's physique may be perplexing in that, despite his weakness, his muscles may appear unusually well developed, a **pseudohypertrophy** resulting from infiltration and replacement of muscle fibers by fat and connective tissue. As the disease progresses, muscle fibers increasingly appear abnormal microscopically, and others disappear. The upper extremities are affected later but in the same fashion as the pelvic girdle and lower limbs. Smooth muscle (e.g., intestinal tract, bladder) is not affected. Subnormal stress on the developing skeleton from the weak musculature delays ossification of long bones, and the mineral content of bones is deficient. Once weakness has resulted in confinement to wheelchair or bed, contractures of extremity joints and **kyphoscoliosis** (deformity of the vertebral column) supervene. A moderate degree of **mental retardation** frequently is an associated problem. Death generally results from **respiratory failure** before age 20.

The defective gene of DMD was identified in 1986. Researchers discovered that this genetic abnormality causes a deficiency of a protein – dystrophin – in the membrane of muscle fibers. Although this substance constitutes only 0.002 percent of total muscle protein, its deficiency is detectable and can serve as a specific diagnostic test.

At the other extreme of severity from DMD is **facio-scapulo-humeral dystrophy** (FSHD), described by French neurologists Louis Landouzy and Joseph Déjerine in 1884. Onset usually occurs during adolescence but can be much later. Incidence has been estimated as from 5 to 50 percent of the incidence of DMD. Inheritance is autosomal dominant, and FSHD occurs equally in both sexes. As the name indicates, muscles of the face and shoulder girdle are affected first. Sometimes only facial muscles are involved. An affected person may be unable to close the eyelids completely or to purse the lips. Muscular involvement progresses

downward to the pelvic girdle and legs but may become arrested at any time. Reproduction is not impaired. Death from sudden **heart failure** occurs in some cases. So far there is no effective treatment for the underlying abnormality of any of the muscular dystrophies.

Thomas G. Benedek

97. Myasthenia Gravis

Myasthenia gravis is a disorder of skeletal muscle characterized by weakness and easy fatigability resulting from autoimmune destruction of the acetylcholine receptor in the postsynaptic membrane of the neuromuscular junction.

Characteristics

The disease has a worldwide distribution and is the primary cause of death in 1.5 cases per million annually in the United States. It attacks whites and nonwhites equally and seems to be uniformly distributed around the globe. There appears to be a twin-peaked incidence, with females peaking between ages 15 and 24, and males peaking between 40 and 60. The death rate is slightly higher for women than for men. Morbidity data in surveys of the United States, Canada, England, Norway, and Iceland over a 10-year period using retrospective analysis show that the incidence of myasthenia is probably 0.2–0.5 per 100,000, with prevalence being 3–6 per 100,000. In other words, the prevalence is approximately 10 times the incidence.

The overwhelming evidence is that myasthenia gravis results from an **immune system dysfunction** that produces an autodirected antibody against the acetylcholine receptor in the postsynaptic membrane of the neuromuscular junction. The evidence is clinical, laboratory, serologic, and therapeutic. The clinical evidence that myasthenia is an autoimmune disease is based on the association of myasthenia with vaccination, insect sting, infection, and trauma and its association with autoimmune diseases such as **hypothyroidism, systemic lupus**, and **polymyositis**. Laboratory abnormalities pointing to an immune-system dysfunction include serologic abnormalities, increased incidence of a specific human leukocyte antigen (HLA-B8) in certain types of disease, histologic abnormalities of thymus and skeletal muscle, and abnormal responsiveness of lymphocytes to mitogens. Antinuclear antibodies are positive in uncomplicated myasthenia in about 18 percent of cases and in 54 percent of myasthenic patients who have **thymoma**, a tumor derived from elements of the thymus. Antistriated muscle antibodies are present in about 11 percent of patients with uncomplicated myasthenia and in all patients who have myasthenia associated with thymoma. Perhaps the most important serologic test in myasthenia is the IgG antibody directed against the acetylcholine receptor. This antibody is probably positive in 70–95 percent of clinically diagnosed myasthenic patients and is the cause of the weakness and easy fatigability in the disease.

The single most important feature of myasthenia gravis is weakness of skeletal muscle worsened by exercise and relieved by rest. Weakness with easy fatigability is the only constant in this disease; all other features are variable. For instance, the weakness is usually worse in the afternoon and evening, although some patients are weaker in the morning when they first awaken. Usually the muscles supplied by the cranial nerves are the first and most severely affected, with resultant **diplopia, ophthalmoplegia, dysphagia, dysphonia, dyspnea**, and **dysmimia**. The disease may involve proximal lower- and upper-extremity muscles. In rare instances, however, proximal muscles weaken first. Involvement of individual muscles may be symmetrical but is often asymmetrical with a dominant leg and arm usually weaker than a nondominant counterpart. Myasthenia gravis can also present as weakness of a single muscle (for example, the external rectus or superior oblique in one eye) or as a single complaint (for instance, jaw **ptosis** from inability to close the mouth). It can also present as a symptom seemingly unrelated to the neuromuscular system – for instance, burning eyes from exposure to **keratitis**, from incomplete eye closure during sleep, or a sore throat on awakening from mouth breathing during sleep. The disease may affect people of any age and either sex and varies in severity from mild nonprogressive disease involving the eyes only (ocular form) to severe cases that may be rapidly fatal such as acute myasthenia gravis afflicting older men.

No two myasthenic patients look alike or have the same signs and symptoms. The classical appearance is unmistakable and is usually associated with bilateral ptosis, weakness of the face, and difficulty in smiling, chewing, and talking. The consistent pathology found in every patient is autoimmune destruction of the postsynaptic receptor, simplification of the postsynaptic membrane, widening of the synaptic gap, and reduction in the acetylcholine receptor numbers and efficiency. Thymic pathology is also present; approximately 80 percent of patients have germinal centers and enlarged thymus, and about 10 percent have a thymoma.

History

Although myasthenia gravis was not described as a clinical entity until the late nineteenth century, a mention by seventeenth century English clinician Thomas Willis indicates that he knew the disease and recognized its chief symptom. His description of strangely weakened patients occurs in his 1672 work on the physiology and pathology of disease. Willis noted that such patients developed general albeit partial paralysis and that they were unable to move their members strongly or bear any weight. This seems to be a description of myasthenia gravis, although, of course, we will never really know.

Nearly 200 years passed before myasthenia gravis was again mentioned in medical literature. The next recorded observation appears to have been made by English physician Samuel Wilks in 1877. He discussed a woman who could scarcely walk and had defective extraocular movement. Her speech was slow and deliberate, and she fatigued easily. Subsequently, she developed trouble swallowing, was unable to cough, and died of respiratory paralysis. This incomplete discussion is the first fatal case of myasthenia gravis ever described. Wilks's report was of some importance because the patient was autopsied and no nervous system abnormality found, indicating that the trouble was caused by some functional defect.

The first really complete report of myasthenia gravis was by Wilhelm Erb in 1879. His first patient's illness developed over 4 months, and the first principal symptoms, which were clearly described, included ptosis, neck weakness, and dysphagia. Some atrophy was noticed in the neck muscles. The patient, who seemed to respond to induced current (he was probably one of the first to be treated by Erb with electricity), went into remission, and it was natural for Erb to attribute the improvement to his electrical treatment. Erb's second case had symptoms of double vision, ptosis, dysphagia, and weakness. She died suddenly at night, and no autopsy was done. She had clear-cut exacerbations and remissions. The third patient reported by Erb had difficulty holding his head up, and showed bilateral ptosis and facial weakness.

Subsequently, a score more cases were reported by 1893, when Samuel Goldflam provided a detailed study of myasthenia gravis, mentioning all the currently accepted signs of the disease: (1) The disease occurs in early life; (2) both sexes are equally affected; (3) it attacks the motor system; (4) chewing, swallowing, and eye movements are most affected at first, followed by involvement of trunk extremity; (5) trunk involvement is usually but not always symmetrical; (6) most patients are worse in the afternoon and evening and are improved by rest.

Goldflam also mentioned that daily exacerbations and remissions may occur, and that death may suddenly occur from respiratory impairment. His article in many ways is the most important ever written in the history of myasthenia gravis.

The next major advance occurred in an 1894 paper by F. Galle. He was first to analyze the

reaction of muscles in myasthenia gravis to electrical stimulation and to name the disease. He also suggested physostigmine as drug treatment but does not seem to have pursued this important point; 40 years later, the therapeutic value of physostigmine was demonstrated.

Modern studies of the pathological physiology of myasthenia gravis started in the 1940s with a series of illustrious researchers, who recognized the characteristic response of evoked muscle action potential to repetitive stimulation of nerve, thereby localizing the defect of myasthenia gravis to the neuromuscular junction. Evidence accumulated of an immunologic disorder in myasthenia. This was first suggested in 1959 by recognition of the histological parallel between the thymus in myasthenia and the thyroid gland in **thyroiditis**. The following year, attention was drawn to the increased frequency, in myasthenia gravis, of other diseases regarded as autoimmune, especially **rheumatoid arthritis**. But the major advance occurred in 1973, when rabbits were injected with acetylcholine receptors. The process induced experimental autoimmune myasthenia gravis in the animals, which led to experiments indicating the nature of the human disease. We now know that the disease is caused by a circulating antibody directed against the acetylcholine receptor and that treatments directed against the abnormal antibody are effective in modifying myasthenia gravis.

Bernard M. Patten

98. Nematode Infection

The thousands of species in the phylum Nemathelminthes, the **nematodes** or "roundworms," include both free-living forms and important parasites of plants and animals. Many species of nematodes parasitize humans, and several of them are major public-health problems in poor countries, especially in the tropics. Some species reside as adults in the intestine; others are found in the blood and tissues.

See: **Ascariasis, Dracunculiasis, Enterobiasis, Filariasis, Onchocerciasis, Strongyloidiasis, Trichinosis,** and **Trichuriasis**.

K. David Patterson

99. Onchocerciasis

Onchocerciasis is caused by a **filarial nematode**, the roundworm *Onchocerca volvulus*. Humans are infected by larval microfilariae transmitted by blood-feeding female flies of the genus *Simulium*. Symptoms include skin damage, extreme itching, and ocular lesions that can lead to permanent blindness. Synonyms include "river blindness" in West Africa, *sowda* in Yemen, and *enfermedad de Robles* in Latin America.

Characteristics

Onchocerciasis is widely distributed in sub-Saharan Africa, especially in the savanna grasslands from Senegal to Sudan. Its range extends southward into Kenya, Zaire, and Malawi. The region encompassing the headwaters of the Volta River system in northern Ghana, northeastern Ivory Coast, southern Burkina Faso (Upper Volta), and adjacent territories has been a major center for the disease. Onchocerciasis was almost certainly indigenous to Africa, but it has been transmitted to the Arabian Peninsula (Saudi Arabia and Yemen) and to the Caribbean basin, where scattered foci exist in Mexico, Guatemala, Colombia, Venezuela, Ecuador, and Brazil.

The disease has a patchy distribution within its range; infection rates in particular villages may range from zero to virtually 100 percent. In the Volta Basin alone, the World Health Organization estimated in the 1970s that 1 million of 10 million inhabitants were infected, with about 70,000 classified as "economically blind." In northern Ghana, surveys in the early 1950s determined that about 30,000 people, roughly 3 percent of the population, were totally blind because of onchocerciasis. In some West African villages, adult blindness rates of 10–30 percent

have been observed. Conversely, dermatologic symptoms predominate in Arabia, and ocular involvement is rare.

O. volvulus, one of several filarial worms that are important human parasites, lives in the cutaneous and subcutaneous tissues. Humans are the only definitive host; there is no animal reservoir. Numbers of adult worms, the females of which may reach a length of 50 centimeters, live in large coiled masses, which usually become surrounded by fibrotic tissue generated by the host. In these nodules, which may reach the size of a walnut and are often easily visible on head, trunk, hips, or legs, the adults live and breed for as long as 16 years. Thousands of larvae, the microfilariae, emerge from the nodules and migrate in the tissues of the skin.

Host immune reactions to dead or dying microfilariae cause various forms of dermatologic destruction, including loss of elasticity, depigmentation, and thickening of the skin. These changes are complicated by the host's reaction to the extreme **pruritis** caused by allergic reactions to worm proteins; the victim may scratch incessantly in a vain attempt to relieve the tormenting itch. This condition is sometimes called *craw-craw* in West Africa. Wandering microfilariae can also cause damage to the lymphatic system. Microfilariae that reach the eye cause the most damage. Larvae dying in various ocular tissues cause cumulative lesions that, over a period of one to several years, can lead to progressive loss of sight and total blindness. Distinct geographic strains appear to exist, which helps explain different pathological pictures in parts of the parasite's range.

Diagnosis is by detection of nodules, by demonstration of microfilariae in skin snips, and, in recent years, by immunologic tests. Therapy includes surgical removal of nodules, which has been widely practiced in Latin America to combat eye damage, and various drugs to kill microfilariae. A number of such drugs, however, may cause serious side effects in heavily infected people.

The vectors and intermediate hosts of the pathogen are flies of the genus *Simulium*, especially *Simulium damnosum*. These annoying and appropriately named insects, sometimes called "buffalo gnats," are close relatives of the "black flies" of the northern United States and southern Canada. The females bite people, cattle, goats, wild animals, and birds to obtain blood meals. Flies feeding on infected humans may ingest microfilariae. These undergo about a 1-week developmental process before migrating to the salivary glands. Here, as infective larvae, they await the opportunity to enter a new host when the fly feeds again. Once this happens, the larvae wander briefly in the skin before settling down in clumps to mature, breed, and produce microfilariae.

Simulium females lay eggs on rocks and vegetation in swiftly flowing, richly oxygenated water. Ripples around rocks, bridge abutments, and dam spillways provide favorable conditions for the larval development of the vector. There is no transovarial transmission, so newly emerged adults must acquire onchocerca in a blood meal. Adult flies have extensive flight ranges: Infected females aided by winds and weather fronts can move hundreds of kilometers to establish new foci of disease. However, because of the vector's breeding preferences, most flies and hence most onchocerciasis cases are found within a few kilometers of a stream with suitable breeding sites. The term "river blindness" accurately reflects the geographic distribution of the disease.

Onchocerciasis often has dramatic effects on human activities and settlement patterns. In many heavily infested areas, notably in the headwaters of the Volta River, swarming flies, tormenting skin infestation, and progressive blindness among a significant proportion of the population have resulted in progressive abandonment of rich, well-watered farmlands near the rivers. Depopulation of river valleys because of onchocerciasis has transpired for some time in northern Ghana, with people forced to cultivate crowded and eroding lands away from the streams. In many areas, land-hungry people were settling river valleys in the early twentieth century, but in recent decades the line of settlement has retreated from the rivers.

It is possible that a cycle of colonization and retreat, with farmers caught between malnutrition and land shortages on one hand and the perils of onchocerciasis on the other, has been going on for centuries in parts of the Volta basin.

History

Onchocerciasis is almost certainly a disease that originated in Africa and has spread to Arabia and the New World as an unintended by-product of the slave trade. Skin lesions caused by onchocerciasis were first described in the Gold Coast (modern Ghana). The organism was first described in 1893 by eminent German parasitologist Friedrich Rudolf Leuckart. In 1916, the disease was first recognized in the Americas by Guatemalan investigator Rodolfo Robles. Robles linked nodules to eye disease and suggested that the distribution of infection implicated two species of *Simulium* as vectors. D. Blacklock, working in Sierra Leone, showed in 1926 that *S. damnosum* was the vector.

In 1931, J. Hissette, working in Congo, linked onchocerciasis with blindness for the first time in Africa, but despite confirmation in the Sudan a year later, colonial doctors generally considered onchocerciasis only a skin disease. Just before World War II, French doctors in what is now Burkina Faso began to link the disease with mass blindness and river valley abandonment. Their colleagues across the frontier in the British Gold Coast did not make a similar discovery until 1949.

Although British physicians and administrators were aware of river valley depopulation, onchocerciasis, and substantial blindness in the northern part of the colony, they did not link these phenomena, partly because doctors who became interested in the problem in the 1930s were repeatedly distracted by other duties or transferred. After the war, the association was finally made. A series of investigations in the 1950s confirmed the widespread incidence and serious consequences of the disease in a number of African countries, and Latin American foci were delimited.

In 1975 the World Health Organization began the Onchocerciasis Control Programme, an ambitious and expensive 20-year effort to eliminate onchocerciasis in the entire Volta Basin. The basic strategy was to kill fly larvae by aerially spraying temephos (an organophosphate) over breeding sites throughout a huge and repeatedly extended portion of West Africa. The absence of an effective agent to kill adult flies has not prevented tremendous success in reducing and sometimes eliminating *Simulium* populations.

Although treatment of victims was less successful until recently because existing drugs were too dangerous for mass use, the vector control program, though costly and constantly faced with the problem of reintroduction of adult flies from places beyond its limits, has resulted in dramatic declines in biting rates, infection, and blindness in most of the region. Recently, treatment of thousands of victims with ivermectin, a safe and effective microfilaricide, has helped to reduce blindness among infected persons and has reduced the chances that a feeding fly would ingest infective microfilariae.

The absence of an agent to kill adult worms and the logistical and financial difficulties of the massive larviciding campaign make total eradication unlikely, but vector control and microfilaricidal treatment can reduce the number of infected persons and lessen or eliminate severe clinical symptoms. Success at this level could help make thousands of square kilometers of valuable farmland safe for use in many regions of Africa. It is, however, clear that there must be a long-term commitment to the campaign for many years into the future, or river blindness will reconquer its old haunts.

K. David Patterson

100. Ophthalmia (Trachoma, Conjunctivitis)

In its broadest sense, **ophthalmia** is an inflammation of the eye, especially of the conjunctiva.

The term derives from the Greek *ophthalmos* ("eye"), and almost any eye disease was called ophthalmia until the twentieth century. The problem for historians of past disease is that "ophthalmia" meant any of a number of eye ailments and that blindness from "ophthalmia" had many possible causes. Historically, two of the most important "ophthalmias" were **trachoma** and **conjunctivitis**.

Trachoma

Trachoma (also called **granular conjunctivitis** and "Egyptian ophthalmia") is caused by *Chlamydia trachomatis*. It is characterized by inflammatory granulations on the inner eyelid that severely scar the eye, eventually causing blindness (but not in all cases). It was a leading cause of blindness in the past and still blinds millions in Asia, the Middle East, and Africa. Two estimates place the number of victims worldwide at between 400 and 500 million, with perhaps 2 million totally blinded.

Because a dry climate seems to affect incidence, some of the highest rates of infection are found in the countries of North Africa and the Middle East, from Morocco to Egypt and Sudan and from the Red Sea to Turkey and Iran. It is also widespread in Asia, with 20–50 percent of the population infected in Burma, Pakistan, India, China, Indonesia, and Borneo. Such rates also occur in sub-Saharan Africa (excepting West Africa, where incidence falls below 20 percent). Similar trachoma rates continue along the Mediterranean coast of Europe, in Eastern Europe, Russia, Korea, Japan, Australia, New Zealand, and Oceania. In the Western Hemisphere, Brazil and Mexico have the highest incidences, but trachoma also infects Indians and Mexican-Americans in the U.S. Southwest. Sporadic cases appear in Europe, the Philippines, and some Central and South American countries. Trachoma is practically extinct in Canada, Switzerland, Austria, and northern Europe – areas with high standards of living and sanitary conditions and without extreme poverty. Where living conditions have improved, trachoma has declined or disappeared.

Trachoma generally requires prolonged contact in filthy and overcrowded conditions for transmission. In endemic areas, infection first occurs in childhood as a result of close family contact. Transmission may be from mother to baby, from eye to eye, by fingers, and by eye-seeking flies. In urban slums and poor villages where people live crowded together in unsanitary conditions, garbage and raw sewage attract flies that breed copiously. As the insects swarm on the faces of infants and children, they feed on the infected eye discharges of those with trachoma and carry it to the eyes of other victims. Most children in endemic areas have trachoma at an early age, but hosting the disease in childhood does not provide a lifelong immunity.

Trachoma transmission may also occur by direct touch, by contamination of clothing or bedding, possibly by bathing in communal pools, and by sexual means. Factors contributing to trachoma are ocular irritants and **bacterial conjunctivitis**. It is most prevalent in hot, dry climates – low humidity can excessively dry the conjunctiva. Wind, dust, and smoke further irritate the eyes. Bacterial infections often cause the worst cases.

The clinical features of trachoma are usually divided into four stages: Stage 1 (**incipient trachoma**) is characterized by increasing redness of the conjunctiva lining the upper lids. As the organism proliferates, pale follicles appear. Both features spread across the conjunctival surface. Minimal exudate occurs but may be more profuse with secondary bacterial infection. The upper part of the cornea becomes edematous and infiltrated with inflammatory cells, and pannus appears. Stage 1 lasts several weeks to months.

Stage 2 (**established trachoma**) marks the increase of all Stage 1 symptoms and is often termed the "florid stage." The pannus increases toward the apex of the cornea, and the red vessels in the cornea are visible to the naked eye. In severe cases, a secondary bacterial infection may worsen the appearance of the eye. Duration is 6 months to several years.

Stage 3 (**cicatrizing trachoma**) is the scarring and healing stage. Scar tissue forms on the undersurface of the eyelids. A new infection of *C. trachomatis* may occur at this stage and start the process all over again. Thus Stages 2 and 3 may coexist for many years and may be further complicated by repeated infections. Each new attack forms more scar tissue, and an ever-increasing pannus covers the cornea. This phase may be several years in duration.

Stage 4 (**healed trachoma**) is the final stage in which healing has been completed without inflammation, and the disease is no longer infectious. Trachomatous scarring remains, however, and may deform the upper lid and cause opaqueness in the cornea. When the eyelid inturns, the lashes rub on the cornea (**trichiasis**), irritating, tearing, and scarring the corneal surface. Ulcers may develop, and bacterial infection of the ulcers can lead to blindness. Another complication may be drying of the conjunctiva and cornea. Many combinations of complications may account for impaired vision and blindness.

Conjunctivitis

Simple acute conjunctivitis is a common eye infection, caused by a variety of microorganisms and characterized by a red or bloodshot eye. Mild cases may present with feelings of "roughness or sand" in the eye, but serious cases produce pain and photophobia. After some days, discharges may become so purulent that they gum the lids together. The infection often begins in one eye before spreading to the other. An acute conjunctivitis may last up to 2 weeks.

Bacteria often infect the conjunctiva simultaneously with trachoma (causing acute bacterial conjunctivitis), and the two in combination may blind many individuals. Viruses can also cause conjunctivitis; historical descriptions of mild ophthalmia may indicate bacterial or **viral conjunctivitis**. By contrast, more severe ophthalmias – producing eye-scarring or permanent blindness – were often trachoma. Even today, forms of bacterial and viral conjunctivitis are still confused with trachoma. Severe forms of conjunctivitis include **ophthalmia neonatorum**, from infection in the birth canal;

follicular conjunctivitis, often confused with early trachoma; **phlyctenular conjunctivitis**; and **hemorrhagic conjunctivitis**.

Gonococcal conjunctivitis, caused by *Neisseria gonorrhea*, infects newborns as well as children and adults but is now transmitted mainly by sexual intercourse. Ocular gonorrhea infection was one of the principal causes of blindness in Europe until the 1880s, when a silver nitrate solution came into use in newborns. The consequent decrease in blindness has been described as "one of the great victories of scientific medicine." In contrast to gonococcal conjunctivitis, which has declined in the developed world, chronic follicular conjunctivitis and acute conjunctivitis in newborns have been on the increase along with other sexually transmitted diseases.

History

Trachoma was known in China in the third millennium B.C. and in Egypt in the second. The *Ebers Papyrus* clearly described a chronic ophthalmia with discharge, **leukoma** of the cornea, and trichiasis – all suggestive of trachoma.

By the time of the ancient Greeks, eye inflammations were frequently described, and about 60 A.D. the term *trachoma* ("roughness") was first used by Dioscorides. Although the Hippocratic books do not define ophthalmia precisely, Galen defines it as "an inflammation of the conjunctiva." An important Hippocratic reference to trachoma describes not the disease but its treatment: scraping the eyelids, cutting away the fleshy granulations, and cauterization with a hot iron. Another Hippocratic text describes an operation for trichiasis. The concern with trachoma in the Hippocratic corpus may have arisen from an apparent outbreak of the disease among the Athenians during the Peloponnesian War (431–404 B.C.).

For treatment of trachoma, Greek physicians stressed scraping thickened eyelids with fig leaves or the rough skins of sea animals such as sharks. In the first century A.D., Celsus described trachoma and recommended treatment for trichiasis. About 45 A.D., a younger contemporary of Celsus wrote a book of remedies for many diseases, including several for trachoma.

The Romans were also well acquainted with trachoma. Troop movements must have dispersed the disease throughout the Mediterranean region and beyond. In France, England, and Germany, the stone-seals of Roman oculists name remedies used for trachoma. Roman medical books also include remedies for the ailment. In the fourth century, Theodorus Priscianus used garlic juice to anoint the conjunctiva.

In the sixth century, Aetius of Amida in Asia Minor distinguished four stages of trachoma, whereas in the seventh century, Paul of Aegina, an Alexandrian physician, provided descriptions of trachoma treatments as well as different phases of the disease. Like his predecessors, Paul recommended eyelid scraping. Trichiasis patients were operated on with needle and thread, a procedure "reinvented" in 1844. To prevent eye inflammation, he recommended burning the forehead and temples – a treatment later used on Saint Francis of Assisi in Italy. Paul and Aetius were also familiar with eye diseases in newborns.

Later Arabic authors continued to study trachoma. In the ninth century, Ibn Masawaih mentioned pannus and trichiasis. His pupil, Hunain ibn Is-haq, distinguished the four forms of trachoma. In the eleventh century, a Christian oculist in Baghdad, Ali ibn Isa, distinguished 13 diseases of the conjunctiva and 13 of the cornea. He clearly described trachoma and was the first to make the connection between trichiasis and trachoma. His is the best description of trachoma and its treatment written in antiquity, and probably the best until the work of J. N. Fischer of Prague in 1832. Most subsequent works in Arabic copied Ali ibn Isa's chapters on trachoma. One exception is by Cairo oculist Sadaqa ibn Ibrahim al-Sadhili in the fourteenth century, who meticulously noted his own informed observations of the disease, including (for the first time) its high incidence in Egypt.

Thus the Greeks and Arabs knew far more about trachoma than did their counterparts in Europe until the nineteenth century. They recognized the stages of trachoma, the scars, the contagiousness, and the danger of reinfection. The Arabs also knew the connection of trichiasis and pannus with trachoma, and their treatments were superior to those in the West.

In contrast, medieval Europe was poorly prepared to confront trachoma when it appeared, often accompanying returning Crusaders. However, frequent mercantile and military traffic between Italy and the Middle East meant that Italy (especially Salerno) became a center of eye-disease knowledge. Arabic and Greek writers, translated into Latin, influenced Italian concepts of trachoma and its treatment. (Latin translators, garbling the Arabic, called trachoma "scabies.") A possible trachoma victim was Saint Francis of Assisi, who certainly had some kind of ophthalmia acquired on a trip to Egypt. He returned to Italy in the early stages of the disease and sought treatment at an ophthalmia center in Rieti. He later underwent the ancient temple-cauterization treatment and was finally blinded shortly before his death.

In the fourteenth century, French surgeon Guy de Chauliac provided a description of trachoma, whereas in England, one medical tract on eye disease (by John of Arderne in 1377) survives from the period. Some of its references suggest trachoma, although a form of conjunctivitis is more likely. Trachoma usually was poorly identified, but possibly remained established in Europe until the sixteenth century onward, when notable epidemics of "ophthalmia" coincided with troop movements. A well-known epidemic, described by Forestus, occurred in 1556. A little later, Jean Costoeus mentioned the treatment of trachoma by cautery. Epidemics similar to that of 1556 occurred at Breslau in 1699 and 1700 and at Westphalia in 1762. In the later 1700s, trachoma epidemics swept through Sweden and Finland.

Trachoma was again imported after Napoleon Bonaparte's campaign in Egypt (1798–1801). An ophthalmia epidemic swept Europe, and many returning French troops lost their sight. Trachoma and conjunctivitis were still endemic in Egypt; indeed, European travelers referred to Egypt as the "land of the blind." It has been suggested that eye disease there had increased under Turkish rule, with 2 million peasants living in misery. Perhaps poverty combined with the arrival of foreign armies to trigger the terrible epidemics of "ophthalmia" that tormented Europe for half a century.

When Napoleon's troops invaded Egypt in 1798, they suffered from a contagious ophthalmia, probably the conjunctivitis prevalent in Egypt during the summer months. By September, few soldiers had escaped. Some were suffering from gonorrheal conjunctivitis and trachoma; many were completely blinded by swollen eyelids. Of one group of 3,000 men, 1,400 were unable to fight because of "ophthalmia." Thousands suffered, and those blinded were hospitalized, sent home, or massacred in battle. Many veterans suffered from eye problems for years after their return to Europe.

Turkish and British troops in Egypt also contracted ophthalmia. British surgeon George Power described the disease as a purulent conjunctivitis that had been prevalent in Ireland about 1790. He regarded it as infectious and related to Egyptian ophthalmia. "Egyptian ophthalmia" accompanied British troops on their return home. As early as 1802, Patrick MacGregor described granulations on the conjunctivae of 56 veterans who had returned from Egypt. Reaching grave proportions by 1806, this epidemic may have been gonorrheal ophthalmia rather than trachoma. When British troops attacked Egypt in 1807, they again contracted "ophthalmia," then spread it when they moved on to Sicily. Ophthalmia continued to ravage the British army for another decade. By 1818, over 5,000 men had been invalided out for blindness.

Probably the eye diseases that afflicted the French, Turkish, and British forces were the same two forms of conjunctivitis that prevail in Egypt, sometimes complicated by genuine trachoma in its various stages. When trachoma occurs along with acute conjunctivitis, it tends to be more severe and contagious. Lack of sanitation in the armies and among the local population would have facilitated the rapid spread of the ophthalmias.

The epidemics, of course, had spread to other armies. In 1801, Italian troops were infected at Elba and Leghorn by the French. This epidemic lasted until 1826. The Italians carried the disease to the Hungarian (1809) and Austrian (1814) armies. A severe epidemic struck the Prussian army from 1813 to 1817, with 20,000–25,000 men affected. From there it passed to Swedish troops in 1814 and to the Dutch in 1815. More than 17,000 suffered in the Russian army between 1816 and 1839, and by 1834, 4,000 Belgian troops had become completely blind. In fact, in 1840 one in five Belgian soldiers still suffered from "ophthalmia." When the epidemic hit Portugal in 1849, it affected 10,000 soldiers over an 8-year period. In 1813, it even reached Cuba, where it devastated 7,000 soldiers; reports claimed that "most" were blinded.

But although the Napoleonic Wars had doubtless furthered the transmission of endemic Egyptian and European ophthalmias, other epidemics may have had different points of origin. As the nineteenth century progressed, "ophthalmias" continued to afflict European troops around the world. By the end of the nineteenth century, the disease had become known as **military ophthalmia**.

Yet civilians carried the disease as well. Immigrants and slaves brought ophthalmia to the Americas, and British reports identified trachoma among immigrants from Ireland, Poland, Finland, Russia, and Armenia. The United States and Canada declared trachoma dangerous and prohibited entry to those infected, but many escaped detection. "Ophthalmia" also was among the most feared diseases of the slave trade, as it could spread quickly through a slave ship, blinding the entire cargo and crew. Such ships were occasionally discovered drifting helplessly on the open sea. In the 1830s and 1840s, slave ships from Angola and Benguela repeatedly introduced the disease into Brazilian port cities, from where it spread to the surrounding plantations. But historians cannot attribute all ophthalmias to trachoma. Along with conjunctivitis, other eye-affecting diseases such as **smallpox, measles, leprosy, tuberculosis, syphilis**, and **onchocerciasis** doubtless also blinded slaves.

By the nineteenth century, the term ophthalmia had come to cover an extraordinary variety of eye diseases. Hence, qualifiers such as cachectic, senile, menopausal, abdominal, and scrofulous were attached to the word ophthalmia. Only in the twentieth century were the actual causes of eye diseases isolated and accurate descriptions of trachoma and conjunctivitis made possible.

Mary C. Karasch

101. Osteoarthritis

Osteoarthritis (OA) is the most common rheumatic disorder afflicting humankind and vertebrates in general. The most common alternative terms, **osteoarthrosis** and **degenerative joint disease**, are used because of divergent concepts of the nature and cause of the disorder. One school maintains that OA is a family of systemic inflammatory disorders with similar clinical and pathological results. Another supports the use of the term "osteoarthrosis" because inflammation is not present. Still another uses the term "degenerative joint disease" because it is held that aging and "wear-and-tear" are responsible for its occurrence.

OA is a multifactorial systemic inflammatory disorder with clinical symptoms of pain and stiffness in movable joints, showing radiographic evidence of cartilage loss and bony overgrowth. The anatomic changes – cartilage loss and a kind of bony overgrowth and spurs – may occur physiologically without clinical symptoms. The disease is classified as **primary osteoarthritis** when there is no known predisposing factor, or **secondary osteoarthritis** when there is a clearly defined, underlying condition contributing to its etiology, such as trauma, metabolic diseases, or **gout**. Several symptom complexes are grouped as variant subsets such as **generalized osteoarthritis** or **erosive inflammatory osteoarthritis**.

Characteristics

Osteoarthritis spares no race or geographic area. In most – especially younger – patients, the disease is mild and causes no significant disability. However, in older patients, it is more severe, often producing disability, loss of time from work, and thus economic loss. The disease occurs with increased severity and frequency in older populations as a result of prolonged exposure to pathophysiological processes responsible for its development.

OA occurs with more frequency and severity in women than in men. There is a sex difference in distribution of the joints involved. Lower spine and hip disease are more common in men, whereas cervical spine and finger arthritis are more common in women. The most commonly affected joints are the distal interphalangeal joints **(Heberden's nodes)**; the proximal interphalangeal joints of the fingers **(Bouchard's nodes)**; the first metatarsophalangeal joints of the feet ("bunions"); and the spine, hips, and knees.

Studies of the incidence of osteoarthritis produce divergent data because of differences in definition and diagnostic techniques. For example, when the definition includes only pathological anatomic changes (cartilage loss and bony growth), investigators find evidence for the disorder in 90 percent of persons over age 40. Only about 30 percent of persons with radiographic changes of degenerative joint disease complain of pain in relevant joints. The frequency and severity of symptoms of the illness increase with age so that osteoarthritis is a major cause of symptomatic arthritis in the middle-aged and elderly population.

The first epidemiological studies on osteoarthritis were reported during the first half of the twentieth century in England, using only questionnaires and clinical examination to evaluate incapacity and invalidism caused by the disease. These methods, however, lacked diagnostic reliability, and classification of the disease was difficult. Later, use of roentgenograms to detect changes allowed for the classification of OA ranging from mild to severe, depending on the loss of cartilage and the presence of bony overgrowth. The cartilage loss is seen as joint space narrowing, whereas bony overgrowth can be one or more of the following: osteophytes, bony eburnation, or increased bone density. Early physical findings such as Heberden's nodes may precede radiographic changes.

Surveys of skeletal remains of contemporary white and black Americans, twelfth-century Native Americans, and protohistoric Alaskan Eskimos showed that those who underwent the heaviest mechanical stresses suffered the most severe joint involvement. Climate does not influence the prevalence of OA. Hereditary predisposition to Heberden's nodes has been found in half of observed cases. Remaining cases are considered traumatic.

Differences in patterns of affected joints occur in different ethnic groups. Heberden's nodes, for example, are rare in blacks, as is nonnodal generalized osteoarthritis. Occupational factors may play a role in incidence, especially in males. Studies from Britain, the United States, and France show osteoarthritis to be a major cause of incapacity, economic loss, and social disadvantage in persons over age 50. **Hip disease** is more common in white populations than in blacks and Native Americans. Asian populations have a low incidence of hip disease, but incidence of OA of the fingers in Asia is high, as in Europeans. **Knee disease** shows less difference among ethnic groups, being similarly prevalent in whites and blacks in South Africa and Jamaica.

The popular concept that osteoarthritis is a single disease resulting from attrition of cartilage due to age and wear-and-tear is not tenable in light of modern experimental studies. Osteoarthritis can be regarded as the result of aberrations in a complex pattern of biological reactions whose failure leads to anatomic changes in joint structure and function. One or more biological feedback loops may lead to malfunction of the complex system. Biological modifiers induce variable effects, depending on the target mechanism. One hypothesis proposes that OA is a multifactorial metabolic inflammatory disorder in which too little cartilage and too much bone are synthesized because of impaired liver function in processing growth hormone and insulin. **Hepatic dysfunction** results in altered neuropeptide levels: too little insulin-like growth factor 1, which is required for cartilage growth, and too much insulin, which accelerates bony growth and osteophyte formation.

Osteoarthritis usually has an insidious onset depending on the specific joints afflicted and the patient's tolerance to pain. The characteristic symptoms are pain and stiffness localized to the involved joints. In early disease the pain occurs with use of the joint; later pain occurs during rest. Morning stiffness is usually of short duration, less than 30 minutes. Frequently it is related to changes in the weather. The affected joint creaks on movement, and its motion is reduced.

The affected joint is enlarged, owing to bony overgrowth and to **synovitis** with accumulation of fluid. It is tender and painful. Late in the disease, **subluxation** and muscle atrophy occur. Rarely is there **ankylosis** or fusion with complete loss of motion. Radiographic examination shows cartilage loss, causing joint-space narrowing with bony overgrowth.

History

Since prehistory, vertebrates have presumably suffered from osteoarthritis. Dinosaur bones show bony spurs and ankylosed spinal segments that mark the disease. The same changes occurred in prehistoric humankind as well as in animals, modern and ancient, such as horses and dogs. Clinical descriptions of arthritis date back to the fifth century B.C., to Hippocrates, who described the Scythians as having markedly lax or hypermobile joints. The disorder was attributed to divine retribution for the destruction of the Temple of Ashkelon, which the Scythians wrought during an invasion of Palestine. Severe shoulder OA, **deform-ing arthrosis**, was found in a Scythian skeleton derived from the Hippocratic period. Evidently, shoulder OA was common among the Scythians despite treatment.

Over the centuries, the names of disorders encompassing OA have changed and have included terms such as **rheumatism** and **lumbago**, which are no longer scientifically used. Today we recognize dozens of forms and subsets of OA.

The prevalence of OA and the pattern of joint involvement show wide geographic differences. In a worldwide study, OA was most prevalent in the north of England, where 67 percent of men and 73 percent of women had OA. The lowest incidence was in Nigeria and Liberia. Prevalence of OA was also low in Soweto, South Africa, and in Piestany, Czechoslovakia. The incidence of OA also varied with the specific joint being studied. Data on Heberden's nodes revealed the highest frequency (32 percent) in the population of Watford, England; 30 percent in the Blackfeet Indians of Montana; and 26 percent in the people of Azmoos, Switzerland. All black populations had low prevalence, as did inhabitants of Oberholen, Germany. The Pima Indians of Arizona had an 11 percent incidence in women, whereas in men 20 percent were affected, a reversal of the normal sex distribution.

Factors influencing osteoarthritis prevalence in populations include heredity, occupation, and possibly diet and resultant body build. Comparison of populations living in different parts of the world indicates no correlation with latitude, longitude, or any type of climate. No significant differences are found among different groups in the prevalence of osteoarthritis.

Charles W. Denko

102. Osteoporosis

Osteoporosis is defined as a proportional decrease of both bone mineral and bone matrix, leading to fracture after minimal trauma. It differs from **osteomalacia**, which presents a normal amount of bone matrix (osteoid) but decreased mineralization. There are two clinical syndromes of osteoporosis. Type I (**postmenopausal osteoporosis**) occurs in women aged 51–75, involves primarily trabecular bone loss, and presents as **vertebral crush fracture** or **distal radius fracture**. Type II (**senile osteoporosis**) occurs in both men and women, particularly after age 60, involves trabecular and cortical bone loss, and commonly presents with **hip fracture** and **vertebral wedge fracture**. Postmenopausal osteoporosis is associated with decreased serum levels of parathyroid hormone and a secondary decrease in activation of vitamin D, whereas senile osteoporosis is associated with a primary decrease in activation of vitamin D and increased parathyroid hormone.

Characteristics

Osteoporosis is an enormous public-health problem, responsible for at least 1.2 million fractures annually in the United States. Fractures of the vertebral bodies and hip comprise the majority, and complications of hip fracture are fatal in 12–20 percent of cases. Nearly 30 percent require long-term nursing home care. The direct and indirect costs of osteoporosis in the United States are estimated in billions of dollars annually.

Age-related bone loss or **involutional osteoporosis** begins about age 40 in both sexes at an initial rate of about 0.5 percent per year. The bone loss increases with age until slowing very late in life. In women, accelerated postmenopausal loss of bone occurs at a rate of 2–3 percent per year for about 10 years. Over their lifetime, women lose about 35 percent of cortical bone and 50 percent of trabecular bone, whereas men lose about two-thirds of these amounts. The skeletal bone mass is comprised of 80 percent cortical and 20 percent trabecular bone. Trabecular or spongy bone has much higher turnover – nearly eight times that of cortical or compact bone.

The process of age-related osteoporosis is universal, although certain populations are affected to a greater degree or at an earlier age. Osteoporosis in the elderly is exceedingly common and involves multiple factors of age, sex, endocrine system, genetics, environment, nutrition, and physical activity. Age-related factors include decreased osteoblast function, decreased intestinal calcium absorption, decreased renal activation of vitamin D, and increased parathyroid hormone secretion combined with decreased clearance of the hormone by the kidney.

In women, decreased estrogen production in menopause accounts for 10–20 percent loss of total bone mass. Although men have no equivalent of menopause, gonadal function declines in many elderly men and contributes to osteoporosis. Multiple pregnancies and extended breastfeeding in premenopausal females may also produce negative calcium balance and subsequent bone loss. Underlying medical conditions or medications can contribute to osteoporosis, particularly **hyperthryoidism**, **hemiplegia** or paralysis, alcoholism, use of glucocorticoid steroids, and smoking.

Population and familial studies implicate both genetic and environmental factors in causing or inhibiting osteoporosis. Blacks, for example, tend to have greater initial bone mass or bone density than whites. Even with similar bone loss, osteoporosis begins at a later age in blacks. Among whites, women of British ancestry had a higher incidence of osteoporosis than those of other national origins.

Nutrition, particularly calcium intake, plays a role in inhibiting osteoporosis. Long-term trials of calcium supplementation, however, have had mixed results in postmenopausal women. Such supplementation may be more effective if initiated years before onset of menopause. A high-protein diet increases urinary excretion of calcium and may induce a negative calcium balance. Decreased renal activation of vitamin D with age may also be a factor in populations without vitamin D supplementation or with the elderly confined indoors.

Physical activity decreases the rate of bone loss in the elderly. Skeletal stresses from weight bearing and muscle contraction stimulate osteoblast function, and muscle mass and bone mass are directly related.

Osteoporosis was defined as a clinical entity in 1941. Since then, many studies have attempted to evaluate the varying rates of osteoporosis and osteoporosis-related fractures in different populations. The process of age-related and post-menopausal bone loss occurs in all populations. It appears to start earlier for women in Japan and India compared to women in Britain and the United States. It occurs later in Finnish women, and age-related rates of bone loss in women between 35 and 64 are lower in Jamaica and the four African countries studied than in other countries examined.

Relating the differing rates to calcium intake correlates well with populations in Japan, India, and Finland but not Jamaica or the African countries. Other factors such as genetically determined initial bone density or increased physical activity may also be involved. The rate of hip fracture varies according to the age distribution of osteoporosis in all countries. Incidence of hip fracture is higher in white populations in all geographic areas, compared to indigenous populations. For example, low incidence is noted among Maoris in New Zealand and the Bantu in South Africa compared to white populations in both areas. In the United States, over 90 percent of all hip fractures occur in individuals over 70. By age 90, a third of all women have sustained a hip fracture. Vertebral fractures occur in 25 percent of women over 70.

History

Age-related bone loss has been examined in prehistoric skeletal populations. Skeletons of hunting-and-gathering archaic Indians (c. 2500 B.C.) showed differential rates between females and males as well as overall rates of osteoporosis quite similar to those of a modern hospital population. A more recent Hopewell Indian population showed greater age-related bone loss, probably resulting from genetic or nutritional factors. Study of three ancient Nubian populations found that osteoporosis occurred earlier in life among these women as compared

to modern Western samples, perhaps secondary to inadequate calcium intake or extended lactation.

R. Ted Steinbock

103. Paget's Disease of Bone

Paget's disease of bone was described as **osteitis deformans**, a "chronic inflammation of bone" by Sir James Paget in 1876. His original description was masterful and thus has withstood the test of time. Paget's disease of bone describes an abnormal osseous (bony) structure whereby isolated and sometimes contiguous areas of the skeleton undergo changes leading to clinical deformity for some of those affected. Clinically affected people may have the appearance of enlarged bone, bowed extremities, shortened stature, and simian posturing because the body's usual system for maintaining strong and healthy bone malfunctions. Normal bone turnover is altered in the affected areas. The resorption process accelerates, and the repair process responds by building a heavy, thickened, and enlarged bone. Although the new bone contains normal or increased amounts of calcium, the material of the bone is disorganized, and the bone is structurally weak. The result may be pain, deformity, fracture, and **arthritis**.

Characteristics

The disease apparently has its greatest prevalence in Europe and the neo-Europes, such as Australia, New Zealand, and areas of South America. For no apparent reason, it is uncommon in African blacks, Orientals, and inhabitants of India and Scandinavia. Where studied, incidence ranges between 3.5 and 4.5 percent of the population in high prevalence regions, with a high of 8.3 percent in Lancashire, England, and a low of 0.4 percent in Sweden. In a U.S. survey, incidence was 3.9 percent among Caucasians residing in Brooklyn and 0.9 percent among Caucasians residing in

Atlanta. Similarly, another study revealed no Paget's disease in Lexington, Kentucky, and 1.1 percent Paget's disease in Providence, Rhode Island.

Males are more at risk than females by a 3:2 ratio. There is evidence of heritability: A survey, for example, revealed that 13.8 percent of Pagetic patients had relatives with Paget's disease. Approximately half were from successive generations and half from siblings. Familial cases had earlier onset than others. An autosomal dominant pattern was suggested.

The etiology remains unknown. Paget named the disease "osteitis deformans" believing that it was inflammatory and of infectious origin. Recent ultrastructural studies have revealed nuclear and cytoplasmic inclusions – found in no other skeletal disorders except **giant-cell tumor of bone**. Morphologically, the nuclei resemble ones infected with paramyxoviruses such as **parainfluenza, mumps**, and **measles**, and the cells resemble ones infected with **respiratory syncytial virus** (RSV). This finding suggests the possibility that Paget's disease is a slow virus infection of bone. Other such infections have similarly demonstrated long latent periods, a lack of acute inflammatory responses, a slowly progressive course, restriction to a single organ system, patchy distribution, and genetic predisposition.

Studies have demonstrated both measles and RSV antigens in Pagetic bone. The suggestion of different RNA viruses (measles is genus *Morbillivirus*; RSV is genus *Pneumovirus*) seems incompatible. It has been proposed that Paget's disease stems from a previously uncharacterized virus, perhaps a *Pneumovirus*. According to this hypothesis, Pagetic patients are infected at an early age, probably under 30. The slow virus isolates to particular skeletal areas, and as the metabolic activity of the skeleton decreases with age, the infested osteoclasts increase their metabolic activity, eventually producing diseased bone some decades after initial infection.

Estimates indicate that 80 percent of people with Paget's disease are asymptomatic. When symptomatic, findings may include any of the following: frontal bossing, scalp-vein dilatation, angioid streaks, simian posture, short stature, flexion contractures at hips and knees, anterior and lateral bowing of long bones, warmth of involved extremity, periosteal tenderness, and compressive neuropathy. Pagetic bone pain is uncommon, but when present it is aching, deep, and often aggravated by pressure or weight bearing.

The following deformities may develop: (1) The involved skull may become soft, thickened, and enlarged; (2) femora tend to migrate, deforming the softened pelvis; (3) enlargement of vertebrae alters the spine; and (4) affected long bones soften and bow from weight-bearing or from the force of surrounding muscles.

Pathological fractures can also occur. Low-back pain is the most common clinical presentation of Paget's disease and is often related to **secondary osteoarthritis. Sarcomatous degeneration**, although uncommon, occurs in 1 percent of Pagetic patients – a fortyfold greater risk than that of the general population.

History

Paget's disease is not a new disease, having been suspected in a Neanderthal skull. Although isolated reports in the mid-nineteenth century described it, the classical clinical description by Paget and a pathological description by Henry Butlin clarified the entity in 1876. Paget was a major figure in the medical community, having been knighted at 43. He is also credited with defining diseases such as **Paget's disease of the breast, rectum, and skin; carpal tunnel syndrome**; and **trichinosis**. Paget's disease of bone affects only adult humans; reports of it in animals are not convincing. A childhood osseous condition called **juvenile Paget's disease** appears to be a separate entity.

It is difficult to reconcile the geographic isolation of the disease to Europeans (exclusive of Scandinavians) and their descendants. Theories of a slow virus infection in susceptible individuals seem dubious, for theoretically the disease would then have a more widespread distribution. Temperature cannot be implicated, as high-prevalence areas include disparate climatic regions of Italy, Spain, Germany, and Russia. Similarly, occupation and physical activity seem unrelated, as the geographic areas involve all types of lifestyles. Interestingly, U.S. blacks apparently sustain a higher frequency of Paget's disease than might be expected. An explanation partly involves intermarriage with those of European ancestry.

Roy D. Altman

104. Paragonimiasis

Several species of the genus *Paragonimus*, the **lung flukes**, can parasitize humans. The most important, *Paragonimus westermani*, is found in China, Japan, Korea, Southeast Asia, New Guinea, and parts of India and Africa. It was first discovered in the lungs of tigers in European zoos in 1878. Other species occur in Asia, Africa, Central America, and South America. Wild and domestic members of the cat and dog families and other carnivorous animals are hosts, and in many places humans are accidental hosts of worms that normally reside in other mammals. Adult worms produce eggs in the lungs; these reach fresh water either in the sputum or by being coughed up, swallowed, and passed in the feces.

Motile larvae hatch, penetrate an appropriate snail, undergo two reproductive cycles, and emerge to seek their second intermediate host, a crab or crayfish. Here they penetrate between the joints of the crustacean's exoskeleton and encyst to await ingestion by humans or other definitive hosts. They then burrow through the intestinal wall and the diaphragm and enter the lungs, where they may survive for many years. Slow, chronic lung damage may become serious in heavy infestations. Lost migrating flukes sometimes wander widely and reach atypical (ectopic) sites like the brain, where they cause a variety of neurological symptoms and may prove fatal.

Treatment of the lung form of the disease is usually effective but may be prolonged. The disease can be prevented by avoidance of raw, poorly cooked, pickled, or marinated freshwater crabs and crayfish.

K. David Patterson

105. Parkinson's Disease (Parkinsonism)

Parkinson's disease, or **parkinsonism**, is a syndrome with four cardinal features: resting tremor, **bradykinesia** (physical and mental sluggishness), rigidity, and impaired postural reflexes. Diagnosis is based on finding any three of the four.

Characteristics

Parkinsonism occurs throughout the world; no population is protected. Most studies have investigated Caucasian populations of northern European or Anglo Saxon descent. Prevalence exhibits no geographic patterns and no clusters of increased incidence. Two studies seem to indicate a lower prevalence in blacks; this has been the clinical experience as well, probably indicating decreased risk for blacks. Annual incidence varies from 5 to 24 per 100,000 of the white population.

Parkinsonism usually occurs in late middle life or beyond. The mean age of onset is 58–62. Onset before 30 is rare, but a juvenile form also exists. The greatest incidence is in the 70–79 age group, with 1–2 cases per 1,000 annually. Later, incidence of parkinsonism seems to decline, a finding that – if true – suggests the disease is not simply a result of an aging nervous system. No apparent difference prevails between the sexes in regard to risk. Parkinsonism was known before 1817, when James Parkinson published his famous manuscript, but prevalence studies have been possible only since the 1960s; they indicate no substantial change in incidence.

In 1917, an **encephalitis lethargica** epidemic started in Vienna and spread throughout the world. Following this illness, about half the victims developed parkinsonism with tremor, bradykinesia, and rigidity, often associated with **oculogyric crises, parkinsonian crises** (sudden episodic worsening of symptoms), behavioral abnormalities, **cranial nerve palsies**, and a host of other central nervous system abnormalities. The age of onset of **postencephalitic parkinsonism** is early compared to other types of Parkinson's disease.

Parkinsonism mortality varies from 0.5 to 3.8 per 100,000 population, and duration averages about 10 years depending on age of onset, rate of progression, the patient's general health, and treatment. Treatment with levodopa increases the quality of life, decreases symptoms, and reduces excess mortality. Genetic studies have failed to show significant familial risks of parkinsonism, and analysis of monozygotic twins indicates a lack of concordance for the disease.

Symptoms of parkinsonism are caused by decreased striatal dopamine from loss of dopaminergic neurons in the substantia nigra of the midbrain. Environmental agents are the primary known cause of parkinsonism: exposure to manganese, carbon disulfide, carbon monoxide, and other substances can produce the disorder. Drugs that interfere with dopaminergic pathways or receptors can also produce the syndrome, and the same may be true of multiple head traumas.

History

Tremor was mentioned in the writings of Hippocrates, Celsus, and Galen, but the real history of parkinsonism started in 1817 with publication of Parkinson's essay on what he called the "shaking palsy." He provided a Latin name as well: **paralysis agitans**. He reported on six patients. The first was personally observed; two others were noticed casually in the street; case 4 had an abscess on the chest wall but was lost to followup; case 5 was evidently seen at a distance, and no details of that patient are available; case 6 was a 72-year-old man who was visually inspected but evidently not examined.

By modern standards, Parkinson's essay was scientifically slipshod. The information he conveyed was drawn from visual inspection, not examination. However, his paper was well received, and subsequent clinicians have added to his description.

In 1859, Armand Trousseau lectured on parkinsonism, discussing rigidity and bradykinesia. The great French neurologist Jean Charcot considered parkinsonism a **neurosis** because no causative central nervous system lesion could be identified, and the condition worsened with stress or emotion. Charcot frequently commented that everything possible was employed to treat parkinsonism but with little effect. He recommended belladonna alkaloids, especially hyoscyamine, now called scopolamine. Modern biochemical understanding of parkinsonism indicates that this agent should partially improve the symptoms.

In 1893, Paul Blocq reported a case of **hemiparkinsonism**. Autopsy revealed a lesion in the inferior peduncle with complete destruction of the substantia nigra. This suggested that the neuroanatomic substrate of parkinsonism was the substantia nigra and probably is the first description of a lesion producing parkinsonism. Many other descriptions merely added to the fundamental and original observations of Parkinson.

The road to effective therapy was paved in the 1960s by A. Carlsson, who showed that bradykinesia could be reversed by administration of L-dopa, a dopamine precursor. Further studies reported a marked decrease in dopamine in parkinsonism patients. Small doses of L-dopa were tried, both orally and intravenously, with possible temporary benefits. Other studies, however, failed to confirm any major effect until George Cotzias and colleagues showed that much larger oral doses of L-dopa resulted in dramatic improvement in many patients – so dramatic that the efficacy of levodopa treatment was established beyond doubt, and a new era in the management of parkinsonism began.

Bernard M. Patten

106. Pellagra

Pellagra is a nutritional disease principally caused by dietary deficiency of niacin, a B complex vitamin. The disease is usually associated with deficiencies of other B vitamins and nearly always with poverty and diets based on maize. Pellagra is characterized by **dermatitis**, **diarrhea**, and **dementia** and is nicknamed the "disease of 3 Ds." If untreated, a fourth "D" – death – may ensue. In the past, mortality sometimes reached 70 percent, but as knowledge about the disease increased, mortality rates were substantially reduced.

During the early twentieth century, the U.S. Public Health Service, working in the South, linked pellagra to the inadequate "3-M" (meat, meal, and molasses) diet of the region's poor. Cornmeal bread constituted the bulk of dietary intake, although occasionally flavored with "meat" (usually only fat back) and molasses (cane syrup). Widespread pellagra was found among agricultural laborers, mill workers, and institutionalized individuals. The diet of pellagrins was always both monotonous and cheap, and systematic analysis of diet in relation to income showed that pellagra appeared wherever income was marginal and variety in diet was limited.

Even the realization that pellagra was a **dietary deficiency disease** – and the discovery of niacin as the pellagra-preventive (or "P-P") factor – failed to explain everything about pellagra. For example, why does milk (a poor source of niacin) prevent pellagra? Why does a diet based on corn (with more niacin than milk) cause pellagra? The first question was answered by the discovery that the liver converts tryptophan, of which milk is a rich source, into niacin. The answer to the second question lies in the chemical form of niacin contained in maize.

Niacin is found in many foods, but its presence does not mean that it is available to the body. It may appear in a chemically "free" form (ready to be absorbed) or in a biologically unavailable "bound" form. In maize, niacin is chemically bound and is released only after the grain is treated with an alkali. In Central America, pellagra has seldom been a problem – even though corn is the dietary staple – because the grain is soaked in lime and heated before being baked, thus releasing the niacin content.

Pellagra usually appears in winter or spring and seems to disappear a few months later, only to recur the following year. In the early stages, patients feel weak, lose appetite, and cannot sleep. Dermatitis is the classic symptom of pellagra. Reddened skin (sometimes confused with sunburn) is an early sign. Symmetrical lesions appear on the hands, arms, feet, ankles, neck, and face. Later the skin crusts and peels. Lesions usually (but not always) occur on parts of the body exposed to the sun and in acute cases may blister and rupture.

Pellagra also affects the gastrointestinal tract. Symptoms include nausea, excessive salivation, a reddened tongue, and burning sensations. Diarrhea, sometimes intense, is characteristic.

Particularly distressing are neurological symptoms, including insomnia, apprehension, and peripheral **neuritis**. Mental aberrations are varied. Some patients suffer only mild depression, confusion, or memory loss. Others manifest severe psychotic changes. Some are suicidal. All these symptoms are caused by biochemical changes still imperfectly understood. Electrical rhythms of the brain also change, even if mental symptoms are not present. These changes may be related to altered metabolism of serotonin (synthesized from tryptophan), a substance that modulates behavior.

History

Pellagra has always been associated with maize, the staple food of American Indians. Carried to Europe by Christopher Columbus, maize was at first of interest chiefly to herbalists, and one of these, in the middle of the seventeenth century, observed that the grain might have a deleterious effect if consumed in quantity. Despite this caveat, the advantages (ease of cultivation and prolific yields) of maize ensured its spread beyond the botanical garden and into the field. By the end of the eighteenth century, maize was widely grown in Italy and spreading into Yugoslavia, France, Austria, and Hungary.

Pellagra was first identified by Gaspar Casal, a royal physician of Spain. In 1735 in the town of Oviedo in Asturias, he first noticed a skin disease that the peasants called *mal de la rosa.* He described the disease and noted that its victims lived primarily on maize. Casal emphasized that the "rose" could be treated by consuming milk or cheese, foods seldom seen by the poor. French physician François Thièry read Casal's manuscript and wrote a brief description of the disease for a French journal, published in 1755, although Casal's own work was not published until 1762. Within 10 years, the disease was noted in Italy and named "pellagra" ("rough" or "dry skin") by Francesco Frapolli.

By the nineteenth century, pellagra was rampant in northern Italy. An estimated 5 percent of the population of Lombardy was affected, and 20 percent in the worst areas. In Milan in 1817, 66 percent of inmates in a mental institution were pellagrins.

French physician Théophile Roussel, visiting Spain in the 1840s, determined that pellagra was endemic but often misdiagnosed. The French benefited from the work of Roussel, who strongly believed that pellagra was caused by eating maize. He encouraged improvement of diets and the living conditions of peasants. He wrote two books on pellagra, the second appearing in 1866, stating that the problem would be solved not by scientific discovery but through social progress. His arguments were sufficiently persuasive that the French government decreased maize cultivation for food and encouraged animal husbandry. By the twentieth century, pellagra had virtually disappeared from France.

Few people wanted to believe that pellagra was caused by economic conditions, but many associated it with maize. Italian physician Giovanni Marzari suggested that the grain molded in storage. He also believed that corn lacked a nutritive element. For years,

researchers searched for a toxin. Lodovico Balardini thought he had found it in certain corn-grown molds, and Cesare Lombroso spent a quarter of a century studying these. The spoiled-corn theory was advanced when pellagra broke out in Yucatan in 1882 and later; crop failures meant corn had to be imported from New York. The grain spoiled en route, but the poorer classes ate it anyway, and pellagra followed. Not everyone was convinced that corn caused pellagra. Some thought that heredity, bad air, or an unseen organism was responsible. But when governments were persuaded to curtail maize consumption, as in France, success was possible.

For a century and a half after pellagra was first described, the magnitude of the problem outside Europe was not appreciated. Not until the 1890s, with reports by British epidemiologist Fleming Sandwith, was anything written about pellagra in English. In Egypt, Sandwith found many patients with pellagra. He noted the disease as "country-bred" and associated it with a maize diet. Later, during the Boer War, he found pellagra among poor Bantus living on maize in South Africa.

In the United States, pellagra suddenly drew attention in 1907 as an epidemic ravaged an Alabama hospital with 64 percent mortality. In succeeding months, thousands of cases were identified. Some researchers thought the cause might have an insect vector, like the recently discovered vectors of **malaria, yellow fever**, and **Rocky Mountain spotted fever**. Others blamed foodstuffs other than corn, notably cane sugar and cottonseed oil.

The U.S. Public Health Service began work on pellagra soon after the first Alabama cases were diagnosed, but not until 1914 was real progress made: Joseph Goldberger identified the cause of the disease as a dietary deficiency of some essential substance. He introduced a new diet into selected institutions to see if the disease would disappear. Succeeding in that experiment, he then induced pellagra with a poor diet in a population of volunteer prisoners. Goldberger next attempted to infect several colleagues, including himself. Neither he nor anyone else got pellagra, which strongly indicated that the cause was not a contagious infection.

Goldberger also studied the relationship of pellagra to economics. He noted that rural victims were sharecroppers and laborers caught in a cycle of poverty tied to one-crop agriculture. Few grew foodstuffs or kept a cow, and diet was restricted to the inadequate but affordable "3-M" items mentioned previously. Most were chronically in debt. Millworkers suffered similar poverty. In South Carolina mill villages, Goldberger demonstrated that poverty begets disease. His multiyear epidemiological study conclusively proved that pellagrins were sick because they were poor. The study itself became a model in epidemiology.

In the 1920s, Goldberger began to search for the specific element missing in the pellagrin's diet. Almost accidentally, his team found a rich source of the unknown P-P factor. They added yeast to the daily ration of their experimental animals, and the results were magical. Four days after a pellagrous dog was given yeast, its condition had markedly improved. Distribution of yeast became a standard feature of emergency and economic aid to people. Goldberger was studying liver extracts at the time of his death in 1929, and it was from yeast and liver (another effective pellagra preventive) that the missing dietary element was finally isolated.

After Goldberger's death, the next breakthrough in conquering pellagra occurred in 1937, when Conrad A. Elvehjem isolated nicotinic acid (later named niacin). It was found to be the pellagra-preventive factor, and subsequently Tom Spies used nicotinic acid to treat pellagra patients with considerable success at various hospitals. Commenting on the work of Elvehjem, Spies, and others, the New York Times noted that "an ailment which has baffled medicine for centuries has at last been relegated to the curable diseases."

The disappearance of pellagra from large areas of the world is due as much to social factors as to medical advances. In the U.S. South and elsewhere, enrichment of staples with vitamins has certainly helped to eliminate the disease, but so has burgeoning prosperity. The example of France in the nineteenth century showed that government encouragement of varied agriculture resulted in important benefits. Pellagra was brought under control in Italy by the 1930s, probably because of a rising standard of living. At the end of the twentieth century, the disease appeared in only isolated pockets in Egypt, Lesotho, and India.

Elizabeth W. Etheridge

107. Periodontal Disease (Pyorrhea)

The word **pyorrhea** comes from the Greek *pyon* ("pus") and *rhoia* ("to flow"), a graphic description of the disease in which an outflowing of pus proceeds from the gingival (gum) tissues of the oral cavity. The term "pyorrhea" has been used in Europe since the mid-1500s and in America since the late 1800s. In 1937, however, the term was abandoned in favor of **periodontal disease**.

Periodontal disease means any ailment of the supporting structures of the teeth, including gingiva, periodontal ligament, and alveolar bone. In simplest terms, periodontal disease can be divided into two distinct, but not mutually exclusive, disease processes. The first involves inflammation of gingival tissues, called **gingivitis**, and the second, a destructive loss of bone and connective tissue attachment termed **periodontitis**.

Characteristics
Epidemiological research during the past 25 years indicates that periodontal disease is one of the most common diseases affecting humankind. There is a direct cause-and-effect relationship between the bacterial colonization on the surface of the tooth and the inflammation (and often consequential destruction) of the tooth's supporting structures. The rate of destruction varies and depends on the individual's response to the bacterial irritation.

Periodontal disease is a widespread chronic disease and remains the primary reason for teeth loss in the adult population throughout the world. In fact, virtually all individuals in any population exhibit manifestations of the disease. The prevalence and severity of periodontal disease increase with advancing age, tend to be greater in nonwhites than whites, and are greater for males in both groups. There appears to be an increasing trend in the prevalence and severity of periodontal disease in the over-35 age group. This increase is most pronounced in lower socioeconomic groups and is highly correlated with differing levels of personal and professional oral hygiene.

Many individuals in the older population have had fewer teeth extracted as a consequence of lower **caries** ("cavities") incidence, which results from fluoride use, improvements in dental care, and better public-health education. Paradoxically, this increase in the retention rate of teeth in the aging population provides an increase in the number of teeth at risk of periodontitis. The only improvement noted since the 1970s has been a slight reduction in the incidence and severity of gingivitis among the under-35 age group.

Numerous studies have firmly established the primary etiologic agent in periodontal disease as **plaque**. Plaque is a colorless, soft, sticky film of bacteria that constantly forms on the teeth. Plaque is composed primarily of different and numerous types of microorganisms as well as adherent mucin (a protein and polysaccharide combination), foodstuffs, and cellular debris. One gram of dental plaque contains more than 10^{11} bacteria. Plaque can calcify to form a local tissue irritant – **calculus** ("tartar") – to which new colonies of plaque can readily adhere. The microbial population of plaque is variable and is determined by its location on the tooth surface, the intraoral environment at the time of the plaque formation, and the length of time the colony has been present in the mouth. When plaque is removed, a new plaque may form, having different characteristics in its quantity, quality, and spatial arrangement. The

microorganisms in plaque produce metabolic products and cellular constituents that affect underlying periodontal tissues. These include exotoxins, endotoxins, antigens, and enzymes.

Any microbial plaque within the gingival crevice causes at least gingivitis. In some areas of the mouth, plaque and gingivitis lead to a destructive periodontitis. Periodontal disease is not caused by the intraoral invasion of foreign pathogens, but rather by colonization of microorganisms of the normal oral flora that exists even in the absence of disease. Certain species of this bacterial plaque play a more significant part in the development and progress of disease because they increase in relative proportions as well as in absolute numbers. These species are also relevant in that their virulent mechanisms act to disrupt the host's defenses.

Inadequate or improper oral hygiene techniques must be considered one of the etiologic factors in the development of periodontal disease. Other causative influences include food impaction between teeth, defective dental restorations, malposed teeth, physiological gingival stress due to high frenum attachment, effects of dry mouth, and, to a minor extent, heredity. Of course, there is a strong relationship between all of the etiologic factors and the host's resistance. The capacity to resist or repair depends on many factors such as adequate nutrition and assimilation, antibody production, hormonal influences, white cell defenses, and formative cell capabilities.

The pathogenesis of periodontal disease must be considered in four stages: colonization, invasion, destruction, and healing. During colonization, plaque accumulates on the teeth and microbial growth ensues. If the plaque is not removed through adequate oral hygiene, the formation of calculus may begin, and the early stages of microbial invasion into the adjacent gingival tissues commence. Clinical signs may consist of gingival tissues that are tender, swollen, and red. This tissue may bleed upon probing or during brushing. However, periodontal disease usually progresses over the course of many years, and discomfort is a rarity. It is because of this asymptomatic evolution that persistent bacterial invasion and local irritation can progress into the destructive phase of the disease in which loss of connective tissue and loss of alveolar bone take place. Signs and symptoms of the destructive stage can include pocketing around the tooth within the gingival crevice, gingival recession, suppurative exudate (pus) from the gingiva, and looseness or separation of the permanent teeth.

The healing phase is the least understood of the four stages of the disease. However, studies reveal that periodontal disease is episodic, and undergoes periods of remission and exacerbation. Although colonization, invasion, and destruction are interrelated and overlapping, this fourth stage, healing, is clearly distinct in that it is characterized by reduction of inflammation, repair of gingival tissues, and **sclerosis** and remodeling of the alveolar bone.

History

Although periodontology began being practiced as a specialty only during the twentieth century, the recognition of periodontal disease in various forms has persisted for millennia. The dental structures of teeth and bone of our ancestors have been revealed through examination of skulls discovered in archaeological excavations, evidencing that periodontal disease existed in some of the earliest members of humankind.

Egyptian mummies show signs of dental caries and periodontal disease as well as primitive, yet valiant, attempts at repairing these dental pathoses. Indeed, it is believed that the *Ebers Papyrus*, written around 1550 B.C. by Egyptians, contains the earliest written record of dentistry as a distinctive branch of the healing arts. The Greek historian Herodotus described Egypt as being the home of medical specialties, including dentistry.

About 1300 B.C., Aesculapius, the mythical physician, supposedly recognized the importance of dental hygiene by recommending cleaning of the mouth and teeth. The physician to the king of Babylon, Arad-Nana, in the sixth century B.C. suggested removing "film" and "deposits" from the teeth with a cloth-covered index finger. More aggressive periodontal therapy appeared when first century A.D. Roman physician Celsus treated gums and loose teeth with gold wire and seared the gingiva with red-hot iron. Oral hygiene techniques can also be traced to the Mayan culture and others in Central America between 200 B.C. and 800 A.D.

Roman writer Pliny in the first century A.D. described the prevalence of periodontal disease among the Romans as well as various remedies for its prevention and care. The most notable prescriptions were dentifrices, mouthwashes, and toothpicks. The first mention of "toothbrushing" seems to have been by Roman poet Ovid in the same century. The *siwak*, a fibrous wood product that preceded the toothbrush, was used by the Arabians since the ninth century and is still in use in some areas today. The modern toothbrush, however, was invented in China only in 1498.

In 1530, Zene Artzney wrote about dental therapeutics, discussing the formation and prevention of calculus. In 1575, Ambroise Paré coined the term **pyorrhea alveolaris** and described the attachment of teeth to the jaw by their roots.

Pierre Fauchard, the founder of modern dentistry, in 1728 suggested that teeth and gums might suffer from the same diseases. In 1820, Eleazar Parmly recommended that all deposits on teeth be removed. He later became known as the "apostle of dental hygiene." In the latter half of the nineteenth century, John Riggs, who was to become the "father of periodontology," described periodontal disease as a "progressive process from marginal gingivitis to the final exfoliation of the teeth." He developed preventive as well as surgical treatments for what he called "scurvy of the gums." For decades, any such condition was called **Riggs' disease**.

Our understanding of periodontal disease, including its etiology and pathogenesis, grew enormously during the 1900s. Periodontal disease is currently under attack on several fronts, through preventive care, improvements in oral hygiene techniques, mechanical and chemical plaque inhibitors, nutrition, surgical interven-tion, drugs, and immunology. Much work, how-ever, remains ahead, especially in the relation-ship of the disease to the host's immune system.

Jeffrey Levin

108. Pica

Pica usually means a pathological craving for nonfoods, although it can mean a craving for foodstuffs as well. Although pica is not a dis-ease, it is often a symptom of disease and is frequently associated with nutritional deficien-cies – especially of minerals. In addition, psychi-atry and psychology find that pica is often con-nected with mental problems. Anthropologists study it as a cultural phenomenon, as it has been associated with some religions and also perhaps because the use of nonfoods is indicative of food shortages in the distant past.

The word "pica" comes from the Latin for "magpie," a bird that eats practically anything. Ambroise Paré first employed the term in the 1500s, although references to the practice can be found in many ancient and medieval writ-ings. In 1638, M. Boezo distinguished between pica, an appetite for "absurd things," and **mala-cia**, a voracious desire for normal foods.

Probably the type of pica that has received the most scrutiny is the consumption of earth, called **geophagy** ("dirt eating"). Unlike other types of pica, geophagy has occurred on nearly all continents, and at nearly all times. Through-out history, various humans have consumed dirt, clay, mud, chalk, and other earths for nu-tritional, cultural, and psychological reasons.

Another form of pica – although that is de-batable – is **papophagia** (ice eating). Chewing or sucking ice is sometimes recommended as a method of appetite control, or as a smoking substitute.

Amylophagia means consumption of laun-dry starch and is almost exclusively associ-ated with women. It was first observed in the American South and may have originated as clay consumption, with its practitioners later switching to starch. Although the flavors of clay and starch are different, the texture is similar. Research indicates that pregnant women eat starch because it relieves nausea, vomiting, and morning sickness.

Trichophagia is the ingestion of hair and is al-most always associated with young females who habitually chew their long hair. Trichophagia is closely related to other "mouthing" behaviors. Over time, ingested hair can form "hairballs" in the stomach, causing gastrointestinal problems.

Other harmful forms of pica include **lithophagia** (eating rocks or pebbles). Indeed, many picas are dangerous; consumption of paint chips by children, for example, can result in **lead poisoning**.

Pica has been closely associated with women and pregnancy since classical times. It was long believed that pregnancy caused mental insta-bility, provoking the mother's craving for both foods and nonfoods. Recent studies, however, indicate that changes in taste are not a constant in pregnancy, despite a desire for sharp-flavored foods.

Most medical investigations of pica are con-cerned with children. The practice is usually as-sociated with those in poverty, especially black children in rural areas and urban slums. Re-ports conflict as to whether pica in this group is nutritionally motivated. No difference in preva-lence has been found between males and fe-males. However, during adolescence, girls are more likely than boys to begin or continue the practice.

Babies put many things in their mouths. The ingestion of nonfood substances may begin at 6 months of age, but declines with a devel-opmental increase in hand/mouth activity and drops sharply after 3 years of age. After that age, the possibility of mental disturbance is often explored.

Pica is usually described as rare among adult males, although some claim that it is merely un-derreported. The most common picalike prac-tice among men – chewing tobacco – is not gen-erally viewed as pica.

Causes of pica are unclear and have been the subject of medical speculation since antiquity. Most modern physicians view pica chiefly as a means of alleviating nutritional deficiency. Similarly, past scholars stressed good nutrition and recommended fresh fruits and vegetables as a remedy. However, no definite connection has been established between pica and dietary imbalance. Nutrients in which pica practitioners may be deficient include vitamins C and D, phosphorus, calcium, zinc, and especially iron. Investigation into the relationship between **iron deficiency** and pica continues today.

Mental specialists suggest that nutritional deficiencies and psychological disorders are linked in pica patients. A 1971 study of 90 children demonstrated that those who practiced pica after infancy generally were slower to develop than the others. Other studies have found that black children are more likely than white children to exhibit pica, which has been linked to lower income levels rather than to any racial cause. Numerous studies indicate that the pattern of pica in youngsters is very close to that of addiction. Often, pica seems an emotional or psychological defense mechanism. Most children who practice pica exhibit other oral activities, such as thumbsucking or nailbiting.

There is also a "cultural" etiology for pica. Anthropologists have long sought to explain why certain cultures require consumption of nonfood items. Symbolic geophagy was practiced in ancient times in Europe, the Middle East, and even among early Christians. In parts of Africa, belief holds that clay eating promotes female fertility and lactation. Pregnant women in Nigeria consume clay as "loaves" purchased in the marketplace, gaining needed calcium and magnesium.

A last reason for pica is pharmacological. Individuals engaged in pica may be attempting to medicate themselves for real or imagined illness. Physiological causes of pica might include gastrointestinal malaise, stress, hunger, parasitic infestations, and **toxicosis**.

History

Pica was well known to the ancients. Aristotle discussed earth eating, and as early as 40 B.C. in Greece, the sacred "sealed earth" was used as a "cure-all." Clays from Samos, Chios, and Selinos were said to be especially effective. Galen transported 20,000 clay lozenges from Lemnos to Rome to treat victims of poisoning. Pliny described how residents of Campania mixed chalk with their porridge, adding color and texture. He also noted a region in northern Africa, where a similar porridge was made with gypsum mixed in.

Many early researchers concentrated on the pica habits of pregnant women. In the sixth century, Aetius of Amida claimed that the urge to consume nonfoods was caused by suppression of menstrual flow. He recommended exercise and fresh fruits and vegetables. Avicenna described pica (although not by that name) and employed various iron preparations in treatment, among them iron dross steeped in fine wine and strained through a plant known as "Hippocrates'-sleeve." Avicenna believed that pica in pregnant women was treatable, but if the children of that pregnancy began practicing pica, they could not be cured of it. This disorder must have been fairly widespread, because Avicenna wrote of the need to control it in young boys, recommending imprisonment if necessary. Pregnant women, however, were to be treated more gently, for fear of damaging their infants.

Medical writers of medieval Europe tended to view mental instability and food as important causes of pica. J. Ledelius, for example, stated that leftover food in the stomach rotted, emitting humors that ruined an individual's sense of taste and caused cravings for odd substances. H. Betten, by contrast, argued that the cause of pica was not foul humors in the stomach but weakness of the mind. He concluded that this was why women exhibited pica more often than men. He recommended that nonpregnant women receive stern lectures to strengthen their will and prescriptions to strengthen their stomachs.

Famine was often a cause of pica, as in China, where starving people consumed varicolored clays instead of rice. Usually, grass, foliage, weeds, and tree bark became famine food, but in truly desperate times, such as the 1640 famine in Hunan, people ate not only clay but also shoes, leather, and wood. Similarly, in Europe during the Thirty Years' War, with armies plundering village and countryside, the peasants of Pomerania baked bread of dough mixed with powdered earth. The practice was repeated in Germany during the War of the Austrian Succession, not only in peasant villages but also in the castle of Wittenberg.

As Europeans explored Africa, Asia, and the Americas, they discovered that pica existed on almost every continent of the globe. The Otomac Indians, living along the Orinoco River in South America, were particularly fond of an iron-rich clay in the neighborhood. Pica was also observed among natives of Peru, where powdered lime mixed with coca leaves was sold in the marketplaces. The Indians of the Rio de la Hacha, however, preferred to consume lime without additives, usually carrying it about in small boxes.

In Central Africa, David Livingstone reported that some tribes were clay eaters. Africans called the practice *safura*; it was most prevalent among pregnant women but was also practiced by males. Availability of food seemed unrelated to the prevalence of clay consumption.

The literature of India indicates that geophagy was practiced in ancient times, yet no early European accounts mention it. By the end of the nineteenth century, however, British colonial physicians believed that earth eating was universal in India. At the beginning of the twentieth century, a native-born Indian physician thought it was a racial characteristic. He wrote that although clay eating was practiced in many areas of the world, the Aryan and Dravidian races were unique in using clay for food on a regular basis, whereas other races ate it only occasionally for sustenance, or for pharmacological reasons.

Plantation managers in all slaveholding areas of the New World were concerned about pica because slaves who consumed earth appeared to become addicted to it, and the addiction was thought to be fatal. Planters referred to pica as a disease, calling it *mal d'estomac, cachexia Africana*, or "stomach evil." Contemporary authors described the practice as widespread in the West Indies. The dirt eaters usually became sick, with stomach pains and difficult breathing, often followed by nausea, **diarrhea**, depression, and listlessness. Death followed within months. Slaveholders tried every means at their disposal to break the habit but were generally unsuccessful.

In 1843, physician John Imray in Dominica wrote that pica became much rarer in the West Indies after emancipation. He noted that slaves had been expected to feed themselves from their provision grounds, but had been overworked by the planters; thus, they had little energy left for their own crops. In desperation, they turned to earth eating. Freedom gave them more time to grow their food.

Iron deficiency and earth eating, associated since ancient times, remain so today. Over time, physicians have increasingly believed that **anemia** causes geophagy. Moreover, during the twentieth century, pica in its various forms was more systematically studied than previously, leading to a greater appreciation of its mysteries – and its dangers.

In 1924, it was suggested that lead poisoning arose from pica, specifically the consumption of paint chips by children. In the early 1940s, the U.S. government limited lead content in paints and plasters. Unfortunately, pica continued to be a major cause of lead poisoning in children. In New York City alone, there were about 52 reported cases every year, with mortality ranging from 13 to 27 percent.

In the late 1940s and early 1950s, the practice of clay eating in the United States was examined in articles by a number of physicians and nutritionists. A 1942 survey of black children in rural Mississippi found that of 209 children, 25 percent of the girls and 26 percent of the boys had eaten either dirt or clay in the previous 2 weeks. In 1947, the practice was observed among pregnant black women in North Carolina. There were no reports of clay eating by males, and it was concluded that the practice was related to gender. The same year, another study examined the types of clays consumed and among them identified soot from stovepipes. (Subjects did not eat the soot directly but placed it in bags that were subsequently soaked in water, making a sort of tea.)

In the 1950s, questionnaires to 47 health agencies and 91 individual health workers in the southeastern United States revealed that superstition and oral tradition played a large role in the selection of pica materials. A subsequent study discovered that women who ate clay and cornstarch had diets that were otherwise low in calories, calcium, iron, thiamine, and niacin. In 1957, a book-length study appeared, which included the history of pica and its association with mental and physical illness and nutrition. It argued that pica becomes established in children because they lack an understanding of dietary taboos. Poor nutrition leads them to practice pica with any number of substances. Another major work appeared the following year, which focused on the geography of the disorder, scrutinizing geophagy in Indonesia and Oceania as well as among blacks in Africa and America.

Throughout the twentieth century, most studies assumed that nutritional deficiency leads to pica. Although iron deficiency is assumed to be the major cause, other elements, especially zinc, have also been investigated. Yet, despite the fact that **iron-deficiency anemia** and pica have been associated for centuries, the question of whether pica is a cause or an effect of the anemia is still debated. Moreover, although both children and pregnant women practice pica, there is no clear understanding of the mechanisms causing the behavior. Pica has been recognized by physicians since the beginning of history, but medicine has yet to understand its causes.

Brian T. Higgins

109. Pinta

Pinta (meaning "spotted") is also called *mal de pinto* and *carate*. It is the least destructive of the human **treponematoses**. Although the taxonomy of the treponemes is by no means resolved, pinta is sufficiently distinctive to argue for a separate causal species, *Treponema carateum*. As a specific treponemal variety, it was not described until 1938. The disease is chronic, predominantly affects the skin, and is now found only among isolated rural groups in Central and South America and Mexico, where it is endemic. Local names for the illness are *tina, empeines*, and *vitiligo*.

Characteristics
According to one historian, pinta may have had a considerable world distribution at the end of the Paleolithic period, some 10,000 years ago. However, its past geographic distribution is in some doubt, and an alternative view suggests that it evolved purely in Amerindian communities of the New World as a final microevolution in the treponematoses there. It is not greatly destructive and remains untreated in many Latin Americans. As many as a million individuals may have the disease.

Pinta is caused by *T. carateum*, which cannot be distinguished from *Treponema pallidum* (the causative agent of **endemic syphilis** and **venereal syphilis**). These treponemes are found mainly in the lower Malpighian layers of the epidermis and may be present for years before the skin lesions eventually become inactive and depigmented. Large areas may be infected, and the disease may remain infectious for a long period. It is unusual for other areas of the body, such as the genitals, to be involved. In contrast to the other human treponematoses, the skeleton is never affected.

This chronic clinical condition usually begins in childhood and lasts into adulthood, if not for most of the infected individual's lifetime. Social and hygienic factors result in differential incidence of the disease in varying components of Latin American societies, with native Indians, mestizos, and blacks being most affected. Infection seems most likely to be by skin contact. Insect vectors have also been suggested as a means of transmission, but this has not been substantiated. Serologic reactions are positive early, then increase in degree. Experiments show that there is cross-immunity to a varying extent in individuals infected with *T. carateum, T. pallidum,* and *Treponema pertenue.*

There is no chancre. The condition begins as an extragenital papule, usually situated in the lower extremity (and perhaps associated with damage to the skin surface). Within 3 weeks, the papule has expanded into a reactive patch of circinate form, termed a pintid. In the next few months, a more general rash occurs on the face and limbs, which can be similar in appearance to diseases such as **psoriasis, ringworm,** and **eczema**.

Histologically, **hyperkeratosis** and intercellular **edema** are evident, with an increase of lymphocytes and plasma cells. In adults, there are usually pigmentary changes in the later stages. Bluish patches are perhaps most characteristic, but lesions may be white. Pigmentary function is clearly disturbed, and in the white patches pigment is absent. It should be emphasized that other treponematoses can start out to some extent like pinta, but the others progress beyond purely skin changes. The disease is not transmitted to the fetus.

History

Pinta is believed to be most prevalent in Mexico, Venezuela, Colombia, Peru, and Ecuador. It is an "old" disease in the Americas, clearly present before the arrival of Europeans. Although relatively mild, it has tended historically to evoke a variety of social responses. In some instances the *pintados* or "spotted ones" have been shunned, much like lepers in the Old World. Yet in other circumstances their distinctive appearance brought them high status. For example, Montezuma, the Aztec emperor, selected such individuals to bear his litter, and they were apparently frequently formed into special elite battalions in Mexican history.

It appears, however, that the earliest recognizable description of pinta as a separate disease was not recorded until 1757 in Mexico. Because of the possible similarities to **leprosy** in regard to skin changes, it is not so surprising that a medical commission in 1811 reported on it as leprosy. In 1889, pinta was viewed as perhaps linked to syphilis and was thought to be transmitted by venereal contact. Indeed, this hypothesis seemed to support accounts that reported the efficacy of mercury in the treatment of pinta and the fact that infected individuals who worked in mercury mines felt better. The positive Wassermann reaction was demonstrated in 1925, but the true nature of this distinctive treponemal condition was not recognized until 1938.

Don R. Brothwell

110. Plague of Athens

The Greek historian Thucydides interrupts his history of the Peloponnesian War between Athens and Sparta to describe a virulent epidemic in 430 B.C. Expanding rapidly in early summer, it was far more lethal than other epidemics Thucydides had known, and he claimed that the novelty of the disease left Greek physicians powerless to deal with it. The epidemic was said to have begun in Africa, south of Ethiopia, spreading first to Egypt and Libya, then Persia, then Greece.

Characteristics

The stricken initially complained of "violent heat in the head," **coryza**, swollen and inflamed eyes, throat, and tongue, proceeding to violent coughing. Then the victims usually began to vomit, the disease bringing on "all the vomits of bile to which physicians have ever given names." Death claimed many of the sufferers in 7–9 days, a merciful end to wrenching convulsions, intense internal heat, and extreme thirst. Thucydides described an **exanthem** characterizing many cases: The skin, not hot to the touch, took on a livid color, inclining to red, and breaking out in pustules and ulcers. However, he did not offer clear comment about the distribution of the rash, thus permitting much disagreement in the literature.

Causing almost equal difficulty for medical observers today is Thucydides' description of the behavior of sufferers, hurling themselves into wells and cisterns in order to assuage the "inner heat" and satisfy their thirst. Thucydides does not identify any age group, sex, or socioeconomic category among those most at risk, rather emphasizing that the previously healthy were as likely to suffer and die as those previously debilitated by illness. He claims that 1,050 of 4,000 adult male soldiers perished in the epidemic – a high mortality rate even if all were afflicted. Pericles, the great orator and leader of Athens, apparently perished from the sickness, but Thucydides and Socrates did not. Thucydides assumes that the disease was contagious, and no one has questioned that assumption.

The epidemic lingered for 4 years in southern Greece, killing up to 25 percent of the population (if one accepts the highest mortality estimates). No subsequent epidemics in the Hellenic and Hellenistic Greek hegemony are comparable to this epidemic in magnitude. Because the epidemic, according to Thucydides and to many later historians of ancient Greece, was responsible for Athenian military losses to Sparta, many have judged the **Plague of Athens** to be a "turning point" in the history of Western civilization.

Historiography

Although many have speculated on causal questions surrounding the Plague of Athens and are convinced of their retrospective diagnoses, no consensus is likely to emerge. Fairly well-supported arguments have advanced **epidemic typhus, measles**, and **smallpox** as candidates because all produce some of the clinical and epidemiological features of Thucydides' description. Less frequently, **bubonic plague, ergotism, streptococcal infection**, and,

most recently, **tularemia** have found scholarly proponents.

The facts that (1) the Plague of Athens occurred during wartime; (2) the severe clinical course lasted 7–10 days; and (3) the fever was accompanied by first respiratory, then gastrointestinal complaints, and finally delirium associated with a rash – all have led several physician-historians to a diagnosis of epidemic typhus. Typhus is a louse-borne disease, and severe cases could lead to circulatory collapse, accounting for the loss of distal extremities (fingers and toes) as well as damage to the optic nerve.

Insofar as Thucydides mentions vision loss as well as crippling of the extremities among some survivors, William MacArthur and Harry Keil, writing in the 1950s, both found more support for this diagnosis of the clinical symptoms than for that of smallpox. By contrast, Hans Zinsser – author of the 1935 work, *Rats, Lice, and History* – was not persuaded that the description Thucydides offered bore any resemblance to the typhus that cost many lives in the two world wars. Yet other clinicians, citing their clinical experiences in wartime, have been equally persuaded that the description of Thucydides does suggest typhus.

J. F. D. Shrewsbury, however, has argued against a diagnosis of typhus, pointing out that Thucydides made no mention of either cloudy mental state or depression, both among the typhus symptoms most frequently reported over the last 500 years. Shrewsbury emphasizes the generally good personal and domestic cleanliness of the ancient Greeks, in order to argue that they were not lousy and thus could not have transmitted typhus with ease. Yet Keil has provided an extensive survey of the words for lice found in Greek texts of the fifth century B.C., which indicates that they were hardly uncommon. Even so, Shrewsbury argues that typhus is too mild a disease to have killed a quarter of those who fell ill, and consequently, he holds that some **virgin-soil epidemic** of a viral nature was the more probable cause of the Plague of Athens.

Indeed, Shrewsbury favored a diagnosis of measles, as did classicist D. L. Page. Shrewsbury points to similar levels of mortality in the severe virgin-soil epidemic of measles in the Fiji Islands in 1876, where more than 25 percent of the native population died. He considered the most significant passage in Thucydides to be the description of sufferers plunging themselves into cool water for relief. The Fiji Islanders displayed identical behavior. Because even in the twentieth century, measles in adults could be malignant, causing severe **diarrhea** and **pneumonia**, he argued that the Plague of Athens might have been measles in an early virulent form, not the "emasculated" modern virus. Page agrees that the Plague of Athens was measles, feeling that the clarity of Thucydides' account was such that little support can be found in the text for other diagnoses; that is to say, Thucydides, although a layman, was not guilty of omitting crucial diagnostic details that medical contemporaries would have noted.

Robert J. Littman and M. L. Littman, however, have more recently argued for smallpox as the disease called the Plague of Athens, on the basis of the specific terms used by Thucydides to describe the exanthem or rash of the infection in question. Using Page's careful retranslation, the Littmans emphasize terms meaning "small blister" or "pustule" and "ulcer" or "sore," contending that the description could refer only to a vesicle-forming eruption. In other words, Thucydides' description suggests a diagnosis of smallpox, because neither measles nor typhus typically forms vesicles in the exanthem. Moreover, the description hints strongly at the centrifugal spread of the rash, from face and trunk to extremities, again confirming a diagnosis of smallpox. The fact that Thucydides does not mention pockmarks among the survivors is found by the Littmans to be without import because they believed he was more concerned with the military impact of the disease than long-term effects on the survivors. In addition, the Littmans point to the absence of reference to pockmarking even in some modern medical accounts of smallpox.

Edna Hooker and many predecessors inclined toward a diagnosis of bubonic plague. Littman and Littman, however, argue against bubonic plague, dismissing any possibility that the terms Thucydides chose could refer to buboes (**lymphadenopathy** associated with plague).

Another hypothesis suggests that ergotism, caused by fungal toxins in grain, explains the Plague of Athens, even though Athenians rarely ate rye, the grain on which ergot usually grows. The occurrence of **gangrene** in extremities of victims who survived is, supporters maintain, an important symptom, which does not support other diagnoses but does support one of ergotism.

John Wylie and Hugh Stubbs have provided a review of those infections with a wide host range that might have caused this level of human mortality 2,400 years ago, and thus they consider zoonoses other than plague and typhus. Alexander Langmuir and colleagues have revived a pre-twentieth century diagnosis of **influenza**, but emphasize that concurrent or subsequent **staphylococcal infection** could easily have created a **toxic-shock syndrome**, with severe respiratory symptoms, bullous (or vesicular) skin infections, and violent gastrointestinal symptoms. As staphylococcal infection heightened the mortality from influenza in 1918, so a similar combination of viral and bacterial infection could explain the great Plague. On the other hand, Holladay takes issue with this latter explanation.

Study of the epidemic briefly described by Thucydides has inspired discussions of how diseases in the distant past can be identified, and thus discussions of the methods of historical epidemiology. Three difficulties emerge in the literature of the Plague of Athens that are illustrative of problems in retrospective diagnostic efforts. The first has to do with virgin-soil epidemics. Although Thucydides only implies that all members of society were at risk of contracting the sickness, that no one was immune, and that immunity was conferred on the survivors of infection, he does specifically state that the disease was previously unknown to lay and medical Athenians. Some scholars hold that a new disease among a population immunologically virgin to the microorganism in question need display neither the expected seasonal onset characterizing the disease nor the case-fatality rates usually seen. Those who oppose this methodological stance hold that this principle of retrospective analysis calls into question all diagnostic precepts. Many assume that supramortality would cause a breakdown in normal nursing care and hygienic services, leading to excess mortality; therefore, they stress the need for distinguishing the socioeconomic effects of a virgin-soil epidemic from discussions of the virulence of the disease or the immunologic vulnerability of the population.

The second difficulty pertains to the changing epidemiology (or even clinical presentation) of diseases over time and thus is a variation of what is called "virgin-soil epidemics argument": that infections of the past may have been caused by an organism known today but that the organism behaved quite differently in past individuals and populations. From a historical standpoint, this can be a particularly pessimistic argument, and in fact James Longrigg has disallowed the possibility of ever discovering the cause of the Plague on much these grounds. Poole and Holladay go even further in denying any possible resemblance of the Plague of Athens to an infectious disease known in more recent times, whereas Langmuir and colleagues suggest that the discussion abandon altogether the hope for a one-to-one correspondence with a modern infectious disease and look instead to a physiological understanding of the processes involved.

The third difficulty focuses on the intent and fidelity of Thucydides' account to actual events. Of the authors discussed here, only Watson Williams argues that Thucydides himself might not have been terribly well informed about the epidemic, because he did not write his history until after 404 B.C., approximately 25 years after the epidemic occurred. Williams further suggests that even if Thucydides wrote from notes or consulted one of the few physicians who survived (the account claims that most died early in the epidemic), individuals tended to believe that their own experience with an infection was characteristic of all those who suffered from it.

Most assume, however, that Thucydides' account of events lacks some crucial details from a modern point of view but is otherwise accurate. Since Page's review, which offers abundant detail that Thucydides was particularly well versed in medical terms and ideas, most have come to believe that the account was informed by contemporary medical knowledge. Longrigg agrees, but skeptically. Jody Pinault, however, tracing an ancient legend that Hippocrates himself devised the successful remedy of building fires to combat the epidemic at Athens, argues that Thucydides's failure to mention Hippocrates's achievement is compelling evidence that he was not at all well versed about the Plague.

Clearly, discussions of the cause of the Plague of Athens form an important and instructive example of the study of the history of human infectious diseases. In addition, such a study reveals the many pitfalls connected with this type of integration and points to the need for still more sophisticated methods and techniques.

Ann G. Carmichael

111. Pneumocystis Pneumonia (Interstitial Plasma Cell Pneumonia, Pneumocystosis)

This form of **pneumonia** is caused by *Pneumocystis carinii*, a **protozoan** in the class Sporozoa. An extracellular parasite of the lungs of humans, dogs, rodents, and other mammals, the organism occurs worldwide. It appears to have low virulence and almost never causes disease except in weak or immunosuppressed individuals. *P. carinii* was discovered in guinea pigs in 1909, but human disease was first recognized in the 1940s in malnourished and premature infants. Victims of **leukemia, Hodgkin's disease**, and other immunosuppressive diseases, or organ-transplant recipients and others whose treatment requires suppression of immune responses, are also vulnerable to infection. In the early 1980s, **pneumocystis pneumonia** achieved prominence as the most common opportunistic infection afflicting patients with **acquired immune deficiency syndrome** (AIDS). Over half of AIDS victims suffer from the disease, and it frequently is the proximate cause of death.

Transmission is usually by airborne droplets, although transplacental passage resulting in fetal death has been reported. Latent infection may be common, with clinical disease and droplet transmission developing only in weakened hosts. The parasite damages the alveolar walls and induces an abundant foamy exudate and **fibrosis**. Death results from asphyxiation by the exudate. Although initial response to chemical therapy is common, treatment is difficult because of drugs' side effects and patients' debilitated state.

K. David Patterson

112. Pneumonia

Pneumonia is an acute inflammatory condition of lung parenchyma (lung tissue excluding the airways) caused by a variety of infectious agents and toxins and favored by aspects of the environment and/or the general physical status of the patient. The term "pneumonia" is derived from a Greek word meaning "condition about the lung" and refers to a clinicopathological state that arises in several different yet specific disease patterns. All of these are characterized by some degree of fever, cough, chest pain, and difficulty in breathing. Technically speaking, **pneumonitis** ("inflammation of the lung") is a synonym for pneumonia, but the former is usually reserved for benign, localized, and sometimes chronic inflammation without major **toxemia** (generalized effects). Many modifiers are applied to the term pneumonia to reflect cause (e.g., **embolic pneumonia**) and localization (e.g., **bronchopneumonia**). The classic form is **lobar pneumonia**, an infectious but not particularly contagious condition usually localized to part or all of one of the five lobes of the lungs, and caused by a pneumococcus, *Streptococcus pneumoniae* (formerly *Diplococcus pneumoniae*). Untreated lobar pneumonia has a mortality of about 30 percent, but the advent of antibiotic treatment has improved survival rates.

Several other pathogens (bacterial, viral, fungal, and parasitic), chemical irritation, exposure to or aspiration of noxious substances, and hypersensitivity are also recognized causes. In many cases, pneumonia is only one manifestation of another specific disease such as the **acquired immune deficiency syndrome** (AIDS), **ascariasis, cytomegalovirus, influenza, Legionnaire's disease, plague, pneumocystis, Q fever, rickettsial diseases, tuberculosis, tularemia**, and **varicella**.

Characteristics

Many pathogens have been associated with **infectious pneumonia**. However, despite the large number of possible pathogens, pneumonia develops only if other host or environmental conditions are met. Normally the airways and lung tissue distal to the throat are sterile. Occasionally, organisms that are always present in the upper airway, in the digestive tract, or on the skin enter the lung. Ordinarily they are rapidly eliminated either by mechanical means, such as coughing and the microscopic action of cilia, or by immune mechanisms. Infection and the resultant inflammation of pneumonia can occur in healthy individuals but are often associated with a breakdown in one or more of the usual defense mechanisms – or, more rarely, with exposure to a particularly virulent pathogen or an unusually high aerosol dose of organism (as in Legionnaire's disease). Occasionally, **bacterial pneumonia** will occur as a result of septicemic spread from an infectious focus elsewhere in the body.

Immune defenses are altered by underlying debility, be it nutritional (starvation and alcoholism), infectious (tuberculosis and AIDS), neoplastic (**cancer** or **lymphoma**), or iatrogenic. Iatrogenic causes of immune depression are becoming more important with the increasingly frequent use of immunosuppressive or cytotoxic drugs in the treatment of cancer, autoimmunity, and organ transplantation. One special form of immune deficiency resulting from absent splenic function leads to an exaggerated susceptibility to *S. pneumoniae* infection and lobar pneumonia. This condition, called **functional asplenia**, can arise following splenectomy or as a complication of **sickle-cell anemia**. Thus a relative predisposition to **pneumococcal infection** can be found in the geographic regions containing a high frequency of hemoglobin S.

Controversy surrounds the ancient etiologic theory about cold temperatures, but two factors do tend to support an indirect correlation between cold and pneumonia: Predisposing viral infections are more common in winter, and some evidence suggests that the mechanical action of cilia is slowed on prolonged exposure to cold.

Lobar pneumonia appears in all populations. Incidence and mortality are higher in individuals or groups predisposed to one or more of the factors described above. Elderly patients frequently develop pneumonia as the terminal complication of other debilitating illness, hence the famous metaphor "friend of the aged."

Mortality rates for pneumonia are difficult to estimate because of its multifactorial nature and complication of other diseases. With antibiotics, fatalities are reduced to a varying extent depending on the underlying condition of the patient, but in persons over age 12, mortality is at least 18 percent, and in immunocompromised persons much higher. Atmospheric pollution may have contributed to the apparent rise in pneumonia mortality in Britain during the last half of the nineteenth century. Toward the end of that century, William Osler saw pneumonia as one of the most important problems of his era and applied to it John Bunyan's metaphor (originally intended for tuberculosis): "captain of all these men of death." Contemporary pneumonia mortality combined with influenza is still the sixth most common cause of death in the

United States, where mortality is estimated to be approximately 0.3 per 1,000.

The incubation period for pneumonia is variable, depending on the causative organism, but **pneumococcal pneumonia** has a fairly uniform pattern. A brief prodrome of cold-like symptoms may occur, but usually onset is sudden, with shaking chills and rapid rise in temperature, followed by a rise in heart and respiratory rates. Cough productive of "rusty" blood-tinged sputum and **dyspnea** are usual. Most patients experience pleuritic chest pain. In severe cases, there can be inadequate oxygenation of blood, leading to **cyanosis**. If untreated, the fever and other symptoms persist for at least 7–10 days, when a "crisis" may occur consisting of sweating with defervescence and spontaneous resolution. With antibiotic treatment, the fever usually falls within 48 hours. Untreated, or inadequately treated, the disease may progress to dyspnea, shock, abscess formation, **empyema**, and disseminated infection. When empyema occurs, surgical drainage is essential.

History

Lobar pneumonia has probably always afflicted humans. Pneumococcal organisms have been found in prehistoric remains, and evidence of illness has been observed in Egyptian mummies from 1200 B.C. Epidemics of this disease have probably been less common than previously thought. Pre-germ-theory observations cited sixteenth to late-nineteenth century reports of epidemic outbreaks of "pneumonia" in numerous places on six continents, emphasizing "malignant" and **typhoid**-like symptoms. But these qualifiers raise doubts about whether such outbreaks were truly pneumonia. It is probable that most, if not all, were caused by organisms other than pneumococcus. Conditions now called by other names and known to have pneumonic manifestations, like plague and influenza, are far more likely candidates for retrospective diagnosis.

Pneumonia is not only an old disease but also one of the oldest diagnosed diseases. Hippocratic accounts of a highly lethal illness called *peripleumonin* give a readily identifiable description of the symptoms, progression, and suppurative complications of classic pneumonia and localize it in the lung. This disease was a paradigmatic example of the Greek theory that all illness progressed from *coction* (approximately, incubation and early illness) to crisis and lysis ("breaking up"), while certain days in the sequence were "critical" to the outcome. Auscultation was recommended to confirm the presence of pus in the chest. Variant pneumonic conditions of the lung were also described, including lethargy, **moist pneumonia**, and **dry pneumonia** (also called **erysipelas of the lung**). Therapy included bleeding, fluids, expectorants, and, only if absolutely necessary, surgical evacuation of empyemic pus.

In the first century A.D., Aretaeus of Cappadocia distinguished this disease from **pleurisy**, and four centuries later Caelius Aurelianus recognized that it could be confined to only certain parts of the lung. Except for a few subtle modifications, little change occurred in the clinical diagnosis and treatment of pneumonia until the early nineteenth century.

Eighteenth century anatomists drew attention to the microscopic appearance of the lung in fatal cases of lobar pneumonia. This work, however, had little impact until 1808, when Jean-Nicolas Corvisart at the Paris Clinical School translated and revised the 1761 treatise on percussion by Leopold Auenbrugger. This technique made it possible to detect and localize fluid or consolidation in the lung and to follow its evolution. Eight years later, Corvisart's student, René Laennec, carried this one step further by inventing the stethoscope. In calling his technique *médiate auscultation*, Laennec readily gave priority to Hippocrates for having practiced the "immediate" variety by direct application of the ear to the chest. Laennec recommended both percussion and auscultation of the breath sounds and voice to confirm the physical diagnosis of pneumonia. With this combination he was able to distinguish consolidated lung from pleural fluid or pus in the living patient. He introduced most of the technical

terms for pathological lung sounds – including "rale," "rhoncus," "crepitation," "bronchophony," "egophony" – some of which became pathognomonic for disease states. Percussion and auscultation changed the concept of pneumonia from a definition based on classic symptoms to one based on physical findings. This conceptual shift was endorsed by the advent of the chest X-ray at the turn of the twentieth century.

The Italians Giovanni Rasori and Giacomo Thommasini had recommended high-dose antimony potassium tartrate (tartar emetic) as a treatment for pneumonia, and Laennec used the new method of statistical analysis with historical controls to suggest that this was an effective remedy. Yet in spite of its potential utility, the extreme toxicity of the drug guaranteed its unpopularity. Benjamin Rush, an American, and Laennec's contemporary, Jean Baptiste Bouillaud, were proponents of copious phlebotomy. Until the late nineteenth century, when salicylates became available for fever, pneumonia therapy consisted of the ancient remedies: emetics, mercury, and especially bleeding.

Germ theory had a major impact on the concept of pneumonia, but it was rapidly apparent that despite its fairly homogeneous clinical manifestations this disease was associated not with a single germ but with a variety of pathogens. This situation cast some doubt on the imputed role of each new pathogen. In December 1880, Louis Pasteur isolated the organism that would later become the pneumococcus. Carl Friedlander discovered the first lung-derived pneumonia organism, *Klebsiella pneumoniae* (Friedlander's bacillus) in 1883. Albert Frankel identified the pneumococcus (*D. pneumoniae*) in 1884, and Anton Weichselbaum confirmed his findings in 1886. *Klebsiella* was found to be quite rare and seemed to favor the upper lobes, whereas the pneumococcus favored the lower lobes; however, there was some overlap between the pneumonic states induced by these organisms. Specific diagnoses could be made only by isolation of the pathogen.

Gradually many other organisms and viruses came to be associated with pneumonia, usually in clinical settings that deviated more or less from classic lobar pneumonia. Moreover, it is likely that new pathogens will be recognized as antibiotics and vaccination alter the ecology of the lung.

Knowledge of the pneumococcus led to improvement in treatment and reduction in mortality from pneumonia, but it also had a major impact on the broad fields of immunology, bacteriology, and molecular genetics. Study of the capsule – its antigenic properties and capacity to transform – provided key information about drug resistance in bacteria.

Treatment and prevention of pneumonia have been dramatically improved in the twentieth century. Oxygen therapy was introduced during the 1918 New York influenza epidemic. Typing of pneumococci led to the 1912 introduction of antisera; it was claimed that, by 1929, this therapy dramatically reduced mortality in some populations. Antisera, however, were effective only when the exact type of pneumococcus was known. Pronotosil (sulfanilamide) was not particularly effective against pneumococcus but did control other predisposing conditions. Its successor, sulfapyridine, was more effective. The advent of penicillin in the mid-1940s led to further reduction in mortality; however, it also led to the evolution of penicillin-resistant strains of pneumococci and the now seemingly endless chase after effective derivatives against so-called new organisms.

Pneumonia-control programs relied at first on antipneumococcal serum therapy, but as early as 1911, vaccination trials were conducted on thousands of black South African gold miners. These trials (conducted before the diversity of capsular types was fully appreciated), were inconclusive. Not until 1945 was unequivocal protection against type-specific pneumococcal infection in humans demonstrated using a tetravalent vaccine. Contemporary vaccines contain at least 23 capsular antigens and are 80–90 percent effective in immunocompetent persons but may be useless in some forms of immunodeficiency.

Jacalyn Duffin

113. Poliomyelitis

Poliomyelitis is a disease of inflammation and destruction of motor neurons caused by a poliovirus. Sensory functions are not affected. Although frequently asymptomatic, the infection may cause fever and a number of other general symptoms, described as **abortive polio** or minor illness. Occasionally, however, these prodromal symptoms are followed by a central nervous system infection and fever, with **meningitis**, or **paresis** (weakness) or **paralysis** of one or more muscles. Many patients recover use of affected muscles in subsequent months, although some have permanent paralysis or paresis. When respiratory muscles are affected, death may follow. In the past, cases of abortive polio and temporary paralysis were often included in polio statistics. Today, only cases with paralysis or paresis after 3 months are recorded as **paralytic polio**.

Poliomyelitis was known by different names (such as **infantile paralysis** and "Heine-Medin disease") until the 1870s, when it became known as **acute anterior poliomyelitis**. Poliomyelitis – inflammation of the gray marrow – eventually became the name of choice and is often shortened to **polio**.

Characteristics

There are three immunologic types of poliovirus, with strain differences in each. Each type has a wide range of ability to cause paralysis, from the highly virulent type 1 Mahoney strain to avirulent wild and vaccine strains. Wild strains may paralyze only a few individuals while immunizing others. The introduction of a new virulent strain, however, may cause an epidemic, as in Malta in 1942. Strains differ widely in their transmissibility: In Malta, the pattern of cases suggests that everyone was rapidly infected. But many small epidemics have spread no further than those initially afflicted.

The virus spreads from person to person via the fecal-oral route, although a few epidemics may have resulted from contaminated milk. Ingested virus replicates in the gut and lymphoid tissue. The level of **viremia** correlates with virulence; there is little viremia with avirulent strains. Animal experiments indicate that the protecting antibody level is below the detection threshold. Exposure leads to lifelong immunity against viruses of the same type. People who are immune may still be infected but have no viremia. Humans are the only natural host and reservoir.

Since 1910 it seemed that immunization might be feasible, but first attempts in 1935 ended with deaths attributed to the vaccines. Many vaccines were made for experimental use, but a human vaccine was not possible until the virus could be grown in quantity, the number of types established, and cheap methods of testing for viruses and antibodies developed. J. F. Enders, T. H. Weller, and F. C. Robbins grew poliovirus in 1948 and solved all three problems. In 1954, Jonas Salk's inactivated polio vaccine (IPV) was given to 400,000 children in a successful field trial involving 1.8 million children. The 1980s produced a purified and more antigenic IPV that required two doses instead of three.

In the 1950s, A. B. Sabin produced an oral polio vaccine (OPV), which has been used extensively throughout the world. The Sabin vaccine has many advantages: (1) It can be administered by nonmedical staff; (2) it induces gut immunity; (3) it is inexpensive; and (4) immunity spreads to nonvaccinated individuals. Yet it also has disadvantages: (1) Three doses are required; (2) it is inactivated by heat; and (3) it causes some vaccine-associated cases (VAC). Purely as a precaution, the Sabin vaccine is not given to pregnant women. About one child in a million given OPV develops paralysis. A very small number of contact VACs occur, mainly among mothers of OPV-vaccinated children.

Oral polio vaccine is successful in temperate climates but less so in many warmer developing countries, largely because cold-chain facilities and organization are lacking. The most effective method of immunization is the semiannual "polio day." Vaccine is distributed to local immunization posts a few days in advance, reducing

potential problems of the cold chain. On the day of immunization (which is heavily advertised), all available children 2 years and younger receive OPV. The flood of virus shed by vaccinees then vaccinates any who did not receive OPV.

Inactivated polio vaccine is more stable and may be combined with other vaccines, thus simplifying immunization schedules and reducing cost. The latest IPV is very safe, highly purified, and antigenic.

Epidemics of polio are difficult to assess because several polioviruses of different virulence and type may be circulating. Thus the extent of circulation of virulent viruses will not be known, and cases will not necessarily correspond to the geographic boundaries used for reporting. Consequently, our epidemiological knowledge of the disease depends on the study of virgin-soil epidemics in islands and isolated communities with definite boundaries.

Until the early twentieth century, most polio cases occurred in young children. Beginning in the 1930s, however, there was a shift to older children and adolescents, first in Scandinavia and the United States, and then in Europe. Older children suffered less paralysis, and fatality rates were low. By contrast, young adults had paralysis and fatality rates like those of small children. In many severe epidemics, case rates for 2-year-olds have been about 2 percent, with increasing rates up to 10 years of age, when the rate stabilizes at 25 percent.

Early epidemiological surveys included all cases whether there was residual paralysis or not. From the late 1930s, however, statistics were increasingly restricted to those with paralysis, and later only those with residual paralysis. In countries with universal immunization and very few cases, every suspected case is investigated.

For reasons unknown, there are more male than female cases of polio at any age; however, pregnant females have higher incidence than nonpregnant females of the same age. Fatality rates of males and females are similar. Studies of afflicted pregnant women show no increase in miscarriages and no affected births. Yet when mothers suffered paralysis between 7 days before and 10 days after birth, 40 percent of babies suffered concurrent paralysis, with a 56 percent fatality rate. By contrast, babies born of mothers who had experienced paralysis earlier in the pregnancy (nonconcurrent) had a less than 0.01 percent chance of polio in the month after birth and only a 10 percent case-fatality rate.

There are two theories as to how virus reaches the central nervous system (CNS). The first suggests that virus crosses the blood-brain barrier and travels along neuronal pathways in the CNS. However, postmortems reveal that lesions in the CNS can be discrete and separate, suggesting that virus enters at motor neurons in the muscles and reaches the CNS at many different places. The time taken to reach the CNS from any muscle depends on the length of the nerve to be traveled, during which time the virus would be shielded from antibody.

Leg muscles are more often affected than arms. In general, the larger the muscle, the greater the chance of paralysis; the smaller the muscle, the greater the chance of paresis. Muscles are not affected at random. The neurons serving them lie in adjacent and overlapping bundles in the CNS: Damage in one bundle often spills over into the next, so there is a high probability that both muscles will be affected.

Up to 60 percent of the neurons serving a muscle may be destroyed before loss of function occurs; thus patients with past nonparalytic CNS infection can have considerable damage. Many survivors suffer **late effects of polio** (LEP) more than 30 years later. Previously unaffected muscles become weak; already affected muscles become weaker; generalized fatigue occurs. Most commonly affected are those muscles that recovered well from the initial attack and have been used strenuously ever since. Loss of motor neurons continues with age, and LEP may indicate normal aging superimposed on previous polio loss.

In the acute stage, the condition resembles a **host-versus-graft reaction**. Infected neurons are destroyed, although the inflammation does not correspond with the location of virus. In animal experiments, however, it was observed that 75 percent of infected neurons recover. Second attacks by another poliovirus presumably should occur; yet only 44 have been reported – far less than expected. This does suggest, however, that second attacks are not blocked by antibodies.

History

Polio may be as old as humankind, but few early indicators of the disease exist. An Egyptian stele (c. 1400 B.C.) shows a priest with a deformed foot in the typical equinus position of polio. During the 1830s, three small epidemics were reported from England, the United States, and St. Helena. In the 1890s and early 1900s, greater epidemics were reported in Scandinavia, Massachusetts, and Vermont, and then the New York epidemic of 1916 occurred, with over 9,000 cases in the city itself. Almost all patients in the New York epidemic were under 5 years of age. After this, polio cases in the United States fell to a low level, then exhibited peaks and troughs, and then rose again to some 40,000 cases annually in 1951–55.

After 1955, with widespread use of IPV in the United States, Canada, South Africa, Australia, and some countries in Europe, cases fell dramatically. Not all children were immunized, and small epidemics still occurred among the poorest classes. But soon almost all countries in temperate climates were using vaccine, and vaccine potency was improved. Nonetheless, by 1960 many doubted that IPV would eliminate polio.

By the end of 1960, however, Sabin's OPV, given to more than 115 million people in Russia and eastern Europe, had practically eliminated polio there. Gradually, opinion favored routine use of OPV instead of IPV, although Scandinavia and Holland continued to use IPV. With these exceptions, beginning in 1961, OPV was increasingly used in temperate countries, and the number of cases fell even lower. But small epidemics still struck communities that refused immunization or lacked primary health care. The United States now has about 10 cases a year, roughly half of which are vaccine-associated.

By contrast, in Holland there is a large community that rejects immunization on religious grounds and has suffered eight epidemics since 1960. Polio has not, however, spread to the immunized population. The epidemic that occurred in 1978 produced 110 cases with 79 paralytic (one baby died). During that outbreak, the virus was carried to Canada. Cases occurred in Alberta, British Columbia, and Ontario, after which polio reached Pennsylvania, then Iowa, Wisconsin, and Missouri, and then returned to Canada, causing 21 cases and three nonparalytic attacks in North America. Genomic sequencing confirmed that the same virus was involved for over 15 months on both continents. It may well have originally come from Turkey.

Polio was previously thought to have low incidence in developing countries, although it occurred in such diverse and remote places as St. Helena, Greenland, and Nauru, which suffered severe epidemics. Despite outbreaks among Allied troops in the Middle and Far East and India during World War II, little attention was paid to the disease, epidemics in Singapore, the Andamans, and Bombay notwithstanding.

Early data from developing countries were based on hospital admissions and seriously underestimated the true number of cases. Even in the 1980s, country statistics sent to the World Health Organization represented perhaps only 10 percent of the true number. By way of illustration, in Nigeria in 1977 more children attended one clinic than the official number of polio cases for the entire country. Truer estimates are yielded by lameness surveys of schoolchildren and seeking out disabled children who do not attend school. Unfortunately, such investigations always produce outdated data and do not include deaths.

Very promising immunization programs are under way in Central and South America, which reach more than 80 percent of children below 1 year of age. By contrast, in central Africa few countries achieve even a 50 percent immunization rate of children under 1 year of age. Similarly, India, with 22 million children born

annually, immunizes fewer than half, and lameness surveys show rising prevalence among older children despite increased use of vaccine. Indeed, in India, surveys of all kinds reveal a steady increase in prevalence since 1945. This increase, however, may merely reflect better reporting and investigation.

H. V. Wyatt

114. Protein-Energy Malnutrition

Protein-energy malnutrition (PEM) – or, as it is still sometimes called, **protein-calorie malnutrition** – is a term of convenience that refers to a range of syndromes among infants and children of preschool age in whom manifestations of growth failure occur because of protein and energy deficiencies. In most instances, this condition besets those in the less-developed world of Asia, Africa, and Latin America, where dietary factors are thought to be a crucial part of the etiology. PEM thereby tends to exclude what is conventionally known as "failure to thrive" in Europe and North America, in which the vast majority of cases result from organic disorders such as **cystic fibrosis** and **congenital heart disease** and are not so directly associated with diet as such.

Characteristics

PEM is best described in its two clinical versions of **kwashiorkor** and **marasmus**. In the former, **edema** is always present, whereas extreme wasting (below 60 percent of normal weight for height) identifies the latter. However, cases purely of one or the other are the exception rather than the rule; most display both edema and extreme wasting, plus a variable mix of other symptoms, and are designated by the term **marasmic kwashiorkor**. Far more common than these three clinical entities are numerous subclinical syndromes usually referred to as **mild-to-moderate PEM**. A frequent analogy for PEM, therefore, is an iceberg; only a small proportion of the total is clearly visible.

Most cases remain below the surface and go undetected except under close analysis.

Numerous attempts have been made to develop a logically ordered, comprehensive classification of PEM, but several problems have prevented the achievement of one satisfactory to both clinicians and field workers. A particular dilemma is that the various syndromes are not static. Mild-to-moderate cases fluctuate considerably and can move in the direction of kwashiorkor, marasmus, or marasmic kwashiorkor. Moreover, clinical conditions may not remain constant: Kwashiorkor can become marasmus, and vice versa.

Traditional interpretations have stressed the predominant role of diet in the etiology of PEM, with protein singled out as the most important missing ingredient. Critical shortages of protein alone, it was believed, led to kwashiorkor – and when combined with severe energy deficits, to marasmus or marasmic kwashiorkor. Mild-to-moderate syndromes simply reflected lesser shortages of the two essential dietary requirements, protein and calories.

The behavioral variables deemed most critical in the past were duration of breast-feeding and subsequent food habits. Too-early weaning onto poor-quality substitutes for mother's milk such as rice water, sugar water, diluted milk or formula, and cornstarch was associated with marasmus. These substances are often contaminated with bacteria because of polluted water supplies and unsanitary utensils; consequently, repeated bouts of **diarrhea** were seen to accentuate nutritional shortages. Later-age weaning onto predominantly bulky carbohydrate/low amino acid foodstuffs, notably cassava and plantains, was seen as the pathway to kwashiorkor. Abrupt weaning was believed especially hazardous, particularly if children had to compete for food from a "common pot" with older siblings and adult males who often monopolize high-quality protein foods such as meat, fish, eggs, and milk. With kwashiorkor, the problem was the balance of protein and energy, not the quantity of food consumed, which generally appeared ample.

This portrayal has proved not so much erroneous as somewhat oversimplified. Clinical research has verified that kwashiorkor is always associated with low serum proteins, but considerable variation has been found in energy intake. Some cases show deficits, whereas others have adequate and occasionally even excessive energy levels. **Protein deficiency** is clearly secondary to **energy deficiency** in marasmus and probably marasmic kwashiorkor. Indeed, if energy were not so severely restricted, it is unlikely that signs of protein shortages would be observable.

An extremely important finding is that diet does not seem to play quite the overarching role in PEM that was initially believed. What is critical is availability of nutrients to the cells, and thus infections can act as an equal if not more important limiting factor. Included in these infections are not only the various diarrhea-producing gastrointestinal disorders but also widespread childhood diseases such as **pneumonia, measles, tuberculosis**, and **malaria**. All can imitate symptoms of PEM by inducing **anorexia** and lowering amino acid levels, and it is clear that malnourished children are more susceptible to serious episodes of infection. The various syndromes of PEM, therefore, are best construed as resulting from complex **nutrition-infection interactions**. Based on current knowledge, it would appear that how they develop depends on how the life history of a child unfolds within a particular environmental context.

Many cases undoubtedly begin in the uterus. Because of widespread maternal malnutrition, low birthweights are common throughout Asia, Africa, and Latin America. Breast-feeding on demand during the first 4–6 months of life tends to compensate for any fetal growth deficit and provides important disease immunities, but infants who are not breast-fed are well along a pathway to PEM. If a serious infection should ensue, then marasmus may very likely develop. If not, then – at the least – growth failure continues, and the child remains at risk.

After about the first 6 months of life, breast-feeding alone no longer provides adequate nutrition, and at this point many children begin to show signs of mild-to-moderate PEM. Food supplies might be limited generally, or perhaps there is little knowledge of proper supplements. In any event, the course of PEM depends on the severity of the food shortage – a "hungry season" seems especially dangerous – and once again on infections to which the child is exposed. When **nutrition-infection stress** is extreme, then overt clinical symptoms of PEM can be expected.

Weaning is frequently a time of stress, and when it occurs at 18–24 months of age, symptoms of kwashiorkor tend to predominate over marasmus, assuming no gross deficiency of energy in the new diet. However, weaning by itself does not appear to produce kwashiorkor; this is true even if staple foods are overwhelmingly starchy. The child must already be nutritionally disadvantaged or otherwise in poor health before discernible symptoms of kwashiorkor emerge.

The overriding etiologic issue, of course, is poverty, and PEM is a problem only where poverty is pervasive. Poverty means that local food shortages cannot be overcome by purchases, that living conditions foster recurring infections, that education for effective intervention is inadequate, that proper parental supervision of the feeding of infants and young children is likely to be lacking, and that preventive and curative health services are not readily available. In a real sense, then, PEM is the outcome of "total deprivation." Acceptance of this has led to recent shifts in policies designed to combat it. For many years, officials emphasized providing protein-fortified and energy-rich food substitutes or developing meat and dairy industries, but these approaches have proven too costly for most people in need and address only part of the problem. PEM must be attacked on a broad front, including economic and political as well as nutritional intervention.

In the earliest stages of PEM, the child simply appears smaller than he or she should be for that age. If the condition deteriorates further, however, clinical symptoms begin to emerge.

The edema that defines all cases of kwashiorkor varies. It can be mild and localized on the extremities and sacrum or more severe and general. Although muscle wasting is discernible, subcutaneous fat is usually retained, and consequently the child takes on a bloated appearance, called the "sugar-baby" look in the West Indies. Some growth retardation in head length and circumference may also occur.

More often than not, the skin develops ulcerating areas, open and healed sores, **scabies**, or "flaky-paint" **dermatosis**, in which removal of the flakes reveals lighter patches of skin. When kwashiorkor persists, the hair is affected; it loses its luster, and dark hair becomes lighter. Curly hair straightens, and eventually the hair becomes brittle and falls out, leaving bare areas of scalp clearly visible.

Upon examination, the liver and spleen frequently are found to be enlarged, and a range of other symptoms includes **anemia** and **vitamin-A deficiency**, with some vision impairment; a range of micronutrient deficiencies; plus tendencies to **hypothermia**, higher bilirubin, **hyponatremia, hypoglycemia**, and low plasma albumin.

Behavioral changes are marked. Vomiting and diarrhea become persistent; without resolution, anorexia usually sets in. As the child's strength wanes, motor skills regress, and eventually he or she becomes almost totally apathetic to external stimuli. This withdrawal makes treatment difficult outside of a clinical setting where the child can be fed intravenously.

The overt symptoms of marasmus are far fewer and less medically unusual. Wasting of both muscle and subcutaneous tissue, along with stunting, is marked. Because the victim is so emaciated, the head appears abnormally large, especially the eyes. The skin tends to be dry and patchy, but neither dermatosis nor any significant hair changes appear. Anorexia is uncommon, and in fact appetite is usually good, which helps simplify therapy. As in kwashiorkor, there is likely to be hypothermia and a tendency to hypoglycemia. Dehydration is a problem as marasmus worsens, and behavior changes from fretfulness and irritability to a semicomatose state immediately preceding death.

With severe PEM, mortality is high – over 20 percent. Seldom, however, is starvation the final cause of death; rather it is one or more of the infections that brought on the condition, and these usually run their fatal course in just a few days. Onset of hypothermia and hypoglycemia probably signals the need for immediate treatment.

For those who have recovered, the question of long-term effects remains. Available evidence supports a relationship between chronic PEM and some permanent stunting. But much more importantly, areas of chronic-PEM prevalence also have a high incidence of **cephalopelvic disproportion** among women, leading to miscarriages, stillbirths, and heightened maternal mortality. Investigators suspect that PEM interferes with calcium metabolism, producing incomplete pelvic development, but this has not been conclusively proven. There is also some suggestion that later-age **cardiovascular disease, hepatic ailments**, and **pancreatic conditions** may be connected with childhood PEM.

The issue that has stimulated the most interest and controversy, however, is the effect of PEM on the brain. Research has shown that subnormal mental and psychomotor functioning tends to follow PEM, and during the 1960s and 1970s, direct causal connections were commonly made. Some investigators even hypothesized that severe PEM resulted in permanent mental disabilities. But once again important reassessments have been forthcoming: Earlier tests generally failed to control for the learning environment of their subjects. Currently, the prevailing view is that neither mild-to-moderate nor acute clinical PEM seems to be associated with long-term intellectual and psychological disabilities. The matter of permanent injury caused by chronic PEM, notably of the marasmic variety during the first year of life, however, remains unresolved. Irreversible **brain damage** may well occur in more serious cases, as is strongly suggested by research on laboratory animals.

History

PEM is undoubtedly as old as humankind. The term marasmus has referred to starvation for centuries. However, medical literature fails to mention PEM specifically until about the mid-nineteenth century, when concepts of **malnutrition** were developing, especially among pediatric specialists in France and Germany, who treated numerous childhood illnesses. One disorder, in particular, received considerable attention. Called **mehlnährschaden**, it was attributed to diets based excessively on flour, usually breads or thin gruels, with little milk or meat included.

At the same time, in the wake of colonial expansion, doctors began to report similar disorders in many tropical areas. Although such diseases were initially blamed on parasites, by the 1920s a dietary etiology gained some acceptance. A proliferation of terms ensued, such as "infantile pellagra," "nutritional edema," "infantile edema," "starchy dystrophy," and "fatty-liver disease" – all describing, of course, what is now designated kwashiorkor, a term first used in the 1931–32 *Annual Medical Report of the Gold Coast* (now Ghana). The term was taken from the local Ga language and refers to an ill child who has been "deposed" from the breast because of a new pregnancy.

Although terminological and etiologic arguments continued, by the 1950s the concept of kwashiorkor was firmly entrenched in nutrition literature and accepted by the medical community as a certifiable human disease resulting from a deficiency of protein. Continuing research led to discovery of other syndromes and to formulation of the more general concept of protein-calorie malnutrition. The word "calorie," however, was subsequently replaced by "energy" in the 1970s, when the international system of unit measures was adopted by the United Nations.

A rough regional patterning of PEM has been attempted by two studies using both weight-for-age information and weight-for-height (wasting) calculations. What emerges from these efforts is a focus of PEM in Southeast Asia. Some

52 percent of preschool children are estimated to fall below 80 percent of the weight-for-age standard, led by Bangladesh with 91 percent and India with 75 percent. No country in the region shows a prevalence of wasting among 12- to 23-month-olds under 10 percent. Once again, Bangladesh and India are at the upper extreme, with 53 percent and 43 percent, respectively.

Both African and eastern Mediterranean regions show 35 percent deficient by weight-for-age criteria. Of the countries included, only Yemen and Mali stand above 50 percent. Wasting totals are generally in the vicinity of 10 percent, but there are two countries that register exceptionally high totals: Malawi (36 percent) and Somalia (66 percent).

On both measurement scales, the less-developed countries in the Americas fare much better. The regional below-weight-for-age average is 21 percent, and all countries except one show a less than 10 percent incidence of wasting. That lone exception is Haiti, where the figure is calculated at 18 percent, still far lower than figures for many places in Asia and Africa.

Limited trend data suggest some lessening of the incidence of PEM since the 1960s, an observation supported by declining infant and child mortality rates. This is true even in Africa, where scenes of famine have created the image of spreading malnutrition. Still, there is little room for complacency, given the magnitude of the problem that remains and the fact that poverty has proved to be intractable in many areas.

James L. Newman

115. Protozoan Infection

Protozoa are one-celled animals or animal-like eukaryotic (having an organized nucleus) organisms. Older classifications treated the Protozoa as a phylum in the animal kingdom, but modern taxonomists generally consider them members of a distinct kingdom, the Protista, along with other simple eukaryotes. Three phyla

or classes of Protozoa have species pathogenic for humankind. The Sarcomastigophora (the flagellates and amebas) include trypanosomes, leishmanias, and parasitic amebas. The Ciliophora (the ciliates) have only one human pathogen, *Balantidium coli*, an intestinal parasite of wide distribution but, usually, little clinical significance. The Apicomplexa (the sporozoans) include many pathogens, including the four species of *Plasmodium* that cause **malaria**.

K. David Patterson

116. Puerperal Fever

Historically, the terms **puerperal fever** and **childbed fever** meant any acute fever occurring in puerperae during the first few days after delivery. Less frequently, the terms were also applied to similar diseases occurring during pregnancy or even in the newborn. From a modern point of view, what was formerly called puerperal fever includes a range of disorders, most of which are now called **puerperal sepsis**. Typically, puerperal sepsis involves postpartum infection in the pelvic region, but it can mean disorders in other areas, such as **mastitis**. In modern usage, the term puerperal fever occurs mainly in discussing the great fever epidemics that afflicted maternity clinics in earlier centuries.

Characteristics

A wide range of microorganisms have been associated with acute pelvic inflammation and other postpartum inflammations identified as puerperal fever, but a principal cause is **streptococcal infection**. Group A streptococci (pyogenes) were probably the leading agents in most puerperal fever epidemics during earlier centuries. However, since the 1970s, group B streptococci (agalactiae) have become the most prevalent causal agents.

Among puerperae, the clinical manifestations of puerperal sepsis include acute fever, profuse lochial flow, and an enlarged and tender uterus. Onset is generally 2–5 days after delivery. Normally there is inflammation of the endometrium and surrounding structures as well as the lymphatic and vascular systems. One also finds pelvic **cellulitis**, septic pelvic **thrombophlebitis**, **peritonitis**, and pelvic abscesses. Among neonates, infection usually becomes apparent in the first 5 days after birth, but onset is sometimes delayed by several weeks. Symptoms include lethargy, poor feeding, and abnormal temperature. Infection by group B streptococci is often clinically indistinguishable from other bacterial infections.

History

The Hippocratic corpus contains case histories of puerperal fever. Various epidemics were recorded in the sixteenth and seventeenth centuries. The disease was first characterized and named in the eighteenth century when serious epidemics began appearing with regularity in the large public maternity clinics of Europe. In the late eighteenth and early nineteenth centuries, various English and American obstetricians concluded that puerperal fever was sometimes contagious. Alexander Gordon and Oliver Wendell Holmes argued that physicians transmitted the disease from one patient to another, and they recommended measures to limit such accidents. By the early nineteenth century, the disease was responsible for mortality of 5–20 percent of maternity patients in most major European hospitals. Smaller hospitals had outbreaks in which, over several months, 70–100 percent of maternity patients died. The etiology of puerperal fever was unclear, although seasonal patterns and high incidence in maternity clinics suggested that it resulted from a local poison conveyed through the atmosphere. By the middle of the nineteenth century, the disease attracted much attention in medical literature, and cases were reported worldwide.

In 1847, Ignaz Semmelweis became assistant in the Vienna maternity clinic. Incidence of puerperal fever in the Vienna hospital was about 7 percent, which compared favorably with other hospitals around Europe. However, the Vienna clinic consisted of two divisions, one for obstetricians and the other for midwives; the former consistently had a mortality rate three to five times greater than the latter. After months of investigation, Semmelweis concluded that the difference was caused by decaying organic matter (usually from autopsied corpses) conveyed to patients in the first division on the hands of medical personnel. He introduced washing in a chlorine solution for decontamination, and mortality in the first clinic dropped below that in the second. However, incidence of the disease had always been seasonal, and most obstetricians were unpersuaded.

By 1850, Semmelweis was convinced that decaying organic matter caused all cases of puerperal fever – even the relatively few occurring in the second clinic. Indeed, he provided an etiologic characterization of puerperal fever in which it became true by definition that all cases of the disease resulted from contamination. Given Semmelweis's definition, it also followed that puerperal fever was not a unique disease but only a form of sepsis. Semmelweis had virtually no evidence for this position. His critics cited cases of women dying from puerperal fever without any exposure to decaying organic matter. Semmelweis responded that in such cases the decaying matter was produced internally, perhaps by decomposition of blood or placental fragments. Even physicians who accepted his initial results rejected this bold and apparently unwarranted claim.

By the 1860s, Louis Pasteur's work on fermentation and putrefaction heralded the possible significance of microorganisms in disease processes. Building on Pasteur's work, and certainly aware of Semmelweis's theories, Carl Mayrhofer examined vaginal discharges from more than 100 patients at the Vienna maternity clinic. In 1865, he described various microorganisms that appeared only in discharges from puerperal fever victims. Using the techniques he had available, Mayrhofer isolated these organisms, cultured them in solutions of sugar, ammonia, and water, and then reproduced the disease by introducing the organisms into healthy test animals.

Mayrhofer's work was unimpressive to his Vienna colleagues but received considerable attention in Berlin. Within a few years, many investigators pursued the discoveries of Semmelweis and Mayrhofer, studying the microorganisms identified in puerperal fever and other forms of sepsis. Through the middle decades of the nineteenth century, most of those who wrote about wound infections, including Edwin Klebs, Robert Koch, and Pasteur, gave prominence to puerperal fever. In 1879, Pasteur identified the streptococci that principally caused the disease. By this time, it was apparent that puerperal fever was actually a form of sepsis. In this sense, therefore, puerperal fever ceased to exist as a diagnostic or theoretical entity.

Studies in the early twentieth century led to serologic classification of streptococci and to recognition that group A strains were the most prevalent agents in puerperal fever. Group B streptococci were first reported in puerperal sepsis in 1935 and in recent decades have displaced group A strains as the most prominent agents in puerperal sepsis in the United States and Britain. Infections of group A streptococci are generally exogenous and affect puerperae, whereas infections of group B pathogens are usually endogenous and, although the mother may be affected, generally strike the fetus or neonate. The change has had important ramifications in clinical manifestations, prophylaxis, and therapy. Development of antibacterial agents has obviously revolutionized the management of puerperal sepsis. Improved care for delivering mothers has also had an important impact, and liberalization of abortion laws has reduced incidence of puerperal sepsis associated with illegal abortions. However, control of sepsis is now recognized as more difficult and complex than previously believed; it remains particularly difficult in Third World countries, where medical care is not readily available. Therefore, although incidence of puerperal sepsis has been dramatically reduced, the various forms of this disorder continue to be a leading cause of maternal and neonatal death throughout the world.

K. Codell Carter

117. Q Fever

The "Q" in **Q fever** stands for "query," the designation applied by E. H. Derrick to an acute illness with fever and severe headache of unknown cause occurring in abattoir workers and dairy farmers in Queensland, Australia, in 1935. Despite the discovery of the causative agent, a rickettsia-like organism, this unenlightening name has remained current, although an alternative is **abattoir fever**. Q fever, occurring in epidemics in military personnel stationed in the Balkans and Italy during World War II, was known as "Balkan influenza" or "Balkan grippe."

Q fever is caused by infection with *Coxiella burnetii*, the sole member of genus *Coxiella*, family Rickettsiaceae. It was initially confused with viruses, but though *C. burnetii* is an intracellular parasite, it has a true bacterial cell wall.

Q fever is a zoonosis of worldwide distribution. Many animals, birds, ticks, and other insects are natural hosts. In animals, naturally acquired infection appears to be asymptomatic. Transmission to humans occurs via inhalation of contaminated dust while infected animals, carcasses, or animal products are being handled; via laboratory accidents; and sometimes via tick bite or consumption of unpasteurized milk. Asymptomatic infection is common. Illness may take two forms. **Acute Q fever** is usually a self-limiting febrile flu-like illness or atypical **pneumonia** lasting up to 4 weeks. Untreated, mortality is less than 1 percent. **Chronic Q fever** presents as **endocarditis** and/or **hepatitis**. Endocarditis usually occurs in those with preexisting **heart-valve disease**; untreated, it is usually fatal.

Characteristics

The distribution of acute Q fever is worldwide, but chronic Q fever appears more limited, most cases being reported from Britain, Australia, and Ireland. Surveys of British livestock suggest that 3–5 percent of dairy cattle and 2–6 percent of sheep are infected. In other countries, it is still rare, which may result from underdiagnosis or perhaps differences in strain virulence. Acute

Q fever affects predominantly adult men, and association with farmers, abattoir workers, and veterinarians is well recognized. Q fever often occurs in seasonal spring and autumn peaks associated with lambing and calving.

In the United States, Q fever was recognized as endemic in dairy herds throughout the country by 1960. Reports of human cases were uncommon but increased steadily from 1948 to 1977. Over this period, 1,164 cases were reported to the Centers for Disease Control and Prevention. Fully 67 percent of cases occurred in California, which has a high prevalence of infection in cattle and consequently a high proportion of cattle excreting organisms in milk.

Coxiellae differ from other rickettsiae in not needing an arthropod vector for transmission. Two cycles of natural infection have been recognized. In the wildlife cycle, transmission between wild animals and birds occurs from tick bites, from inhalation of dust, and possibly (in carnivores) from ingestion of infected placentas and meat. Ticks are infected from the blood of an infected host, but transovarial spread has also been documented. Coxiellae multiply in the tick gut and salivary gland, and transmission occurs by biting or when tick feces contaminate broken skin. In the domestic animal cycle and in human infection, tick-borne infection is less important, and transmission occurs usually from inhalation of contaminated dust and possibly from direct contact with infected animals. Cows, sheep, and goats are the main reservoirs for human infection. In these animals, coxiellae localize in the genital tract and udder and are excreted in vast numbers in milk, birth fluids, and placentas without usually causing disease or decreased milk yields in cows, although abortion may occur in sheep and goats. Investigations have also implicated rabbits and parturient cats as possible sources of human infection.

Coxiellae are very resistant to environmental conditions, surviving for months or years in dust and animal litter. Experiments have shown that they can survive – among other harsh conditions – temperatures of 63°C for up to 30 minutes, an observation of importance because it places coxiellae at the border of resistance to high-temperature/brief-interval milk pasteurization. However, some experts dispute whether symptomatic Q fever can be acquired from drinking contaminated milk, although antibody prevalence is raised in raw milk drinkers. Person-to-person spread has been documented but is unusual.

The vast number of organisms excreted by infected animals, their dissemination in dust by wind, their hardy nature, and the low infective dose for humans (said to be one organism) explain a characteristic feature of Q fever – the occurrence of explosive, localized outbreaks often without an obvious source of infection. Moreover, even when the source of infection is identified, such as sheep used in medical research institutions, human cases occur in people only indirectly exposed by being in the vicinity of the animals.

Subclinical infection is common. Only 191 of 415 newly infected persons were symptomatic in an outbreak in Switzerland in 1983, caused when infected sheep were driven from mountain pastures through several villages on the way to market. The clinical features of acute Q fever are similar to other infectious agents. Illness begins 2–4 weeks after exposure, with incubation possibly varying with the dose. There is sudden onset of fever, sweating, shivering, rigors, malaise, joint and limb pains, severe frontal headache, retro-orbital pain and photophobia, and a mild nonproductive cough. Rash is uncommon. Untreated fever usually lasts 1–2 weeks, but pneumonia may persist considerably longer. **Jaundice** is less common, and severe respiratory symptoms are unusual. Rarer complications of acute Q fever are **meningoencephalitis, cerebellar ataxia**, coma, **myocarditis, pericarditis**, infiltration of bone marrow by granulomas leading to **marrow failure, orchitis**, and **placentitis**. There may be **splenomegaly** and **lymphocytosis**.

Chronic Q fever is usually considered a rare occurrence, particularly but not exclusively affecting patients with preexisting aortic or mitral valve malformations or disease and occurring months to years after acute infection. However, the lack of a history of acute illness or preexisting heart-valve disease or exposure to infection does not exclude the possibility of chronic Q fever. Illness begins as a low-grade fever with night sweats, **anemia**, joint pains, finger clubbing, heart murmur, and developing heart failure. There is usually **hepatosplenomegaly**. Coxiellae can be isolated from vegetations on damaged or prosthetic heart valves. Abnormal liver function tests are usual, and chronic Q fever may sometimes present as chronic liver disease.

Acute Q fever can be treated successfully, but chronic Q fever is difficult to treat. Eventually, heart-valve replacement may be unavoidable. Reinfection of prosthetic valves has been described, possibly occurring as a result of persistent extracardiac infection.

History

In 1935, E. H. Derrick investigated an outbreak of a febrile illness among meat workers in Australia. In 1937, he published the first report of a new disease that he called Q fever. He went on to show that guinea pigs could be infected by inoculating blood or urine from febrile patients and that extracts of guinea pig liver and spleen could transmit infection to other guinea pigs. In collaboration with Derrick, F. Burnet and Mavis Freeman searched for a virus in extracts of guinea pig liver using animal inoculation experiments and identified a rickettsia-like agent that was named *Rickettsia burnetii*. In 1938 in the United States, G. Davis and H. Cox reported an organism isolated from ticks collected in Montana, which they called *Rickettsia diaporica*. It was later proved to be identical to *R. burnetii*, and its infectivity for humans was unhappily demonstrated by laboratory-acquired infections. Cox showed that the Q fever agent differed significantly from other rickettsias, and it has been placed in a separate genus, *Coxiella*.

Derrick had speculated that transmission was via blood-sucking insects and that the organism had an animal reservoir; he identified the bandicoot as such a reservoir. However, the wildlife cycle has not proved a significant source of human infection. The domestic animal cycle is far more important and explained the epidemic of Q fever during and after World War II, when thousands of troops in the Balkans and Italy were infected.

The epidemic began in Yugoslavia in 1941 and involved more than 600 troops. Further outbreaks occurred in Yugoslavia, Crimea, Greece, Ukraine, and Corsica. Risk of illness was associated with sleeping on hay or straw. Further outbreaks in 1942, 1943, and 1944 were noted in German troops exposed to sheep and goat flocks. Following the Allied invasion of Italy, Allied troops shared the Q fever epidemic. In 1945, other outbreaks occurred in Italy, Greece, and Corsica.

The epidemics of Q fever were militarily significant. The attack rate among exposed troops was very high and illness was prolonged. For example, of 160 men billeting in a hay barn, 53 (33 percent) developed Q fever. Of 900 men on a training exercise, which included sitting in a barn loft to watch training films, 267 (30 percent) became ill. After the war, outbreaks occurred from 1946 to 1956 among Greek and Swiss troops, in 1951 among U.S. servicemen in Libya, and in 1955 among French soldiers in Algeria. Factors contributing to epidemics among troops were the sudden exposure of susceptible people to infection, particularly by sleeping on straw and hay (the local indigenous population was apparently unaffected), the rapid movement of flocks during wartime, and the mixing of infected and uninfected flocks. This was well illustrated in 1974–75 on Cyprus. An outbreak of abortion affected sheep and goats herded together to escape the Turkish invasion. In a nearby camp, 78 British soldiers developed Q fever.

The importance of domestic animals as the reservoir for human infection was further emphasized by outbreaks in the United States, where the first naturally acquired cases were reported in 1941 in Montana. In March 1946, 55 of 132 livestock and meat handlers in a plant in Texas developed Q fever, and 2 died.

In August of the same year, a similar outbreak occurred in Chicago. Further studies revealed sporadic cases, particularly in California. During outbreaks that occurred in 1947, city residents living near dairy farms were infected, probably by dust carried in the wind.

Laboratory-acquired infection was one of the earliest problems caused by Q fever. During 1938–55, 22 incidents involving more than 250 cases were recorded. In one military institution, 50 cases were recorded during 1950–65. In 1940, an outbreak occurred in the U.S. National Institutes of Health in which 15 workers were infected. In this and other laboratory-associated incidents, infections occurred not only in those directly handling the organism but also in those who worked near or walked through the laboratory buildings, an observation that emphasized the importance of the respiratory route of infection. In the 1970s, attention was drawn to the serious risk of working on infected animals in research institutions, and interest in developing a safer and more effective vaccine was restimulated in the United States. In the 1980s, in both the United States and Britain, large outbreaks were associated with operative procedures on pregnant sheep.

The first vaccines for Q fever were developed principally to protect laboratory workers from infection. Used in the late 1940s and early 1950s, they had the drawback of provoking severe skin reactions. In 1956, the unique phenomenon of *C. burnetii*'s phase variation was reported, which has proved of great value not only in diagnosing chronic Q fever but also in developing an effective vaccine. In the 1970s in Australia, an upsurge of infection in abattoir workers led to renewed efforts in vaccine development.

Following the original work in Australia, the United States, and the Mediterranean area, many other countries quickly identified cases. Surveys by the World Health Organization revealed that by 1956, 51 countries on all continents were infected. Only Scandinavia, Ireland, New Zealand, and the Netherlands were said to be free of infection. Since then, in Ireland

there is good evidence that infection was introduced through importation of infected sheep from England in the 1960s, with the first indigenous cases being identified, retrospectively, in 1962. Today Q fever is known to be global in distribution, and it is likely that any patchiness in distribution reflects as much the differing levels of awareness of the disease as differences in disease incidence.

S. R. Palmer

118. Rabies

Rabies is a viral inflammation of the brain and spinal cord of humans and other mammals. The disease is nearly always transmitted to humans in the saliva of biting animals and is almost invariably fatal. The terms "hydrophobia" and *la rage* illustrate two common symptoms.

Characteristics

Rabies occurs in Africa, Asia, the Americas, and most of Europe. It has never occurred in, or has been eliminated from, Britain, Ireland, Sweden, Norway, Japan, Australia, New Zealand, Hawaii, and many islands in the Pacific and Caribbean. Rabies is a disease of wild carnivores, particularly canids such as foxes, wolves, jackals, and coyotes. Skunks and raccoons are also common hosts, as are bats. Virtually any mammal can contract the disease when bitten by an infected animal. Domestic dogs are the major threat to humans; cats are a growing danger in North America. Cattle, horses, sheep, and other livestock may also be affected, but **bovine rabies** and **equine rabies** usually pose little danger for humans.

Rabies is relatively uncommon in humans, occurring sporadically as isolated cases or in small clusters. Persons working alone in remote areas are vulnerable to attack by infected animals. Wolves are especially dangerous because their size and strength allow them to inflict multiple bites. Most human cases result from the bites of "mad dogs," which were themselves victims of such attacks by feral animals. Vampire bats in parts of South America are a source of rabies in cattle and occasionally humans. Other bats can infect people and animals, but this is uncommon.

Human rabies has become a rare disease in developed countries. There were 236 cases in the United States in 1946–65. No cases at all have been reported in many of the subsequent years. Canada reported only 21 cases in 1924–86, but Mexico recorded 157 fatalities in 1985–86. In Africa, Ghana had 102 cases in 1977–81, whereas Ethiopia had 412 in 1982. In the early 1980s, India reported the highest annual number of cases (20,000) as well as the highest rate of infection – 28.8 per million individuals.

Rabies is caused by a virus of the rhabdovirus group. Large concentrations of virus are present in the saliva of sick animals. The virus is neurotrophic; it migrates along nerves to the brain, where it multiplies, causing grave damage manifested in part by behavioral changes.

Rabies circulates primarily in wild carnivores and only incidentally attacks domestic ones. Humans are accidental and terminal hosts. The spread of rabies in skunks and raccoons, two species that have adapted with great success to suburban habitats, has caused concern in the United States, but thus far no human cases have occurred.

In the wild, rabies tends to occur in irregular waves and may spread over thousands of miles in a few decades. Control of rabies by population reduction is generally unsuccessful, and vaccines for wild mammals are still experimental. Monitoring reservoir hosts can alert public-health authorities to possible cases among dogs and cats and provide warning of wild animals. In the United States, where **canine rabies** steadily declined for decades, cases in cats began to exceed cases in dogs in 1980, resulting in widespread campaigns to vaccinate felines.

Animals exhibit either **furious rabies**, with agitated, aggressive behavior preceding paralysis and death, or **dumb rabies**, with lethargy and progressive immobility. The classic "mad

dog" (foaming at the mouth and wandering the streets) does exist, but not all sick dogs display such dramatic symptoms. In northern Canada, rabid foxes and wolves may become "crazy," invading settlements, mingling with sled dogs, and attacking dogs or their owners. Nocturnal animals like skunks and raccoons may wander through inhabited areas in daytime and exhibit little fear of people or other animals. Unfortunately, such abnormal behavior can deceive; many people have undergone a series of rabies shots after handling "friendly" raccoons.

Although people commonly contract rabies via virus-laden saliva, two other mechanisms have been reported: inhalation of virus in dust and contamination in surgery. High concentrations of virus may occur in dust in bat-populated caves, and spelunkers have died of rabies after inhaling the virus. Laboratory inhalation of virus-laden aerosols has also caused infections. Cornea transplants from undiagnosed rabies victims have caused at least two deaths, but immunologic testing of donors should prevent future incidents.

If infected saliva enters a break in the skin, viruses are carried from the wound through the nerves to the brain. Incubation takes up to 16 weeks, depending on severity and location of the wound and the size of the viral inoculation. Severe bites on the face and head are the most dangerous and have the shortest incubation periods, because the virus does not have far to travel. Infection results in destruction of cells in the brain and spinal cord and damage to the myelin sheaths of nerves. Clumps of viruses (called "Negri bodies") are often seen on microscopic examination.

Rabies patients show restless, agitated behavior and hypersensitivity, becoming apprehensive or aggressive shortly after onset. Convulsions and excessive salivation are common. Patients often suffer intense thirst but have severe muscle spasms in the throat when they attempt to drink. This frequently develops into extreme hydrophobia, with the sight or even mention of liquids inducing terror and spasms. Within days, this "furious" phase is followed by depression, paralysis, and death. The gruesome symptoms and inevitability of death make rabies one of the most frightening diseases.

There have been a handful of reports of survivors, but even the most intensive supportive care is generally futile, and there are no specific drugs or other therapies. Prevention is the only solution. Vaccinating dogs and cats, controlling strays, monitoring wildlife populations, and education are all essential. A preexposure human vaccine is available for persons at special risk, such as game wardens, veterinarians, and laboratory workers.

Fortunately, persons bitten by a rabid animal can be effectively vaccinated before the disease completes its long incubation period. If the biting animal is rabid, or if grounds exist to suspect it is rabid, prompt treatment is essential. Cleansing of the wound to remove as much virus as possible is followed by injections of a serum containing preformed antibodies to the virus. The key measure, a series of shots with a specific vaccine, is then begun.

In the 1880s, Louis Pasteur developed the earliest vaccines using rabbit spinal-cord tissue. Brain tissue of sheep, goats, or mice is used in some developing countries but is being replaced because it can cause allergic reactions. Duck-embryo cultures were used until human diploid cell vaccine was developed in the late 1970s. This vaccine is cheaper, safer, and requires fewer injections. An improved vaccine was released in the United States in 1988.

History

Rabies possibly was described in Mesopotamian texts as early as 2300 B.C., and it was well known to ancient writers from China to Rome. The first certain reference in Chinese texts dates from the sixth century B.C., and the disease is described in a first century Indian text. Rabies is also mentioned in ancient Greek literature including works by Euripides, Xenophon, and perhaps Homer. Aristotle described rabies in dogs and other animals in his *History of Animals*.

Roman writers of the first and second centuries, such as Dioscorides, Pliny, Galen, and especially Celsus, wrote extensively on rabies and established ideas about the disease that remained influential in European and Islamic medicine well into the eighteenth century. In accordance with prevailing humoral doctrines, it was believed that animals developed rabies from a "corruption of the humors" caused by factors such as stress, cold, heat, or poisoning. Their saliva became poisonous, and bites carried the "virus" to others. Like his contemporaries, Celsus described a wide array of internal and external remedies, none of which (based on modern knowledge) could have done any good but which lasted into the nineteenth century. Pliny's unfounded belief that a canine "tongue-worm" caused rabies lasted as long as the ideas of Celsus.

Rabies interested many writers after the fall of Rome and into medieval times. Jewish authorities wrote about rabies in the *Talmud*. Christian writers in the West and the Byzantine Empire followed the humoral theories of classical times. Islamic authorities such as Rhazes in the tenth century and Avicenna in the eleventh also worked in the humoral tradition and were strongly influenced by Celsus. Avicenna gave good accounts of rabies in dogs, wolves, foxes, and jackals.

As in most medical matters, commentators in medieval Europe had little to add to ancient and Islamic writers. In the thirteenth century, Arnold of Villanova wrote wrongly that dogs became rabid after eating corpses, but he rightly stressed the thorough washing of bite wounds. Once symptoms appeared, many persons resorted to religious healing. In Western Europe, pilgrimages and prayers were directed toward Saint Hubert, patron of hunters. Other saints were invoked elsewhere in Europe and among the Coptic Christians of Egypt.

Early modern medical authorities had little to add. Girolamo Fracastoro, sometimes hailed as a sixteenth-century forerunner of germ theorists, considered rabies one of many diseases caused by "seminaria," something more like a seed or a self-replicating poison than a microorganism. Sixteenth-century French surgeon Ambroise Paré gave a good clinical description and recognized central nervous system involvement.

Perhaps because the disease was more common or because of the growing volume of medical research, literature on rabies became much more abundant in the eighteenth century. Autopsy studies were performed (although without results, as the lesions are microscopic) and many case reports published. The growth of literature was especially notable in France, where considerable interest in rabies existed. About 1750, many physicians believed in "spontaneous" rabies. But within a few decades it was recognized that rabies resulted only from bites of rabid animals and that not all such bites transmitted the disease. Joseph-Ignace Guillotin, inventor of the guillotine, proposed an experimental approach: Condemned criminals would be bitten by mad dogs, whereupon trials of various remedies would be conducted on them.

This scheme was not adopted, but some important experiments occurred around the turn of the nineteenth century. English physician John Hunter proposed saliva inoculation experiments in the 1790s. Italian investigator Eusebio Valli claimed that gastric juice from frogs rendered the "virus" in saliva less virulent. The first saliva inoculation experiments are credited to German investigator Georg Gottfried Zinke, who was aware of Hunter's work and may have been inspired by it. In 1813, French researchers François Magendie and Gilbert Breschet infected dogs and other animals with saliva from a human rabies victim.

Nineteenth-century therapy, however, remained a hopeless melange of useless remedies, many inherited from ancient times. Doctors tried everything possible from drugs and purges to electric shock and immersion in the sea. Sedatives were often employed, and euthanasia may have been practiced.

Modern knowledge of rabies dates from the last half of the nineteenth century and is closely linked to the rise of experimental methodology and germ theory. Rabies was not common

enough to be a major public-health hazard, but it was spectacular enough to attract a fair amount of research. The work of French veterinarian Pierre-Victor Galtier was especially important. In 1879 he published experiments in which he maintained rabies in rabbits. The development of a vaccine was the climax of the career of another investigator, Louis Pasteur.

Pasteur published his first paper on rabies in 1881. Working with rabbits as advocated by Galtier, Pasteur used dried spinal-cord material as a source of infection. By 1884 he had developed a method of attenuating the still unknown agent in the material. The weakened infective agent was injected into dogs. Unlike fresh preparations, it did not cause sickness, but instead provided protection against injections of virulent virus.

The first human trials were conducted in 1885. Pasteur and his associates could not inject a human with the virus to test the vaccine, but rather had to treat a recent bite victim, hoping that the weakened virus in the vaccine would convey immunity before the virulent virus from the bite could cause disease. In July 1885, a 9-year-old boy – badly bitten by a rabid dog – was brought to Paris within 2 days of exposure. Doctors were convinced that he was infected, and Pasteur knew that death would supervene unless the new vaccine was effective. The boy was given serial injections of progressively fresher rabbit spinal-cord vaccine. He lived – and eventually became concierge at the Institut Pasteur. A second victim was treated successfully in October, and 350 others were inoculated over the next several months. Only one died – a girl who received vaccine over a month after exposure.

The treatment was a major breakthrough, causing a public sensation, and people bitten by rabid or suspicious animals flocked to Pasteur's laboratory from all over Europe. Success rates were consistently high, especially if vaccine was promptly administered and if wounds were not on the head. Even with a long train ride to delay treatment, 35 of 38 Russians who had been bitten by rabid wolves were saved. The French government promptly began to fund Pasteur's work, and his institute was expanded. His associates, notably Emile Roux, and others developed methods of vaccine production and treatment. Research suggested a route from the bite through the nerves to the brain, but this was not proven until well into the twentieth century.

In 1903, Adelchi Negri in Italy discovered microscopic bodies in nerve cells of rabid dogs. He thought they were protozoans. Although this proved erroneous, the "Negri bodies" became a useful sign. However, inoculation tests introduced in 1935 and serologic methods have largely replaced histological examination for Negri bodies as tests for rabies. The virus was first seen in 1962; electron microscope studies in 1965 showed that the Negri bodies were clumps of viruses and antibodies.

Rabies epidemics and epizootics are difficult to trace before the twentieth century. In Europe, most descriptions are of isolated cases or small outbreaks. In 1271, rabid wolves invaded towns in Franconia, attacking herds and flocks and killing 30 persons. There was a fox epizootic in Frankfurt in 1563. Rabies became more widespread in Western Europe during the eighteenth and nineteenth centuries, possibly because population growth caused greater contact between feral mammals and domestic dogs. In 1701 Nancy, France, was beset by rabies and enacted laws against stray dogs. Paris responded to rabies cases in 1725 with a leash law, and other European cities followed with similar ordinances. Such restraints, as well as campaigns to rid the streets of strays, were seldom strictly enforced until there was a rabies scare.

A widespread epizootic in 1719–28 involved France, Germany, Silesia, and Hungary, and many cases occurred in Britain in 1734–35. Rabies was common in greater London in 1759–62 and in France, Italy, and Spain in 1763. A major epizootic in French foxes in 1803 apparently lasted until the late 1830s and spread over Switzerland and much of Germany and Austria. Outbreaks among wolves, foxes, and dogs continued throughout the century and caused hundreds of human deaths.

Rabies declined in the twentieth century in wild and domestic animals as well as in humans. The disease was exterminated in Britain in 1922 and became rare throughout Western Europe. In the early 1940s, however, a fox epizootic developed in Poland and spread westward at a rate of 30–60 kilometers a year, reaching France in 1968. Denmark defended itself by intensive fox control in a belt of territory near the German border; Britain is still protected by the Channel.

The history of rabies on other continents is little known. Sporadic cases and scattered epidemics occurred in Ethiopia prior to the twentieth century, a pattern that must have been common in other African and Asian countries. Rabies did not exist in Australia or New Zealand prior to English colonization in 1788 and seems to have been absent from the Pacific islands as well.

The antiquity of rabies in the New World is unclear. It is possible that **bat rabies** existed in pre-Columbian times, and Arctic foxes and wolves could have carried the virus from Siberia to Alaska millennia ago. Oral traditions suggest that the Eskimos were aware of rabies long before European contact. However, early European sources do not mention rabies among the American fauna, and a 1579 Spanish work specifically denied its existence in the "Indies." The first accounts of the disease are from Mexico in 1709, Cuba in 1719, Barbados in 1741, Virginia in 1753, North Carolina in 1762, New England in 1768, Jamaica and Hispaniola in 1783, and Peru in 1803. Because rabies is such an obvious disease, at least when it afflicts domestic animals and people, and because it was so well known to both lay and medical observers, the absence of early reports could indicate that rabies, at least in temperate and tropical America, was a late biological importation from Europe.

Fox rabies was known in the eighteenth century, and the disease was widespread in North American wildlife populations in the nineteenth century. Rabid skunks were described in the Great Plains in the 1830s and in California in the 1850s. Most U.S. cases in the twentieth century were in dogs, but as canine rabies is in decline, greater attention has been given to wild animals.

Raccoon rabies was first described in 1936, and bat rabies, now recognized in 47 states, was detected in 1953. An epizootic among raccoons in Florida in 1955 spread northward into Georgia and South Carolina in the 1960s and 1970s. Sportsmen transported infected raccoons from this focus to the Virginia-West Virginia border in the mid-1970s; rabies has spread in both states and into Pennsylvania, Maryland, and Washington, DC.

Skunk rabies has been spreading slowly from two foci in the Midwest for several decades. Fox rabies is widespread in Appalachia. In Canada, an epizootic was recognized in the far north in 1947 but probably began in the 1930s or earlier. Foxes and wolves are the primary victims, and the epizootic has spread south into Ontario, Quebec, and the United States.

Wildlife rabies represents a potential threat to Europeans and North Americans, but vaccination of pets should prevent more than an occasional human case. In developing countries such as Mexico and India, canine rabies is a real danger, and little attention has been given to wildlife reservoirs of the virus.

K. David Patterson

119. Relapsing Fever

Relapsing fever is a disease characterized by one or more relapses after the primary febrile paroxysm has subsided. Various types of relapsing fever are caused by blood parasites of the *Borrelia* group. There are two chief forms of the disease: **endemic relapsing fever**, transmitted to humans by various ticks of the genus *Ornithodoros* and maintained among a variety of rodents; and **epidemic relapsing fever**, caused by a parasitic spirochete, *Borrelia recurrentis*, which is transmitted by human head and body lice. *B. recurrentis* is less virulent than the tick-borne forms. Under favorable conditions,

mortality is about 5 percent, but in times of distress, as in war or famine, it can reach 60–70 percent.

It is also known as **famine fever** and **tick fever**, and in the past as "yellow fever" (which it is not) because of associated **jaundice**. The term "relapsing fever" was first used by David Craigie in 1843. The disease often was, and is still, confused with **malaria** and **epidemic typhus**, whose symptoms are similar.

Characteristics

Tick-borne relapsing fever is normally contained between tick and rodent host; humans become affected only when they accidentally become involved in that relationship. For example, if human shelters such as log cabins attract rodents, they may in turn become tick habitats. Transmission of relapsing fever is through the infected saliva or coxal fluid of the tick, making it essentially a disease of locality. In the case of **louse-borne relapsing fever**, the only reservoir of *B. recurrentis* is humans, despite the fact that the disease is spread by lice, either in the bite, or by contact with the body fluids of the louse through scratching. The louse is infected by ingesting infected human blood; once infected, it remains so for the rest of its life, which is about 3 weeks. The infection is not congenital in the offspring. As in typhus fever, the febrile condition of the patient encourages the departure of lice because they are sensitive to temperature and, consequently, prefer the temperature of healthy persons.

Tick-borne relapsing fever tends to be more severe than the louse-borne variety, but both types vary greatly in severity and fatality. In 1912, for example, louse-borne relapsing fever was very severe in Indochina and India but very mild in Turkey and Egypt. There are also indications that levels of individual and residual immunity are important. Illustrative are *Borrelia* infections that are severe in European populations in North and East Africa but mild in the local populations. In West Africa, however, the disease is equally severe among Europeans and locals. Case fatality depends not only on the type of infection and availability of treatment but also on the individual's nutritional status and resilience. Thus, after World War II, adult fatalities from the disease averaged 8.5 percent among poorer classes but only 3.6 percent among the well-to-do. Children suffered the most, with death the outcome in 65 percent of cases.

Because mortality varies inversely with living conditions, louse-borne relapsing fever is a true famine fever, generally manifesting itself in times of distress, when overcrowding, diminished hygiene, and undernutrition encourage its spread and increase its deadliness. It is called "the most epidemic of the epidemic diseases," and it rarely occurs except as an epidemic. The factors involved in the survival of the disease between epidemics are still not fully understood.

Endemic foci of tick-borne relapsing fever exist in most parts of the world, but not Australia, New Zealand, and the Pacific islands. Louse-borne relapsing fever has been reported worldwide, but, since 1964, Ethiopia is the only country that has continuously reported large numbers of cases. Foci of the disease appear, however, to be present in other African countries.

As with tyhpus fever, there is a marked seasonal incidence coinciding with the winter months. Warm winter clothes (and in the past, deficient winter hygiene) favor the growth of louse populations, whereas rising heat and humidity in spring and summer cause lice to die.

After incubating some 5–8 days, the disease manifests itself suddenly, with shivering, headache, body pains, and high temperature. Nausea and vomiting are occasionally present. The spleen and liver are enlarged and tender; **bronchitis** is present in 40–60 percent of cases and jaundice in 20–60 percent. In cases with a favorable outcome, there is a crisis of 1–2 hours or longer within 3–9 days, followed by a fall in temperature. **Relapse**, shorter and less severe than the primary attack, follows in 11–15 days. A diminishing proportion of patients suffer up to four relapses. Not all cases relapse, however,

and in some epidemics no more than 50 percent of patients suffer relapse. Death results from liver damage, **lobar pneumonia, subarachnoid hemorrhage,** or rupture of the spleen.

The causal organisms are present in the blood during febrile attacks but absent in intermissions. After one or more relapses, the active immunity produced by the patient is sufficient to prevent further invasion of the blood by the spirochetes. It is doubtful, however, that this represents a true end of the disease for the patient. Rather it would seem that equilibrium is established between host and parasite, and like all equilibria is liable to disturbance.

History

The louse-borne form of relapsing fever was clinically distinguished from typhus and **typhoid** by William Jenner in 1849. Louse-borne relapsing fever was the first of the communicable diseases to have its causal organism identified, when Otto Obermeier made his observations of spirelli during the Berlin epidemic of 1867–68. The louse was identified as the vector in 1907 by F. Mackie, then working in India, and the epidemiology of the disease was finally worked out by Charles Nicolle and colleagues at the Institut Pasteur in Tunis between 1912 and 1932.

Moving back in time, Hippocrates described an apparent outbreak of relapsing fever on the island of Thassus, off Thrace, and it is possible that the **yellow fever** of seventh-century Europe may have been relapsing fever. The disease may also have been among those constituting the epidemics of **sweating sickness** that affected England in 1485–1551. There were probably a series of relapsing-fever epidemics in late eighteenth-century Gloucestershire, and the first reliable observation of the illness was recorded in Dublin by John Rutty in 1739. The disease was observed principally in Britain and Ireland before the mid-nineteenth century, when it became more active. An outbreak in Scotland in 1841 spread south into England, and from there to the United States. The disease was present, with typhus, in Ireland during the Great

Famine of 1846–50. Epidemics also occurred in Prussia (1846–48) and Russia (1864–65), which presaged repeated outbreaks in Germany and Russia during the remainder of the century.

Relapsing fever was reintroduced into the United States by Irish immigrants, resulting in outbreaks in Philadelphia in 1844 and 1869, and in New York in 1847 and 1871. There was an extensive epidemic in Finland in 1876–77. Egypt, Russia, central Europe, and Poland all suffered great epidemics during World War I, and widespread outbreaks occurred in Russia and central Europe in 1919–23. There were further outbreaks in the Middle East, notably in Egypt, after World War II. The disease was shown to be endemic in China along the Yangtse River in the 1930s, and its appearance in Korea after the Korean War suggests that a Chinese focus persists.

Since the 1950s, however, the major continuing focus of louse-borne relapsing fever has been in Africa. In 1910, it was present in Tunisia and Algeria; in 1921, a virulent outbreak appeared in North equatorial Africa and spread across the continent as far as Sudan. In 1943, a serious epidemic in North Africa spread into the eastern Mediterranean and Europe. From the 1950s, at least, the disease has had an endemic focus in Ethiopia, making excursions into neighboring Sudan.

Conditions in Ethiopia and Sudan during the past 10 years have not been conducive to the collection of satisfactory statistical information. Reports from the field, however, suggest a continuing low endemic prevalence of relapsing fever, while at the same time indicating confusion of the disease with malaria and typhus by fieldworkers. It seems likely, however, that any major epidemic escalation would have received attention, and thus fears of an epidemic escalation in Sudan have so far proved unfounded.

The history of tick-borne relapsing fever is less well documented, probably because of the local, nonepidemic character of the disease. It was first recognized in Africa in 1847, and in the United States soon after the West had been settled. Among recent recorded outbreaks are two from the western United States among people occupying tick-infested log cabins. The first took place at Browne Mountain in 1968; of 42 people, 11 became ill. The second – and the largest outbreak known in the Western Hemisphere – resulted in 62 cases on the north rim of the Grand Canyon in 1973.

Anne Hardy

120. Rheumatic Fever and Rheumatic Heart Disease

Rheumatic fever is a noncontagious disease characterized by febrile inflammation, primarily of articular and cardiac tissues, less frequently affecting the skin and brain. The cerebral manifestation (**Sydenham's chorea**) and the superficial manifestations (subcutaneous nodules and **erythema marginatum**) are limited to children and young adults. Rheumatic fever is caused by **streptococcal infection**, usually of the throat. Fever, joint pains, and **tachycardia** typically begin 1–3 weeks after onset of untreated **streptococcal pharyngitis**. However, only 0.1 to 3.0 percent of untreated bouts of this infection result in a first attack of rheumatic fever. Consequently, various largely unidentified factors must participate in initiating the immunologic pathogenesis of the disease.

First attacks of rheumatic fever can be prevented by timely treatment of the infection with antibiotics, but such treatment does not affect the disease once it has begun. Rheumatic fever recurs only as a result of a new infection with a pathogenic strain. Antibiotics diminish but do not eradicate recurrences. The shorter the interval since the previous bout, the greater is the likelihood that a new attack will occur. An infection occuring within 2 years of an attack has a 20–25 percent chance of inducing recurrence. If the first attack spares the heart, a recurrence usually spares it too, but if the heart has been involved, a second bout will likely result in greater damage. Attacks of rheumatic fever usually last several weeks but are rarely fatal. Death usually results from chronic heart failure caused by **heart-valve damage**. In about half the cases, **rheumatic heart disease** develops in the absence of any history of acute rheumatic fever, the infection having slightly initiated the pathogenic immunologic mechanism in the heart.

History

The symptoms of rheumatic fever were first described separately, their relationships not being recognized until the nineteenth century. Thomas Sydenham in 1685 distinguished an acute, febrile **polyarthritis** from **gout**. One year later, he described as "Saint Vitus' dance" the neurological disorder now called Sydenham's chorea. In 1839, Richard Bright connected the condition with rheumatic fever.

In 1797, Matthew Baillie of London noted thickened heart valves in patients with acute **rheumatism**. In 1809, David Dundas, surgeon to George III, described nine cases of "a peculiar disease of the heart." Four years later, William C. Wells published 16 cases of "rheumatism of the heart" (median age 15 years).

Before the introduction of auscultation by René T. Laennec in 1818, rheumatic heart disease was recognized from abnormal pulse and respiration, with fever and joint pain. Laennec described murmurs caused by **heart-valve deformities**. In 1835, James Hope also described **heart-valve murmurs** and concluded that rheumatic fever is the most frequent cause.

In the 1870s, bacteriologic studies were made on blood and joint fluid aspirates. This approach was justified in 1883 by demonstration of the cause of **gonococcal arthritis**. The normal bacterial flora of the throat was not understood, yet contrary to most investigators of the time, a Berlin physician concluded that rheumatic fever must be caused not by a specific microbe but by a peculiar reactivity of susceptible individuals.

In 1916, Homer F. Swift of New York began investigating rheumatic fever. By 1928, he had concluded that an allergic response to repeated streptococcal infections was the most likely cause. Investigations begun by Alvin F. Coburn in New York in the mid-1920s resulted

in the extension of Swift's conclusions and identified the pathogen as the hemolytic streptococcus, serologic type A. The hypothesis that the disease is mediated immunologically was supported by the discovery by E. W. Todd in London of antibodies to streptococci in the blood of rheumatic fever patients.

In the 1880s, it was estimated in London that about 20 percent of patients without symptoms or history of rheumatic fever who were admitted to a hospital for any reason had a sibling or parent who had had rheumatic fever; such familial cases were present in about 35 percent of the patients who were hospitalized because of rheumatic fever. It was also noted in a medical survey that rheumatic fever's greatest prevalence was among the lower classes. The occurrence of multiple cases in a family was at first attributed to inheritance. But as bacteriologic studies expanded, researchers realized that both familial occurrence and the association with poverty could best be explained by the easier spread of an infectious agent in crowded living conditions. (Several modern investigations, however, have suggested that there is a heritable factor that influences susceptibility to rheumatic fever.)

During World War I, crowded living conditions gained further attention because of the prevalence of the disease in military encampments. Between April 1917 and December 1919, for example, 24,770 U.S. soldiers, representing 27 percent of all rheumatologic cases, were diagnosed with rheumatic fever.

The development of epidemiological data about rheumatic fever has been difficult because the acute phase of the disease may be brief or actually imperceptible, so that it may be recognized only from findings of **valvular heart disease**, perhaps years later in an uncertain proportion of the cases. This problem began to be addressed in 1943 by the Cardiovascular Diseases Subcommittee of the National Research Council. Boston cardiologist T. Duckett Jones devised a set of five "major" and seven "minor" criteria for diagnosis. These criteria received international acceptance quite rapidly.

Greater understanding of the causes and effects of rheumatic fever did not immediately affect its treatment because there was no way to eradicate streptococcal infection. Eventually, sulfanilamide was found to prevent recurrences. Penicillin became available in 1945 and quickly proved to be safer and more reliable.

London physician G. B. Longstaff may have been the first to suggest (in 1905) that the prevalence of rheumatic fever was decreasing. Numerous studies over more than a century of data (beginning in the 1880s) in Britain and the United States have confirmed this decline but not explained it. Interestingly, the major declines in morbidity and mortality from rheumatic fever took place before the advent of antibiotics. In the latter half of the twentieth century, such decreases continued at a lesser – albeit still impressive – rate. In the United States, for example, reported incidence of rheumatic fever declined from 10,470 cases in 1961 to 2,793 cases in 1971 and 264 cases in 1981.

Characteristics

Rheumatic fever was at first thought to be rare in the tropics, as judged by English observations from India and Malaya in the nineteenth century. But these observations are somewhat perplexing, for beginning in 1925 many cases of rheumatic heart disease were reported from tropical India. Nevertheless, rheumatic fever has been found to occur less frequently in tropical than in temperate regions despite the fact that poverty is in general more prevalent in the tropics. Climate may be a factor, as a north-to-south declining gradient of rheumatic fever within the United States, suggested during the 1920s, has been confirmed by numerous studies. Moreover, a similar gradient has been reported from China, and an altitude gradient has been demonstrated in Kenya and in Mexico. In both countries, there was significantly more disease in the more temperate highlands.

The "classical" manifestations of rheumatic fever were described in northern Europe, and whether its acute manifestations differ in the tropics has long been debated. If one considers, however, the wide variation in acute manifestations of the disease in temperate regions, it seems doubtful that there are consistent biological differences in the presentation of rheumatic fever in the tropics. Some reported inconsistencies reflect selection biases, whereas others reflect over- or underdiagnosis. For example, the fact that virtually all patients in a series of cases from Nigeria and Uganda had **carditis** probably indicates that cases of lesser severity were simply not seen, rather than nonexistent.

The wide range of occurrence of **arthritis** in rheumatic fever cases may be attributed in part to the differentiation by some authors between objective signs of joint inflammation and mere **arthralgia**. Nevertheless, there can be striking differences in the occurrence of "arthritis," even when rigorous diagnostic criteria may be assumed. But the extreme variations in the occurrence of chorea – ranging from 2 to 52 percent – are the most inexplicable.

The relationship of subcutaneous nodules to carditis may indicate real geographic differences in disease expression. Nodules have occurred in 8–12 percent of several series of cases from temperate regions, whereas they have been less common in others and have consistently been rare in the tropics. In temperate climates, nodules are almost always associated with acute carditis and may be predictive of severe valve damage. In tropical areas there is a weaker association between the occurrence of nodules and carditis and a difference in valvular involvement, or at least this seems to be the case of India. There, carditis not only results in permanent valve injury more rapidly and is more likely to be acutely fatal, but it also has a peculiar tendency to cause pure **mitral stenosis**. Reports from other countries do not resolve the question of whether this finding represents an ethnic difference or is a result of delayed medical care.

The surgical treatment of rheumatically damaged heart valves began in the late 1940s when Dwight E. Harken in Boston performed the first successful mitral commissurotomy, a procedure improved by Charles P. Bailey of Philadelphia a year later. This was "closed" heart surgery. No attempt to repair a damaged valve was possible until an oxygenating system to bypass blood around the heart was developed. The first practical apparatus was employed by John W. Kirklin. The first valve operations to ameliorate **aortic insufficiency** and to correct **aortic stenosis** were performed in 1959, respectively, by Bailey and Donald G. Mulder of Los Angeles. The next technical phase was the replacement of an active valve. This began with the ball valve devised by Albert Starr and Lowell Edwards. Such plastic valves, however, tend to destroy red blood cells, and thus valves were developed with leaflets of pig, cattle, or sheep tissue. This type of prosthesis was first inserted to replace an aortic valve in 1965, and a mitral valve in 1967, both by A. Carpentier in Paris.

By 1983, tens of thousands of valve replacements were performed annually in the United States. However, the cause of the injury, particularly of the aortic valve, has gradually shifted from rheumatic to other varieties of heart disease.

Thomas G. Benedek

121. Rickets and Osteomalacia

Rickets and **osteomalacia** are diseases with multiple etiologies primarily related to abnormal metabolism of vitamin D and secondarily to calcium and phosphate metabolism. Of the many causes, by far the most important relate to **dietary vitamin D deficiency** and the activation of vitamin D precursors by the kidney and sunlight. Rickets and osteomalacia are characterized by a failure of normal mineralization of bone and epiphyseal cartilage resulting in skeletal deformity. Rickets occurs in growing infants and children, and both bone and epiphyseal cartilage are affected. Osteomalacia occurs in adults after closure of the epiphyses, and its manifestations are often much less prominent.

History

Historically, rickets was among the earliest diseases to be described. As early as 300 B.C., Lu-pu-wei described crooked legs and hunchback; however, these can occur with other disorders. More specifc references are found in the separate writings of three Chinese physicians of the seventh and eighth centuries A.D., including enlarged head, body wasting, pigeon breast, and delayed walking. In the tenth century, Chien-i, the father of Chinese pediatrics, described many cases of rickets.

In the second century A.D., Soranus of Ephesus mentioned characteristic deformities of the legs and spine in young children and remarked on the higher frequency in urban Rome compared to Greece. Slightly later, Galen's work included a description of skeletal deformities in infants and young children, particularly the knock-knee, bow leg, funnel-shaped chest, and pigeon breast seen in rickets. Sporadic and somewhat ambiguous references to the disease were made until the mid-seventeenth century, when the classic descriptions of Daniel Whistler and Francis Glisson appeared.

In 1645, Whistler published his medical thesis on rickets. Five years later, Glisson wrote the classic text on the subject, still unsurpassed as a clinical description of rickets. Both physicians considered the disorder of recent origin, and indeed the northern climate, crowded living conditions, and socioeconomic changes may have influenced its prevalence at that time. Glisson noted a number of cases affecting wealthy families, perhaps related to the use of swaddling clothes and the vitamin D-deficient diet of pap and starch.

The word "rickets" was first used in the London Bill of Mortality report for 1634. The derivation of the word has been a source of contention since that time. Possibilities include *rucket* in Dorset dialect, meaning "short of breath"; the verb *rucken*, meaning "to rock or reel"; the Middle English word *wricken*, denoting "to twist"; the Saxon word *rick*, meaning "heap" or "hump"; or the Norman word *riquets*, for hunchback. Glisson suggested the term **rachitis**, derived from the Greek word for "spine," and this term remains in use in many countries today.

Nearly 250 years passed before the specific role of vitamin D and its active metabolites was elucidated via biochemical studies. In 1908, L. Findlay reported inducing the disease in puppies raised in a confined, darkened space. A year later, Georg Schmorl demonstrated the striking seasonal variation of the disease by autopsy findings. In 1917, Alfred Hess and L. Unger described the prevention of rickets by cod liver oil or by ultraviolet irradiation. Shortly thereafter, a number of researchers, particularly Elmer McCollum's group, isolated vitamin D and related compounds. A better understanding of the exact mechanisms and conversion of vitamin D metabolism into more active forms was gained only since the mid-1960s.

Vitamin D is more accurately classified as a prohormone rather than a vitamin. It is formed by interaction of ultraviolet light with a cholesterol derivative in deep layers of the skin, but small amounts of vitamin D may also be derived from dietary sources such as dairy products and fish liver oils. Vitamin D is then hydroxylated – first in the liver and then again in the kidney. It acts upon the target organs, intestine, and bone to regulate serum calcium and phosphate levels and the mineralization of bone.

As a disease producing characteristic skeletal deformities, rickets can be traced back to antiquity by direct examination of the skeletal evidence. As expected, the disease was extremely rare in ancient Egypt. Only one or two possible cases have been described in skeletal remains from North and South America. Most reported examples of ancient rickets come from Europe. A few date back to Neolithic times in Norway, Sweden, and Denmark. Examples become more plentiful during the Middle Ages in cities across northern and central Europe, confirming the central role of inadequate sunlight in causing the disease.

Characteristics

As early as 1890, Theobald Palm gathered data worldwide and concluded that the main etiologic factor in rickets is lack of sunlight. It was much later before scientists linked the variable pigmentation in races of humans with the regulation of vitamin D synthesis. The processes of pigmentation and keratinization of the outer layer of skin (stratum corneum) directly affect the amount of solar ultraviolet radiation reaching the deeper stratum granulosum, where vitamin D is synthesized. White or depigmented skin of the northern latitudes allows maximum ultraviolet penetration. Black or heavily pigmented skin and Oriental or keratinized skin minimize ultraviolet penetration in southern latitudes to maintain vitamin D synthesis within physiological limits. Skin pigmentation or keratinization also plays a role in preventing sun-induced **skin cancer**, a problem among light-skinned people who move to sunnier climates.

Historically, rickets incidence increased with the rise of sunless, crowded urban centers as part of the Industrial Revolution. Indeed, rickets may, among other things, be considered an **air-pollution disease**, because factory-produced smog filters and decreases available ultraviolet light. In 1899, Theodor Escherich reported that in Vienna 97 percent of infants 9–15 months old had clinical evidence of rickets. An autopsy analysis in Dresden by Schmorl showed that 89 percent of children between 2 months and 4 years exhibited evidence of active or healed rickets. Similar high numbers were reported near the turn of the twentieth century for Oslo, Bergen, Berlin, Glasgow, Dublin, Belfast, Edinburgh, Paris, Florence, and Moscow. Some authorities noted a general decrease in rickets at higher altitudes in the Scottish Highlands and Swiss Alps, related to the increased ultraviolet component of solar radiation. However, cases became more numerous and severe at the highest altitudes, presumably related to the practice of keeping infants heavily bundled or indoors nearly year-round.

Large American cities also had a high prevalence of rickets. In 1900, John Morse estimated that 80 percent of all infants under 2 years old in Boston had rickets. Hess reported in 1921 that 75 percent of New York City children had clinical evidence of rickets. Martha Eliot found that 83 percent of infants under 8 months in New Haven had radiographic findings of mild rickets. L. Du Buys noted that rickets was widespread in New Orleans and that clinical manifestations were more marked in blacks than whites.

As **deficiency diseases** involving sunlight and diet, rickets and osteomalacia involve cultural and socioeconomic factors interacting with climate. In general, rickets is uncommon in sunny climates; however, even sun-rich areas may have rickets. For example, nearly 30 percent of children seen at an Ethiopian clinic had clinical evidence of rickets, primarily related to reduced breast-feeding and swaddling of infants to avoid the "evil eye." In many Muslim countries, the custom of *purdah* – the complete shielding of women and young children indoors or with veils – is a major factor in rickets and osteomalacia. A study of 1,482 Muslim girls aged 5–17 showed that 40 percent had evidence of rickets.

Among many Asian groups, the use of *chupatti* flour as a dietary staple also contributes to rickets prevalence. The high phytate content binds calcium and zinc, resulting in decreased intestinal absorption of these minerals. Moreover, the lignin component binds to bile salts and ingested vitamin D, decreasing their absorption. The use of *raghif*, an unleavened bread rich in phytates, is also a factor in osteomalacia among Bedouin women of childbearing age.

With the addition of synthetic vitamin D to dairy products and bread in the United States, there has been a dramatic decline in the incidence of rickets. Vitamin D supplementation is not practiced in Britain, and 9 percent of young children in Glasgow still had radiographic evidence of rickets in 1968. Osteomalacia among the elderly remains a significant public-health problem related to decreased sunlight exposure, intestinal malabsorption, poor diet, and decreased hydroxylation of vitamin D in liver and kidneys. Osteomalacia in combination with **osteoporosis** is an important factor in the occurrence of hip fracture among the elderly.

R. Ted Steinbock

122. Rickettsial Diseases

The **rickettsial diseases** have common characteristics and similar symptoms. The prototype is classic, louse-borne, **epidemic typhus fever**. Most other rickettsial diseases, originally described as "typhus-like," were differentiated from the classic disease during the twentieth century. Those in the genus *Rickettsia* are epidemic typhus, **murine typhus, Rocky Mountain spotted fever** and others of the spotted-fever group, and **scrub typhus** (*tsutsugamushi*). **Trench fever** and **Q fever** are also designated rickettsial diseases, but in recent decades, key differences between the rickettsiae and these two diseases have prompted their classification in separate genera.

Pathological rickettsiae were discovered early in the twentieth century and named after Howard Taylor Ricketts, who lost his life investigating typhus in Mexico after several years of fruitful research into Rocky Mountain spotted fever. Although smaller than most bacteria, rickettsiae are visible under the light microscope. Unlike common bacteria, they are obligate intracellular parasites – that is, they metabolize and multiply only inside living cells, a characteristic shared with viruses. For several decades, this combination of traits caused rickettsiae to be classified as organisms midway between bacteria and viruses. By the late 1960s, however, research revealed that they were true, if highly fastidious, bacteria.

Most rickettsial maladies are "diseases of nature," normally existing as infections of arthropods (insects, ticks, and mites) and their mammalian hosts. Humans are accidental intruders into the natural cycle. Like **bubonic plague** and **yellow fever**, the manifestations of infection are often more severe in humans than in the arthropods and mammals to which the organisms have adapted over eons. The geographic distribution of rickettsial diseases is linked to environments favorable to host arthropods, and the diseases tend to occupy "islands of infection" within favorable environments. This phenomenon has been attributed to ecological conditions (in the case of scrub typhus) and to antigenic incompatibility between pathogenic and nonpathogenic rickettsiae residing in the ovaries of female ticks (in the case of Rocky Mountain spotted fever).

The common clinical manifestations of these diseases reflect their pathological physiology as infections of the human circulatory system. The agents multiply inside endothelial cells lining small blood vessels. Affected cells become swollen and may impede blood flow. Electrolyte imbalance and capillary permeability establish a vicious circle that progresses to circulatory collapse in fatal cases. Blood seeping from capillaries into the skin causes the typical rash, and capillary blockage in the brain contributes to neurological symptoms. Since the introduction of broad-spectrum antibiotics in 1948, the rickettsial diseases are curable if diagnosed before progressing too far.

Victoria A. Harden

123. Rocky Mountain Spotted Fever and Related Diseases

Rocky Mountain spotted fever is an acute rickettsial disease transmitted by ticks and limited to the Western Hemisphere. Its major symptoms are similar to **epidemic typhus**, but its rash covers the entire body, including face, palms, and soles of the feet. Between 20 and 25 percent of untreated victims die, making it the most severe rickettsial infection in the Americas. First identified in the U.S. Rockies, its earliest name has remained even though it is inaccurate and even misleading.

Characteristics

The severity with which Rocky Mountain spotted fever treats its victims underscores its natural existence as an infection of ticks and their mammalian hosts. The microbe causing the disease, *Rickettsia rickettsii*, inhabits ixodid ("hardshell") ticks, apparently causing little harm to the host. Small mammals are susceptible to mild infection and may transmit it, but the principal way the organism is maintained in nature is in the eggs of ticks.

The Rocky Mountain wood tick (*Dermacentor andersoni*) and the American dog tick (*Dermacentor variabilis*) are the most common vectors in the United States, although the Lone Star tick (*Amblyomma americanum*) also transmits the disease in the south central and southeastern parts of the United States. Two other ticks (*Rhipicephalus sanguineus* and *Amblyomma cajennense*) carry the disease in Mexico, Central America, and South America. Usually, less than 5 percent of ticks are infective.

In the western United States, hikers and the like may become subjected to infection when traveling in tick-infested areas, especially during spring. In the East, where most cases now occur, changing land-use patterns have brought humans into the ticks' habitat. Suburban housing developments and the transformation of agricultural land into recreation areas are two examples.

Rocky Mountain spotted fever characteristically appears in "islands" of infection. During early research on a particularly virulent form in Montana's Bitterroot Valley, for example, investigators were baffled by the fact that Rocky Mountain spotted fever appeared on the west side of the Bitterroot River but not on the east side. Recently, Rocky Mountain Laboratory investigator Willy Burgdorfer has shown that this peculiar epidemiological occurrence is related to an antigenic "interference phenomenon." Nonpathogenic rickettsiae in the ovaries of ticks on the east side of the river "interfere" with the establishment of pathogenic rickettsiae in these tissues, thus preventing the pathogenic *R. rickettsii* from being passed on to the next generation of ticks.

Rocky Mountain spotted fever has been identified in Canada, the United States, Mexico, Costa Rica, Panama, Brazil, and Colombia. Before 1940, most cases were reported in the Rocky Mountains, but since then, cases in the U.S. Southeast and Southwest (sometimes called the "tick belt") have far outstripped those in the West. In the 1970s, incidence in the United States began rising, peaking with 1,192 cases in 1981. Oklahoma has the highest infection rate, whereas North Carolina reports the most cases. A few cases continue to occur in Canada. In Mexico and Central and South America, the disease is poorly reported.

After an incubation period of 3–12 days, typhus-like symptoms appear abruptly: headache, joint and back pains, prostration, and high fever. About the fourth day, the characteristic skin rash appears. Usually beginning on wrists and ankles, it spreads to cover the entire body. The fever continues 2–3 weeks, usually subsiding gradually. In fatal cases, neurological symptoms of deafness, delirium, and coma are accompanied by circulatory collapse and kidney failure. The rash may darken and spread, becoming almost black, and confluent in cases. These characteristics contributed to two early names: "black measles" and "blue disease."

If diagnosed early, Rocky Mountain spotted fever may be treated effectively with antibiotics. Patients at risk of dying are usually those not diagnosed in time for this treatment. At special risk are people who suffer from **glucose-6-phosphate-dehydrogenase (G6PD) deficiency**, a genetic disorder especially frequent in black males. Thus Rocky Mountain spotted fever mortality is significantly higher for black males than for the general population.

History

Rocky Mountain spotted fever as a specific disease entity is essentially twentieth century in origin. The first reports differentiating it from other fevers were published in the late 1890s. Travelers in western North America encoun-

tered a disease in the spring variously known as "trail typhus," "spotted fever," "spotted typhus," and other names. Mortality varied from under 5 percent in Idaho to approximately 70 percent in the Bitterroot Valley of western Montana.

In 1901, public outcry against the deadly disease in the Bitterroot Valley stimulated the newly created Montana State Board of Health to launch a scientific investigation. In 1902, pathologists suggested that the wood tick might be the vector of the disease, possibly caused by a protozoan. In 1906, Howard Ricketts of the University of Chicago and Walter King of the U.S. Public Health Service confirmed the tick as the vector. Ricketts continued the investigation, seeking a vaccine. In 1909, when Ricketts's funding was delayed in the Montana legislature, he began studying *tabardillo* (**Mexican typhus**). Tragically, he contracted typhus in Mexico and died in 1910.

Between 1910 and 1920, efforts focused on tick-eradication programs. Modeled on the program that had eliminated Texas cattle fever throughout the South, the campaign failed against Rocky Mountain spotted fever for two reasons. The Texas-cattle-fever tick was a one-host vector, whereas the Rocky Mountain wood tick chose different hosts for each stage in its life cycle, making control difficult. Second, cold spring weather in Montana interfered with livestock dipping when ticks emerged. In 1916, Burt Wolbach at Harvard University described the agent of Rocky Mountain spotted fever. Wolbach originally named it *Dermacentroxenus rickettsi*, the genus name after its vector and the species name after Ricketts. Taxonomists later classified it in the same genus with typhus germs, changing its name to *Rickettsia rickettsii*.

In 1921, the U.S. Public Health Service renewed efforts to prepare a vaccine against Rocky Mountain spotted fever. In 1924, Roscoe Spencer and Ralph Parker produced the first successful vaccine made from arthropod vectors. From 1925 through 1948, when effective antibiotics were introduced, the Spencer-Parker vaccine was the chief weapon against Rocky Mountain spotted fever.

In 1931, the disease was discovered in the eastern United States, and shortly thereafter, pockets of infection were identified in Brazil, Colombia, Mexico, Canada, and other areas of the Western Hemisphere. The original names of the disease underscored its "local" character. For example, it was called *febre maculosa brasiliera* but also "Sao Paulo typhus" in Brazil, "Tobia petechial fever" in Colombia, and *fiebre de Choix* as well as *fiebre manchada* in Mexico. Investigators suggested more appropriate names, such as **tick-borne typhus, tick spotted typhus, American spotted fever**, or **spotted fever**. None successfully supplanted "Rocky Mountain spotted fever."

After introduction of broad-spectrum antibiotics in 1948, Rocky Mountain spotted fever incidence in the United States dropped to about 250 cases per year, with only about 24 deaths. But beginning in 1969 and continuing through the 1970s, incidence rose inexorably. Although this phenomenon was not reported from other countries of the hemisphere, it *was* reported in the Mediterranean basin for **boutonneuse fever**, a related but milder spotted-fever disease. The increase in U.S. cases and deaths stimulated new research into diagnosis and prevention.

Unlike epidemic typhus, Rocky Mountain spotted fever poses no threat of epidemics; however, it is unlikely to be eradicated. If patients and physicians are alert to the possibility of infection during "tick season," effective therapy can avert unnecessary loss of life.

Other Diseases of the Spotted-Fever Group

Three other major tick-borne rickettsioses are known. These "spotted-fever group" maladies are usually mild and fatal only to aged or debilitated patients. All exhibit a distinctive **eschar**, or dark scab, that forms over the initial tick bite.

Boutonneuse fever, named for the button-like eschar, was the earliest to be identified. Described in North Africa in 1910, it has had many local names, including "Mediterranean spotted fever," *fièvre boutonneuse*, "Marseilles exanthematic fever," "Indian tick-typhus," "South African tick-bite fever," and "Italian eruptive

fever." Its usual agent is *Rickettsia conorii*. Several ticks transmit it; *R. sanguineus* is most common. Many Africans apparently gain immunity from childhood infection, for the disease is primarily seen in tourists and new residents. Boutonneuse fever is known from Africa throughout the Mediterranean basin and into India.

Siberian tick-typhus was first documented during the 1930s, when exploitation of Siberia's forests and steppes brought humans into the habitat of its vector ticks. Transmitted by several species of ixodid ticks, it may be far more widespread than reported statistics indicate. The agent is *Rickettsia siberica*. Known also as "North Asian tick-typhus," it is found in China and elsewhere in north Asia as well.

Queensland tick-typhus, caused by *Rickettsia australis*, was reported in North Queensland, Australia, in 1946. Its vector tick, *Ixodes holocyclus*, parasitizes marsupials and rodents. Forest and scrub areas in Queensland are risk areas, and in 1979 an urban focus was reported in Sydney.

A final member of the spotted-fever group, **rickettsialpox**, is unique in not being transmitted by ticks. In 1946, a disease resembling **chickenpox** and exhibiting an eschar was reported in a New York apartment building. New York investigators collaborated with the U.S. Public Health Service, and within 8 months the entire picture of the disease had been elucidated. The agent was a hitherto unknown rickettsia that inhabited the mite *Allodermanyssus sanguineus* (a parasite of the house mouse) and was named *Rickettsia akari*. In 1949–50, the illness was also identified in the Soviet Union and there called **vesicular rickettsiosis**.

Victoria A. Harden

124. Rubella

Rubella ("German measles," "3-day measles") is a common viral infectious disease, principally of children and young adults, with worldwide distribution, frequently characterized as a mild rash illness. Inapparent infection is common, occurring in as many as half the cases. Rubella has special significance when a woman contracts it in early pregnancy because fetal infection can ensue and result in **congenital rubella syndrome** (CRS). Rubella is a vaccine-preventable disease, but the vaccine is not yet widely used on a global basis.

Characteristics

Rubella is caused by the rubella virus, of the genus *Rubivirus*, which contains a single-stranded RNA genome. It is highly contagious, transmitted by contact with nose and throat secretions of infected persons, primarily by droplet spread. Infection also occurs by direct contact, indirect contact through freshly soiled articles, and airborne transmission. No reservoir other than humans exists, meaning that a continuous chain of susceptible contacts is necessary to sustain transmission. Communicability lasts from about 1 week before rash onset to at least 4 days after. Infants with congenital rubella, who may shed virus for many months after birth, are the only carriers. Rubella's incubation period from time of exposure to onset of rash is 16–18 days, with a range of 14–23 days.

In populated areas with no or low vaccination coverage, rubella is primarily an endemic disease of children with periodic epidemics. However, a significant proportion of adults remain susceptible. In remote isolated populations, rubella is not endemic and disease depends on introduction from outside, at which time epidemics may occur, affecting all persons born since the last epidemic. No evidence exists for a sex difference in incidence or severity, although more female cases may be reported because of concern about congenital rubella. No evidence exists for any racial difference in incidence or severity.

The risk of congenital rubella is related to gestational age at the time of maternal infection. Fetal or placental infection accompanies 85 percent of maternal infections during the first 8 weeks of pregnancy. Data from the last major epidemic in the United States, which occurred in 1964–65 and produced 20,000 infants with CRS, showed that the risk of defects was about 50 percent when mothers were infected during the first month of pregnancy, 22 percent during the second, 6 percent during the third, and about 1 percent during the fourth. Infection in the first 8 weeks of pregnancy also produces high rates of abortion and stillbirth.

Rubella has a global distribution. In populated areas where it is both endemic and epidemic, 80–90 percent of adults show evidence of prior infection. In remote populations where rubella is not endemic, a significant proportion of the population can be susceptible. In some countries, such as the United States and Britain, extensive vaccination and notification policies have caused impressive declines in reported cases of rubella and CRS.

Infants usually have a passive immunity to rubella because of maternal antibodies acquired transplacentally from immune mothers. This protects the infant from infection for 6–9 months, depending on the amount of maternal antibody acquired.

Rubella infection in both clinically apparent and inapparent cases induces lifelong immunity. Because a significant percentage of rubella infections are inapparent, persons may develop immunity without recognizing that they have been infected. A single dose of live attenuated rubella virus vaccine confers long-term, probably lifelong, immunity in approximately 95 percent of susceptible individuals.

The prodromal phase of postnatally acquired rubella usually occurs 1–5 days prior to rash onset but may be completely lacking, especially in children. Prodromal symptoms may include headache, low fever, malaise, **conjunctivitis**, mild **rhinitis**, and **lymphadenopathy** (most commonly tender swelling of the lymph nodes behind the ears and at the base of the skull). Next, a reddish, discrete rash, sometimes itchy, usually appears first on the face and then spreads to hands and feet. Although the progression, duration, and extent of the rash vary greatly, it typically covers the whole body within 24 hours and disappears completely by the end of the third day – hence the name 3-day measles.

Complications in postnatally acquired illness may include **arthritis** and **arthralgia**, which are more common in adults and women than in prepubertal children and men. Neurological involvement, including **encephalitis**, is rare.

In congenitally acquired rubella, the fetal infection may result in abortion, stillbirth, congenital malformations, or growth retardation. CRS results from inhibition of cell multiplication in the developing fetus and a chronic infective state that may persist many months after birth. Some consequences of fetal infection may not become apparent until years after birth. Common congenital abnormalities and active infective processes at birth include cataracts, deafness, central nervous system defects leading to **mental retardation**, structural defects of the heart and **myocarditis**, bone lesions, **pneumonitis**, and **hepatitis**.

History

Although it has been suggested that early Arabian physicians differentiated rubella as a form of measles known as *Hhamikah*, the disease appears to have been first described in 1619 by Daniel Sennert, who used the term *Rotheln* (*röteln*), attributing the name, which seems to have been popular in origin, to the red color of the rash. Two German physicians are credited with clinically describing rubella as a separate entity during the 1750s, and it continued to be called *Rotheln* by German investigators from the mid-eighteenth to the mid-nineteenth century. The early interest in the disease by German physicians apparently led to use of the term "German measles" in other countries. It has, however, also been suggested that the word may have actually been "germane" rather than "German," with derivations meaning "closely akin to." In other words, "germane measles" was intended to indicate a disease similiar to **measles**.

In 1866, Henry Veale proposed the name "rubella" for its ease of use in speech and writing. The International Congress of Medicine in 1881 reached a general consensus that rubella was an independent entity. During the next 60 years, medicine focused on the characteristics, symptomatology, and course of rubella, which was considered an inconsequential infection of childhood. In 1938, Y. Hiro and S. Tasaka established that rubella was caused by a transmissible virus.

Then, in 1941, Norman Gregg published his landmark observations of an epidemic of congenital cataracts and other ocular and cardiac abnormalities in infants whose mothers had contracted rubella in the first trimester of pregnancy. Although skepticism at first prevailed, Gregg was confirmed, and other congenital abnormalities associated with rubella in pregnancy were described. In 1953, researchers documented that rubella infection can occur without rash.

The rubella virus was isolated in 1962, leading to the hemagglutination-inhibition test introduced in 1967 and subsequent research and development of vaccines. In 1969, a live attenuated rubella virus vaccine was licensed for use in the United States, and shortly thereafter other strains were adopted for use in the United States and several European countries.

Robert J. Kim-Farley

125. Saint Anthony's Fire

This disease is associated with **ergotism**, which results from ingesting the ergot fungus that grows on rye. Most authorities assume that the name **Saint Anthony's fire** refers to Saint Anthony the Great, third-century hermit and founder of Christian ascetic monasticism, who renounced the world for the deserts of Egypt. However, Saint Anthony of Padua, born in the late twelfth century, may also be connected with the name of the disease. He was a noted preacher, popular for exorcising demons and restoring the insane to health.

Supposedly, the "fire" part of the name refers to the painful skin infections, **gangrene**, and neurological disturbances that occur with **ergot poisoning**. Thus, in French areas where rye was a staple, historians have attributed most cases of *mal des ardents* to ergotism. Sufferers reportedly lost limbs, attributable to gangrenous ergotism, if they survived both the initial inflammation and the generalized famine that accompanied such epidemics. Possibly, however, **erysipelas** and other bacterial skin infections caused the symptoms mentioned, for these diseases also flourish during famines.

Saint Anthony's fire was commonly described in Western Europe from 900 to 1700. During the eleventh century, recurrences of the "sacred fire" (usually associated with erysipelas in classical medicine) resulted in creation of hospitals and also appeals to interceding saints, of whom Anthony was only one. In France, however, Count Gerlin II acquired the relics of Saint Anthony the Great and in 1070 installed them in Vienne. By 1090, healing miracles were attributed to them, and local nobles and lay hospitalers formed a pilgrimage site for "fire" sufferers. By the twelfth century, this hospice was run by regular clergy called "friars of the blue Tau" after the Greek letter symbolizing Anthony iconographically. Wine or water steeped with the saint's bones was the miraculous cure, but food supplements at the hospice of Saint Anthony may have arrested **ergot intoxication**.

During the later Middle Ages, the cult of Saint Anthony spread beyond the regions of southern France and Savoy, where it had gained rapid popularity, through central Europe and into Russia. There, people commemorated cures with votive art that has come to symbolize the disease to posterity. The earliest unambiguous references to ergot fungus occur in the late sixteenth century; by the late seventeenth, ergotism was described independently. The older name – perhaps the older "disease" as well – rapidly disappeared from learned descriptions, partly because of the association of ergot fungus with epidemics of neurological disorders rather than the skin infections and gangrene that characterized "Saint Anthony's fire."

Ann G. Carmichael

126. Scarlet Fever

Scarlet fever is an acute infectious disease, caused by certain types of group A hemolytic streptococci. The disease is characterized by sore throat, fever, headache, and a rash. The term "scarlet fever" was supposedly first used by Thomas Sydenham in 1683, but it appeared in a diary of Samuel Pepys from 1664. From the seventeenth century to the early twentieth, **scarlatina** popularly denoted a mild form of the disease.

Characteristics

Like **streptococcal sore throat** – to which it is closely related – scarlet fever is a disease of temperate climates, prevailing generally in winter months. It occurs principally in young children, although adults may suffer sore throats as a result of the same infection.

Group A hemolytic streptococci are responsible for a range of afflictions other than scarlet fever, including **erysipelas, rheumatic fever**, and the sore throats known as **tonsillitis** in Britain and **pharyngitis** in the United States. Scarlet fever is caused only by certain strains that release a soluble toxin, whose absorption causes the disease's characteristic rash. Different strains of streptococci produce different amounts of toxin. Epidemics vary greatly in severity, with mortality ranging from 0 to 30 percent. Transmission of infection is by intimate contact, such as in overcrowded homes and classrooms. Evidence of airborne or droplet nuclei infection is slight. In the past, scarlet fever occasionally occurred as a hospital infection and was also transmitted in contaminated milk.

Susceptibility to the skin rash differs according to the immune and hypersensitivity status of the individual. Those who experience scarlet fever once are unlikely to do so again but remain vulnerable to streptococcal sore throats when exposed to a new serologic type. Research into susceptibility of different population groups suggests that more than half of young infants are immune to the disease, but by age 2 only some 20 percent remain so.

Thereafter the proportion of immune individuals rises steadily, reaching 77 percent at 10–15 years and 86 percent in adults. Rare second attacks of scarlet fever with rash probably result from a new antigenic erythrogenic toxin. Evidence suggests that the geographic dominance of particular strains of scarlet fever streptococci is long-term, varying from country to country and from time to time. With all types, the disease appears to follow a general pattern of alternate severity and mildness.

Initial symptoms of scarlet fever are similar to those of streptococcal sore throat: sudden onset of soreness on swallowing, fever, and headache. Vomiting and nausea are often early symptoms in young children. The characteristically erythematous and **punctuate rash** appears within 2 days, at first on the upper chest and back, then spreading to the rest of the body. In white patients, the rash does not commonly appear on the face, but in about half of black patients it does. The rash is accompanied by the characteristic "raspberry tongue." In general, the rash is variable in its manifestations. **Desquamation** usually occurs, beginning sometimes as early as the fifth day, sometimes as late as 4–5 weeks after disease onset. A range of complications, principally affecting young children, add to the dangers of the disease. These include **anemia, otitis media**, rheumatic fever, and **meningitis**. In rare cases, scarlet fever appears in severe septic or toxic forms.

History

It is possible that outbreaks of scarlet fever were observed by Near Eastern practitioners of the Arabian school, but the first undoubted account of a disease with a characteristic fiery rash was provided by Giovanni Ingrassia in 1553. The disease was apparently present in Germany and Italy in the early seventeenth century, and we know of a severe outbreak in Poland in 1625. At that time, the disease was variously known as *rossalia, purpurea epidemica maligna,* and *febris miliaria rubra.*

It is clear from observations by Daniel Sennert in 1619, Michael Düring in 1625, and Johann Schultes in 1665 that the scarlatinal manifestations of desquamation, **nephritis**, and **dropsy** were well known before the disease received its modern name. Although in 1683 Sydenham wrote of the disease as having a mild character, he nevertheless established its autonomy, distinguishing it from other acute **exanthema**. By the end of the seventeenth century, the identity of scarlet fever was well recognized, although much epidemiological confusion remained – and still remains – over the respective roles of scarlet fever, streptococcal sore throat, and **diphtheria** (*cynanche maligna*) in contemporaneous epidemics.

During the seventeenth and eighteenth centuries, scarlet fever was epidemic throughout Europe and the United States. It appeared in Copenhagen in 1677, in Scotland in 1684, in the United States in 1735, and in Sweden in 1744. In general, however, evidence suggests that the disease made irregular epidemic appearances, and its mortality varied considerably. During the early 1700s, it seems to have been fairly mild, but by midcentury a quite virulent strain also appears to have been present.

Scarlet fever's character as a relatively new disease may be reflected in age incidences reported during this period. Sydenham noted that it attacked whole families, though especially infants. Nils von Rosenstein observed in 1744 the simultaneous occurrence of sore throat without rash in children in infected households, a pattern observed in adults by Maxmilian Stoll in 1786. In the last years of the century, scarlet fever was extensive and virulent in Europe, with severe outbreaks in Denmark and Finland in 1776–78, and in central Germany in 1795–1805. By 1814 it was again very mild, but continued its global spread, appearing in Greenland in 1847, in Australia and New Zealand in 1848, and in South America in 1892.

During the 1820s and 1830s, however, a more virulent form reappeared, and consequently, the disease was the leading cause of death among infectious childhood maladies until 1875. During the 1880s, scarlet fever continued as widely prevalent but declined as a cause of death, and by the 1890s its character was again relatively mild, although not as mild as it has become today. The decline in severity was first apparent in Britain and Western Europe, although a malignant form was still present in Poland, Russia, and Romania during the 1930s. Observations by Edward Goodall showed that as fatality dwindled, so did the more serious clinical forms.

Streptococci were first isolated from the blood of scarlet fever patients by Edward Klein in 1887, but he failed to reproduce the disease in animals. In 1911, Karl Landsteiner produced a similar disease in monkeys with material from scarlet fever patients, but until about 1922 the streptococci were generally considered secondary invaders.

In the early 1920s, seminal work by George Dick and Gladys Dick proved scarlet fever to be primarily a local throat infection caused by type A hemolytic streptococci. In 1923, the Dicks successfully inoculated volunteers, and in 1924 they developed the Dick test: intradermal injection of a diluted filtrate of a scarlatinal strain of streptococcus, which by the resultant appearance or not of a local erythematous reaction, determines the subject's susceptibility to scarlet fever. In other words, a negative Dick test is an indication of antitoxic immunity.

Anne Hardy

127. Schistosomiasis

Schistosomiasis (also **bilharzia**), with many local names such as "red-water fever," "snail fever," "big-belly," and "Katayama disease," is an immunologic disease caused by eggs of blood-vessel-inhabiting worms of the genus *Schistosoma*. The eggs induce an immunologic response after being trapped in body organs, especially the liver, gut wall, and urogenital tract.

Three major human schistosome species exist. *Schistosoma haematobium* inhabits veins of the bladder area, and its eggs are discharged in the urine. *Schistosoma mansoni* and *Schistosoma japonicum* inhabit the mesenteric veins supplying the intestines. Their eggs are discharged in feces. However, the worms may also be found in the liver and portal system. A few other species also parasitize humans. Another name for the disease is bilharzia (or even **bilharziasis**, a technically unacceptable term) to honor Theodor Bilharz, discoverer of the **trematodes** causing it. But it is more accurately known – especially in America – as schistosomiasis, after its generic name *Schistosoma*.

Characteristics

Schistosomiasis has an almost worldwide tropical distribution but is absent from the Indian subcontinent. *S. haematobium* is endemic in the Nile Valley and is distributed about the Middle East and North Africa, West and central Africa, and along the East African coast from Somalia to Natal. *S. mansoni* is endemic in the Nile Delta and possibly spreading into the Nile Valley. In Africa, it has a similar (although irregular) distribution to that of *S. haematobium*, but *S. mansoni* also occurs in South America and the Caribbean. It was transported to the New World via the slave trade. *S. japonicum* is endemic to the Yangtze Valley and coastal mainland China; it also occurs in Sulawesi and the Philippines, with smaller foci in Malaysia, Thailand, and Japan. Over 200 million people may be infected with the disease, although data are extremely unreliable. However, in the Nile Delta and other areas, prevalence can approach 100 percent. Surveys of 42 affected countries indicated an overall infection rate of 21 percent.

The worm eggs are shed by a human host and hatch, producing a minute larva called a miracidium. The miracidium invades a specific snail host, where it reproduces asexually, eventually producing the final larval stage, the cercaria. These are released from the snail, swim freely, and then bore into the skin of a human host. In the human, the parasite migrates via heart and lungs, eventually maturing in veins of the liver, gut, or bladder. Eggs appear in urine or feces 30–40 days after infection. The disease has a complex epidemiology, partly because of the intricate relationship between parasite and snail intermediate host. Not only are there strains of each schistosome species, but also there are multiple genera of snails, varying in susceptibility, with a taxonomy undergoing constant revision. Historically, this has long created confusion.

Schistosomiasis can be a serious chronic disease in poor rural areas, where humans are regularly in contact with fresh water contaminated by schistosome cercariae. In most endemic areas, prevalence and intensity of infection (i.e., the number of eggs released – an indication of the number of worms carried) peaks in the teenage years. But even in highly endemic areas, the transmission rate is low, partly because of patchy distribution of the surprisingly few infected snails.

Reservoir hosts play an important role in Oriental schistosomiasis. Rodents may be significant reservoirs of *S. mansoni* in South America. Human schistosomes belong to a large family of trematodes (Schistosomatidae) that parasitize birds and mammals. In many regions, particularly the lake country of the central and western United States and Canada, non-human schistosome cercariae penetrate human skin accidentally. Although they are destroyed in the skin, this causes a harmless but irritating rash – "swimmer's itch" or **schistosome dermatitis**.

Embolized trematode eggs induce inflammatory reactions in various body organs, causing symptoms of **chronic schistosomiasis**. The pathology is quite variable and generally related to the intensity of infection. With *S. haematobium*, lesions occur in the bladder and ureter around the entrapped, calcifying eggs, with eventual development of fibrous connective tissue. Symptoms include blood in the urine (**hematuria**), painful and excessive urination (**dysuria**), distension of the ureters (**hydroureter**), and distension and atrophy of the kidneys through blockage of the urethras (**hydronephrosis**). With intestinal schistosomes, gut wall and liver lesions occur, also with deposition of fibrous connective tissue. The resulting venous obstruction causes compensatory increased arterial flow, leading to portal hypertension and the classical enlargement of liver and spleen (**hepatosplenomegaly**). Moreover, eggs of all three species may be trapped in the lungs, and with *S. japonicum*, nervous disorders or **cerebral schistosomiasis** can occur if eggs collect in the brain.

History

Human schistosome worms were first described in Egypt by Bilharz in 1851 and related to disease symptoms by Wilhelm Griesinger shortly thereafter. Both men assumed the worm was a single species, occurring in blood vessels of the gut or bladder. That two Egyptian species existed was suggested in 1907 by Louis Sambon, who named the second species *S. mansoni*. A year later, Piraja da Silva in Brazil gave the first description of *S. mansoni* but assumed it was a third distinct species. A long controversy over the existence of two Egyptian species was finally resolved by Robert Leiper in 1915. Meanwhile, in 1905 Fujiro Katsurada had described eggs and worms from patients in Japan and named them *japonicum*.

The worms' life cycles long remained mysterious, although researchers usually assumed involvement by an intermediate host. In 1894, Arthur Looss, then the foremost authority, argued against any intermediate host, claiming that the miracidia bored directly back into humans. This bizarre theory likewise generated controversy, finally resolved in 1913. Keinosuke Miyairi and Masatsuga Suzuki discovered the snail host entered by the miracidia and described the schistosome cercariae emerging from the snails later. Leiper, sent to China to uncover the mysterious life cycle of the worm, hurried to Japan to confirm the breakthrough. In 1914, he was posted to Egypt and quickly resolved the life-cycle problem in that country, distinguishing the two species by their morphologies, egg types, and different snail hosts. With such problems resolved, interest in schistosomiasis subsided. It was thought curable by the drug antimony tartrate and preventable by the snail-killing chemical copper sulfate.

Between the two world wars, campaigns using these chemicals were undertaken in Egypt, Sudan, Rhodesia, and South Africa, particularly after schistosomiasis was found among children of "poor whites" in Transvaal. In addition, high prevalence among African mineworkers generated interest by the South African Institute for Medical Research. The International Health Division of the Rockefeller Foundation financed an eradication campaign against **hookworm** and schistosomiasis in Egypt between 1929 and 1940.

After World War II, interest in the disease dramatically increased, especially in British, French, and Belgian colonies in Africa. By 1950, schistosomiasis, previously considered unimportant outside Egypt, Sudan, South Africa, and China, was recognized as the most important tropical disease after **malaria**. In America, interest followed from an outbreak among Americans in the Philippines, where in 1944 over 1,000 combat-engineering troops involved in bridge building and road construction came down with the disease. Scientists and physicians posted to Leyte to deal with the problem brought the disease to American attention immediately after the war and initiated the growth in schistosomiasis research.

In British Africa, a helminth subcommittee of the Medical Research Advisory Committee began to stress the danger of schistosomiasis, particularly as new irrigation schemes threatened to spread the disease. The subcommittee initiated testing of a new drug, Miracil D, discovered by the British after occupying the Bayer laboratories toward the end of World War II. The first major British work on the epidemiology of the disease in Africa occurred between 1955 and 1965, when the East Africa Medical Survey was conducted and the South African government initiated surveys and supported research into experimental schistosomiasis in animals.

The 1950s also witnessed the first mass campaign involving more than the introduction

of latrines, drugs, and mollusc-killing chemicals. Utilizing a host of methods including mass reclamation of swampland, the Chinese eradicated schistosomiasis from many areas of their country.

The threat posed by irrigation schemes led to development of better molluscicides. Chemotherapy has now become the favored weapon, particularly after a 15-year experimental control campaign in St. Lucia sponsored by the Rockefeller Foundation. Oral oxamniquine proved effective against *S. mansoni*, and metrifonate against *S. haematobium*, whereas praziquantel is emerging as a "wonder drug" effective against all schistosome species. Today, with support from the McConnnell Clark Foundation, emphasis is on problems of schistosome immunity and development of vaccines.

John Farley

128. Scrofula

Scrofula can be defined only historically. It was a term about which there was some measure of consensus in the past but has now largely been superseded by terms indicating some form of **tuberculosis**. Scrofula is not, however, simply an old name for tuberculosis. Our ontology of disease centers on the tubercle bacillus, and we would commit a grave historical error if we assume that with its aid we can know what underlay old discussions of scrofula. To understand such discussions, we must learn how and why the concept of scrofula was constructed.

The distribution of scrofula (or "scrophula") resulted more from the religious and political convictions of those who saw it than from physical geography, economic conditions, or other circumstances normally considered conducive to disease. In regard to its clinical manifestations, we note, first, that the term itself implies an underlying entity that becomes manifest. But second, scrofula historically was its collection of symptoms and signs. We must understand what went into that collection, and why.

History

"Scrophula," like **scurvy** and **syphilis**, was not a term used by the ancients. Whereas there may be special reasons why the latter two were unknown (a distribution to the north of the ancient Mediterranean and a possible Columbian origin, respectively), there seems no reason to suspect that scrofula was a new disease – or at least so it seemed to Renaissance humanist doctors trying to reconstitute Greek medicine. In fact, the best they could do in the case of scrofula was to claim that one of its chief symptoms, neck tumor, was the *struma* of the classical physicians. But *strumae* in the ancient descriptions were not associated with other features that Renaissance physicians knew were part of scrofula. But how did they "know" this? Where did their picture of scrofula come from?

The answer is that medieval descriptions of scrofula existed. Partly these came from a surgical tradition, which was less Hellenizing than Renaissance physicians' medicine. Partly they came from popular tradition, in which scrofula was identified as the "King's Evil" and was believed curable by a king's touch.

The essence of the medieval ceremony of touching in order to dispel evil was demonstration of the quasi-sacerdotal nature of kingship. The political advantages were clear, for a king, in performing the cure, showed he was king in accordance with God's will. This was the important point in the seventeenth and eighteenth centuries, when scrofula's nature was energetically explored: The power of curing by Royal Touch was vouchsafed by God only to true kings. It could be used to legitimate claim and accession. French kings continued to touch until the Revolution and were emulated by other monarchs.

In France and pre-Reformation England, the ceremony's religious nature cemented the relationships and mutual stability of church and throne. The ceremony was too miraculous for some Protestants, although English Puritans at first tolerated it, and James I, although of Calvinist background, found it increasingly expedient to use the Touch. But by the time of Charles I, his opponents saw it as a justification of absolute rule by a king who claimed to be God's representative. The Stuarts, whether on the throne or in temporary or permanent exile, continued to touch for the King's Evil, and their supporters claimed that their success in curing scrofula was a sure sign of their status as the only legitimate monarchs. The Puritans and Parliamentarians saw the Touch as politically dangerous and tried to suppress it. Queen Anne was the last British monarch to use the Touch. The Hanoverians made no attempt to practice it, and their Whig supporters professed horror at the superstitious medieval ritual.

Conflicts surrounding the issue aroused the strongest passions. Crowds of thousands pressed around the Stuart kings to receive the Touch. Because the King's Evil was intimately bound up with the king's person, if we look for a "distribution" of scrofula – in seventeenth-century medical literature, for example – we find abundant references to it in Britain and France. But elsewhere, texts may not mention it at all. Thus in Holland, recently freed from absolutist Catholic rule, scrofula had no place in medical consciousness. Nor did Italian or German physicians – with no national attachment to a "true" royal dynasty – emphasize scrofula as a disease entity, rather viewing its various symptoms discretely.

By the eighteenth century, some medical works betray Enlightenment embarrassment in identifying scrofula as having a nonmedical cure, the Touch. In discussing the disease, British writers followed a tradition based on the works of Richard Wiseman, surgeon to Charles II. In the nineteenth century, after the disappearance of the French kings, scrofula was still identified, although perhaps more usually in adjectival form applied to a symptom. The notion underlying the name failed to survive germ theory, when attention turned from symptom clusters to causative microorganisms.

Characteristics

We have seen something of the geography and history of scrofula. We next examine what observers saw when describing the disease. The classical description was by Wiseman, a passionate royalist to whom the Restoration seemed an expression of God's will, which had placed the rightful line of kings back on the throne. The king's power to cure by Touch was again triumphantly demonstrated, and if it was good to show that the king cured, it was better to show that he cured where medicine or surgery could not. Thus Wiseman selected only the most difficult cases for the Touch.

Wiseman rejected the identification of scrofula with *struma*, insisting that scrofula included more than *struma*'s tumors-in-their-own-membranes. There was bifurcated swelling of the upper lip; tumors of muscles, ligaments, tendons, and bones; **fistulae** of the tonsils and the lachrymal region; and **ophthalmia**. Cases for the king had characteristic tumors near the mastoid muscle and eye protrusion (**lipitudo**).

Wiseman assembled his description of scrofula partly from descriptions by others, and there must have been some consensus of what the disease was. There would not otherwise have been any perception of the disease or the king's role in its cure among ordinary people, or among their parsons or squires who, we may suppose, encouraged them to go to London for the Touch.

The term "scrofula" remained in use in mainly British and French texts through the eighteenth century, and we can gather more information from medical practice in hospitals. The voluntary hospitals of the time were charitable institutions. Demand for effective use of funds (and the utility of recovered patients for advertising purposes) often meant pressure for rapid patient turnover. As a result, chronic or infectious cases were generally not admitted. So when we see scrofulous patients admitted to an eighteenth century hospital, we can assume that the physician permitting the admissions did not consider the disease chronic or infectious. In practice, hospital admissions show the same ambivalence about scrofula as the eighteenth century medical world at large. Sometimes the term simply did not exist for physician or hos-

pital; other times, scrofulous patients were rejected as incurable or infectious. Often a physician admitted a patient to test for "scrofulous" symptoms, and sometimes admittedly scrofulous patients were taken into hospitals in the belief that a course of mercury sweats would cure them.

From the records, we can see that the physician sought several signs to establish a scrofulous condition: an itch and tumors in the glands, joints, and other tissues. As the disease progressed, the physician saw these tumors change into ulcers, which deepened and ultimately produced **caries** in the bones. Exploratory surgery attempted to discover the stage of disease and what, accordingly, the prognosis was. Sometimes patients were released as incurable, sometimes they were treated with mercury sweats to unblock glands and vessels from the impedimenta held to cause scrofula. Which of these many alternatives was used probably depended on where the doctor had been trained.

The politics of early nineteenth-century Europe no longer supported the idea of the "true line of kings." Without true kings, there was no King's Evil, and scrofula was seen as a disease entity less often than in the preceding century. William Cullen's influential system retained the disease entity, but in fact even he helped destroy the unity of scrofula as a concept by subdividing it into differing conditions: "scrofula vulgaris," "scrofula mesenterica," "scrofula fugax," and "scrofula Americana."

The term "scrofula" survived largely in adjectival form, so that "scrofulous" tumors or ulcers could be described independently without necessarily referencing other "defining" characteristics of the seventeenth-century disease. With new emphasis on postmortem pathological anatomy in the nineteenth century, internal scrofula was often associated with tubercles in the lungs. Discovery of the causative bacillus created an ontology of disease around tuberculosis, thus rendering "scrofula" peripheral to medicine and accessible only to the historian.

Roger K. French

129. Scurvy

Scurvy is a **dietary deficiency disease**, arising from lack of vitamin C (ascorbic acid). It usually occurs in the absence of fruit and vegetables. Scurvy appears in no regularly recognizable way in ancient literature. Its name, derived from northern European vernaculars (for example, *schverbaujck* in Dutch and *scorbuck* in Danish), was Latinized as *scorbutus* in 1541 by Dutch physician Johannes Echthius.

Characteristics

Humans, unlike many other animals, do not synthesize vitamin C, and scurvy has historically appeared under circumstances where diets are circumscribed, especially on long sea voyages. In modern times, **infantile scurvy** has been a problem, occurring mostly in lower socioeconomic groups. Such outbreaks are associated with trends away from breast-feeding, combined with maternal ignorance about substitute foods.

Scurvy occurs in followers of fad diets, and in single, middle-aged men. It is not widely reported from the Third World, perhaps because of comparatively greater availability of fresh plant foods but doubtless also because of a lack of medical services to report the disease.

Generally, scurvy is a disease of northern countries, although the traditional Eskimo diet of uncooked meat is sufficient to prevent it (meat has vitamin C, but heat – as in cooking – destroys the vitamin content). Until recent times, adult scurvy was endemic in Russia, but not infantile scurvy, for suckling infants do better than adults when the diet is scorbutic.

The characteristic features of scurvy have been experimentally monitored. At 12 weeks without vitamin C, a feeling of lethargy appears. At 19 weeks, the skin becomes dry and rough, and hair follicles form lumps. Small hemorrhages in the legs begin at 23 weeks; a bit later, fresh wounds will not heal. A classic symptom – swollen, soft, purple gums – appears after 30 weeks. In a mid-twentieth century study, one volunteer developed a tubercular lesion at

26 weeks, and two others suffered apparent cardiac hemorrhages at 36 and 38 weeks. They were clearly near that stage of the disease that killed an eighteenth-century self-experimenter, not to mention many thousands of sailors. (When volunteers were given large doses of ascorbic acid, all made complete recoveries.) Historical reports of symptoms, involving far more severe cases, add flaccidity of flesh, loosening of teeth, and reopening of old wounds.

History

No doubt scurvy appeared in ancient times and was treated by physicians. The ancients, however, do not seem to have had a name for it. In any event, scurvy could not be found in the writings of Hippocrates or Galen by individuals of the late fifteenth and sixteenth centuries, to whom the disease was so obvious, and for whom medicine was founded on Hippocrates and Galen. As with the other apparently new disease of the Renaissance – **syphilis** – it was important for humanist physicians to believe that, notwithstanding name changes, ancient writers had known the disease. Only then could it be fitted into "classical" theory and practice and effective treatment sought. Attempts were made to show that Hippocrates knew of scurvy, but practical persons, such as ships' surgeons, treated it as a new disease.

Of course, the circumstances surrounding scurvy's appearance during the Renaissance were very different from those surrounding diseases discussed by Galen and Hippocrates. European economic power was growing rapidly, and the desire to trade was matched by technical developments of shipbuilding and navigation. The Europeans' theater of action was the Atlantic, not merely the enclosed Mediterranean, and all these factors meant that ships stayed at sea long enough for scurvy to develop. In 1498, Vasco da Gama, reaching the east coast of Africa, reported many of his men suffering from what was probably scurvy. Twelve weeks at sea on the return journey renewed the disease. Fernando Magellan, too, saw much scurvy among his crew when at sea for 15 weeks in 1519.

Spain and Portugal established control over southern routes to the Far East but were quickly followed by the French and English, who tried to find a northern route. A French expedition of 1534, overwintering on the St. Lawrence River in North America, suffered greatly from scurvy.

The seventeenth century saw expeditions by big trading firms like the East India Company, and the establishment of more colonies by more countries. It also witnessed more sea voyages of long duration. The East India Company, for example, sent an expedition to Sumatra in 1601; it was 29 weeks at sea before reaching the Cape, and scurvy was widespread. The only ship exempted was that of Sir James Lancaster, who provided lemon juice for his sailors.

Observers noted the rapid recovery of scorbutic sailors on reaching a port where fresh food was available. Experience showed in particular the value of citrus fruits. But general acceptance of this knowledge was long delayed. Part of the problem lay in provisioning the ever larger ships and squadrons: Citrus fruits are not native to the countries where merchant fleets were based; these fruits might spoil over long voyages; and attempts to concentrate or preserve the juice must have often reduced its effectiveness. The Dutch East India Company tried to ensure regular supplies by planting orchards at Mauritius and St. Helena, and even experimented with shipboard gardens. Review of company records indicates that, at least in regular trading voyages with known landfalls and provisions for the crews including fruit juice, scurvy was not very deadly.

This did not hold, however, for European navies, particularly during the eighteenth century. Their operations were far from regular. In any such operation, it was expected that lives would be lost, and experience showed that disease would take many. Fully 855 of 1,000 men succumbed – most to scurvy – when Commodore George Anson fulfilled his 1740 commission to capture Spanish treasure shipments.

Naval warfare involved not only long-distance operations but also blockades of long duration. The citrus fruit supply was simply not adequate for such operations: A complement of 500 men for a large warship was not unusual. Some physicians even advised against citrus juice, and generally substitutes were sought. One was cider, to which tradition attributed antiscorbutic properties. In the early 1740s, ship's surgeon Edward Ives was losing the usual large number of men to scurvy when he persuaded his admiral to provision with cider. While it lasted, he lost no crewmen: Scurvy came only afterwards, all other conditions remaining the same.

This was essentially a forced clinical experiment, a technique used more elaborately by James Lind. Lind divided scurvy patients into those taking citrus fruit, those taking cider, and those taking other remedies. The first group improved rapidly, followed by the second; the remainder did not improve. Lind has been much celebrated for this early clinical trial, but doubt has recently been cast on his results on the grounds that modern research shows no vitamin C in cider. Yet cider made in the eighteenth-century manner was high in vitamin C. By 1753, Lind had published his results in the most authoritative argument yet made for the use of citrus to prevent scurvy. But not until the end of the century did administrator Sir Gilbert Blane obtain regular issue of lime juice to British sailors.

Lessons learned at sea enabled control of occasional outbreaks of scurvy in early nineteenth-century prisons. But there was no adequate remedy for the scurvy produced by the great failure of the potato crop in 1845–46. Potatoes are rich in vitamin C, and the population of Ireland depended upon them as food. Scotland also suffered. Later in the century, when conditions precluded access to fresh fruit and vegetables, scurvy appeared: in the California Gold Rush of 1848 and later; in the Crimean War (1854–56); during an American blockade of Mexico in 1846; and during the U.S. Civil War, particularly in prisoner-of-war camps.

Scurvy was a special danger in Arctic regions. Where regular commerce obtained – in Hudson Bay Company territory, for example – scurvy was only a minor threat, and since the seventeenth century the company had shipped lime juice. Fresh meat was also recognized as valuable, a truth learned the hard way in early overwintering disasters. Explorers, however, generally encountered scurvy, particularly when small parties left their ships for exploration on foot.

Perhaps the least expected occurrence was that of infantile scurvy in Europe and America between the 1870s and World War I. The odd feature was that infantile scurvy occurred in the higher social classes, where no economic reason for **vitamin C deficiency** obtained. The reason was that upper-class mothers tended to avoid breast-feeding, and newly available preserved-milk products contained no vitamin C. Scurvy often occurred before children began consuming adult food. Upper-class mothers had also avoided breast-feeding in previous eras, but then infants were breast-fed by wet nurses.

Before the discovery of vitamin C, etiological theories of scurvy were more destructive than helpful overall. Many government officials, trading-company surgeons and officers, and eventually naval and military administrators, were convinced that certain fruits prevented and cured the disease. But advice from educated physicians was sometimes bad: Medical theory had its impact on practice.

The rise of the germ theory of disease in the second half of the nineteenth century, which changed medicine more than anything else had done in the preceding 2,000 years, had an enormous effect on the study of scurvy. Disease was now seen as caused by living microorganisms, and clinical symptoms as secondary. By the end of the century, the new medicine proved spectacularly successful in combatting infectious diseases. For scurvy, the effect of this revolution was to encourage a search for a causal organism, or at least a poison. In other words, the new research ran counter to the previous consensus that incomplete diets caused scurvy, and numerous disputes arose about the nature of the disease.

Over time, the theory of the disease had changed with theories of medicine. In the sixteenth century, humoral theories attributed scurvy to spleen damage from a dietary cause – the salt meat, stale water, and preserved food of long sea voyages. In the seventeenth century, when chemical notions of the body were attractive, some writers distinguished between **acid scurvy** and **alkaline scurvy**. When mechanism was employed in the medicine of the eighteenth century, physicians discussed corrosive particles in the blood. These were still humoral theories, and the humors' vices still derived from diet.

Hermann Boerhaave, the most authoritative eighteenth-century voice, blamed salt; dried and smoked meats, including fish and seabirds; ships' biscuits; dried peas and beans; and old, sharp, salty cheese. Such a diet, he argued, led to the proximate cause of the disease: The blood became thin and sharp. From this all the symptoms could be deduced, and all treatment should be directed to restoring the blood. (The theory of the time held that "disturbance" of the blood caused many diseases.)

Boerhaave mentioned citrus fruits, but only in a list of other remedies, and without explaining how such remedies worked. The value of citrus juice was after all merely an empirical discovery. Boerhaave's rationalist view attributed scurvy not to a lack in the diet but to an excess of things undesirable. His student Gerard van Swieten, however, believed that the cause of the disease was a dietary lack. Scurvy, he argued, appeared more often in besieged cities than in besieging armies, which had access to fresh provisions.

In 1795, Sir Gilbert Blane became commissioner of the Board of Sick and Wounded Sailors. Supported by recent experiments with lemon juice, he persuaded the Admiralty to authorize a daily dose to each sailor. Over the next 20 years, this totaled more than 1.5 million gallons.

Although scurvy virtually disappeared from the British fleet (but not from other fleets), on land the theories of physicians continued to threaten practice. The Siege of Paris (1870–71) produced an outbreak of scurvy, focusing attention on its cause at a time when ideas about contagion and germs were becoming widespread. In 1874, the French Academy of Medicine aired the view that scurvy was a contagious miasma and no more caused by lack of fresh fruit than **malaria** was caused by lack of quinine. A British expedition of 1894 spent three winters in the Arctic, remaining healthy on a diet including fresh meat but little lime juice. Physicians explaining the absence of scurvy stated that the disease was caused by bacterial action in spoiled meat. They realized that no one had studied scurvy in the light of germ theory; such a study was undertaken and seemed to support a germ theory of scurvy. So thoroughly was scurvy associated with germ theory that one physician explained lime juice as simply an antibacterial mouthwash.

The final recognition of scurvy as a deficiency disease is a twentieth-century story. From the last years of the nineteenth century, there had been concern about the incidence of **ship beriberi**. Axel Holst knew about the use of chickens in previous studies of **beriberi** but chose guinea pigs (which, like humans, do not synthesize their own vitamin C) as his experimental animals. Under a restricted diet, the animals developed symptoms of scurvy. By 1913, Holst and his collaborator Theodor Frölich showed that scurvy indeed resulted from a deficient diet.

Meanwhile, in 1912, Casimir Funk in London proposed that scurvy was one of four diseases (along with beriberi, **rickets**, and **pellagra**) caused by dietary deficiency. Each missing factor, he believed, was a nitrogenous base, for which he coined the name "vitamine." The deficiency thesis met opposition from bacteriologists, and in 1916 and 1917 cultured bacteria from scorbutic animals were inoculated into healthy animals, producing signs of scurvy. Related to the bacterial theory was E. V. McCollum's notion that scurvy was caused by bacteria-developed poisons.

Despite these opposing doctrines, the results obtained by Holst and Frölich prompted efforts to isolate the active component. McCollum had already identified a fat-soluble factor "A" and a water-soluble factor "B" in experimental rats, and it was natural to look for a "vitamine C."

From 1918, S. S. Zilva and others attempted to isolate vitamin C, a feat achieved by Hungarian Albert Szent-Györgyi, who was actually working on a different problem involving the sugars in lemon juice. In 1932, Glen King in Pittsburgh published results that combined Szent-Györgyi's findings with his own. Vitamin C had been discovered, and scurvy was vanquished.

Roger K. French

130. Sickle-Cell Anemia

Sickle-cell disease is an inherited disorder resulting from an abnormality in the structure of a protein in the red blood cell called hemoglobin. It represents a spectrum of disorders ranging from the full-blown form, **sickle-cell anemia**, to the carrier state called **sickle-cell trait** or simply **sickle trait**. Also included in this spectrum are several other variant hemoglobin disorders, which all have the sickle hemoglobin. Sickle-cell anemia is the prototype for most molecular diseases and was the first disease to have its cause isolated to a single molecular change in the human genetic structure. This single change is responsible for all of the dramatic physiological changes and clinical events that occur in this disease.

Sickle-cell trait occurs when the individual is heterozygous for the sickle-cell gene and results in abnormal hemoglobin (hemoglobin S) concentrations of less than 50 percent. It generally causes no serious illness, although this has been disputed. Other sickle-cell syndromes occur when hemoglobin S is present in a heterozygous state with other hemoglobin variants – some with similar properties. Common examples of these include hemoglobin C and hemoglobin E.

Characteristics

Sickle-cell anemia is found in up to 4 percent of Africans and 1 percent of black Americans. Upward of 40 percent of Africans carry the sickle-cell trait, as compared to 9 percent of black Americans. The trait is also present in some Mediterranean cultures. Experts believe that sickle-cell gene mutation occurred independently in several areas of Africa, explaining its presence in different peoples.

Hemoglobin S is transmitted as an autosomal recessive gene. So if both parents have sickle-cell trait, the chances are 1 in 4 that their child will have hemoglobin SS and thus sickle-cell anemia; 1 in 4 that it will have hemoglobin AA and be normal; and 2 in 4 that it will have hemoglobin AS and have sickle-cell trait.

The pattern of death in persons who have sickle-cell anemia is bimodal, with the first peak occurring in childhood and the second occurring among people in their late 30s. Deaths during childhood are related to infectious causes, whereas those during adulthood result from organ failure caused by repeated tissue destruction.

Hemoglobin carries oxygen in the bloodstream and is found inside red blood cells. Along with iron, it is composed of amino acids that in turn are built from deoxyribonucleic acid (DNA). In sickle-cell anemia, the DNA molecule is changed through a single genetic mutation, thus changing the amino acid composition of the hemoglobin, which alters its solubility and interactive properties. Under appropriate conditions, this results in a conformational change in the red cell from a flexible biconcaved disk to an inflexible sickled cell. Thus, recurrent sickling can cause the cellular membrane to become permanently calcified, resulting in rigid, irreversibly sickled cells. These cells are found in all persons afflicted with sickle-cell disease and may represent from 5 to 50 percent of the red cell mass.

Hemoglobin S has a lower affinity for oxygen, resulting in early release of oxygen and inability to oxygenate tissues adequately. Sickled cells have difficulty traversing the small vasculature of the capillary bed; vascular occlusion and tissue destruction result. Cell lifespan is also decreased and is manifested as a **hemolytic anemia**.

Indeed, sickle-cell anemia is characterized by chronic hemolytic anemia and recurrent states called "crises," divided into three types: "pain," "sequestration," and "aplastic." **Pain crisis** (the most common) occurs an average of three times annually. It first presents after 6 months of life, when fetal hemoglobin reaches low levels. At this age, early signs often include painful inflammation of extremity bones (**hand-foot syndrome**). Older patients develop recurrent joint, back, abdominal, or long-bone pain lasting approximately 7 days.

Sequestration crisis occurs when a large proportion of red cells become trapped in the spleen, resulting in shock. With age, recurrent vascular occlusion in the spleen causes its functional destruction. Because the spleen eliminates certain bacteria, sickle-cell patients are at increased risk of infection.

In rare **aplastic crises**, the blood-forming bone marrow becomes suppressed for short periods, resulting in acute reduction of red cells. Known as **red-cell aplasia**, this temporary condition may require blood transfusions until the bone marrow recovers.

By contrast, sickle-cell-trait carriers are phenotypically normal in most respects, although sickling is occasionally reported in such individuals at high altitudes or low oxygen, resulting in **splenic infarction**. Kidney bleeding and decreased renal concentrating ability occur more frequently in people with sickle-cell trait. The condition is almost always benign; nevertheless, claims have arisen that sickle-cell-trait carriers are at increased risk for acute muscle destruction and sudden death. These reports are controversial and require confirmation.

History

Sickle-cell anemia has been traced back to at least 1670, when it was noted to be present in the Krobo tribe of Ghana. It was first described clinically by Chicago physician James Herrick in 1910. Thirteen years later, J. Huck reported on 14 patients and first noted the reversibility of sickling. In 1939, J. Bibb and L. Diggs described irreversibly sickled cells, and in 1946, M. Sherman demonstrated the ordered structure of hemoglobin S. Linus Pauling investigated hemoglobin S by electrophoresis and reasoned that the sickling resulted from a single gene. V. Ingram then demonstrated that the condition resulted from the amino acid substitution of valine for glutamic acid. In 1949, A. Raper noted the high incidence of sickle-cell trait in **malaria**-endemic areas and suggested that it protected against infestation. In 1954, A. Allison correlated sickle trait with regions of past and present **falciparum malaria** endemicity.

Further analysis showed that the mutation illustrated a genetic principle termed balanced polymorphism. Generally, a gene such as sickle cell – causing severe morbidity and mortality – dies out unless circumstances create a more favorable survival. Africa and the Mediterranean have areas that are (or were) endemic for *Plasmodium falciparum*, which causes **malignant malaria**. But when persons with sickle-cell hemoglobin are infected with malaria, the infected cells tend to sickle and are selectively destroyed. Therefore, the sickle-cell gene – itself potentially fatal – helps defend against a potentially fatal disease and, paradoxically, prolongs survival. In regions where *P. falciparum* is not endemic, the sickle-cell gene becomes the sole determinant of morbidity and does not prolong life. This explains why sickle-cell frequency has decreased in much of the Americas.

Georges C. Benjamin

131. Smallpox

Smallpox, now existing only in laboratories, is no longer an active infection. It was a viral disease usually transmitted by airborne droplets and entering the body through the respiratory tract. There never was a cure. Closely related are **cowpox** and **monkeypox**, but smallpox probably was an exclusively human infection. Virologists recognized two kinds of smallpox: *Variola major*, with a mortality rate of 25–30 percent; and *Variola minor*, with mild symptoms and a death rate of 1 percent or less. The characteristics of smallpox viruses varied, and strains intermediate between *V. major* and *V. minor* probably existed. The history of smallpox is mostly a history of *V. major*.

Characteristics

As far as we know, the source of smallpox was always an infected human. No animal reservoir existed. Laundry workers occasionally contracted smallpox from clothing and bedding of smallpox patients, but most transmissions were airborne over distances of no more than a few meters. Quarantine was effective, as long as it was applied early (even before the appearance of symptoms) and strictly enforced.

Incubation lasted about 12 days. Onset was abrupt and prostrating: high fever, headache, back and muscle pain, and in children sometimes vomiting and convulsions. In the severest infections, extreme **toxemia** and massive hemorrhaging into skin, lungs, and other organs could cause death swiftly. In most cases, victims experienced the characteristic rash 2–5 days after onset. Generally, it appeared more densely on face, palms, and soles than on the trunk. In another few days, the rash turned to pustules that in extreme cases were confluent, usually indicating a lethal infection. William Bradford observed cases like this among Amerindians in 1633–34. Complications may have been common in these peoples.

Drying and crusting of the pustules began on the eighth or ninth day after the first eruptions. The scabs fell off 3 or 4 weeks after onset, and the victim was well again, barring complications. Among possible sequelae were blindness and male infertility. The probable sequel was a pocked and scarred face, appalling to others as well as the survivor. Literature is full of references to women thus robbed of their smooth skins.

Except in the rarest instances, smallpox infection ended in one of two ways: death or long-lasting immunity. Lacking an animal reservoir and the ability to remain latent within the body, smallpox existed only as an active infection. It was a classic epidemic disease, surviving in many eras and parts of the world only as rolling waves of infection. It achieved endemicity only in large and cosmopolitan populations, where it could infect nonimmune visitors, infants, and children. Where it was endemic, it was usually a childhood disease; trial by smallpox was a prerequisite of adulthood for all but a small minority.

History

Because it persisted only by passing from one human to another, smallpox could not have existed among the sparse populations of the Paleolithic Age. It may have first appeared sporadically among village dwellers of the Neolithic Age.

Smallpox may well have afflicted ancient Egyptians. The face, neck, and shoulders of the mummy of Pharoah Ramses V, who died in 1157 B.C., is disfigured by a rash of elevated pustules, but researchers cannot be sure of the infection that caused them. Dreadful epidemics rolled through the Old World in ancient times, but rarely were symptoms described clearly enough for researchers to make diagnoses. In the second and third centuries A.D., two pandemics devastated the Roman Empire, but we know very little about them. There is some indication of smallpox in China by the fourth century, and stronger evidence of it in Japan in the 730s.

With Rhazes, a ninth-century Baghdad physician, we are finally on solid ground. He differentiated between smallpox and **measles** and revealed smallpox to be a common childhood disease in southwest Asia. The density of population centers suggests strongly that smallpox was prevalent throughout advanced Old World civilizations before the end of the first Christian millennium. In the same period, smallpox may have invaded sub-Saharan Africa, northern Europe, and Indonesia.

Though widespread, smallpox seems not to have been among humanity's chief curses in those centuries. It ranked behind **plague** and **tuberculosis** in the Middle Ages and became a major demographic check in Europe only during the sixteenth and seventeenth centuries.

Smallpox historically acted as a solvent exuded by dense populations. For example, it was an important ally of the Russian invaders of Siberia and of the Hollanders in South Africa. But it was a merciless enemy of barbarians trying to penetrate such populations. The Manchus were obliged to excuse dignitaries from the thinly populated steppes from coming to Beijing to make obeisance to the Emperor. For their safety, special audiences were provided in Jehol, north of the Great Wall.

No later than 1519, smallpox crossed the Atlantic to a New World still free from the disease. It decimated the Arawaks of the West Indies; accompanied the Spaniards to Mexico; and rolled on ahead of them into the Incan Empire. Amerindians had at best no more resistance than did Europeans, and they must have suffered similar morbidity rates. Spanish estimates of Amerindian death rates in this first of many pandemics of smallpox ranged from about one-fourth to one-half – rates comparable to those of afflicted European children. The psychological effect was considerable. The Amerindians quaked in confusion and terror; and the Europeans preened themselves as the chosen people.

In 1789, smallpox appeared among Australian aborigines neighboring the newly arrived English settlers at Sydney Harbor. It destroyed half the indigenes, by English estimate, and spread into the interior. This epidemic was probably the single greatest demographic shock ever dealt the aborigines.

By the eighteenth century, smallpox accounted for 10–15 percent of all deaths in some European countries, 80 percent of the victims being under 10 years of age. Similar rates were probably common in major cities of North Africa and Eurasia. Outside these densely populated areas, smallpox was epidemic, killing high percentages of adults.

Modern techniques of inoculation and vaccination began – no one knows when or where – with variolation (artificial infection with smallpox of healthy people), an effort to produce immunity through mild cases of the disease. In China, smallpox scabs were blown up the nostril, seemingly a dangerous method because it might infect the respiratory tract, but the scabs were apparently aged first, attenuating the virus. Elsewhere, variolation generally involved scratching infected matter into the skin. If variolation was expert, the infection was mild and death rates no more than 4 percent.

Variolation was practiced for a long time, not by trained physicians but by folk healers. For example, Cotton Mather in Massachusetts first heard of it about 1706 from his African slave, who told him that smallpox and variolation were both common in Africa. Peasants in Scotland, Wales, Greece, the Middle East, and elsewhere were "buying the smallpox" long before the rich and wellborn learned of variolation. Lady Mary Wortley Montagu, whose brother died of the disease, was herself attacked as an adult, losing her beauty, even her eyebrows. While in Constantinople, she learned about "ingrafting" the disease, which usually led to a mild infection and yet stout immunity. She had her son variolated in Constantinople in 1717, and her daughter in London in 1721.

The same year, smallpox broke out in Boston, where the people, too few to maintain the disease endemically, periodically suffered epidemic waves of it. Mather knew nothing of Lady Montagu's experiments, but he had heard of variolation from his slave and other sources. He persuaded Zabdiel Boylston to experiment with the new technique in Boston. Despite fierce opposition from those who viewed the practice as dangerous (which it certainly was), Boylston scratched pus from a smallpox pustule into the skins of his son and two slaves. In all, he variolated 244 people, while other physicians variolated 36 more. This was the first large-scale test of the practice, at least in the West. Also –

amazingly – it may have been the first example of careful quantitative analysis of the effects of a medical procedure. Of Boston's population of around 11,000, 5,980 caught the disease, and 844 – or 14 percent – died. But only 6 – or just 2.4 percent – of the 244 variolated by Boylston died.

Variolation, however, was not adopted rapidly. After an initial flurry among the upper classes and their domestics in the 1720s, the spread of the new procedure slowed. British North Americans resorted to it only during epidemics, when contracting the disease naturally seemed more dangerous than embracing it via variolation.

Acceptance of variolation was contingent on several developments: increased fear of smallpox, which a surge of the disease around 1750 stimulated; reduction of fees for variolation; and improvement of the technique to reduce the chances of death. These changes were accomplished by, among others, American James Kirkpatrick and the British Sutton family. The Suttons reduced variolation to a slight pricking of the skin rather than deep incisions. Smallpox hospitals, where variolated patients could be isolated, helped quell fears of artificially triggered epidemics.

From the 1760s onward, variolation became increasingly common in the British Empire and Europe. The smallpox death of Louis XV in May and the variolation of Louis XVI in June of 1774 spurred the practice everywhere. By the end of the century, many thousands had been variolated in Europe and America. Some experts claim that the spread of variolation was among the causes of the population explosion that began in the eighteenth century, but it is impossible to separate this factor from others, such as improved nutrition. Yet we can be sure that in the long run variolation stimulated population growth, at least indirectly.

The greatest windfall of variolation (indeed, the greatest in the history of medicine) occurred in the last decades of the eighteenth century. English variolator and scientist Edward Jenner noticed that variolation failed to produce symptoms in people who had previously contracted a mild pox from cattle. He "vaccinated" (a new word derived from the Latin for "cow") several people with cowpox matter and then attempted variolation. Inoculation with smallpox matter uniformly failed to produce illness.

Jenner published his results in 1798. Vaccination may have been practiced before by common folk, like variolation, but now one of the elite had printed an account of the technique for the whole world to read, and that made all the difference. England led the way – more than 100,000 were vaccinated there by 1801 – and the rest of the world followed. Within 3 years of Jenner's publication, his work was translated into German, French, Spanish, Dutch, Italian, and Latin. In France, 1.7 million were vaccinated between 1808 and 1811; in Russia about 2 million in the decade ending 1814; and so on.

Getting potent vaccine across oceans as scabs or bits of thread soaked in infected matter was problematical. Often, the virus proved useless. The surest way of preserving cowpox virus over great distances was by serial infection: Recruit several unimmunized people and vaccinate one. When his pustules are ripe, transfer the disease to another, and so on in sequence until the destination is reached. This technique was used by Francisco Xavier Balmis, who from 1804 to 1806 led a Spanish-government-backed expedition to the Americas and then on to the Philippines and China, vaccinating thousands as he went. He used young boys – usually orphans – as cowpox reservoirs, the first set obtained in Spain and others as required.

During the 1800s, humanity began to win its battle with smallpox. Vaccination continued to spread, and in some countries was made compulsory for infants. Its benign effect on death rates, unlike variolation, was obvious. Literally millions of children, who would have died without Jenner's discovery, lived to enrich their societies and to fuel the population explosion. In a few advanced and disciplined societies, such as England and Prussia, where doctors, officials, and the public cooperated to smother smallpox, deaths from the disease had declined to near zero by the end of the century. Elsewhere, success was equivocal, even though the effect of vaccination was supplemented by the appearance of *V. minor* toward the end of the century, displacing the more virulent form in some regions.

Jenner realized that his discovery could mean "the annihilation of smallpox," but not until the mid-twentieth century did this seem a practical possibility. By 1950, wealthy societies in the temperate zones with strong governments, skilled medical personnel, and scientifically sophisticated populations were nearly free of the disease. But most of the world's smallpox raged in the tropics, where few of these factors existed and where vaccine lost potency quickly in the heat. Freeze-drying, invented in the 1940s and adapted for vaccine production in the 1950s, solved that problem.

In 1966, the World Health Assembly called for eradication of smallpox from the Earth. An officer of the World Health Organization, Donald Henderson, led the Smallpox Eradication Programme. In 1967, smallpox existed in every continent except North America and Europe, and it was estimated that from 10 million to 15 million people contracted the disease annually. By 1972, it was gone from South America. By 1974, it was restricted to India, Ethiopia, and Somalia. In October 1975, the last case of smallpox in Asia occurred, and in October 1977 in Somalia came the last case of naturally occurring smallpox in the world. In 1978, smallpox virus somehow escaped from a laboratory in Birmingham, England, infecting a mother and daughter. The daughter died; the mother survived; and the laboratory's director committed suicide while in quarantine. These were the last deaths associated with the ancient scourge of smallpox. In 1979 came the official announcement of the demise of the disease. As of 1980, stocks of vaccine sufficient for 200 million vaccinations were being maintained in case smallpox should arise again.

Humanity won the victory against the smallpox virus by displacing it with the vaccine virus.

Almost everyone for more than a century believed that virus to be cowpox, but in 1939 careful comparison of vaccinia virus (which does not exist naturally), cowpox virus, and smallpox virus showed them to be related but clearly distinct. One expert claims that the Jenner strain of vaccinia virus was early contaminated with a mild strain of smallpox and that vaccination was thus actually a continuation of variolation. Decades of variolation, according to this theory, produced attenuated strains of smallpox, and vaccinia virus is one of these tamed varieties. Other experts suggest that Jenner's strain was not cowpox but **horsepox**, which cattle occasionally contracted. Horsepox died out early in the twentieth century, so this hypothesis remains untested. Still others suggest that vaccinia virus resulted from hybridization of other pox viruses. Careful analysis, however, has uncovered little indication of this. The stuff of smallpox vaccination, although a mystery, is perhaps the greatest happy accident in the history of the relationship between humans and pathogens.

Alfred W. Crosby

132. Streptococcal Diseases

Microorganisms of the genus *Streptococcus* are responsible for many common and not so common human and animal diseases. Streptococcal **pharyngitis** and **pneumonia, scarlet fever, impetigo, erysipelas**, neonatal **meningitis** and **sepsis, puerperal sepsis**, and **bacterial endocarditis** all follow infection with streptococci. In addition, some streptococci provoke two postinfectious conditions: acute **rheumatic fever** and acute **glomerulonephritis**.

Characteristics

Streptococci are classified into distinct serologic groups – labeled alphabetically – each with discrete subgroups. Microbiologists further classify streptococci on whether and how they hemolyze red blood cells (alpha: incomplete or green hemolysis; beta: complete or clear hemolysis). Thus, for example, the streptococcus responsible for pharyngitis is known as a "group-A beta-hemolytic streptococcus."

The streptococcus has several biological peculiarities that influence its infectiousness. The genetic insertion of a bacteriophage produces a toxin responsible for the rash of scarlet fever. A group of proteins renders the streptococcus impervious to the normal bodily defense of phagocytosis. Hemolysins and enzymes, when present, help the streptococcus to invade the host. This potential biological variability may be responsible for abrupt changes undergone by streptococcal illnesses in the past.

Streptococcal illness is extremely common. Few have escaped streptococcal pharyngitis or superficial impetigo of the skin. Some forms of streptococcal illness, however, are rare, such as **streptococcal endocarditis**. Most streptococcal diseases are spread through respiratory droplets. Other means include bacterial contamination of food or milk, soiled hands or instruments touching open wounds, or invasion of the bloodstream by normal resident bacteria.

Group A streptococci produce several common illnesses. Streptococcal pharyngitis presents with fever, headache, sore throat, and abdominal discomfort. Before penicillin, the disease was often self-limited, but the streptococci could disseminate to other sites, producing **otitis media, mastoiditis,** tonsillar abscesses, or **osteomyelitis**. Puerperal sepsis, or **childbed fever**, occurs when streptococci, introduced at delivery, invade the internal lining of the uterus. Group A streptococci can cause impetigo (a superficial skin infection), **cellulitis**, and erysipelas (a life-threatening, rapidly progressing soft-tissue infection). Group A streptococci are responsible for two striking postinfectious conditions. The first, rheumatic fever, can include one or more of the following: **carditis (pericarditis, myocarditis,** and/or endocarditis); migratory, nondeforming **arthritis; chorea**; subcutaneous, fibrous nodules; and **erythema marginatum**. The second postinfectious condition is acute glomerulonephritis, a usually temporary form of renal failure.

Group B streptococci form part of the normal flora of the vagina and usually do not produce illness in adult women but can infect babies during delivery, producing meningitis and sepsis. Group C streptococci are usually pathogenic only for animals. Group D streptococci, normal residents of the human body, can produce endocarditis in people with deformed heart valves. Some streptococci cannot be readily grouped, such as *Streptococcus viridans*. These can also cause endocarditis and play a role in the formation of **dental caries**.

History

Women have suffered from puerperal fever, presumably caused by streptococci, since ancient times. Many case studies in the Hippocratic corpus indicate that women suffered from postpartum fever, debility, and death. But childbed fever was probably never common. Oliver Wendell Holmes wrote in the early 1840s that it was rare. When it occurred, it clustered around the practice of an individual physician. Holmes pointed to the need for cleanliness to prevent further victims.

Similarly, in 1861 Ignaz Semmelweis demonstrated that physicians who followed dead patients to the autopsy room and then returned to the lying-in room to deliver babies had more patients die of puerperal fever than did midwives who did not perform autopsies. The observations of Holmes and Semmelweis illustrate the tremendous gulf in personal cleanliness that existed between pre- and post-germ-theory practitioners. Holmes, for example, tells of distinguished obstetricians who carried pelvic organs removed at autopsy in their street coat pockets. Both accounts also underscore the irony in the fact that the most scientifically oriented physicians, the ones who performed autopsies, were responsible for spreading illness! Those accounts, however, treat with silence the plight of infants born of infected mothers.

Erysipelas's role in history was an inevitable accompaniment of wounds, whether accidental or surgical. Any deep cut through uncleansed skin risked injecting streptococci into susceptible tissue. Erysipelas also accompanied other streptococcal-related illnesses, such as childbed fever. Scarlet fever crosses medical history in a number of places. In the latter part of the nineteenth century during the early years of bacteriology, Friedrich Löffler had to sort out scarlet fever cocci from **diphtheria** bacilli (both produced sore throats). Scarlet fever often occurred in epidemics passed both in the usual droplet fashion and in contaminated foods – especially milk.

Streptococcal pharyngitis, with or without rash, provoked postinfectious acute rheumatic fever. For about a century, rheumatic fever injured more hearts than any other disease. It struck children and young adults (usually under 25) in temperate climates. Although mentioned by prominent seventeenth-century writers, such as Thomas Sydenham, rheumatic fever apparently was not a major problem until the late eighteenth and early nineteenth centuries, when carditis emerged as its major component. This may have resulted from a biological change in the body's response to the streptococcus (rheumatic fever is not an infection in the usual sense, but rather an immunologic response) coupled with introduction of the stethoscope, which facilitated diagnosis.

All streptococcal diseases except neonatal sepsis and meningitis have become less virulent since the end of the nineteenth century, a phenomenon yet to be explained. Incidence was clearly declining before the arrival of specific measures to treat these illnesses. The possibility exists that streptococci, with their biological variability, became less invasive in natural fashion. But they did so at the precise time in history (at least in Europe and the United States) when nutrition, housing, and living standards substantially improved. Today, streptococci are usually sensitive to sulfonamides and penicillins; thus most infections are curable with appropriate antibiotics.

Peter C. English

133. Strongyloidiasis

Strongyloidiasis, or **Cochin-China diarrhea**, is caused by a minute **nematode**, the threadworm *Strongyloides stercoralis*. The organism was discovered in 1876 in French troops with severe diarrhea in what is now Vietnam. *Strongyloides* occurs around the world, with a range similar to that of hookworms. Millions of people harbor the organism. Because poor sanitation and bare feet favor transmission, it is especially prevalent in poor tropical countries. Like **hookworm disease**, strongyloidiasis prevalence has declined greatly in the southern United States since the early twentieth century but still has foci in Kentucky and other states.

The worm has a complex life cycle. Parasitic males may not exist, but if they do, they are eliminated from the body shortly after infection. Females burrow in the mucosa of the intestine, where they feed and lay eggs, apparently by parthenogenesis. The eggs pass into the lumen of the intestine, where they hatch into a rhabditiform larval stage. In most cases, these larvae are voided in the feces and either transform themselves directly into an infective filariform larval stage, or, if conditions are favorable, undergo one or more generations of sexual reproduction before filariform larvae appear. Like hookworms, the filariform *Strongyloides* larvae penetrate human skin, often on an unshod foot, enter the venous circulation, and are carried through the heart to the lungs. Here they burrow through the walls of the air sacs, ascend to the throat, and are swallowed. **Autoinfection** is also possible and can maintain the parasite for years after the host has left endemic areas. In this variation of the life cycle, rhabditiform larvae develop into infective filariforms while still in the intestine. These larvae penetrate the mucosa, enter the bloodstream, and are eventually swallowed to continue the cycle.

Migrating larvae may produce itching when they penetrate the skin, and cough and chest pain when they are active in the lungs. Light intestinal infections are often asymptomatic, but heavier worm loads may cause abdominal pain, nausea, alternating diarrhea and constipation, **anemia**, weight loss, and low fever. Autoinfection can produce an enormous number of worms and can be fatal. Persons with immune deficiencies from diseases such as **cancer** or **acquired immune deficiency syndrome**, or whose therapy requires immune suppression, may develop devastating hyperinfections from mild or inapparent strongyloidiasis. Therapy is usually effective, although side effects from drugs are common. Prevention is largely a matter of education and improved living conditions.

Strongyloides fülleborni, a parasite of monkeys, has been found in many people in Zaire, Zambia, and other central African countries; larvae may possibly be transmitted in mother's milk. The same or a similar species has been found in 80–100 percent of infants in a region of New Guinea.

K. David Patterson

134. Sudden Infant Death Syndrome

Sudden infant death syndrome (SIDS) is difficult to define because medical scientists do not yet fully understand its nature. In the typical SIDS case, an apparently healthy infant, who may recently have suffered some minor respiratory ailment, is put to bed in the evening and is found dead in the crib next morning. The baby shows no signs of having been distressed; autopsy reveals no significant findings to explain the cause of death. Physicians diagnose SIDS by excluding other causes of death in infants between one month and one year.

Characteristics

The vast majority of reported and published SIDS cases come from countries and continents in the Earth's temperate zones (e.g., the United States, Canada, Europe, Australia, New Zealand, Japan, Hong Kong, and Israel). But SIDS occurs worldwide, in countries in tropical and frigid zones, in the mountains and at sea level.

SIDS tends to receive less attention in countries with high infant-death rates from problems such as infections and **malnutrition**. Autopsies are rarely performed on adults, much less on children, in these countries, making it almost impossible scientifically to label a sudden infant death as SIDS. SIDS becomes a significant factor in a country when the infant-death rate approaches approximately 15 per 1,000 live births. The lower the death rate from other causes of infant mortality, the higher the proportion of deaths from SIDS.

The occurrence of SIDS has probably not changed much over the centuries. Generally, rates range from 1.5 to 3.5 cases per 1,000 live births per year, though incidence varies from country to country. SIDS accounts for 6,000–7,000 infant deaths per year in the United States. It is the greatest killer of infants between 1 month and 1 year old.

SIDS' outstanding characteristic is the age at which it strikes children. Most deaths occur between 1 and 6 months of age, peaking between 2 and 3 months. Very few cases occur before 1 month; incidence drops significantly after 6 months. SIDS deaths thus occur when babies are undergoing their most rapid systemic development, and when their needs for efficient bodily processes and outside sources of energy to fuel them are greatest. Infants at this time are adjusting, for example, their sleep patterns to changing internal needs and to the outside environment, their gastrointestinal systems to changing foods, their immune systems to new antigens and pathogens, and their nervous systems to a variety of new motor and sensory stimuli. Life outside the womb is very different from life inside the womb.

SIDS strikes children of both sexes, of all social, economic, ethnic, and racial groups, and at all times of year. The distribution of SIDS within these groups and seasons is not equal, however. About 60 percent of SIDS victims are boys. SIDS occurs more commonly, but by no means exclusively, during the colder months of the year (autumn and winter), in both northern and southern hemispheres. Lower socioeconomic groups generally suffer a higher incidence of SIDS than do others. The distribution of SIDS also seems to follow racial lines in the United States: Afro-Americans (blacks) show the highest incidence, followed by Euro-Americans (whites), followed by Asian-Americans. That racial distribution may be deceptive, as it probably reflects the generally lower socioeconomic status (SES) of blacks compared to other groups. Low SES does not always translate into high risk for SIDS, however. Studies show that Hispanics of low SES have a SIDS rate comparable to or lower than that for whites.

Certain other characteristics of babies, mothers, and families appear to be risk factors associated with a higher incidence of SIDS in infants. None of these factors is predictive of SIDS and none are found in all SIDS cases, but all increase the risk in a child vulnerable to SIDS. All can be related to low SES. Both prematurity and low birthweight are important risk factors in SIDS. SIDS occurs more frequently in children of the following: multiple births, younger mothers, mothers who smoke, mothers of greater parity, higher birth rank in the family, single mothers, mothers who abuse drugs, mothers with poor prenatal care, and families in which a SIDS death has previously occurred (slightly increased risk).

At present, the etiology of SIDS remains a mystery. It is not even clear whether SIDS has a single cause, has several causes, or is the result of a combination of factors working together.

Before medicine took an interest in the sudden, unexplained deaths of infants in the eighteenth century, they were attributed to accidental suffocation in bedclothes or accidental smothering and overlaying by sleeping parents. Less charitable people accused parents or nursemaids of infanticide. These theories persisted throughout the nineteenth and early to mid-twentieth centuries concomitantly with medical theories ascribing the deaths to an enlarged thymus or a thymic condition. Since the 1940s, when researchers took a renewed interest in the etiology of sudden unexplained infant deaths, medicine has proposed numerous theories to explain why these children die.

When medical examiners in the 1940s and 1950s tested the blood of infants who had died suddenly and inexplicably, they often found fulminant infections that could easily have caused death. For some years, bacterial and viral infections were considered a major cause of sudden infant deaths. But when deaths from infection were weeded out, there still remained a large number for which pathologists could find no infectious agents. Researchers then found other possible causes of death, including the following: powerful allergic reactions to cow's milk, dust mites, or an unidentified allergen; **botulism** (beginning in 1976 when a number of infants infected with *Clostridium botulinum* were discovered in California); severe undetected respiratory viral infection; response to vaccination; overheating; **hypothermia**; high blood sodium; deficiency of a trace element such as magnesium, zinc, copper, calcium, selenium, or manganese; vitamin deficiency; and high or low levels of thyroid hormones. Some physicians reiterated the old view that a proportion of parents committed infanticide. Further research into these and other proposed etiologies continues.

Most current research relates the "final pathway" of SIDS to malfunction or immaturity of the respiratory or cardiovascular system. Etiologic theories under consideration include preexisting **hypoxia**, heart conduction problems (**arrhythmias**), and **apnea**. Evidence indicates that children who die of SIDS possess physical risk factors such as small size, slower growth rate, fatty changes in the liver, and thymic changes compatible with previous infection. These risk factors are not specific to SIDS but reflect increased risk for all infant deaths. When a young patient possesses enough of these physical and social factors, all that is needed is a trigger to cause SIDS to occur. Presumably, the trigger is activated during sleep, because virtually all SIDS deaths occur during sleep. The nature of that trigger is the mystery of SIDS.

SIDS leaves few pathological footprints in its young victims' bodies. Postmortem examination reveals little for the physician to use in understanding the pathology of the condition. The very definition of SIDS incorporates this fact, stating that negative postmortem findings help to classify an infant's cause of death as SIDS. Pathologists studying large numbers of SIDS cases have, over the years, noted only a few consistent postmortem findings that might at some time help explain the nature of SIDS. The pathological changes so far discovered fail to provide enough information for medical scientists to understand the etiology or mechanism behind SIDS deaths.

History

The medical profession and society did not recognize SIDS until the late twentieth century. And yet people from Biblical times onward described sudden unexplained infant deaths that matched the typical history of a SIDS death today. Because the deaths almost always occurred at home or in private situations, and to seemingly healthy children, most people, including parents and caregivers, generally ascribed the cause of death to accidental or intentional smothering or suffocation. When discovering their infants, with whom they regularly slept, dead next to them after a night's sleep, with no signs of any disease or disturbance, and no cries during the night, parents believed that they had unknowingly overlaid and smothered their children.

Or, if they had not slept with their infant, but found it lifeless where they had put it down for the night or for a nap, parents assumed the child had suffocated in its bedclothes. In either circumstance, parents blamed themselves for the tragedy. Worse, others suspected not just parental negligence but overt infanticide. Because SIDS leaves no telltale marks on its victims, no one could determine if the infant's demise was truly accidental or intentional. As a result, society assumed parental negligence and punished the parents or whoever was responsible for the child's care. Medical people were not consulted in these situations except perhaps to confirm the death. It was purely a societal matter dealt with by religious, and later by secular, authorities.

Perhaps the first recorded Western case of SIDS is found in the Bible story of the two women who went before King Solomon with claims to motherhood of an infant boy. One of the women had awakened, found her son dead, thought she had overlaid him, and secretly switched the child with another.

Medieval church rules enunciated specific punishments for those who overlaid their children, and forbade parents from taking infants to bed with them. As early as the sixteenth century, Florentine craftsmen designed a wooden arch that fit over, and kept blankets away from, the child, thus preventing potential suffocation with bedclothes.

The power of ecclesiastical courts began to wane in the Renaissance. As secular authorities gained power during subsequent centuries, civil courts investigated cases of overlaying and smothering to determine causes of death. At the same time, medicine was learning more about human anatomy and physiology. In 1761, Italian physician Giovanni Morgagni published his treatise correlating specific autopsy findings with disease signs and symptoms during a patient's illness. The resultant development of pathological anatomy in the early nineteenth century helped medicalize the previously nonmedical conditions of sudden unexplained infant death. As autopsies of these children revealed large thymuses (actually a normal finding), physicians explained death on the basis that the thymus gland cut off the tracheal airway or overly reduced the size of the thoracic cavity in which the heart and lungs had to function. Such explanations relieved parents of blame for their children's deaths.

Despite evidence presented by other physicians during the nineteenth and early twentieth centuries that neither an enlarged thymus nor a similar but more complex condition called **status thymico-lymphaticus** could cause sudden infant death, many people, including judges in courts, used thymic death to absolve parents of guilt. By the end of the nineteenth century, medical people were divided over sudden un-explained infant deaths. For example, a Scottish police surgeon in 1892 openly accused parents of neglect, ignorance, carelessness, and drunkenness in overlaying their children, whereas William Osler still discussed thymic enlargement as a cause of sudden infant death in the 1904 edition of his influential and widely used medical textbook.

Recognition of the condition now known as SIDS began to occur in the 1940s and 1950s with studies demonstrating the extreme difficulty of overlaying a child or smothering a child in bedclothes, and the importance of performing full autopsies on these children. As medical scientists and epidemiologists gathered information during the 1960s and 1970s, they better characterized SIDS. Public awareness and political campaigns since the 1970s have succeeded in removing much of the parental stigma associated with sudden infant deaths.

Todd L. Savitt

135. Sudden Unexplained Death Syndrome (Asian SUDS)

Sudden unexplained death syndrome (SUDS) occurs when a relatively young healthy person, usually male and Asian, dies unexpectedly while sleeping. The victim has no known antecedent illnesses and no factors that might precipitate cardiac arrest. At autopsy, no cause of death can be identified in heart, lungs, or brain. Postmortem toxicologic screening tests reveal no poisons.

Characteristics

SUDS has occurred among Southeast Asians in the United States, mainly Laotians, Hmong, Kampucheans, and Filipinos. In Asia, SUDS is described in Japanese and Filipino medical literature and has been observed in Thailand. Incidence of SUDS has decreased since 1983, and evidence indicates that the longer an immigrant has been in the United States, the lower the risk.

The first comprehensive report of SUDS in the United States was published in 1981; it described 38 victims, all Southeast Asian refugees. All but one of the cases were male. Median period of time in the United States was 5 months (range, 5 days to 52 months) before death. Geographic distribution of the deaths reflected the distribution of Southeast Asians in the United States. The deaths occurred between 9:30 P.M. and 7:00 A.M. The victims whose deaths were witnessed appeared to be asleep prior to death or were just falling asleep. None of them complained of illness or symptoms before going to bed, and all were considered in good health.

Witnesses of SUDS deaths become aware of abnormal breathing sounds, in some cases preceded by a brief groan. Victims cannot be aroused. Terminal respirations are said to be labored and deep, irregular and without wheezing or stridor. The victims remain flaccid during these events, although a few are described as having **tonic rigidity**. Some victims are incontinent of urine or feces. Witnesses recall no signs of pain or terrifying dreams. A few victims who are still alive when paramedics reach them are found to be in **ventricular fibrillation**.

The etiology of SUDS remains unknown. Because of differences between these cases and other victims of sudden death, SUDS may involve a new syndrome. The quickness of the deaths is unusual, and extensive postmortem investigation reveals no ascribed cause. A case-control study yielded meager results. No single variable differentiated cases from controls. Victims tended to have been in the country less than 6 months, to have left Laos less than 3 years earlier, to have spent a greater proportion of their income on housing, and to have acquired fewer possessions in the United States than other immigrants. Although cases had similar amounts of English training, they had less job training. Cases had gained weight less frequently than controls and lost weight more frequently. Researchers concluded that factors enhancing emotional stress or resulting from such stress may have been involved.

History

Sudden death in healthy individuals is a phenomenon that has occurred throughout history and in many cultures. Because of their unexpected nature, many such deaths have been attributed to supernatural or psychological causes. Some have speculated that SUDS among Southeast Asians in the United States may be triggered by stress, night terror, evil spirits, or culture shock.

Yet a number of reports in past Filipino medical literature identified a sudden nocturnal death syndrome known as **Bangungut**. Previously healthy males die during the night, making moaning, snoring, or choking noises. *Bangungut* means "to rise and moan in sleep" in Tagalog, reflecting folk beliefs that the deaths are caused by terror from nightmares. The victims are men 20–50 years old. No consistent cause has been found despite extensive autopsy evaluation. The main postmortem finding is **hemorrhagic pancreatitis**, which most observers believe is not a cause of the syndrome but, rather, an effect after death.

Filipino physicians claim to see numerous cases of SUDS every year. The typical victim is a young male adult with a stocky build, usually a poorly educated construction worker who migrated from the Visayan Islands to work in Manila and who had either been on a drinking spree shortly before sleeping or just eaten a fatty meal prior to retiring for the night. The victim is brought to the hospital by fellow workers who are unable to wake him, but who remember his moaning and groaning in sleep.

Similar episodes of sudden death among Filipinos living in Hawaii were described in medical and popular literature during 1930–60. Nearly universally, Filipinos have heard about *Bangungut* and believe in its authenticity. Many describe experiences as children being assigned to watch over their fathers' afternoon naps.

In Japan, a disease called ***pokkuri*** involves sudden death similar to those previously described. A study of autopsies found cardiac death of unknown etiology in some cases. Almost all such deaths occurred in young men who were considered healthy and died suddenly during sleep. Some Japanese pathologists believe that the cause of death is a fulminant deletion of myoglobin from myocardial fibers during a state of acute cardiac failure. In refugee camps in Thailand, certain deaths were quite similar to SUDS deaths occurring among similar refugees in the United States.

Emotional trauma, voodoo, spirits, and magic have all been suggested as important factors for sudden unexplained death in folk cultures. Modern biomedical beliefs prescribe that psychological factors cannot cause death per se but may trigger a fatal event. A different emphasis occurs in cultures where the concept of psychological sudden death has greater currency than in scientific Westernized cultures. For example, in Australia the aborigines believed that a person pointed at with a bone would die as a result. A government surgeon in 1897 reported witnessing several such cases. A phenomenon of wishful dying has been described among rural Bantus in South Africa.

Several studies of the Hmong, the group hardest hit by SUDS in the United States, have proposed psychological triggers as explanations for their deaths. An extensive cultural study of SUDS focused on Hmong religion and health concepts, but no correlation was found between the deaths and religious preference, degree of belief in traditional religion, or anxiety over religious questions. Again, it was concluded that one possible triggering mechanism for SUDS might be overwhelming and inescapable stress. Another study also considered stress as a potential trigger in SUDS, specifically that night terror might have contributed to the deaths. Researchers speculated that such terror was brought on by exhaustion, culture shock, family quarrels, or even violent images found on television.

Neal R. Holtan

136. Sweating Sickness

The **sweating sickness**, or **sudor anglicus**, is one of the great puzzles of historical epidemiology because no modern disease easily corresponds to its principal features. Thus it has generated much speculation and debate over what caused the five English epidemics attributed to the "Sweat."

The first description, written in 1486, indicated that the earliest epidemic occurred (northern England) during June of 1485. Strictly contemporary accounts use the words "plague" and "pestilence" to describe the local mortality crisis. However, most modern authors agree that the initial outbreak began later, in London, on September 19, 1485, brought with Henry VII's mercenaries from France and Flanders.

Once in London, the epidemic displayed some of its most characteristic and consistent features: higher mortality among men than women, peaking during middle adulthood among the economically advantaged, and a sudden, acute fever accompanied by profuse sweating. Its victims generally lapsed into coma and died within 48 hours. Similar outbreaks have been identified: in 1508, 1517, 1528, and 1551. Oddly, the disease preferred Englishmen at home and abroad. In the British Isles, Scots, Welsh, and Irish were spared.

The "Sweat" had no important demographic repercussions, as the numbers affected were always small in comparison to other epidemics of this period. Nonetheless, each recurrence of the disease produced widespread fear. In 1528–29, the Sweat uncharacteristically extended to Calais and many German regions but was clearly associated with severe famine as well as epidemics of **typhus** ("petechial fever") and **plague**. As might be expected, a body of literature on the disease accumulated at the time as well as later, which has fueled interest in the Sweat's identity.

In 1508, Sir Thomas More informed Cardinal Wolsey of the Sweat's progress among young scholars at Oxford and Cambridge, but little discussion was generated. In fact, the 1517 and

1551 epidemics are the only two epidemics for which we have substantial contemporary accounts.

Court historian Polydore Vergil's graphic description of the disease was based on his experience during the Sweat's 1508 and 1517 appearances and written from memory. In addition, some speculate that Vergil had access to reports contemporary with the 1485 outbreak. The earliest description by a physician was not written until 1552. His advice, however timely or expert, was to no avail, for the disease never recurred.

Early nineteenth-century epidemiologist J. Hecker was fascinated by the Sweat's abrupt appearances and disappearances and felt that English methods of therapy were partly responsible for the high case-fatality rates. Writing over a century later, Maurice Strauss concurred, arguing that efforts to encourage perspiration and to stimulate vigorous purging of the bowels would have exacerbated fluid and salt losses associated with a high fever and led to circulatory collapse. Hecker, however, also blamed the English climate and gluttonous habits of Englishmen of the period.

Building on the suggestion that peculiarities of the sixteenth-century English diet might account for the disease, Adam Patrick argued that the Sweat resembled a **shock reaction**, with its hyperacute **pyrexia** (fever) and sweating, occasionally associated with evidence of circulatory collapse. Among the most likely toxins, he passed over bacterial endotoxins and exotoxins in favor of fungal toxins associated with food poisoning. Ultimately, he felt that the sweating sickness was a form of **ergotism**.

Writing in 1891, Charles Creighton, by contrast, denied the possibility that local conditions could alone explain the appearances of the Sweat, and he was loath to identify it with any one known infection. He was, however, convinced that it was introduced by Flemish mercenaries hired by Henry Tudor. An opponent of the germ theory of disease, Creighton believed that the soil of the Seine's lower basin perennially harbored the disease, its epidemic appearances dictated by variations in weather conditions. He contrasted the ability of the French to host the disease and survive, and the partial immunity many Africans displayed when exposed to **yellow fever**, with the susceptibility of the English and drew a parallel with the effect, on unprotected flocks of cattle, of bringing an animal infected with **Texas cattle fever** into the fold.

Most recent authorities concur with Creighton that whatever caused the Sweat, it was a disease that found "virgin soil" in England or among the English. In so doing, they follow Hans Zinsser's assessment that the Sweat was caused by a viral illness to which the uniquely susceptible English population gradually acquired immunity. Zinsser departed from earlier twentieth-century physicians in ascribing the cause of the Sweat to **influenza**, although today there seems to be agreement that the Sweat was not an influenza virus, although it spread in a similar manner.

Finally, John Wylie and Leslie Collier speculate that a novel arbovirus infection, transmitted by an insect vector, accords with most of the clinical and epidemiological information. By the mid-sixteenth century, the disease was becoming endemic in England, affecting children more than adults and in the process losing some of its terror.

Ann G. Carmichael

137. Syphilis

Venereal syphilis was long the most serious and dreaded of the **sexually transmitted diseases** (STD). Caused by *Treponema pallidum* subspecies *pallidum*, a spirochetal bacterium, the only known natural hosts of which are humans, venereal syphilis is one of the **human treponematoses** – along with **pinta, yaws**, and **endemic syphilis**. Predominantly transferred by sexual contact, *T. pallidum* may also be transmitted through other physical contact, intravenously (as in contaminated blood transfusions), and by infected mothers to fetuses during pregnancy (**congenital syphilis**).

Syphilis develops naturally through three clinical stages (primary, secondary, and tertiary or late), separated by subclinical periods. Of the latter, that between the secondary and tertiary stages is most pronounced (**latent syphilis**). Clinical manifestations of syphilis are extremely protean and capable, at the tertiary stage, of affecting any system of the human body.

Syphilis was named from Girolamo Fracastoro's 1530 poem, *Syphilis, sive morbus gallicus*, in which the Italian physician discussed the disease then known throughout Europe as ***morbus gallicus*** (the "French disease"). However, the term syphilis was not widely used until the late eighteenth century, and that usage was vague and applied to many other symptoms besides those of venereal syphilis until the development of the germ theory in the late nineteenth and early twentieth centuries.

Characteristics

Unlike the nonvenereal treponematoses (pinta, yaws, and endemic syphilis), venereal syphilis has established a worldwide distribution, although its incidence patterns are somewhat different in developed and developing countries. For example, it has declined in the West since the 1860s, although major wars have momentarily interrupted this trend. After World War II, congenital syphilis and **late syphilis** almost disappeared, mainly because of public-health measures and penicillin. Since the 1950s, however, both **primary syphilis** and **secondary syphilis** have increased, with peak incidence in the 15–34 age group. A high male/female ratio results from considerable incidence of syphilis in male homosexuals.

In developing countries, the disease remains widespread, although interpretative problems of serologic tests for syphilis make it difficult to estimate the numbers of infected people in those regions. Syphilis is increasing where yaws was previously endemic, as in tropical America and Africa and Southeast Asia. Infected prostitutes are important to the spread of syphilis in

these areas. Congenital syphilis is considerable in many developing countries.

The *Treponema* genus includes several pathogens responsible for four human diseases: (1) pinta, a Central and South American disease affecting the skin, caused by *Treponema carateum*; (2) yaws, a disease of skin and bones occurring in rural populations of the humid tropics, caused by *T. pallidum* subspecies *pertenue*; (3) endemic syphilis, similar to yaws but found only in warm, arid climates, caused by *T. pallidum* subspecies *endemicum*; and (4) venereal syphilis, with no climatic restrictions, affecting any bodily tissue, and caused by *T. pallidum* subspecies *pallidum*. Surprisingly, in spite of the differentiated diseases they produce, the four treponemes cannot be morphologically distinguished. Moreover, they elicit the same immunologic reactions, and all are susceptible to penicillin.

Almost from the time of Columbus's arrival in America, but particularly from the European Enlightenment, the uncertain geographic and historical origins of syphilis have been the object of scholarly controversy. Since the 1950s, however, the rise of molecular biology has pushed anthropologists and historical epidemiologists to frame this problem progressively in terms of the evolutionary origins of all the human treponematoses. At present, two major theories – the unitarian and the nonunitarian – contend with each other in providing an explanation for the surprising similarities of the human treponematoses.

For E. H. Hudson, the most outstanding defender of unitarian theory, there is only one treponematosis, although it assumes different clinical patterns under different epidemiological conditions. Thus, the changing physical and sociocultural environment of humans has caused treponematosis to change into one or another of those four different clinical syndromes already mentioned: pinta, yaws, endemic syphilis, and syphilis. From the unitarian viewpoint, then, it does not make sense to talk about transmission of syphilis from the New World to the Old, or vice versa.

By contrast, C. J. Hackett, the main upholder of nonunitarian theory, maintains that the clinical variety of human treponematoses probably resulted from mutational changes in the treponemal strains themselves. His thesis is that successive mutations have been responsible for the different human treponematoses starting from a lost ancestral **animal treponematosis**. The earliest of the treponematoses seems to have been pinta, which might have extended from Africa and Asia into America about 15,000 B.C.; that is, during the last part of the last glaciation and before the subsequent melting of the polar icecaps that formed the Bering Strait.

By about 10,000 B.C., a warm humid environment caused either the pinta treponemes themselves (hypothesis A) or the lost ancestral animal treponemes (hypothesis B) to mutate in Afro-Asia, bringing forth yaws, a disease that extended through Africa, Southeast Asia, and eventually Australia and the Pacific islands, but that did not reach the Americas.

Around 7000 B.C., in the warm arid climates that developed after the last glaciation, another mutation occurred, this time from yaws to endemic syphilis. The latter appeared in northern and Saharan Africa, southwestern and central Asia, and central Australia, whereas yaws itself remained unchanged in the warm and more humid climates.

Finally, about 3000 B.C., the development of large urban areas and the increasing use of clothing in the eastern Mediterranean and southwestern Asia became selective agents for still another mutation as syphilis changed from a nonvenereal disease of rural children (endemic syphilis) to a venereal disease of urban adults (venereal syphilis).

According to Hackett, by the first century B.C., syphilis had spread throughout the Mediterranean. He suggests, however, that this early venereal syphilis was a "mild" form of the disease – a possible explanation for the lack of evidence of it before the end of the fifteenth century. Then, a new successful treponeme mutation – probably favored by conditions in congested European cities at that time – produced a more serious disease. Initially extremely virulent, this form of syphilis is supposed to have progressively weakened since around the 1530s. Still other scholars, however, trace the sudden epidemic of venereal syphilis to a post-Columbian importation of an American parasite to Europe.

As noted previously, the natural course of syphilis includes three clinical stages separated by latent periods with no visible symptoms. In primary syphilis, *T. pallidum* penetrates mucous membranes and skin. After incubating over a period of 2–6 weeks (average 3 weeks), the primary lesion (**chancre**) appears. It is a small, painless ulcer, usually appearing in the genitalia and less frequently in other regions. The chancre heals spontaneously in 2–6 weeks.

In most patients, after a brief latent period, there is a secondary stage characterized by the appearance of disseminated lesions on the skin and in the internal organs. In women, these are often the first sign of syphilis. Secondary lesions consist of a painless rash, variable in appearance and localization, and usually accompanied by fever, malaise, and bone aches. After a few weeks, secondary lesions and symptoms disappear. In about 25 percent of patients, however, secondary lesions recur during the first 2 years.

The tertiary (late) stage develops only in about one-third of untreated cases, and only after another latent period lasting from 1 to 20 years or even longer. Tertiary syphilis involves progressive destruction of skin, mucous membranes, bones, and internal organs. The typical lesion is the **gumma**, a small, rubbery, benign tumor, developing anywhere in the body. Serious forms of late syphilis attack the cardiovascular and central nervous systems. **Cardiovascular syphilis** may cause **aneurism** and dilatation of valves. **Neurosyphilis** includes a loss of positional sense and sensation (**tabes dorsalis, locomotor ataxia**) or a form of insanity (**general paresis** [GPI], **dementia paralytica**). Since the introduction of antibiotics, tertiary syphilis has almost disappeared.

History

Historians usually identify today's venereal syphilis with *morbus gallicus*, first mentioned in European writings of the late fifteenth century. The disease erupted in Europe in the 1490s, although neither its geographic origins nor its precise date of appearance is certain. These issues have been the object of a continuous and unresolved controversy between defenders of an American origin of syphilis and those who claim that syphilis existed in the Old World long before Columbus's voyages. The most varied documental proofs (medical and lay writings, iconography) and – increasingly since the late nineteenth century – material proofs (paleopathological remains) have been wielded in this debate. It is an unfinished debate, however, for in claiming that present-day venereal syphilis was already known and had been described under several names before or after the Europeans' arrival in America, historians have produced the kind of contradictory conclusions that serve only to keep it alive.

Another approach to the history of syphilis by studying it in the context of the development of human treponematoses has already been mentioned. It has yielded some promising hypotheses but no definitive conclusions.

Thus, a third approach – examining the history of the concept of syphilis rather than the history of the disease itself – seems appropriate. This third way requires contemplating the disease entity called syphilis within the strict historicocultural context it occupies, and from which it receives its true significance. Put plainly, every disease entity is an intellectual construction that is peculiar to some form of medicine; and every form of medicine is nothing but a historical variable in any human community. Venereal syphilis took shape in Western medicine only because of intellectual and social changes in the latter nineteenth and early twentieth centuries, foremost among them the formulation of germ theory. Let us consider the development of the concept of syphilis in this light. Our departure point is an epidemic in late fifteenth century Europe.

The term *morbus gallicus* became dominant in designating a disease generally considered new in 1490s Europe. It was incurable and loathsome, consisting of sores – usually beginning in the genitals but eventually covering most or all of the body – and other symptoms. Contemporaries included it among the numerous calamities that befell Europeans at this time. Sources indicate that the "French pox" spread in Italy in 1494–95, after the armies of France and Spain clashed over the question of the kingdom of Naples. The notoriety the phrase *morbus gallicus* achieved throughout Italy was closely associated with the tragic impact of the French invasion on the fragile Italian political equilibrium. Similarly, the acceptance in early sixteenth century Italy of *morbus gallicus*'s reputed American origins may be explained by the fact that Spaniards were regarded as the newest *barbari stranieri* to devastate Italy. The prestige of Renaissance Italy and its cultural hegemony were important in ensuring the rapid popularization of both the term *morbus gallicus* and the theory of its American origin.

Through the sixteenth century, "French pox" achieved overwhelming dominance over other names for the disease. Only French physicians seem – understandably – to have rejected this name and offered others. For example, in 1552, Thierry de Héry of Paris suggested *maladie vénérienne* or *grosse vairolle*; in 1553, Auger Ferrier of Toulouse proposed *pudendagra* or *lues hispanica*; in 1560, Antoine Chaumette of Paris tried *morbus venereus*; and in 1563, Leonardo Botallo of Paris used *lues venerea*, as did Jean Fernel's 1579 publication.

During the seventeenth century, the term *lues venerea* ("venereal infection") was adopted all over Europe, sharing leadership with *morbus gallicus*. In the eighteenth century, *lues venerea* eventually superseded *morbus gallicus*, and use of the latter declined dramatically.

Two points may be raised about the expression *lues venerea*. The adjective *venerea* stressed the direct relationship between the French pox and the pleasures of Venus, and thus the individual's responsibility for contracting the disease. Applied to *morbus gallicus*, this adjective seems to have appeared for the first time in 1527 in a work by French physician Jacques de Bethencourt, entitled *Nova poenitentialis Quadragesima, nec non Purgatorium in Morbum Gallicum sive Venereum*. Both the title and contents of this book evoke the climate of religious exaltation and of moral rearmament present in Reformation Europe. The second point has to do with the name *lues*, which underscores the perception of the disease, at that time, as a contagious and calamitous one from a physical, and even from a moral, viewpoint.

The dominance exerted by the expression *lues venerea* on eighteenth century medicine is exemplified by French royal physician Jean Astruc's 1736 work, *De Morbis Veneris*, reissued several times and translated into many European languages. It argued that *lues venerea* was caused by a specific virus – *venereum* – and attempted to classify all supposed "venereal" infections under this general rubric.

Until the mid-eighteenth century, most European medical thought defended the unity of *lues venerea* on the basis of a specific virus. However, after 1750 the unified concept was challenged by pathologists, who began to question whether *lues venerea* was a single disease entity after all. This challenge resulted in the progressive disappearance of the expression *lues venerea* from the literature. Although it entirely disappeared only in the nineteenth century, it was increasingly replaced by the plural expression *morbi venerei* ("venereal diseases"). Around the same time, specific denominations for each of the *morbi venerei* (chancre, **gonorrhea, bubo**, and syphilis, among others) appeared with increasing frequency. From the early nineteenth century, medical works specifically devoted to certain among these diseases – mainly gonorrhea and syphilis – began to proliferate.

During the period 1750–1850, specialized hospitals emerged, including those for the treatment of venereal disease, and dermatovenerology was born as a medical specialty. Enlighten-

ment controversy over *lues venerea* eventually concentrated on whether blennorrhagic discharge (usually called gonorrhea) constituted a different disease entity or was just a peculiar clinical stage of *lues venerea*. The beginning of this process of disease differentiation may be found in the work of Giovanni Battista Morgagni, published in 1761. He found that patients with blennorrhagic discharge and no evidence of chancre rarely had hidden chancre, which was supposed to provoke the discharge in the first place.

During the following decades, physicians argued the single or dual nature of *lues venerea*. This controversy lasted well into the nineteenth century, in part because tremendous ambiguity existed in the vocabulary of venereal complaints. The term "syphilis" became almost dominant after the 1820s but nonetheless sometimes appeared as alternative or complementary to "venereal disease."

The controversy over whether venereal disease was a single disease entity or several illnesses was ended in the 1830s by French venereologist Philippe Ricord, who had developed a vast clinical and experimental program in Paris and in 1838 published his experiments demonstrating the existence of the *virus syphilitique*, so that chancre and **blennorrhagia** could be definitely separated. Moreover, he distinguished primary lesions from others, and primary symptoms from secondary symptoms. Ricord proposed the division of syphilis symptoms into primary, successive, secondary, transitional, and tertiary.

Ricord's concept of syphilis was gradually reshaped as other sexually transmitted disease entities (gonorrhea, **chancroid, lymphogranuloma venereum, genital herpes, venereal warts**, and others) emerged. If most of these were first shaped according to clinical criteria, each eventually got its definitive "identity card" when the relevant germ was isolated.

Gonorrhea and chancroid are two illustrative examples. Ricord had definitely separated chancre and blennorrhagia, but the clinical picture of gonorrhea was completed only in 1879, when Albert Neisser discovered the gonococcus germ. Chancroid or "soft-sore" emerged as a disease entity in 1852, when Ricord's pupil Léon Bassereau demonstrated that the two kinds of luetic chancre – one hard, painless, and unique; the other soft, painful, and frequently multiple – resulted from exposure to a like lesion. In 1889, August Ducrey identified the bacillus responsible for it.

As for the concept of syphilis, it changed profoundly during the second half of the nineteenth century as the disease became a major research area in Western medicine. French venereologist Jean-Alfred Fournier perhaps contributed most in developing the concept of syphilis during this period. Fournier propounded the idea of latency in both acquired and congenital syphilis, established the relationship between syphilis and parasyphilitic affections, and began a social campaign against the disease.

The syphilis germ, however, was not discovered until 1905, when Fritz Schaudinn and Erich Hoffmann isolated it from a secondary lesion. In 1906, August von Wassermann, Albert Neisser, Carl Bruck, and others made possible the first serologic procedure to diagnose syphilis: the complement-fixation test, later known as the Wassermann reaction. In subsequent years, *T. pallidum* was also found in tertiary lesions, verifying Fournier's theory. Karl Reuter, for example, in 1906 found the germ in a syphilitic aorta, whereas Hideyo Noguchi in 1913 proved its presence in brain tissue from paretics.

By way of conclusion it should be emphasized that, as has been the case with many other disease entities, a crisis of a disease-entity concept based on its specific biological cause has also ensnared venereal syphilis. In 1935, as most researchers still claimed specificity of a causal microorganism to be the definitive criterion for an infectious disease, Ludwik Fleck lucidly stressed the essential incompleteness of the concept of syphilis.

Time has confirmed Fleck's insight. Put plainly, it should be obvious from the foregoing that Western medicine has had enormous

difficulties in establishing scientific criteria that delimit precisely the so-called venereal syphilis from the remaining human treponematoses.

Jon Arrizabalaga

138. Syphilis, Nonvenereal

Nonvenereal syphilis has apparently occurred in many forms and places, and one interpretation of this phenomenon is that **venereal syphilis** can revert to nonvenereal transmission. Others see it as a discrete disease with its own etiologic epidemiology. The most common and enduring form of the disease is called *bejel*; it occurs in the arid regions of North Africa, the Middle East, and the eastern Mediterranean, and seems to have antedated venereal syphilis by a considerable period of time. It is one of the **treponematoses** caused by spirochetes, bacteria belonging to the genus *Treponema*. Other diseases in this group are **yaws** and **pinta**. Like yaws, *bejel* is essentially a disease of children, although those who escape the illness as children are likely to acquire it as adults, often from their own children. Its specific cause seems to be *Treponema pallidum*, the same agent as that of **syphilis**, although it may be an intermediary form between *T. pallidum* and *Treponema pertenue*, the agent of yaws. Although treponemal disease has been transferred experimentally to animals, humans appear to be the only natural reservoir.

Characteristics

Because the treponemas that cause yaws, nonvenereal syphilis, pinta (an American disease), and syphilis are morphologically and serologically indistinguishable, it is believed that at least the Old World diseases may represent an evolutionary continuum running from south to north. Yaws, thought to be the oldest, spreads by skin-to-skin contact and flourishes in the hot, moist regions of sub-Saharan Africa where individuals have historically worn little clothing. Syphilis, by contrast, seems to be the newest of the treponematoses. Venereal transmission allows it to spread among peoples of colder climates whose clothing would frustrate skin-to-skin transmission.

Bejel or nonvenereal syphilis seems to be intermediate between the two both bacteriologically and geographically. It has been conceived of as yaws modified by a desert environment, and as juvenile, nonvenereal syphilis. It is not transmitted congenitally. The disease spreads from child to child in dry, mostly rural areas where lack of cleanliness facilitates transmission. The spirochetes of nonvenereal syphilis, like those of yaws and syphilis, perish in the presence of atmospheric oxygen, soaps, detergents, and antiseptics, and are sensitive to drying. *T. pallidum* can penetrate mucous membranes, but intact skin is a formidable barrier. The primary lesion is often in the region of the mouth, probably from sharing drinking vessels or utensils or direct mouth-to-mouth contact. It can also spread via direct nonsexual contact. Flies, lice, and fleas may also have a role in transmission.

The stages of the disease – primary, secondary, and late or tertiary – are not so pronounced as those of syphilis. In the case of *bejel*, the primary lesion is soon followed by the appearance of moist papules in skin folds and by drier lesions on the trunk and extremities. Late lesions, when they occur, can be ugly. Huge ulcers may form, and ulceration of the palatal and nasal bones can cause them to erode. Other possible physical symptoms are changes in pigment distribution and the deformity of other bones, especially long bones such as the tibia.

Although pinta has been given experimentally to syphilitics, a high degree of cross-immunity between *T. pallidum* and *T. pertenue* seems to exist. Thus, one who has suffered nonvenereal syphilis is not only safe from another attack but is also at least partially protected against syphilis and yaws.

The pathogenic mechanisms in this and other treponemal infections are not fully understood. The pathogens kill no cells and produce no known toxic substances. Thus it seems that much of the pathology stems from the immune response of the host. Nonvenereal syphilis or *bejel* is similar to yaws in some respects, among them, juvenile acquisition, absence of **chancre**, and congenital transmission. Moreover, both diseases rarely involve the cardiovascular and central nervous systems. Yet nonvenereal syphilis resembles syphilis in its affinity for the mucous membranes and in many of its pathological aspects. And, like syphilis, it occurs outside the tropics. Finally, the usual serologic tests for syphilis are positive in nonvenereal syphilis.

History

The story of *bejel* is intimately bound up with the work of physician and medical historian Ellis Hudson. He described the disease in 1928, after observing it among Bedouins. In 1937, he summarized all available information on the disease and stated that the Arab word *bejel* had been introduced into the literature to distinguish this nonvenereal and endemic form of syphilis from the venereal variety. In 1946, he emphasized the intermediary nature of *bejel* between yaws and syphilis and presented a unitarian concept of treponematosis, which stressed an evolutionary relationship among yaws, **endemic syphilis**, pinta, and venereal syphilis, and held that they were all varieties of a single disease caused by one parasite, *T. pallidum*.

Not all agree. Some, for example, argue that the various treponemal infections arise from changes in the treponemal strains themselves – mutations. Others feel that the treponemal infections are essentially different diseases, caused by different parasites. One hypothesis argues that venereal syphilis has reached villages (in the Sudan at least) from towns, only to become endemic (i.e., nonvenereal) in a rural environment.

There is, however, general agreement that nonvenereal syphilis is an old disease. Hudson argued that it flourished in villages during the early Neolithic period and that it was the "venereal leprosy" of the Middle Ages, the "sibbens" of Scotland, the "button-scurvy" of Ireland, the *radesyge* of the Scandinavian countries, and the *skerljevo* of the Balkans. Apparently, it never took root in the Americas.

Because endemic syphilis fades in the face of the cleanliness associated with civilization, and because of the high efficacy of penicillin as a cure, the disease has withdrawn from most of Europe. But the *bejel* of the Middle East has its counterparts in the *njovera* of Rhodesia, the *dichuchwa* that plagues the Bushmen, and the *irkintia* of the Australian aborigines.

Kenneth F. Kiple

139. Tapeworm Infection

Tapeworms are flatworms in the class Cestoda of the phylum Platyhelminthes. The body of an adult worm consists of a small head or scolex, usually armed with hooks or suckers to attach the animal to the wall of its host's small intestine, and a chain of segments or proglottids. New proglottids arise by budding from the scolex region. As they mature, they are pushed away from the head by formation of new proglottids and develop both male and female sex organs. After fertilization, eggs or gravid proglottids are excreted with the host's feces. Tapeworm life cycles are complex. In general, the eggs must be ingested by an intermediate host, where they typically become saclike larvae in the tissues. When the host of the adult form (the definitive host) eats an infected intermediate host, adult worms develop in its intestine. Some species have two or more intermediate hosts and can use several species as the definitive host. Serious clinical disease often occurs when a parasite becomes established in an atypical host or when larval forms are able to develop in what is normally a definitive host.

History

Because tapeworms can exceed 30 feet in length and strings of segments are often passed in the feces, it is not surprising that they were described by ancient writers in China, India,

and the Mediterranean world. Encysted larvae – bladderworms or cysticerci – have been known in beef and pork for millennia, but their relationship to adult worms was not suspected until the eighteenth century and not proved until 1855, when F. Küchenmeister fed larval tapeworms concealed in food to condemned criminals and recovered adult worms on autopsy. The three large species that infect humans were not clearly differentiated until 1782. The notion of spontaneous generation of adult tapeworms in the human intestine – a theory consistent with the then known facts – was widely accepted until about 1820.

Characteristics

Intestinal infections are discovered when proglottids are passed or when eggs are found by microscopic examination of feces. Diagnosis of larval infections is more difficult and depends on serologic tests or surgery. Drugs are effective against adult tapeworms, but larval infections are more difficult to treat and may require surgery.

Five species are important parasites of humans: *Echinococcus granulosis* and *Taenia solium* are dangerous as larvae; *Taenia saginata, T. solium, Hymenolepsis nana*, and *Diphyllobothrium latum* live as adults in the intestine. Several other species can infect humans but usually have other hosts. For example, *Dipylidium canium*, the **dog tapeworm**, can spread to children who accidentally eat fleas. Larval stages of several species of *Spirometra*, normally parasitic in other vertebrates, can cause a dangerous condition called **sparaganosis** if a person swallows them in their copepod hosts. The Oriental custom of treating wounds or inflamed eyes with a poultice of fresh frog flesh can permit larvae to become established in the patient.

T. saginata, the **beef tapeworm**, inhabits human intestines around the world, although it is no longer common in developed countries. Cattle and other bovids are the intermediate hosts. If a cow or water buffalo eats grass contaminated with feces and eggs, the eggs hatch in the animal's intestine into a larva that migrates through the intestinal wall and forms a bladderlike sac, a cysticercus, in the muscles. Humans acquire the worm by eating raw or poorly cooked beef, as in steak tartare. Infections are sometimes asymptomatic, but many people experience mild to severe abdominal discomfort and a few have convulsions and develop problems of malnutrition. As with many other parasites, higher prices for fuels in poor countries are often accompanied by increasing incidence because of undercooking.

T. solium, the **pork tapeworm**, is much less common than the beef tapeworm but potentially considerably more dangerous. It occurs around the world, except where Islamic or Jewish customs restrict pork consumption. The life cycle resembles *T. saginata*, except that wild and domestic swine are the intermediate hosts. Human infection usually results from eating poorly cooked pork; sausages can be especially dangerous. People can also serve as intermediate hosts if they ingest eggs in food or water or from soiled hands. The resulting larval infection, **cysticercosis**, can be serious and even fatal, especially if cysticercoids develop in the brain. Adults cause symptoms like those of the beef tapeworm. Inspection and thorough cooking or freezing of pork are important for prevention, and adult infections should be treated to avoid the danger of cysticercosis.

H. nana, the **dwarf tapeworm**, is only $1-1\frac{1}{4}$ inches long. It occurs around the world, including the southern United States, and is a common parasite of domestic mice was well as humans. Infection results from eating larvae in fleas or in the grain beetle *Tenebrio*. **Autoinfection** is also common. In this direct life cycle, eggs hatch in a person's intestine, and the larvae attach to the intestinal wall to mature. Heavy infection can cause severe **diarrhea**, abdominal pain, and convulsions, especially in young children.

D. latum, the **broad fish tapeworm**, was described in 1602 and recognized as a distinct species in 1758, but its complex life cycle was not fully explained until 1917. *D. latum* is an old parasite of humankind; eggs have been dis-

covered in pre-Christian archaeological sites in Germany. This large tapeworm is found in the Baltics, the Alps, the lower Danube, European Russia, Central Asia, the Far East, Africa, Alaska, and the Great Lakes area of North America. The worm was probably introduced into the United States and Canada by Scandinavian immigrants. *D. latum* has a complex life cycle, with the first larval stage in small freshwater crustaceans and the second stage, the pleurocercoid, in the muscles of fish of the trout, pike, and perch families. People become infected by eating raw or undercooked or undersalted fish. Adult worms produce as many as a million eggs a day. If the host defecates in or near water, motile larvae emerge that seek a crustacean to complete the cycle. A related species with a life cycle involving marine fish and sea lions has afflicted inhabitants of coastal Peru and Chile since pre-Columbian times.

D. latum may exceed 35 feet in length and, like the beef and pork tapeworms, can thrive for many years in its host's gut. Symptoms are similar to those of other tapeworms, but in rare cases this worm can produce a form of **anemia** by robbing the host of vitamin B_{12}. There seems to be a genetic component to this complication, with Finnish populations most vulnerable. Treatment is effective. Better sanitation and appropriate cooking of fish – to kill pleurocercoid larvae – are preventive.

K. David Patterson

140. Tay-Sachs Disease

Tay-Sachs disease (TSD) is the best known of the **sphingolipidoses**, a group of genetic disorders including **Niemann-Pick disease, Gaucher's disease**, and others. Specifically, TSD is G_{M2}**(beta) gangliosidosis**. Affected individuals (recessive homozygotes) produce virtually no hexosaminidase A (hex A), an enzyme necessary for normal neurological development. TSD is rare in most populations but is about

100 times more prevalent among Ashkenazi Jews. This indicates that TSD gene frequency is about 10 times higher in the Ashkenazi population. Persons with TSD usually show symptoms of neurological degeneration by 6 months of age. Their condition steadily deteriorates, and they seldom live beyond age 4. There is no cure, but heterozygous "carriers" of the defective gene can be identified, and amniocentesis can detect an affected fetus.

History

In 1881, British ophthalmologist Warren Tay first reported some early clinical signs of TSD. In 1887, the American Bernard Sachs further documented the disease he later called **amaurotic family idiocy**. Sachs first noted the familial nature of TSD and its seemingly exclusive occurrence in Jewish families. However, reports of non-Jewish cases soon appeared. In the 1930s, D. Slome surveyed population characteristics of TSD and confirmed the disease's autosomal recessive mode of transmission as well as the gene's higher frequency among Jews. E. Klenk discovered that nerve cells of TSD victims contained what he called "ganglioside." L. Svennerholm later described the specific G_{M2} ganglioside. In the 1960s, D. Robinson and J. L. Stirling discovered that the hexosaminidase enzyme had two components (A and B), and S. Okada and J. S. O'Brien found that **hex A deficiency** was associated with high G_{M2} ganglioside in TSD patients. More recently, the hex A gene has been mapped to chromosome 15, and different variants (alleles) of the gene, each of which causes TSD, have been discovered.

Characteristics

Between birth and age 6 months, children with TSD may display apathy, **hypotonia**, and exaggerated startlement at noise. Between 6 and 12 months, the characteristic cherry-red spot in the eye appears; psychomotor retardation, spasticity, and rigidity are displayed. From 12 to 18 months, children may drool excessively and undergo bouts of unmotivated laughter, and

convulsions. Between 18 and 24 months, **megacephaly**, cortical blindness, and **quadriplegia** commonly occur. After age 2, victims are in a vegetative state, and most die sometime during the next 2 years. Until then their condition steadily worsens.

Though the role of gangliosides in neural physicology is not completely understood, the basic biochemical cause of TSD remains straightforward. In persons with TSD, unusually large amounts of G_{M2} ganglioside accumulate in brain tissues, disrupting normal development and function. This accumulation results from lack of a functional specific enzyme, hex A, that breaks down the G_{M2} ganglioside. Heterozygous carriers of the TSD gene have roughly only half the hex A activity of individuals homozygous for the normal allele. This is apparently enough, however, for normal catabolism of the G_{M2} ganglioside.

TSD and other genetic disorders present an enigma. How can a lethal gene reach a high frequency in a population? How is that frequency maintained? Why is that gene found at a relatively high level in a particular population? In addressing such questions, one examines the basic evolutionary forces that change gene frequencies: mutation, gene flow, genetic drift, and natural selection.

Mutations are the original source of all genetic variability, occurring at generally low but constant rates. Mutation created the TSD gene variants found among both Ashkenazim and non-Ashkenazim, but it cannot explain the high frequency of the TSD genes in the Ashkenazim. No evidence of an unprecedentedly high mutation rate of this gene in Ashkenazi Jews has been found.

Gene flow, the movement of genes from one population to another, plays a greater or lesser role in various explanations of high TSD gene frequency. One intriguing scenario suggests that the Ashkenazim are descended from members of the Khazar Empire, which existed north of the Caucasus from the seventh to the tenth centuries. During that time, some Khazars converted to Judaism. After the empire's fall, such converts could have moved into central Europe, where Jews from Western Europe were also immigrating. If the Khazars carried the TSD gene, they may have delivered it as part of their contribution to the Ashkenazi gene pool. Little evidence of this exists, however, and as with mutation, gene flow by itself cannot account for the high frequency of TSD genes among Ashkenazi Jews. Natural selection and genetic drift are more likely causes.

In 1962, it was suggested that heterozygote carriers of the TSD gene may have a selective advantage over the normal homozygote. Researchers calculated that a selective advantage of about 1.25 percent on the part of the heterozygous carrier of the TSD allele would be sufficient to maintain the allele at its present frequency of approximately 1.3 percent among the Ashkenazim, despite the loss of TSD genes through the deaths of recessive homozygotes afflicted with TSD. They then showed that over the course of 50 generations (roughly from the time of the Diaspora to the present), a heterozygote-selective advantage of about 4.5 percent would increase the TSD allele frequency from 0.13 percent to 1.3 percent, again despite losses of TSD alleles through the deaths of recessive homozygotes. In order to provide support for their hypothesis, they compared sibship sizes of the parents of TSD offspring to the sibship sizes of a control group. They found the former to be slightly larger than the latter. Although the differences were not statistically significant, they indicated a heterozygote advantage sufficient to result in the observed present-day TSD gene frequency in the Ashkenazi population (assuming that the heterozygote advantage had remained more or less constant over time).

Two conditions are essential for a natural selection explanation: (1) a selective agent of sufficient magnitude to affect negatively the reproductive success of individuals; and (2) a physiological basis for the advantage one genotype has over the others. In 1972, it was suggested that heterozygous carriers of TSD were less susceptible to **tuberculosis** – especially common in urban centers during the nineteenth century. However, a negative association found between TSD estimates and tuberculosis prevalence was too small to be statistically significant. Furthermore, no physiological basis was offered to explain why heterozygote TSD carriers might have such an advantage in the face of tuberculosis. The nature of the hypothesized selective forces has yet to be fully elucidated.

It has also been suggested, however, that founder effect and genetic drift (rather than heterozygote advantage and natural selection) better explain high Ashkenazi TSD gene frequencies. Genetic drift refers specifically to random changes in gene frequencies from one generation to the next ("sampling errors"). Sampling error is most pronounced in small populations in which, simply because of chance combination of a relatively small number of gametes, the offspring generation's gene pool may not exhibit the same frequencies as the parental generation. Thus, gene frequencies "drift" up or down through time.

Founder effect, related to genetic drift, is the random genetic impact of one or a few individuals on the genetic structure of a new population after either migration or population decline. Because of the chance factor, founder effect is usually considered in the context of genetic drift.

One investigation of the population history of Ashkenazi Jewry finds that the conditions most conducive to genetic drift may well have been present throughout much of Europe for hundreds of years. However, others have calculated that even in such a situation, the probability of occurrence of present discrepancies in TSD gene frequencies between the Ashkenazim and non-Ashkenazim is low.

Up to now the difference between Ashkenazi and non-Ashkenazi Jews (and non-Jews) in TSD prevalence and gene frequencies has been emphasized. However, considerable geographic disparity in TSD prevalence exists among Ashkenazi groups as well. These differences are also important in assessing reasons for the overall high frequency of TSD genes among the Ashkenazim. Studies have found that the ancestors of the majority of Jewish TSD cases in the United States came from the northeastern provinces of Poland and the Baltic states.

Such findings can be incorporated into both the natural selection hypothesis and the genetic drift hypothesis. The former is facilitated because a selective agent favoring heterozygotes needs only to be shown to exist in a delimited geographic area. TSD genes spread out from there via gene flow, and it would be some time before their removal in appreciable numbers through the deaths of recessive homozygotes; by then the carrier frequency may become rather high. The case for genetic drift is strengthened because the Ashkenazim no longer need to be viewed as a large interbreeding population, but instead can be viewed as a subdivided population made up of semi-isolated groups, in each of which genetic drift is more likely. The TSD genes spread from areas of high frequency to those of low frequency through gene flow.

In the absence of much substantive data, and given that evolutionary forces usually work in concert, some experts have concluded that a combination of heterozygote advantage and genetic drift is the most probable explanation of high Ashkenazi TSD gene frequencies. Other possible explanations include inbreeding, genetic "hitchhiking," epistasis, or a wider combination of factors acting together.

In recent decades, there has been some debate about whether the incidence of TSD is increasing. Despite various arguments attempting to verify or deny such an increase, it must be remembered that modern "high" levels of TSD may result from better diagnosis and case reporting. Aside from continuing study and debate, more immediate concerns exist. At present, there is no cure for TSD. However, because heterozygote carriers and affected fetuses can be identified, individuals have available some important options.

Bradford Towne

141. Tetanus

Tetanus is an acute disease caused by a neurotoxin produced by the bacterium *Clostridium tetani* when its spores enter a wound and develop into their toxin-producing vegetative form. The case-fatality rate averages 50 percent in adults and is higher in neonates (especially in developing nations) and patients over 60 years old.

Characteristics

C. tetani is an obligate anaerobe, a spore-forming, motile rod. The terminal spore caused the organism to be called the "drumstick" rod. The protein toxin, tetanospasmin, blocks acetylcholine release at motor end-plates. The toxin travels up the nerve trunks, as well as fixing directly on nerve cells. The spinal cord is the primary target organ, with **chromatolysis** of the motor neurons and inhibition of antagonists accounting for the spasm and rigidity that characterize the disease. Toxin fixation to central nervous system neurons may lead to seizures; involvement of the sympathetic nervous system may evoke vascular irregularities.

Humans are accidental interveners in the life cycle of the organism, which is a soil saprophyte and a harmless inhabitant of the intestines of many herbivores. The organism requires a wound to invade mammals. Traumatic, surgical, dental, umbilical, burn, and cosmetic wounds are the most common causes of infection in humans. "Skin popping" of drugs, insect bites, and nonmedical abortions are less common causes. The organism can reproduce and produce toxin only when local oxidation-reduction processes reduce tissue oxygen to near zero; deep, infected wounds are thus ideal culture media. There may be 300,000–500,000 cases of tetanus a year worldwide, of which perhaps 120,000 are neonates whose umbilical wounds become infected.

There is no special characteristic or diagnostic pathology. Incubation ranges from 2 to 14 days after wounding. Cases of "dormant" tetanus have been reported after several months, probably because spores remained in a closed wound as a silent abscess. Diagnosis is based entirely on history and clinical findings; there are no specific laboratory findings. Clinical manifestations are usually classified into four forms:

1. **Localized tetanus** presents with spasm near the site of injury, usually in an extremity. The fatality rate is 1 percent or less.
2. **Generalized tetanus**, the more common form, is marked by the classic **trismus** ("lockjaw"), fixed grin (**risus sardonicus**), and backward arching of the trunk (**opisthotonos**). **Tonic seizures** of muscle groups occur in spasms, lead to rigidity, and are very painful. **Pneumonia** may follow respiratory muscle involvement or laryngeal spasm with aspiration. Cardiovascular disturbances are common, especially **vasoconstriction** and a labile blood pressure. Severe spasms may cause vertebral fractures. The course of this form, in survivors, is 1–2 weeks.
3. **Cephalic tetanus**, an uncommon form of the disease, follows facial wounds, involves the facial nerves, and may be followed by generalized tetanus.
4. **Neonatal tetanus** following infection of the umbilical cord (discussed in another chapter) usually begins 3–10 days after birth and then progresses to generalized tetanus.

Death usually results from respiratory failure with **hypoxia** or pneumonia, and occasionally from circulatory collapse, especially in patients over 60 years old. Treatment involves measures to decrease the organism's presence: debridement of the wound; antibiotics; neutralization of the toxin by antitoxin; and control of toxic effects by drugs with specific neuropharmacological effects. Curarization and artificial respiration have been used in severe cases. Careful continuous nursing care is essential.

History

Hippocrates recorded tetanus cases and discussed the condition in general terms as well, providing details of symptoms, the course of the disease, and treatment. Treatment regimens were many and varied, and largely ineffective. Aretaeus, writing some 700 years later, believed that onlookers' prayers for the death of the patient were useful; he pitied the attending physician's inability to afford relief. After an excellent clinical description of the disease, Aretaeus too urged a wide variety of therapeutic maneuvers.

Ancient clinical descriptions have not been bettered. Therapy has changed, but it is possible that the number of survivors "after the fourteenth day" may not have improved markedly. William Osler, writing in 1892, found 80 percent mortality within 4 days. Therapy had improved: The nasogastric tube enabled feeding and hydration; morphine provided sedation, and chloroform provided muscle relaxation. Osler emphasized antiseptic care of the wound. It is fair to say that from Hippocrates to Osler – and to today – there have been no changes in diagnostic techniques, and there has been only a small reduction in mortality rates in established cases. Tetanus is a disease that must be prevented, and prevention had to begin with isolation of the organism and advances in immunology.

The discovery of the tetanus organism was part of the microbiological revolution that proved the theory that specific organisms caused specific diseases. In 1884, Arthur Nicolaier produced tetanus-like symptoms and death by injecting soil samples into animals. He isolated a rod-shaped bacillus and suggested that it secreted a toxin resembling strychnine in its action. He did not isolate the organism in pure culture. Neither did D. Rosenbach in 1886, although he was able to produce classic tetanus in guinea pigs by injecting tissue from a fatal human case. He described the "drumstick" shapes and correctly deduced that these were terminal spores. It remained for Shibasaburo Kitasato to isolate the organism in pure culture, in 1889, from a fatal case in Berlin. He described the anaerobic culture requirements, confirmed

Nicolaier's observations, and concluded that the clinical effects were caused by a toxin. The study of tetanus toxin and antitoxin followed directly and in parallel with the research of Emil Behring and Kitasato on **diphtheria** toxin, a much more important disease.

Tetanus and diphtheria investigations provided the framework on which Behring built his understanding of the principles of serum therapy. In an 1892 paper, he argued that the serum of a patient should contain material protective and curative for another individual with the disease. In a series of studies, he and others proved this point in animals but did not recommend serum use in humans until its mechanism was better understood. They noted that even if treatment of the animal began very early, at least 1,000 times as much antitoxin was needed to cure as to protect before infection, and that, as the symptoms became general, the antitoxin was useless in any amount.

The availability of horse antitoxin soon led to clinical trials, with widely varying results. Analysis eventually showed that antitoxin had to be given very early in the disease; that dosage – empirical at first – was critical; and that it was essentially useless once the toxin was fixed to neurons and the patient was symptomatic. Better understanding of wound care and more aseptic surgery accompanied the rising rate of successful use of antitoxin and a decreased death rate, especially in selected populations like soldiers.

Given that soldiers often have fought in well-manured farmland and do not have clean skins, and that until very recently armies lived in close proximity to horses used for transport and cavalry, it is not surprising that tetanus was a common problem in wounded soldiers. In 1808, for example, the rate of tetanus before immunization was 12.5 per 1,000; by contrast, the rate was only 0.04 per 1,000 in World War II.

World War I saw the general introduction of early, near-universal use of antitoxin, accompanied by meticulous debridement of wounds. The effect of these measures may be seen in the British army. Incidence was 8 per 1,000 wounded from August to October 1914. As improved wound management and routine antitoxin use developed, the rate fell to 1.5 per 1,000 wounded. World War I patients, perhaps because the antitoxin produced a *forme fruste*, had a syndrome of "local tetanus" – not fatal, and usually confined to one extremity. U.S. forces, entering the war in 1917, had the advantage of the experience of their allies and thus had an incidence of only 0.16 per 1,000 wounded. Allergic reactions to horse serum occurred, more commonly after repeated doses of antitoxin.

The practical use of formaldehyde to produce a toxoid (a formalin-inactivated antitoxin) was introduced for tetanus in 1927. As opposed to the passive immunity conferred by antitoxin, the toxoid produced an active immunity that would protect against tetanus. Later, the duration of immunity and the timing and effect of booster doses was worked out.

A fluid toxoid was in use because of its harmlessness and efficacy (although it caused more local reactions than does the modern aluminum phosphate absorbed vaccine). This toxoid, a combined diphtheria-tetanus toxoid vaccine, was given to infants in parts of France in the late 1920s and, by regulation, to French soldiers in 1931.

Immunization with the much more epidemiologically important diphtheria toxoid began in the 1920s in parts of the United States and just before World War II in Britain. The absorbed tetanus toxoid was used by the armies of Britain, France, and Canada by 1939; the United States began its use in 1941. During World War II, the American army had 5 fatal tetanus cases (2 in nonimmunized patients) and 7 nonfatal cases (all in immunized patients) in over 500,000 wounded soldiers. The reaction rate to the immunization series of three doses was 21 per 100,000, none fatal.

After World War II, routine use of a combined vaccine of diphtheria and tetanus toxoids (DT) was urged for childhood immunization. Soon the triple vaccine, with **pertussis** added (DPT), became legally required for school admission in the United States. Childhood immunization programs in Europe vary but tend to be on similar schedules and under similar laws. Non-fatal anaphylactic reactions occur at a rate of 1–1.5 per 2 million doses. The benefit/risk ratio for tetanus immunization is thus extraordinarily good. A worldwide infant and child immunization campaign, coupled with a booster upon injury, would essentially eliminate the disease as a clinical entity.

Robert J. T. Joy

142. Tetanus, Neonatal

Neonatal tetanus is a form of **tetanus** confined to newborns. It is characterized as a neurological disease resulting in severe muscle spasms, which can persist for at least a week, and commonly results in death. The agent is *Clostridium tetani*, which usually enters the bloodstream or motor nerves through an infected umbilicus.

Characteristics

C. tetani produces two toxins, one of which is tetanospasmin, the extremely potent neurotoxic component causing spasms. This toxin reaches the nervous system and eventually becomes fixed in the ganglion cells of the spinal cord or cranial nerves. Neonatal tetanus differs from numerous other bacterial diseases in that it is not transferred from person to person; instead, *C. tetani* is found in soil and is introduced into the body through an exposed area. The disease has had various names, including *tetani neonatoria, trismus nascentium,* "lockjaw," and the "9-day illness" or "fits" because it normally occurs during the first 9 days of life. Its association with filth and rural conditions means that neonatal tetanus is still common in Third World nations and is one of their greatest public-health problems. Mortality rates are high, even with modern treatment, and preventive measures are essential to avoid the disease.

Neonatal tetanus today is confined primarily to Africa, Asia, and the West Indies, although before the twentieth century, it was global in occurrence. The bacillus, found in soil, water, intestines, and the feces of animals and humans (where it can survive for years if not exposed to sunlight) is ubiquitous. Although it was once common in rural areas like much of Ireland and the southern United States, the disease is virtually unknown anywhere in North America and Western Europe today. Its incidence depends on soil conditions, type of agriculture, level of economic development, available health services, and quality of obstetrical procedures.

The most important reasons for the decline of neonatal tetanus in the twentieth century were improved standards of living, urbanization, and an understanding of **sepsis**. Efforts are being made by the World Health Organization to educate women and birth attendants on preventive measures and to bring obstetrical procedures and concepts of cleanliness to areas where the disease still exists. Statistics have shown that higher standards of obstetrical hygiene significantly decrease the chance of infection.

Neonatal tetanus occurs when *C. tetani* enters the body as a result of a dirty dressing or poor care of the umbilicus. Where the disease is common, the umbilicus is often cut with an unclean instrument such as a knife, razor, sickle, or piece of sharpened rock or bamboo. Often the umbilicus stump is covered with ashes, charcoal powder, cow dung poultices, ghee, powdered pepper, snail saliva, turmeric, or other contaminated substances, and is dressed with leaves or dirty rags, or is left exposed. Rural tribes might blame evil spirits for the disease, but efforts to keep spirits away from a new baby often increase unhygienic postnatal procedures.

Observers have found the disease to be more common among male newborns than among females, although this reported difference may reflect greater parental concern for the health of sons than daughters in some cultures. There is a question of whether race affects the frequency of neonatal tetanus, but unclean habits and living conditions of certain populations are probably much more important reasons why some peoples seem to suffer more than others. It seems to occur more often in warm months, perhaps because during these times babies are more exposed to soil and possible infection. All infants are susceptible unless they receive passive immunity from mothers who have been previously immunized.

Next to prematurity, neonatal tetanus is the most frequent cause of infant death in poor communities where traditional birth attendants serve mothers. Current estimates are that it kills some 10 percent of those born alive in such areas. It has taken an enormous toll in developing nations and, during the first half of the nineteenth century, accounted for many infant slave deaths in the southern United States.

Mortality rates from the disease vary up to 80 percent of infants in Third World nations, although accurate statistics are difficult to obtain because many infants are delivered outside hospitals or clinics, and numerous deaths are never registered. Current estimates are that 750,000 newborns die annually from neonatal tetanus. Mortality is often as high as 90 percent if it is contracted by newborns during the first week after birth, and 50 percent if contracted during the second.

One of the paradoxes concerning neonatal tetanus, and a major problem in eradicating the disease, is that immunization is more difficult in areas where the illness is most common. Such populations are often suspicious of modern obstetrical procedures or are located far from clinical care. Yet the actual cost of preventing the disease is minimal.

Because neonatal tetanus is usually caused by an infection of the umbilicus (though circumcision leads to a few cases), it does not occur as an epidemic. It strikes individuals rather than communities and, therefore, is difficult to study and does not generate the public interest that epidemics do. Consequently, the disease has not yet received the attention it deserves.

C. tetani is an obligate anaerobe (i.e., it grows only in the complete absence of molecular oxygen), a nonencapsulated slender, motile rod. It is introduced into an injured area as spores.

The disease develops if the spores are converted to vegetative organisms, producing the potent toxin, tetanospasmin. The toxin reaches the nervous system via the bloodstream or by traveling along the axon cylinders of motor nerves, eventually becoming fixed in the spinal cord and cranial nerves. Reflex convulsive activity follows.

A baby with neonatal tetanus is beset with symptoms that are easy to recognize and usually appear 3–10 days after birth. Signs include difficulty with feeding and swallowing, generalized stiffness, spasms, and convulsions. The newborn can develop special problems relating to ventilation, hydration, and sedation. The first and most distinctive sign of neonatal tetanus is **trismus**, or a stiffening of the jaw, resembling a smile. The mouth will not open fully, resulting in a condition that has become known as **risus sardonicus**. Patients often have legs and arms partially flexed, arms crossed over the abdomen, hands clenched, excessive flexion of the toes, stifled cry, and wrinkled face.

Body temperatures can reach 100°F or higher. Sucking is impaired, thus making regular nursing impossible. That and general fussiness are the first symptoms most mothers notice. Respiratory complications commonly arise. Infants who die within 48 hours generally succumb to uncontrolled spasms or intense congestion of liver, lungs, or brain. Newborns who die from the disease after 2 days generally die from **bronchopneumonia**. Other complications include **aspiration pneumonia**, acute **gastroenteritis**, and umbilical hernia.

The best means of controlling the disease are those that prevent the organism from entering – namely ensuring sterile conditions for the birth. The umbilicus should be treated conservatively and cleaned with hydrogen peroxide; foreign objects should be removed, and thimerosal (Merthiolate) applied. The transfer of maternal tetanus antibodies across the placenta has been found to be effective in conferring passive immunity to the neonate for several months, though it is better if the mother is immunized before, rather than during, pregnancy.

History

The term "tetanus" is from the Greek verb *tano* ("to stretch"). Hippocrates described three varieties of the infant disease. Aristotle noted infant convulsions that occurred before the seventh day. Moschion (Muscio), writing about three centuries after Galen, claimed that it was caused by stagnant blood in the umbilical cord, as did André Levret and others some 1,500 years after Galen. Indeed, in the early nineteenth century, doctors were still attributing neonatal tetanus to this cause as well as a variety of others, including irritation within the intestinal canal, poverty, filth, poor diet, falls, impure atmosphere, rough handling, a vaginal disease, cold or sea air, costiveness, smoke from chimneys, and mismanagement by midwives.

In 1793, M. Bartram ascribed the disease to the umbilicus, and his theory generated much debate. Some physicians urged cleanliness and washing the umbilicus with a weak solution of silver nitrate and dressing the area with an ointment formed of lard and lead acetate. But attention strayed again from the umbilicus. A 1782 study at a Dublin hospital noted that of 17,650 infants born, 2,944 died within a fortnight from neonatal tetanus. The institution's impure atmosphere and poorly ventilated chambers were blamed for the high rate. In 1846, Marion Sims concluded that a depression of the occipital bone during birth caused the disease and urged colleagues to observe bone formation closely in newborns.

In 1818, however, Abraham Colles first noted the similarity between neonatal tetanus and tetanus and attributed its incidence to inflammation and ulceration of the umbilicus. He suggested that air be purified, that the umbilicus be dressed with spirits of turpentine, and that the baby be plunged into cold water. Efforts were made to bleed patients to remove the noxious influences and produce relaxation. During the nineteenth century, accounts demonstrate a 99 percent fatality for those who were affected. No disease of infancy was more fatal, and few parents saw any reason to call a doctor.

The bacterial theories of Louis Pasteur and Robert Koch were important in eradicating the disease in the twentieth century. In 1884, Arthur Nicolaier found the bacillus in soil and produced the disease in animals. He found the same bacillus in human wounds. Shibasaburo Kitasato obtained the germ in pure culture. The tetanus toxoid was first used effectively during World War II. Immunization, along with the benefits of urbanization and industrialization, and a rise in the standard of living, have helped eradicate the disease from developed nations.

In 1923, another preventive measure evolved when investigators showed that tetanus antitoxin could cross the placenta. Some suggested that this could protect the newborn from tetanus by providing passive immunity. Later, it was proved that immunizing a pregnant woman with two or three injections of tetanus toxoid would decrease incidence of the disease. Unfortunately, it is difficult to provide such medical services to the people who need it most.

The World Health Organization continues to monitor the incidence of neonatal tetanus, to survey mortality rates of home and clinic deliveries, and to hold worldwide conferences to discuss means for improving the care of newborns. Its goal is to eradicate neonatal tetanus.

Sally McMillen

143. Tetany

Tetany is a symptom complex characterized by painful and prolonged contractions of the (generally smooth) muscles. These often appear as convulsions and are usually triggered by **hypocalcemia**. Adult varieties of the condition include **maternal tetany, parathyroid tetany, osteomalacic tetany, magnesium tetany, gastric tetany**, and **hyperventilation tetany**. Another form of the disease – **grass tetany**, caused by magnesium deficiency – is found in cattle. Despite these many forms, however, the disease occurs chiefly in infants (**neonatal tetany**) and young children (**infantile tetany**), in whom it is normally associated with **rickets**. It affects males far more than females and, in the absence of proper treatment, frequently proves deadly.

Characteristics

Tetany has often been confused with **tetanus**. It probably occurs worldwide in temperate zones, with the highest frequency of neonatal tetany among bottle-fed, black, and prematurely born infants. Abundant vitamin D from year-round sunshine may reduce the incidence of infantile tetany in the tropics.

Tetany's etiology is incompletely understood. It was originally associated with calcium deficiency and more recently with magnesium deficiency, although it can also be produced by **alkalosis**. The disease can follow the removal or incapacity of the parathyroid glands and can be a complication of alcoholism and a consequence of prolonged **diarrhea** and vomiting. **Protein-energy malnutrition** may also precipitate the disease.

As a rule, neonatal tetany strikes during the first 14 days of life, producing spasms, twitches, rigid body, and turned-down mouth corners ("carp mouth") nearly identical to the symptoms of neonatal tetanus. Full-term newborn infants generally have significantly higher levels of serum calcium than their mothers. However, these levels fall rapidly during the first days of life, and perhaps the high phosphorus content of cow's milk places the bottle-fed baby at special risk from tetany because it impairs alimentary absorption of calcium. Another contributing factor is, doubtless, parathyroid immaturity, whereas still another can be the poor nutritional status of the mother. Maternal tetany can develop in malnourished and multiparous mothers whose serum calcium falls with each succeeding pregnancy. Thus, frequent pregnancy, maternal dietary deficiency, and **hypocalcemic convulsions** or **hypomagnesemic convulsions** in infants have a positive correlation.

At greatest risk are infants born prematurely, born with low birthweights, and born of multiparous or diabetic mothers as well as those who are products of difficult labor. The greater susceptibility of males suggests the involvement of an androgen. The peak incidence of neonatal tetany for full-term infants occurs about the sixth day of life, and the disease seldom appears before the third day. In those born prematurely or whose mothers suffered a difficult birth, the condition frequently develops within the first 24 hours.

Infantile tetany, the most common form, occurs chiefly between 6 months and 2 years of age and is most prevalent between 4 and 8 months. Males again predominate among victims, and bottle-fed babies are at substantially greater risk than their breast-fed counterparts. In neonatal tetany, vitamin D has the paradoxical effect of raising the incidence of hypocalcemia, perhaps because of its suppressive effect on the parathyroid glands. But a deficiency of vitamin D to promote absorption of calcium is strongly implicated in the etiology of infantile tetany, and indeed, rickets is nearly always evident. The disease is much more frequent during winter months when sunlight and, thus, vitamin D are in shortest supply. Because of pigment, black children in temperate zones have in the past proved the most susceptible to rickets during these months. Doubtless they are also more susceptible to infantile tetany than their white counterparts.

Tetany is often signaled by a tingling sensation in the fingers, and it may become impossible to open and close the hands. **Carpopedal spasms** are common, as are stiffness, pain, and spasms in other muscles. Vomiting is also common. Infants in particular may develop a rigid face and body. Mental symptoms include hallucinations, dullness, and distortion. Cardiac spasms may develop, and coma, along with respiratory failure (following asthma-like attacks), leads to death. Mortality from neonatal tetany is low today in developed countries because of treatment with calcium. However, in the 1950s and previously, it has been suggested that over half of victims died.

History

It is probable that tetany caused by mineral (and perhaps vitamin D) deficiencies has always plagued humankind to some limited extent. In children, the convulsions of tetany in the past were often attributed to "teething." Not until the nineteenth century, with increased bottle-feeding, was a syndrome resembling tetany described in England. François Corvisart gave the syndrome its name in 1852, and in 1854 Armand Trousseau described tetany in lactating women. In 1881, H. Weiss observed that tetany appeared occasionally in patients after **goiter** removal, and in the 1880s the disease appeared in near-epidemic proportions in Vienna.

In 1913, E. Kehrer described neonatal tetany and suggested treatment with calcium salts. However, the first satisfactory chemical study may have been that by J. Howland and W. Marriott in 1918. It distinguished rickets from tetany and reported a substantial reduction of serum calcium in infantile tetany patients. It also reported that calcium salts relieved the symptoms.

In 1929, Alfred Hess pointed out that incidence of tetany peaked in early spring, that cases seldom developed in summer, and that black youngsters were highly susceptible. This suggested a role for vitamin D, given its shortage during winter months in temperate climates and the difficulties blacks have had historically with vitamin D while wintering in those climates.

During the 1950s and 1960s, much attention was focused on the disease. Subsequently, however, as more has been learned about mineral metabolism and as the disease has declined, so has the name "tetany." Although it is still in the literature, since the 1960s experts tend to write of hypocalcemic and hypomagnesemic, rather than tetanic, convulsions.

Kenneth F. Kiple

144. Toxoplasmosis

The agent of this disease, the sporozoan **protozoan** *Toxoplasma gondii*, is a common parasite of many birds and mammals. The organism was first seen in 1908 in the tissues of a Tunisian rodent, the gundi, and described in 1909. Human disease was first described in 1923, and congenital neonatal disease reported in 1939, but the parasite's complex life cycle was not elucidated until 1970. Serologic tests show that humans around the world harbor *T. gondii*, but almost all infections are asymptomatic. The protozoan is an intracellular parasite of a variety of tissues in warm-blooded vertebrates. It multiplies by binary fission in a host cell, eventually rupturing the cell and releasing parasites to attack other cells. Sexual reproduction occurs only in felines. These definitive hosts release oocysts, the stage infective for herbivores, in their feces. Asexual intracellular replication takes place in the herbivore, and, if the tissues containing *T. gondii* are eaten by a carnivore, asexual reproduction may also occur in its tissues. Humans become infected by eating poorly cooked or raw flesh, by ingesting oocytes from cat feces, or congenitally.

Human infections are usually inapparent, although they sometimes lie dormant for years and flare up in weakened or immunodeficient hosts. Most cases in otherwise healthy people are mild and cause vague symptoms like fever and weakness. The disease often mimics **infectious mononucleosis**. Chronic cases can cause **diarrhea**, headache, and eye damage. Rare fulminating infections cause severe symptoms and may affect the brain. Uterine transmission of **toxoplasmosis** often has grave consequences: 5–15 percent of cases result in fetal death; 18–23 percent result in brain and eye abnormalities. Some apparently normal infants later develop severe retinal disease or mental retardation. **Cerebral toxoplasmosis** is a fairly common and serious complication of AIDS.

The highest known prevalence rate, 93 percent, was found in Parisian women who enjoy eating raw beef. By age 25, roughly

70 percent of El Salvadorans and 30 percent of white residents of New York City harbor antibodies against *Toxoplasma*. Estimates suggest that about 3,000 babies with congenitally acquired toxoplasmosis are born annually in the United States.

K. David Patterson

145. Trematode Infection

Trematodes or **flukes** are flatworms of the class Trematoda of the phylum Platyhelminthes. They have complex life cycles that usually involve a snail as an intermediate host. The definitive host of the adult worms, generally a mammal, acquires the parasite by ingesting an encysted form in a second intermediate host or on vegetation. Many species can infect humans, but most normally parasitize other mammals, and humans are accidental hosts.

K. David Patterson

146. Trench Fever

Trench fever is a nonfatal acute disease first described in 1915 during World War I, when it afflicted at least 1 million soldiers on both sides of the conflict. Although initially known by several names, including "Polish fever," "Meuse fever," and "Russian intermittent fever," the term "trench fever" – assigned by British troops in France – has endured.

After incubating 14–30 days, trench fever elicits typical typhus-like symptoms: sudden onset, chills, headache, dizziness, and aches and pains. Two of its descriptive names, "shin fever" and "shank fever," recall characteristic leg pains. Although also known as "5-day fever" or "quintan fever," the disease usually disables its victims for 5–6 weeks. About half of those afflicted suffer only one bout of fever, but others may have several relapses. Although trench fever is never fatal, it caused greater loss of manpower during World War I than any other malady except **influenza**.

Also known as "Wolhynian fever" and "His-Werner disease," trench fever occurred in Russia, England, France, the Middle East, Italy, Germany, and Austria. It is carried by body lice; hence it follows the pattern of its more deadly relative, **epidemic typhus**, in plaguing armies where hygiene is substandard. The disease became quiescent after World War I but reappeared on the eastern European front during World War II.

The etiological agent of the disease, *Rochalima quintana*, was first studied during World War I by a commission of the American Red Cross, which reported that the organism, unlike other rickettsiae, passed through porcelain filters. Later, in another departure from typical rickettsial characteristics, the trench fever organism was cultivated on lifeless blood-agar media. Such differences prompted its removal from the genus *Rickettsia* to a separate genus, *Rochalima*, in 1961.

Victoria A. Harden

147. The Treponematoses

According to most medical texts, the members of genus *Treponema* – family Treponemataceae, order Spirochaetales – include *Treponema pallidum*, which causes **syphilis** and **nonvenereal syphilis**; *Treponema pertenue*, which causes **yaws**; and *Treponema carateum*, which causes **pinta**. The three pathogens, however, may actually be only one, for although they produce different pathological processes, the pathogens themselves are virtually indistinguishable under the microscope, and the diseases they cause respond to the same treatment. The origin of this infamous family and the relationships among its members have been considerably debated since the 1970s, largely because such questions bear directly on the centuries-old debate about whether the Americas bestowed syphilis on the rest of the world.

Many agree that the treponemes probably evolved from microorganisms that originally parasitized decaying organic matter, and which later – perhaps hundreds of thousands of years ago – came to specialize in human hosts, but probably only after first parasitizing another animal host. Few disagree that the first treponemes to parasitize humans did so by entering their bodies through traumatized skin and were subsequently passed on to other humans by skin-to-skin transmission. Real disagreement begins, however, over questions of where the first humans were infected, and the identity of the disease that infected them.

E. H. Hudson argued that the first of the treponemal infections was yaws and that it probably emerged in central Africa, where it quickly became endemic. Then, about 100,000 years ago, it accompanied humans migrating from Africa and spread around the globe. C. J. Hackett, however, portrays pinta as the first treponemal disease, arising only about 20,000 years ago in Eurasia to spread throughout the world.

At issue here are two different concepts of **treponematosis**. Hudson feels that the distinctions among the treponematoses are artificial. In this so-called "unitarian" view, all of the **human treponematoses** actually constitute a single disease, but one that has different manifestations depending on climate and culture. Hackett, however, argues that the distinctions are quite real – the consequence of mutations of the treponemal strains themselves. T. A. Cockburn has shown along Darwinian lines how human geographic isolation, especially after the Ice Age, could have led to treponemal speciation. Similarly, Don Brothwell has also speculated on the evolution of the treponemes and suggests that there may have been six lines of *Treponema*, which underwent separate microevolutionary development to reach the four in existence today.

Historically, yaws has been prevalent in hot and moist regions of Asia and Africa where little clothing is worn, facilitating transmission from skin to skin. By contrast, nonvenereal syphilis has flourished in hot but dry regions, where it spreads mostly from mouth to mouth. Both of these illnesses are normally rural, fostered by unsanitary conditions, and are usually endemic and thus diseases of children. **Venereal syphilis**, however, is a disease of adults, seems to have first become manifest in urban areas of temperate climates, and has been portrayed by Hudson, Cockburn, and others as a consequence of improving hygienic conditions. Put succinctly, in colder climates where people were better clothed and washed, the treponemes were denied their established patterns of skin-to-skin or mouth-to-mouth transmission among youngsters. Consequently, persons reached sexual maturity without exposure to them, and sexual intercourse became another means of transmission for the treponemes, particularly in urban areas where promiscuity and prostitution were common.

The historical gradation of treponemal infections – from the yaws of warm, moist sub-Saharan Africa, through nonvenereal syphilis in hot and dry North Africa, to venereal syphilis in cooler, urbanizing Europe – has constituted a compelling geographic model for both Hudson and Hackett and their followers. They point out nonetheless that yaws and both nonvenereal and venereal syphilis may all prevail in a relatively small geographic area, with yaws and perhaps nonvenereal syphilis dominating the rural area surrounding a city, which harbors syphilis. Moreover, both views hold that venereal syphilis was present in Eurasia long before the voyages of Columbus, but its symptoms were lumped with other disfiguring illnesses (including yaws and nonvenereal syphilis), usually under the rubric of **leprosy**.

Needless to say, this challenge to the long-held notion that syphilis was introduced from the Americas has encountered some heavy opposition. Yet we know that pinta was present in the Americas when Columbus arrived, and both the unitarian and the mutation hypotheses accommodate the notion that other treponemal diseases could have developed there as well. In fact, Brothwell has argued that Asia was probably the cradle for the evolution of human treponemes and that they diffused from there to the Americas via the Bering Straits land bridge to the New World, as well as throughout the Old World. In other words, it is conceivable that all the pathogenic human treponemes were present in each of the major landmasses of the globe by 1492. Yet Hudson believes that endemic syphilis and yaws reached the Americas via the slave trade and there evolved into syphilis; Francisco Guerra holds that all four treponemal infections were present in the New World, but only endemic and venereal syphilis resided in the Old World until yaws, not syphilis, was imported from the Americas; whereas Corinne Wood, after reviewing the arguments and evidence, finds the Columbian hypothesis for the origin of syphilis the most plausible.

Much evidence underlying this last conclusion is skeletal in nature, embracing both negative and positive findings. Most negative findings have to do with the Old World, where it appears that those buried in leper cemeteries were mostly lepers and not syphilitics, as those who placed syphilis in Europe prior to the Columbian voyages felt would be the case. Moreover, there is a dearth of evidence in Old World skeletal remains that would testify to the presence of syphilis in Eurasia prior to 1493, although the presence of yaws and endemic syphilis has been occasionally reported.

In the New World, by contrast, there is a great deal of positive skeletal evidence of pre-Columbian treponematosis. This evidence is not, however, of pinta, which causes changes in pigmentation but does not affect the bones as the other treponemal illnesses are capable of doing. Thus yaws, endemic nonvenereal syphilis, and syphilis are all possibilities for the American infection in question, as is perhaps some other treponemal infection now extinct. Of these candidates, however, venereal syphilis seems least promising, because of an apparent absence of **congenital syphilis** in the skeletal material.

Brenda Baker and George Armelagos, in providing us with an extensive review of literature on the treponematoses, have also provided the latest hypothesis as to their origin and antiquity. Given the scarcity of skeletal evidence of treponematosis in the Old World, and its abundance in the Americas, they suggest that treponematosis is a relatively new disease that arose in the Americas as a nonvenereal infection that spread by "casual contact." However, after the men of the Columbian voyages contracted the illness and carried it back to Europe, the circumstances of urban environments transformed the nonvenereal American disease into the venereal syphilis that raged across Europe and much of the globe for the next century or so before subsiding into the considerably more tame disease we know today.

Clearly, then, despite decades of debate about the nature of the treponematoses, there is still no agreement on their locational origin or their antiquity. It seems to be generally accepted that a transition in methods of transmission of treponemal syndromes can be, and was, rather swiftly brought on by changing environmental and social circumstances, and thus, that syphilis is the youngest of these syndromes. But like other surveys of the treponematoses, this one, too, must end with the hope that more evidence will be uncovered to shed light on the many paradoxes posed by this fascinating family.

Kenneth F. Kiple

148. Trichinosis

Trichinosis, also known as **trichinellosis, trichiniasis**, or **trichinelliasis**, is a disease of humans and other mammals infected with the **nematode** worm *Trichinella spiralis*. The pathological changes and symptomatology of *Trichinella* infection are manifestations of three successive stages in the life history of the worm: (1) penetration of adult female worms into the intestinal mucosa; (2) migration of juvenile worms; and (3) penetration of juvenile worms and subsequent encystment in muscle cells.

Characteristics

Although trichinosis occurs worldwide, in humans it is found principally in the United States, Canada, and Eastern Europe. It is also well known in Mexico, parts of South America, Africa, southern Asia, and the Middle East. People acquire trichinae by ingesting uncooked or poorly cooked meat, especially pork. Homemade sausages have caused many recent outbreaks in the United States. Hence, the prevalence of trichinosis is less in the tropics and subtropics, where less meat is consumed. Trichinosis does not occur among Hindus, Jews, and Moslems, for whom there are religious bans on eating pork.

Although the prevalence of trichinosis in human populations is low (probably 2.2 percent or less in the United States, based on autopsy surveys), epidemic outbreaks are not infrequent. Incidence of infection is likely to be higher than suspected because of the vagueness of symptoms, which usually suggest other conditions.

T. spiralis is unusual in that a single individual animal serves as both intermediate and definitive (final) host, with the juvenile and adult worms located in different organs.

Humans acquire infections by ingesting infective juveniles, which are encysted in striated muscle of swine or other animals. The worms are freed from their cysts by gastric juices and invade the intestinal mucosa where they copulate. Males die shortly after copulation, and females migrate through the intestinal epithelium, each giving birth to as many as 1,500 live young over 4–16 weeks. Spent females eventually die and are absorbed by the host.

Young juveniles are carried throughout the body via the arterial system. They finally reach skeletal muscle, where they penetrate individual fibers and grow in a spiral fashion, eventually becoming encysted by a blunt, ellipsoidal capsule of host origin. The time required for complete encapsulation is about 3 months. Calcification of the capsule begins as early as 6 months and may take up to 2 years to complete. Eventually the worms also become calci-fied, although they may remain viable for several years prior to calcification.

Not all striated muscles are parasitized to the same degree. Among muscles most heavily affected are the diaphragm, tongue, and masticatory muscles, intercostals, and muscles of the arms and legs.

Most mammals are susceptible to *Trichinella* infections. Infections are maintained in nature by flesh-eating animals. Humans are regarded as accidental hosts because, barring cannibalism or the consumption of cadavers by other mammals, the infection reaches a dead end. Most human infections result from eating pork or pork products, but numerous fatal cases of trichinosis have been recorded among people eating undercooked or underfrozen bear or walrus meat.

Cooking meat is of importance in preventing trichinosis. Pork should be cooked until the pink color turns to gray. Alternatively, freezing of meat at −15°F for 20 days destroys all parasites.

Trichinella infection results in development of serum antibodies and cell-mediated immune responses. Resistance to reinfection has been demonstrated by an allergic inflammatory response that expels adult worms from the intestine. Eosinophils may also play a role in immunity to *Trichinella* because experimental depletion of eosinophils has been shown to result in increased numbers of larvae recovered from infected animals.

The first symptoms of *Trichinella* infection occur 1–2 days after ingestion of infected meat. Initial symptoms are vague and often misdiagnosed, if apparent at all. As a host reacts to waste produced by the worms, lesions develop and enteric bacteria are introduced into them. Nausea, toxic **diarrhea**, sweating, and vomiting may occur, mimicking an acute food-poisoning syndrome. Respiratory symptoms may follow between the second and sixth day and last for 6 days. In addition, there may be red blotches erupting on the skin.

During the period of migration of juveniles, there are muscular pains as inflammatory processes develop in the muscles. Difficulty in breathing, chewing, and swallowing develops. **Edema** around the face and hands results from endovascular and perivascular inflammation. Edema around the eyes is a common early sign. Lymph nodes become enlarged and tender. Enlarged parotid or sublingual glands often lead to misdiagnosis of mumps. **Eosinophilia** may be present but often does not occur, even in the most extreme cases. **Myocarditis, peritonitis, pneumonia, encephalitis, pleurisy, meningitis**, and eye damage may result from migrating juveniles. Death from myocarditis may occur at this stage.

Penetration by juveniles into muscle cells, and subsequent encystment, may result in toxic edema, **cachexia**, or dehydration. Blood pressure drops rapidly, and the patient may display nervous disorders such as defects of vision, altered or lost reflexes, hallucinations, delirium, and encephalitis. Severe cases can result in death 4–6 weeks after infection. Death may occur as a result of **toxemia**, myocarditis, **nephritis**, peritonitis, or other complications.

Most cases of trichinosis, however, go undetected, and in milder cases no special symptoms may be present. There is no thoroughly effective treatment.

History

Although knowledge of the parasite causing trichinosis dates from 1835, knowledge of the disease goes back to antiquity. Dietary laws prohibiting consumption of swine may have been engendered by the observation that human illness sometimes followed the eating of such flesh. Historians have surmised that Muhammad – recognizing the possible cause of certain epidemics as ingestion of pork – followed the example of Moses in prohibiting pork consumption.

The first person to actually see trichinae was James Paget, a 21-year-old freshman medical student in London. In 1835, Paget noted a curious pathological condition in a cadaver brought in for study. The cadaver had "spicules of bone" in the muscles – so hard that they blunted the scalpel. Others had seen these gritty particles previously, but Paget had natural history training and the intense desire to observe new things, and thus was the first to note that the particle was a worm in its capsule. Paget did not have a microscope but eventually secured the use of one. Specimens of the worm were taken to Richard Owen, who would become England's greatest comparative anatomist. Owen subsequently presented a paper on the worm and named it.

Although Paget's discovery was overshadowed by Owen's detailed and complete report, Paget retained his intense spirit of scientific inquiry and published many papers on medical subjects. Later, he became Sir James Paget, one of the most distinguished surgeons of his time.

Trichinae in animals other than humans were first noted in 1846. Joseph Leidy in Philadelphia found worms in the extensor muscles of a hog's thigh. Leidy had previously seen trichinae in human bodies in a dissection room, and he perceived no distinction in the worms from the two hosts. In 1850, Ernst Herbst, working in Göttingen, established that trichinae from meat eaten by an animal may invade its muscles. The significance of Herbst's experiments, as well as Leidy's observations, was not appreciated at the time because leading authorities believed that the trichinae from nonhumans were of a different species than those from humans. Herbst himself believed that trichinae were actually the larvae of filarial worms.

The problem of determining the life cycle of trichinae soon caught the attention of two of the leading researchers of their time, Rudolf Virchow of Berlin and Rudolph Leuckart of Giessen. Leuckart, in 1850, observed that female intestinal trichinae are viviparous, but he believed that the trichinae were derived from the intestinal nematode *Trichuris trichiura*. Virchow, in 1859, fed encapsulated trichinae from a human to a dog, where the worms reached sexual maturity. Virchow thus refuted Leuckart's claim that the trichinae were identical with *Trichuris*.

Verification of the life cycle of trichinae and the discovery of the pathogenesis of trichinous infections represent monumental contributions by Friedrich Zenker in 1860. Zenker autopsied a 20-year-old servant girl in Dresden whose illness had been diagnosed as **typhoid fever**. He examined muscle fibers from the arm and was startled to see "dozens" of live trichinae. Other skeletal muscles were likewise inhabited by the worms. Upon examining intestinal contents, Zenker saw sexually mature worms. It was apparent to him that the parasite underwent its entire life cycle in one and the same host.

Zenker subsequently investigated the servant's household and found the parasite in sausage prepared just prior to the girl's illness. Furthermore, other members of the household who had eaten the meat had become seriously ill with the same symptoms.

Following establishment of the life cycle and pathogenesis of trichinae, several outbreaks were recorded. Some 140 epidemics of trichinosis were noted in Europe in 1860–77. In 1863, examination of pork for trichinae began in parts of Germany, and in 1879 a Prussian law required such examination for all pork. In the same year, ordinances were passed in Italy, Austria, and Hungary forbidding importation of swine or pork products from the United States, and other countries followed with similar bans. Subsequently, the U.S. Department of Agriculture, although not requiring specific examination for trichinae, did specify methods of processing pork products customarily eaten raw. Such procedures destroy the infectivity of any trichinae present. Public education and heat treatment of garbage used to feed hogs have also helped to reduce the incidence of the disease in North America and Europe.

Donald E. Gilbertson

149. Trichuriasis

The **nematode** *Trichuris trichiura*, the whipworm or threadworm, is a common parasite that occurs worldwide but is most abundant in warm, moist climates. It still exists in the southern United States but in recent decades has declined there and in other developed countries with improved sanitation; it is now found mostly in poor tropical countries. Adult worms range up to 2 inches long, so whipworms were probably seen by ancient observers, but they were first clearly recognized by an early Portuguese writer on tropical medicine, Aleixo de Abreu, in 1623. Several scientists described the species in the mid-eighteenth century. Archaeological evidence shows that the worm infected people in the Americas prior to the voyage of Columbus.

Trichuris attaches itself to the wall of the large intestine and passes its eggs in the host's feces. Eggs require 10–14 days in the soil to mature or "embryonate." Embryonation is most successful in warm, moist soils in shady places. Like *Ascaris*, which has a similar range, *Trichuris* infects people who have swallowed embryonated eggs in soil or in contaminated food or water. Unlike *Ascaris*, however, the whipworm does not require an elaborate period of larval migration in the host. The eggs hatch in the small intestine, where the larvae spend some time before moving to their home in the cecum.

Trichuriasis rarely causes much harm unless there is a heavy worm load. Severe infections can cause abdominal discomfort, bloody or mucoid **diarrhea**, weight loss, weakness, and **anemia**. Masses of worms can cause **appendicitis**, and prolapse of the rectum can occur in children. Symptoms, including anemia, tend to be more severe in children. Drug treatment is effective, and improved sanitation is preventative.

K. David Patterson

150. Tuberculosis

Tuberculosis is most commonly associated with the lungs but can affect almost any bodily tissue or organ. Caused by a bacillus (*Mycobacterium tuberculosis*), it is usually a chronic infection, lingering for months and sometimes years, although acute forms, which most commonly strike infants and young children, can prove fatal in weeks or days. One acute form is called **miliary tuberculosis** because of the small grain-like tubercles it creates simultaneously in almost every organ of the body. Since ancient times, tuberculosis was endemic in most populations of Eurasia, North Africa, and possibly the Americas, affecting relatively small numbers and maintaining low prevalence rates. But with modern urban and industrial development it became epidemic in much of the globe. In some places, tuberculosis prevalence rates have approached 100 percent of the population. Tuberculosis killed millions over the centuries, placing it on a historical par with other great epidemic diseases: **plague, cholera, smallpox**, and the like. In 1944, researchers discovered streptomycin, which effectively inhibited the disease. In combination with streptomycin, two newer drugs – para-aminosalicylic acid and isoniazid – provided further potent therapy. Today, all but the most advanced cases are curable.

Characteristics

Over 30 species of genus *Mycobacterium* have been identified, more than 15 of which can cause disorders similar, but not identical, to tuberculosis. Human disease typically is caused by members of the species *M. tuberculosis*. In addition, mycobacteria can cause disease in a wide variety of animals, including birds, fish, rodents, elephants, and cattle. Of its animal forms, only **bovine tuberculosis** can infect people. Some bacteriologists consider the bovine form a separate species of the tubercle bacillus, whereas others group it with several variants that they classify together as the "*M. tuberculosis* complex."

The human bacillus has also been divided into three types according to immunologic responses (phage types), which show marked variations in virulence. **Type I tuberculosis** is found in India; **type A tuberculosis** is found in Africa, China, and Japan as well as in Europe and North America; and **type B tuberculosis** is found exclusively in Europe and North America. Type I is the least virulent of the three, making Indians more susceptible to disease when infected with type A or B. These differences probably result from the evolution of widely separated organisms over long periods of time. However, all forms of *M. tuberculosis* show a strong resistance to mutation, and thus it is unlikely that an increase in virulence caused the disease to become epidemic, or that a decrease in virulence prompted the decline in tuberculosis mortality rates that occurred in England, the United States, and other Western nations before the introduction of streptomycin and other specifics.

Except for bovine forms, tubercle bacilli reach human hosts almost exclusively through aerial transmission. Talking, coughing, sneezing, spitting, singing, and other respiratory actions produce airborne particles called droplet nuclei; these, when emitted by tubercular individuals, can contain up to three bacilli – one is enough to establish an infection if inhaled. Once airborne in a closed space, droplets disperse, and some remain suspended, like smoke. Larger ones fall, presenting little threat, although dry tubercle bacilli can remain viable for months. Bovine bacilli are ingested in milk and usually cause intestinal disease but infrequently **pulmonary tuberculosis** or miliary tuberculosis.

After entering the body, tubercle bacilli are remarkably durable. They can remain viable throughout the host's lifetime, dormant until resistance fails, whereupon they can cause disease even if they never did so when first entering the body. Whether or not tubercle bacilli cause immediate disease upon infection depends on several factors: age, gender, and immunogenetics ("host-dependent" factors), along with environmental factors such as crowding, nutrition, and working conditions. A population's genetic pool is important as well. For example, long inhabitation of urban environments has apparently increased Jews' resistance to the disease. By contrast, lack of prior exposure can lead to acute epidemics, such as among the New Zealand Maori and Alaskan Eskimos.

Some epidemiologists assert that natural selection determines the course of tuberculosis epidemics, based on the idea that genetic background and resistance to the disease are of paramount importance. Mortality rates drop, they say, as the susceptible are weeded out. Others oppose this theory, noting that although natural selection has doubtless reinforced resistance to tuberculosis, it has not strongly affected the decline in epidemics. Rather, economic and social changes seem to constitute the most important factors in declining tuberculosis mortality rates until the 1940s, when cures became available. Numerous studies indicate that lowest-income groups suffer most from the disease and also that rising incomes greatly reduce tuberculosis mortality. This means that industrialization alternatively exacerbates and improves tuberculosis rates. An early-stage industrial economy subjects many to crowded and impoverished living conditions. Eventually, however, material benefits improve housing and nutrition, reducing risks of infection and lowering disease rates.

Tuberculosis frequently causes disease in the meninges, intestines, bones, lymph system, skin, spine, kidneys, and genitals. Most of these forms (excepting **tubercular meningitis**) are chronic, sometimes lasting years before either recovery or death. Miliary tuberculosis affects most vital organs concurrently. Pulmonary tuberculosis, however, is the most common form, its most familiar symptom a frequent, violent cough producing purulent sputum and sometimes blood. But symptoms are not universal. Indeed, until the disease becomes advanced, many victims are completely free of symptoms or experience only mild respiratory symptoms. In the past, many developed mild, asymptomatic cases and recovered unknowingly, as autopsies and X-rays later revealed. In early stages, the unalarming symptoms and myriad manifestations of tuberculosis make diagnosis difficult even today. A tuberculin test usually indicates whether a person has become infected. But although tuberculin testing is highly reliable today, false-positive responses do occur.

The tubercle bacillus does not itself damage the body. Rather, cellular and tissue damage arises from an allergic reaction or hypersensitivity to the bacillus. In other words, after the body has become allergic to invading tubercle bacilli, the immune system destroys them. This process, however, releases proteins and fatty substances that in turn cause inflammation and can damage surrounding tissue and cells. The same process also creates the illness's distinctive tubercles. Individual resistance to tuberculosis fluctuates markedly: Quiescent infections rekindle with depressed resistance only to capitulate when resistance returns. Acquired resistance to the tubercle bacillus confers no durable protection (such as in **measles** and smallpox). To the contrary, it can assist the development of active disease. Antituberculosis vaccination usually consists of BCG (bacillus Calmette-Guérin), an attenuated strain of bovine bacillus first isolated in 1921. Tests indicate that it offers some degree of immunity to uninfected recipients.

History

Archaeological evidence of tuberculosis afflicting prehistoric humans dates at least from the Neolithic period. Stone Age skeletons with apparently tubercular lesions have been unearthed in Europe, and **spinal tuberculosis** has been found in Egyptian mummies dating from the third millennium B.C. In China, a mummified body from the second century B.C. has tuberculosis scars on the lungs. Trade and migration ensured dissemination of China's diseases throughout East Asia during the first three centuries A.D. Skeletal evidence strongly suggests that native Americans suffered from tuberculosis as early as 800 B.C., and pulmonary lesions have been discovered in Chilean mummies from 290 A.D.

This evidence suggests two important points concerning the prehistory of tuberculosis. First, the disease quite possibly evolved with humans from earliest times. Second, tuberculosis afflicted most people worldwide from prehistoric times, save for small groups such as the Maori, who lived in isolation for centuries. Most epidemics therefore resulted not from the introduction of foreign pathogens into virgin populations but from changes in host populations and their environments.

Until the present concept of tuberculosis – as a single disease caused by the tubercle bacillus – emerged during the nineteenth century, its various forms were often considered different diseases. For example, pulmonary forms were commonly called **phthisis** or **consumption**; lymph infections were termed **scrofula**, and skin infections **lupus vulgaris**. This confusion makes identification of tuberculosis from historical texts difficult. Consequently, conclusions concerning tuberculosis based on most sources up to the nineteenth century necessarily engender some skepticism.

Nevertheless, classical Hindu, Babylonian, Assyrian, Chinese, Greek, and Roman sources all describe symptoms of tuberculosis. Hindu texts dating from 1200 B.C. and perhaps earlier, along with Mesopotamian texts from the seventh century B.C., described treatments for pulmonary tuberculosis and scrofula. The first description of tuberculosis in Chinese may date from 2700 B.C., and texts from around 400 B.C. clearly describe the symptoms. The first Greek mention of what was probably tuberculosis is by Homer (c. 800 B.C.). Hippocratic writings from approximately 400 B.C. discuss *phthisis* (the Greek term for consumption), which was attributed to evil airs. "Phthisis" became the standard European term signifying a symptom-cluster similar to pulmonary tuberculosis. Other Greek and Roman writers used the term extensively, including Galen, who during the second century A.D. recommended a change of climate as therapy for consumption. Researchers have noted that the ancient cultures that described the signs and symptoms of the disease were primarily urban, whereas pastoral cultures make scarce mention of the disease. Biblical literature, for example, makes scant reference to it.

Medieval Europeans suffered from tuberculosis, although contemporary documents mention it more often in its glandular form –

that is, as scrofula. This was because of the custom of the "king's touch": French and English kings were believed to cure scrofula simply by touching its victims. The custom originated in the twelfth century and continued through the eighteenth.

Chinese texts providing detailed treatments of tuberculosis were written during the Sui (581–617) and Tang (618–907) dynasties. Japanese physicians, using the Chinese texts, clearly described symptoms of tubercular diseases in their own country. By the twelfth century, Taoist priests attributed phthisis both to evil airs and to animalculae, which attacked exhausted individuals. In positing a systematic "germ theory," the Chinese anticipated Western medicine by centuries. In the sixteenth century, Girolamo Fracastoro became the first Western physician to propose such ideas. Unlike the Chinese, however, Fracastoro believed that phthisis was only one of many diseases caused by animalculae.

During the sixteenth century, tuberculosis mortality increased noticeably among urban populations. In England, for example, it caused about 20 percent of all deaths, with the greatest concentrations in London. A similar phenomenon occurred in Japan: Observers in the early seventeenth century noted that phthisis was widespread in the rapidly growing capital of Edo. During the eighteenth century, however, the great epidemics of tuberculosis began and were well under way by the beginning of the nineteenth. The nations that suffered most severely from tuberculosis were experiencing intense urbanization and industrialization. Thus reports of phthisis were common in England, the United States, Italy, and France.

Autopsies showed that close to 100 percent of some urban populations, such as those of London and Paris, developed tuberculosis sometime during their lives, even if they died from another cause. Tuberculosis mortality rates in American cities during the early nineteenth century ranged from 400–500 per 100,000. Women textile workers generally led other groups in tuberculosis mortality in every country where textile factories appeared. When statistics became available for most industrial countries after 1860, they showed that tuberculosis epidemics were declining. In developing countries (including Japan), however, epidemics were just starting at the end of the century.

Beginning in the seventeenth century, European physicians gave increasing attention to tuberculosis, partly because of major changes in medical theory and partly because of growing mortality from phthisis and scrofula. In 1685, Richard Morton became the first Westerner to publish a monograph on phthisis, a term he used to embrace several diseases, including **pulmonary consumption** and scrofula. By the eighteenth century, however, physicians were redefining their concepts of disease and seeking new explanations of causes, and the nineteenth century became a period of intense research into tubercular diseases. In Europe and the United States, investigators sought to identify lifestyle and environmental factors that made people "susceptible." Among such factors were dissolute living, alcohol and tobacco consumption, and developmental life crises such as puberty and childbirth. In addition, damp soil and filth could make an individual susceptible to consumption. Others, however, believed that pulmonary consumption was a hereditary affliction – a belief that became a powerful social stigma. Indeed, throughout the nineteenth century, popular (and some medical) concepts of tuberculosis held that it expressed a person's inherent nature, instead of just being something one had.

A major break with previous theories occurred in the early nineteenth century, which transformed the tubercular diseases' classification by the 1880s. From the early 1800s, the French "clinical school" compared the course of disease symptoms with autopsy observations. Eventually, René Laennec, a leading physician of this school, postulated that all tubercular phenomena including phthisis, scrofula, and miliary tubercles constituted a single disease.

German physicians of the "physiological school" vigorously attacked Laennec's theory of tuberculosis. A leading theoretician of this school, Karl Wunderlich, asserted the impossibility of drawing a meaningful distinction between, for example, **dysentery** and **enteric diarrhea**. Wunderlich thought of disease names only as conveniences, not as linguistic symbols for specific entities. In his views of tuberculosis, Wunderlich echoed his contemporary, Rudolph Virchow, one of the greatest medical theoreticians of the nineteenth century. He also repudiated Laennec's idea that all tubercular phenomena manifested a single, specific disease. Rather, he divided them into separate categories of inflammatory and neoplastic phenomena and thought that some forms fundamentally resembled **cancer**.

Despite Virchow, the tradition of combining clinical and pathological investigation continued in France, most notably by Jean-Antoine Villemin, who followed Laennec's principles and demonstrated in practice what Laennec had postulated. In 1865, Villemin caused tuberculosis in rabbits by injecting them with matter from human tubercles. Although his work had a negligible impact on German ideas, tuberculosis was established as a specific disease by Prussian bacteriologist Robert Koch.

Using clearly defined bacteriologic methods, Koch proved in 1882 that animals contracted tuberculosis from inoculations of bacteria (not simply tubercular matter) isolated from human tubercles. Although many problems remained (such as the identity of scrofula, which some still maintained was a separate disease), Koch's work finally showed tuberculosis to be a single disease entity. For several years, some circles disputed Koch's methods and conclusions. Nonetheless, his discovery of the tubercle bacillus changed the way most people viewed the disease.

Koch's discovery had little effect on treatment but important implications for prophylaxis. Observers concluded that dry tubercle bacilli in dried sputum presented the greatest threat. They recommended general removal of dust from all buildings, restrictions on spitting and the use of spittoons everywhere, and disinfection or destruction of the belongings and surroundings of tuberculosis victims. In some places, such procedures were already "on the books." Not until the 1930s did researchers demonstrate that tuberculosis mainly resulted from airborne infection and that other forms of contact played little role in transmission.

Most practicing physicians, however, were primarily interested not in ascertaining the etiology of tuberculosis but in treating it. Hundreds of thousands of victims created an unbounded demand for remedies, creating opportunity for both physicians and quacks. Popular cures for tuberculosis included creosote, carbolic acid, gold, iodoform, arsenic, and menthol – administered orally, inhaled, or injected directly into lungs. More unusual treatments ranged from drinking papaya juice to enemas of sulfur gases. Starting during the late nineteenth century and continuing well into the twentieth, physicians practiced surgical therapies, including collapsed-lung treatments and surgical removal of ribs to diminish the thoracic cavity.

The search for a remedy (rather than his discovery of the tubercle bacillus) brought Koch international fame. In 1890, under pressure from the German government, he announced a cure for tuberculosis, which attracted thousands to his Berlin laboratory. Soon, however, many questioned the efficacy of "Koch's lymph" (a tubercle extract); indeed, it proved harmful in advanced cases. But it soon became the extremely important diagnostic tool known as tuberculin – the primary means of determining tuberculosis infection.

After 1895, the X-ray too helped change the way people thought about tuberculosis. It displayed tubercular lesions long before symptoms became noticeable, allowing physicians to start treatment much earlier in the disease than before. X-ray photographs together with tuberculin became the basic tools of mass screening programs implemented by governments and antituberculosis associations from the 1920s to the 1950s.

As diagnostic techniques improved but medicinal cures remained ineffective, therapies based on climate and regimen evolved. From the mid-nineteenth century, open-air and rest therapies became increasingly popular throughout Europe and the United States. Systematic integration of these therapies with other forms of treatment culminated in the sanitorium. From the 1880s, luxury sanitoria for the wealthy drew patients from around the world. About 1900, state-sponsored sanitoria began to appear throughout Western Europe, North America, and Japan. Where sanitoria were not feasible, such as in inner cities, public-health officials developed alternatives that offered open-air treatment as well as preventive regimens.

Many sanitoria and prevention programs were sponsored by antituberculosis organizations, established in most of Western Europe and North America from the 1890s and in much of the rest of the world during the next few decades. Their educational programs, which became a mainstay of tuberculosis control, informed the public about disease transmission and encouraged people to secure frequent checkups and early treatment. However, the most commonly afflicted groups – industrial workers and the urban poor – rarely could afford treatment even if they received an early diagnosis.

Tuberculosis declined dramatically from the late nineteenth century onward, and researchers, officials, and volunteers understandably concluded that the decline was the direct result of their efforts, especially in Britain, Germany, and the United States. Yet other experience contradicted such claims. For example, during the early twentieth century, the Japanese implemented Western tuberculosis control measures including extensive legislation, state-sponsored sanitoria, intensive education programs, and mass screenings and BCG immunizations. However, Japan's tuberculosis mortality rate, initially hovering around 200 per 100,000, actually increased from the early 1930s. Not until the late 1940s did rates begin a sustained fall. In Japan's case, the prevention movement was much less important than later improvements in living standards and working conditions, and even later nationwide treatment with modern drugs.

Since the 1950s, the countries with the highest tuberculosis mortality have been those with low standards of living, poor working conditions, and inadequate treatment programs. Medicine has learned that the mere availability of specifics is insufficient to stem the disease; their administration must be coordinated with reforms that raise living standards and improve working conditions. As late as the 1970s, over 20 developing countries had new-case tuberculosis rates over 150 per 100,000 per year.

Thus although many have long envisioned the eradication of tuberculosis, it remains a major health problem in many countries. Even in developed nations, when social conditions deteriorate, the incidence of tuberculosis rises quickly. Clearly, tuberculosis remains far from eradicated and can be a significant health problem during times of depression, war, and unrest.

William D. Johnston

Postscript

The 1990s saw a sharp increase in tuberculosis (TB) cases in the United States and in the world. The number of U.S cases, which had been falling at around 5 percent annually since 1953, suddenly rose from fewer than 23,000 in 1988 to peak at some 27,000 cases in 1992, before falling to around half that number by the end of the century. In the larger world, however, where there was no such reversal, the picture was much bleaker. In the mid-1990s, the World Health Organization (WHO) declared TB a global emergency, with the magnitude of that emergency made clear in 1996 estimates indicating that (1) one in every three of the world's citizens was infected with *M. tuberculosis* (although the majority had not developed active cases); (2) eight million new cases were developing each year; and (3) some three million persons were dying of TB annually. The situa-

tion has continued to deteriorate. The year 1998 was declared to be the *worst* TB year in human history, and it was expected that between 1995 and 2005 some 300 million new TB cases would occur, almost exclusively in developing countries, most of which are ravaged by poverty, and many of which are under siege from **AIDS**.

A good share of the new TB cases has been attributed to the simultaneous rise and diffusion of AIDS, which cripples the immune systems of its victims (indeed, TB and HIV form a lethal combination, with each hastening the progress of the other). But it has also been the case that poorly supervised drug therapy for the disease has helped to create drug-resistant strains that facilitate the spread of TB. Tourism, migration, and international travel do the same, and the WHO has called attention to developing countries that act as facilitators. These include those of the former Soviet Union, whose health systems are in shambles.

But developed countries are not blameless in this regard. Made complacent by the steady reduction in TB rates since the 1950s, their health systems have been slow to react. It was a complacency rooted in the notion that modern medicine had conquered all of the important infectious diseases and therefore could and should turn its attention to the chronic illnesses. Forgotten was that TB had not been subdued in the developing world (meaning most of the world), that pathogens can develop defenses against drugs (as well as vice versa), and that it was possible for new diseases – like AIDS – to emerge that would act in concert with TB. For Western medicine, then, tuberculosis has become "the disease that never went away."

Kenneth F. Kiple

151. Tularemia

Tularemia is primarily a specific infectious disease of rodents and lagomorphs. The causative organism, however, has been isolated from over 100 species of mammals, 9 species of domestic animals, 25 species of birds, 70 species of insects, and several species of fish and amphibians. In humankind, tularemia is an acute, infectious, moderately severe, febrile disease, with mortality of approximately 7 percent in untreated cases. The causative agent, *Francisella* (*Pasteurella*) *tularensis*, is a tiny pleomorphic coccobacillus. Tularemia is also known as "deerfly fever," "Pahvant Valley plague," "rabbit fever," **Ohara's disease**, *yatobyo*, and "lemming fever."

Characteristics

Two variants (biovars) of the causative organism are recognized. *F. tularensis* biovar *tularensis* (type A) has been isolated in nature only in North America and is the most virulent in humans. The second, *F. tularensis* biovar *palaearctica* (type B), is found in all areas where tularemia is endemic in the Northern Hemisphere.

Tularemia is unique in the number of ways humans can become infected, and the clinical picture of the disease depends on the infection route. The most common route is via the skin, either by insect bite or by direct passage through intact skin by contact with infected carcasses or a scratch from an infected animal. Of numerous insects that transmit the disease, the tick is most important. The wood tick (*Dermacentor andersoni*) and three species of rabbit tick are especially important in the United States. Biting insects such as the deer fly (*Chrysops discalis*) and the stable fly (*Stomoxys calcitrans*) also carry the disease to humans. Of several species of mosquitoes that harbor the organism, only two act as human vectors: *Aedes cinereus* and *Aedes excrucians* in Sweden and the former U.S.S.R. Infection of the intestinal canal follows ingestion of contaminated water and undercooked meat. Humans can also contract infection via the respiratory route by inhaling the organism from sources such as contaminated hay and wool.

Susceptibility to tularemia is independent of age, sex, race, and health status. That men are more often infected is related to their intrusion into the transmission cycle through hunting and handling infected animals. Human-to-human transmission is extremely rare, and the disease is largely confined to rural areas. It may occur in any season but is least prevalent in winter when insect vectors are least abundant and small animals are not much hunted.

The fatality rate in North America, prior to widespread use of streptomycin in the late 1940s, ranged up to 9 percent. Today that figure has been reduced to less than 1 percent. In Europe, the mortality rate has always been much lower – in the realm of 1 percent – because of lower virulence there. An attack confers relatively solid lifelong immunity. A live attenuated vaccine is now available that reduces the severity of the **ulceroglandular infection** and reduces incidence of **typhoid**-type tularemia. However, the vaccine is still being investigated and used primarily for laboratory workers who are always at high risk in working with the tularemia organism.

Tularemia in humans is confined to the Northern Hemisphere with three main areas of epidemicity: North America, Europe (especially Eastern Europe and Russia), and to a lesser extent Japan. It is not found in nature in the British Isles. Tularemia has been reported everywhere in the United States except Hawaii. In Canada, the disease is endemic in the central and western provinces as well as the Northwest Territories but seldom is reported from the eastern provinces. Other countries that have reported the disease include Mexico, Norway, Sweden, Belgium, France, Germany, Poland, Czechoslovakia, Austria, Yugoslavia, Turkey, and Tunisia. Sporadic cases have been reported from northern South America including Venezuela, Ecuador, and Colombia, but these have not been confirmed.

In the United States, tularemia became a reportable disease in 1927 and rose to peak incidence in 1939 with 2,291 reported cases (17.5 per million population). Since the 1950s, the disease has undergone a dramatic decline. In 1984 in the United States, only 291 cases were reported (1.2 per million). Since 1931 in Canada, nearly 400 cases have been reported but with a steady decline over the years. In Russia, a similar decrease has been observed. In the mid-1940s, 100,000 cases per year were reported; yet these were reduced to a few hundred cases per year by the mid-1960s. The reasons for this worldwide decline are controversial. The reasons advanced range from ecologically induced selection against the more virulent strains of *F. tularensis* and reduction of the organism circulating in wild reservoirs, to an increased awareness of the disease through mass education, to a failure to detect and report cases.

Tularemia manifests an extremely variable clinical picture depending on the inoculation site and the extent of spread. In general, incubation averages about 3 days. The disease begins with headache, chills, vomiting, and fever, with generalized aches and pains. An ulcer develops at the site of initial entry, while associated lymph nodes become enlarged and tender. The disease lasts 3–4 weeks, with sweating, weight loss, and general debility. Convalescence requires 2–3 months. Several clinical types of the disease have been described:

1. In ulceroglandular **cutaneous tularemia**, an inflamed papule develops at the inoculation site, which soon breaks down, leaving a punched-out ulcer. Associated lymph nodes painfully enlarge, which may last 2–3 months. The usual signs of infection, fever, and prostration are common.
2. Oculoglandular **ophthalmic tularemia** occurs when the bacterium enters via the conjunctival sac. Local inflammation occurs with enlargement of neck lymph nodes. Permanent impairment of vision may occur.
3. **Pleuropulmonary tularemia** develops secondary to other forms. Milder forms resemble atypical **pneumonia** and may include shortness of breath, malaise, chills, and pleuritic pain.
4. Oropharyngeal **gastrointestinal tularemia** is contracted from the ingestion of contaminated food and water and may be

accompanied by acute abdominal symptoms such as pain, vomiting, and **diarrhea** with ulcerative lesions in the intestinal mucosa.
5. **Glandular tularemia** develops without a primary lesion but with enlargement of regional lymph nodes.
6. Septicemic **typhoidal tularemia** develops without a primary lesion and without enlargement of the regional nodes. Infection arises via the respiratory route or is the late result of local infection.
7. **Meningitic tularemia** is rare in North America but not infrequent in Asia, under certain conditions of insect transmission.

In all these types, subclinical infections may be more common than previously supposed.

History
Tularemia enjoys a unique place in medical history as it is the first disease to be identified and entirely described by American investigators. In 1910, G. McCoy, while studying plague in California ground squirrels, reported a "plague-like disease of rodents" in these animals. The following year, he and C. Chapin, using a special nutrient medium, succeeded in culturing the causative organism and named it *Bacterium tularense* after Tulare County, California, where infected squirrels were first discovered. W. Wherry and B. Lamb were first to diagnose a human case of the disease in 1914. The infected patient showed **ulcerative conjunctivitis** and **lymphadenitis**.

Earlier, in 1911, R. Pearse had described several cases of deer fly fever and suggested that the disease was caused by the bite of *Chrysops discalis*, the common deer fly. Edward Francis pieced together the complicated etiologic connection among deer fly fever in humans, the plague-like disease of rodents in California, and similar illnesses in small mammals of Utah and Indiana. Francis isolated the organism in 1921 and proved that it was indeed spread by the bite of the deer fly as well as by direct contact with infected meat. The role of the tick in the spread of tularemia was determined in 1924. It was also Francis who coined the term "tularemia" after finding the organism in the blood of infected individuals. In the late 1950s, the genus name of the organism was changed to *Pasteurella* because of a supposed relationship to the causative organism of **plague**. In 1974, the genus name was changed to *Francisella* to honor Francis who, through more than 30 years of investigation into tularemia, was the man most responsible for sorting out its complexities and many manifestations.

Beginning in 1925, Hachiro Ohara, a Japanese scientist, published studies of a disease of wild rabbits and described how an illness that would become known as Ohara's disease was successfully transmitted to humans. Other papers by Japanese scientists soon followed, but none made reference to American investigations of tularemia. Francis and a colleague, recognizing that Ohara's disease seemed similar to tularemia in every way, requested sera from convalescent Japanese patients, examination of which quickly confirmed that Ohara's disease and tularemia were actually the same illness.

Although tularemia is often described as a "new disease," it is perhaps new only in terms of discovery. Evidence suggests that tularemia was endemic in the United States, Scandinavia, and Russia in the eighteenth and nineteenth centuries. Travelers in Russia as early as 1741 noted a disease with all the characteristics of tularemia and termed "Siberian ulcer."

In the United States at least three written records survive describing the disease, including one from California in 1904 and another from Arizona in 1907. In fact, the wide distribution of the disease and its adaptation to a wide variety of animals suggest that the disease is ancient, perhaps dating from the latter Miocene or early Pliocene periods.

Despite the dramatic decline in the incidence of tularemia since the 1950s, it appears that tularemia will remain a hazard to humans for many years to come. In spite of the great amount of research over the past 70 years, numerous questions remain unanswered because of the complex interactions among hosts, vectors, and varied environments. Such complexity makes eradication of tularemia unlikely.

Patrick D. Horne

152. Typhoid Fever

Typhoid fever is a systemic infection caused by the bacterium *Salmonella typhi*, usually manifested by slow onset of a sustained fever and other symptoms including headache, cough, digestive disturbances, and profound weakness. In a minority of sufferers, specific diagnostic symptoms such as spleen or liver enlargement or a characteristic "rose-spot" rash are found. Untreated, the illness lasts 3–4 weeks; it kills about 10 percent of victims and leaves 2 percent as permanent carriers of the organism. Three-quarters of the world's population live in typhoid-endemic areas; 1 in 300 contracts the disease annually. Each year, typhoid kills 1 million people, mostly children. A variant, **paratyphoid fever**, has similar features but is caused by different *Salmonella* species. Typhoid and paratyphoid are sometimes lumped together under the term **enteric fever**.

Characteristics

The microorganism responsible for typhoid fever belongs to one of the largest and most widespread families of bacteria on Earth, with over 1,700 serotypes recognized. Salmonellae are rod-shaped bacteria that have a cell wall and flagella, which provide motility.

Salmonellae can colonize the gastrointestinal tracts of a broad range of animal hosts, including mammals, birds, reptiles, amphibians, fish, and insects. Some types of salmonellae are highly adapted to specific animals; others have a wide range of hosts. Because of this versatility and the consequent enormous animal reservoir, the eradication of all **salmonellosis** would be essentially impossible.

Salmonellosis is generally a mild disease in humans, characterized by a few hours or days of vomiting and **diarrhea** followed by weeks to months of shedding the organism in feces. The disease is usually acquired by ingestion of contaminated foods, but other means are possible. In the 1970s in the United States, more than 10 percent of salmonellosis was acquired from baby turtles, then a favored children's pet.

By contrast, and almost unique among the salmonellae, typhoid bacilli are adapted to humans alone. They possess a protective envelope that helps resist the host's immunologic defenses. Fortunately, *S. typhi's* adaptation to humans permits control through public-health measures.

Typhoid spreads via the fecal-oral route: Bacteria shed by infected persons are ingested by others, usually through contaminated food or water. Control depends on separating sewage and drinking water. In certain regions, as many as 3 percent of adults may be shedding *S. typhi*. Thus the population is continuously exposed, and the disease constantly present. Many less-developed areas are highly endemic for typhoid fever.

In contrast, where effective sanitation barriers are suddenly breached, transmission becomes epidemic. For example, typhoid is almost unknown in Switzerland; yet in 1963, water contamination caused 280 cases in a brief period. Ten years later, a similar problem in Florida suddenly produced 222 cases, apparently originating with a single carrier.

Though denied another animal host, *S. typhi* also grows well on foods, which has been responsible for large-scale outbreaks. In 1964, 500 cases of typhoid fever in Scotland were traced to imported canned beef that – after processing under sterile conditions in Argentina – had been cooled in a sewage-laden river, where microscopic cracks in the seams of the cans permitted contamination.

The percentage of persons who develop typhoid fever after exposure depends on several factors, including the virulence and number of organisms ingested, and the host's health and immune status. The attack rate of the disease depends directly on the number of organisms

ingested. In experiments using human volunteers, illness was produced in about 25 percent of those ingesting 100,000 bacilli each; ingestion of 10 million bacilli caused illness in 50 percent; and ingestion of 1 billion organisms virtually guaranteed the development of typhoid fever. However, some strains can produce disease at very low numbers, and most epidemics in the developed world appear to be initiated by exposure to only a few hundred or thousand organisms.

A distinctive feature of the epidemiology of typhoid is the existence of a large number of asymptomatic carriers. Normally, fecal excretion of the organism persists for some weeks, but about 2 percent of infected persons never clear the bacillus from their stools. In such persons, the organism appears to colonize the biliary tract; *S. typhi* seems to have a particular affinity for bile and gallstones. Once a stone is infected, it forms a focus of infection sheltered from antibiotics and the host's immune system. The likelihood of becoming a carrier increases with age, peaking at age 55, with female carriers outnumbering males 3 to 1 – a pattern similar to that of **biliary disease** but contrasting sharply with acute typhoid fever, which is a disease of the young and affects both sexes equally. The lack of symptoms often makes carriers difficult to identify, and sequestration of the bacillus on gallstones makes its eradication difficult or impossible.

Since the beginning of the twentieth century, typhoid fever has been largely a disease of the developing world. Estimates suggest that global incidence averages 300 cases per 100,000 persons annually or 15 million cases each year. In endemic areas, 75 percent of cases occur in persons 3–18 years old. Typhoid is only rarely described in children younger than 2 years, although studies indicate that it can be present yet unsuspected clinically. No susceptibility by race has been identified, but poverty, usually associated with poor sanitation and health care, does constitute a risk factor for typhoid. For example, blacks in South Africa have four times the incidence of typhoid – with eight times the mortality rate – of whites. In Israel, the rate for the Jewish population is similar to that for Europe; for the non-Jewish population, it is similar to that for the Middle East.

In endemic areas, typhoid tends to peak in the summer months. Whether this pattern results from greater consumption of water or enhanced proliferation of the bacteria in food is unknown. In the developed world, to judge by the United States, seasonality reflects foreign-travel patterns, with peaks in January and February and again in the summer months.

Most ingested typhoid bacilli are killed by stomach acid. Surviving bacilli enter the small intestine, penetrate the mucosal lining, and are ingested by white cells located in gut lymph nodes. Perhaps because of its protective envelope, *S. typhi* resists digestion and multiplies within the cells that normally destroy bacteria. As bacteria multiply and pass into the bloodstream, they are absorbed by white cells located in the liver and spleen, but there, too, the bacilli multiply and reenter the bloodstream. During this second period of **bacteremia**, the symptoms of typhoid begin. Lymph nodes in the small intestine become laden with bacilli, occasionally to the extent that the tissues die, leading to intestinal hemorrhage or perforation – the major causes of mortality in typhoid. Delirium, heart inflammation, and shock may occur and are caused not by direct infection, but rather by toxins released by the bacilli or by the white cells. Over several weeks, the immune system recognizes the bacillus, and the host destroys the invader.

If the disease is untreated, mortality ranges between 10 and 20 percent; 1 in 5 persons experiences gastrointestinal hemorrhage, and 1 in 50 suffers perforation of the gut. Relapse occurs in about 10 percent of patients, usually after a week free of illness, but symptoms are frequently milder and duration shorter than during the original attack.

In 1896, Fernand Widal determined that most persons develop O and H antibodies to *S. typhi*. Since then, the Widal test for antibodies in the blood has been used extensively to diagnose typhoid fever, although it is not always reliable. Persons with typhoid fever may never show a rise in antibody levels, and past exposure to *S. typhi* (which is common among adults in endemic areas) can mean a positive Widal test, whatever the patient's current ailment. In unimmunized children in endemic areas, however, the Widal test may be of value.

Until 1948, little other than supportive treatment was possible, but with discovery of the antibiotic chloramphenicol, mortality was markedly reduced. For 20 years, chloramphenicol was entirely effective, but resistance emerged in the 1970s. Soon, 75 percent of all *S. typhi* isolates in Vietnam, for example, were resistant. In developed areas, the percentage of resistant strains remained below 5 percent. Trimethoprim, sulfamethoxazole, and ampicillin are now among the drugs of choice for typhoid fever.

Exposure to the typhoid bacillus appears to confer some degree of immunity. However, the immunity is relative, seeming to decay after some years, and can be overcome by administration of sufficient bacilli. Nevertheless, a relative immunity is better than none, and attempts to induce it began almost as soon as the bacillus was isolated in the last decades of the nineteenth century. Most vaccine trials indicate a protective effect of about 75 percent. Although control of typhoid fever is best accomplished with improvement of sanitary conditions, immunization may play an important public-health role in developing countries.

History

Typhoid fever has surely been a human disease since prehistory, but for ancient physicians its nonspecific symptoms did not distinguish it from other illnesses. Hippocrates described a possible case of typhoid, and Augustus was cured of a typhoid-like fever by cold baths, a remedy that persisted well into the twentieth century.

Meaningful reports from ancient and medieval times are lacking. However, early European mercantile and colonial enterprises were clearly affected by typhoid epidemics. In the early seventeenth century, 6,500 colonists at Jamestown, Virginia, died most likely from typhoid fever. About the same time, Belgian anatomist Adriaan van den Spieghel (Spigelius) described lesions in lymphoid tissue of the small intestine, the first report of the characteristic findings of typhoid. Later, British physician Thomas Willis cataloged the course of what he called "putrid malignant fever," which was clearly typhoid.

In the eighteenth century, François Boissier de Sauvages of France consolidated several ailments (including Willis's putrid malignant fever) under the rubric **typhus**. In the 1830s, Pierre Louis, dissatisfied with the "typhus" concept, proposed isolating a particular symptom cluster under the name "typhoid" (typhus-like) fever. Later, William Gerhard in Philadelphia established typhoid fever as an entity independent of typhus. In the 1840s, the Englishman William Budd virtually inaugurated the science of epidemiology by demonstrating that typhoid spread from infected individuals to new hosts through water and food. Unfortunately, Budd was actively opposed, and little came of his public-health recommendations. As a result, the annual incidence in Europe at that time remained as high as 1 per 200 persons.

Finally, however, in 1875, the British Public Health Act was passed, radically improving sanitary practices. Within a decade, typhoid mortality was cut in half. Other developed nations enacted sanitary laws of their own. Since then, typhoid incidence in the developed world has steadily declined.

This profound revolution in public health began before the microbial etiologies of any diseases were established. Yet just 2 years after the Public Health Act was passed in England, the German Robert Koch demonstrated that a microorganism caused **anthrax**, and 3 years later his countrymen Carl Eberth and Edwin Klebs identified the typhoid bacillus. The next 2 decades saw an explosion of knowledge about the organism, and in 1884 Georg Gaffky cultured the bacillus from lymph nodes. Shortly

thereafter it was isolated from blood and stool.

Despite these rapid advances, therapeutic interventions against typhoid were lacking. During the Spanish-American War of 1898, one-fifth of the American army contracted typhoid fever, with a mortality rate six times the number of combat deaths. About this time in England, Almroth Wright developed a vaccine that reduced attacks among Indian soldiers by 75 percent. Despite these impressive results, the vaccine was little used 2 years later in the Boer War, and the disastrous experience of the American army was virtually repeated among British troops in South Africa.

Early in the twentieth century, both British and American forces ordered mandatory typhoid immunization and better sanitation. The effect a decade later was dramatic: During World War I, the typhoid rate was reduced from 1:5 to 1:2,000. Since then, typhoid has been insignificant in armed conflicts.

In 1906, New York sanitary engineer George Soper investigated an outbreak of typhoid in Oyster Bay, a well-to-do town where the disease was unknown. Yet 6 of 11 people in one house had become ill. Soper determined that 3 weeks earlier a new cook had been hired but had left after the first persons began falling ill. Her name, Mary Mallon, was destined to become inextricably linked with typhoid fever.

Koch had proposed that a person might chronically shed the typhoid bacillus and thus infect others yet remain unaffected by the disease – a hypothesis doubted by many. Soper, however, realized that the perplexing cases in Oyster Bay might be explained if the cook were a carrier. He discovered that over 10 years, inexplicable typhoid outbreaks had occurred in seven of the eight families for whom Mary Mallon had worked. A year later, Soper located her working once again in a house stricken with typhoid fever. Mallon was removed against her will to a hospital, where culture of her stool proved that she was indeed shedding *S. typhi* in great numbers. After a 3-year detention on North Brother Island in Long Island

Sound (which raised many civil-liberty questions), she was released with the proviso that she never again handle food. Five years later, however, she was identified as the source of an epidemic at Women's Hospital in Manhattan. She was arrested and spent the rest of her life on North Brother Island. "Typhoid Mary" had established beyond scientific doubt that a carrier state existed in typhoid.

The 1948 discovery of antibiotics against *S. typhi* converted typhoid from a rare but dreaded disease to just a rare one in the developed world. Despite the advances of the past century, however, on a global scale little evidence indicates that typhoid is fading into obscurity. Although inexpensive vaccines make typhoid control affordable for nations with limited resources, the huge reservoir of carriers and the continuation of poor sanitation in endemic areas suggest that some time must pass before developing nations can significantly reduce typhoid fever.

Charles W. LeBaron and David N. Taylor

153. Typhomalarial Fever

Typhomalarial fever as a specific disease is not recognized by medical authorities today, but in the last half of the nineteenth century it was a frequently useful diagnostic category of diverse and often imprecise meaning. Joseph Woodward defined the term during the American Civil War for those camp diseases "in which the malarial and typhoid elements are variously combined with each other and with the scorbutic taint." Woodward considered the disease distinct, both clinically and at postmortem, from **malarial fevers** and **typhoid fevers**.

Characteristics

William Osler once wrote that typhomalarial fever existed "in the minds of doctors but not in the bodies of patients." If so, it existed in the minds of many American doctors in the South, Midwest, and western regions of the country as well as in the minds of military and other European physicians practicing in unsanitary, malarious regions of the globe, particularly the Mediterranean, British India, and some areas of China. It was primarily an Anglo-American phenomenon, although some reports from southern Europe indicate that the possibility of the diagnosis was at least considered.

Typhomalarial fever was generally regarded as a noncontagious, infectious disease resulting from exposure to atmospheric or environmental infections or toxins that caused malarial fevers and typhoid fevers. Most commonly, patients were previously debilitated, or their vital powers were depressed in some way. In Woodward's classic formulation, this was the result of the depression produced by army camp life and **malnutrition** – particularly incipient **scurvy**. The disease required an area of endemic malarial fever, frequently a marsh, into which the animal causes of typhoid fevers – crowding and improper sanitation – intruded. The debilitated individual in such an environment was almost sure to contract typhomalarial fever.

The clinical course of the disease was extremely varied, depending on whether the malarial or typhoid elements predominated. When the malarial element was dominant, the symptoms were those of **periodic fever** – usually of the **remittent** rather than the **intermittent** variety. It was frequently **quotidian** but could be **tertian, quartan**, or irregularly remittent. However, the patient was more than usually depressed; there were frequent central nervous system symptoms, commonly stupor or coma, as well as gastrointestinal complaints, most commonly **diarrhea**. The disease had more rapid onset than classic **typhoid fever**, but if the typhoid elements dominated, the disease would clinically resemble typhoid fever except for a definite periodicity, frequent hepatic tenderness, and a greater degree of **splenomegaly**, often with pain on palpitation. Convalescence was more rapid than typical typhoid fever.

History

Woodward's concept was born of the frustrations of mid-nineteenth century medicine, particularly in America. At the beginning of the nineteenth century, diagnosis was based almost entirely on patient descriptions of complaints – that is, the perceived functional derangements that resulted in consultation with the physician. The physicians placed these complaints in the context of their own experience and knowledge, made diagnoses, and offered patients their professional advice. Diseases were collections of symptoms appearing in known orders in particular locations; adjectives were frequently part of a diagnosis, providing further refinement to a relatively limited array of disease nouns.

The most common disease was "fever," of which fever was the chief symptom. The fever symptom was essentially the subjective sensation of chill and heat and was related by the medical profession to a quickened pulse. Elevated body temperature was related to fever but was not objectively measured by most physicians until the last third of the nineteenth century. If a cause of fever was observed – particularly an inflammation – then the fever was symptomatic. Both **pneumonia** and **erysipelas** were associated with **symptomatic fevers**. Without an observed cause of fever, then the fever was essential – that is, a disease itself. **Essential fevers** were categorized by symptom variation, severity, location, pathological associations, and so forth.

The two main categories were periodic fever and **continued fever**, but they were also categorized by terms such as malignant, pernicious, epidemic, putrid, spotted, and bilious, based on the understandings of the physician observing a particular case. Periodic fevers – intermittent and remittent fevers, which had a classic periodicity – were believed to be caused by atmospheric contamination of vegetable decomposition associated with marshes and other well-recognized areas of periodic fever endemicity. During the nineteenth century, this poison came to be called **malaria**, and the fevers it caused were "malarial" fevers. Continued fevers were more variable: Some were of short duration and only an inconvenience to the patient, whereas others were long and grave of prognosis. Continued fevers with coma or stupor and of severe aspect were frequently called **typhus** by the Anglo-American medical world of the late eighteenth century. The adjective "typhoid" was applied to fevers that were typhus-like but not true typhus.

During the first half of the nineteenth century, a group of research-oriented, urban-hospital-based physicians began to define disease on the basis of the postmortem findings as correlated with the clinical course. This hospital-based medicine was most strongly associated with the pathologists of Paris, particularly René Laennec, Jean Corvisart, and Pierre Louis. In Britain, Irish clinicians William Stokes and Robert Graves and London physicians Richard Bright, Thomas Addison, and Thomas Hodgkins were part of the same movement. This approach to medicine spread through the world but did not fully replace the purely clinical approach, particularly among those whose chief interests were in medical practice. In 1829, Louis described a specific fever with lesions of "Peyer's patches" of the small bowel and named it "typhoid" because he thought it was the disease British authorities of the previous generation had called "typhus." This is, of course, the disease known today as typhoid fever.

All of this nosographic confusion was reflected in North American medical literature. Daniel Drake, the great medical geographer of the interior valley of North America, wrote about the typhoid stage of "autumnal fever," by which he probably meant what we might call **pernicious malaria**. Louis's American students brought his view of typhoid to America, and one of them, James Jackson, demonstrated that what was commonly called "autumnal fever" in New England was the same disease Louis called typhoid. Another student of Louis, William Gerhard, proved that the disease his mentor had termed typhoid was distinct from the disease usually called "autumnal fever" in Philadelphia.

Based largely on his New England practice and experience, Elisha Bartlett described typhoid fever as the most common disease in the United States. By 1847, however, he realized that malarial fevers were the dominant concern of physicians in the South and Midwest, but not enough people learned of the revised opinion. Support for almost any interpretation could be found in the medical literature of the period.

In the 1850s, as the American South became increasingly isolated culturally, there arose a campaign for a distinctively southern medicine. In part, this desire reflected real geographic differences in disease, but in part it was a result of the increasingly strident southern nationalism that led to the Civil War. As a result of this campaign and the preexisting nosological confusion, there was, by 1860, a belief in a "southern typhoid fever" that was occasionally periodic and frequently cured by quinine therapy.

Etiologic theories of the mid-nineteenth century also contributed to the confusion. Urban diseases, like typhus and typhoid, were believed to be the result of the unsanitary conditions of life in the early industrial city. Crowding, general lack of cleanliness, and a combination of animal and human waste gave rise to a distinct and unpleasant odor in the cities. Where the smell was worst was also frequently the area of greatest morbidity, and it was believed that some animal miasmas caused urban fevers, much like the marsh miasmas (malaria) that caused rural fevers. If the two causes were simultaneously present, a combined or composite disease state should be expected. In the camps of the Civil War, that is exactly what was experienced, and typhomalarial fever was the name officially sanctioned for the camp disease that was not obviously a malarial or typhoid fever.

During and immediately after the war, an era when disease theory was changing and the diagnostic precision of the profession was limited, physicians found the concept of typhomalarial fever to be very useful and flexible in diagnosis. There were, however, serious doubts on the part of leading medical theorists concerning the specific nature of typhomalarial fever. In the 1870s,

these doubts increased, but so did the utilization of the diagnosis. By the late 1870s, the specificity, in pathological terms, of typhomalarial fever was an idea of the past, but the clinical reality remained, and the name seemed to explain the etiology of the symptom complexities so described.

For the same reasons, physicians in other parts of the world began seriously to consider the American diagnosis in the 1870s. In the 1860s, British army surgeons stationed on Malta had identified a new disease originally called **gastric remittent fever** and later "Malta fever." We know it today as **brucellosis**. In 1875, W. Maclean suggested that Malta fever might be typhomalarial fever. James Donaldson, on the other hand, suggested the name "faeco-malarial fever" to reflect more accurately the current understanding of dual causes. By the 1870s, the special role of human fecal matter in the propagation of typhoid fever was becoming accepted in Britain, largely because of the work of Charles Murchison and William Budd. Similar new diseases reported by British doctors overseas were also considered typhomalarial fever by some authorities.

In the 1880s, miasmatic etiologic speculations began to give way to the new germ theory of disease based in medical microbiology. Alphonse Laveran observed the malaria plasmodium; Georg Gaffky isolated *Salmonella typhi*. David Bruce discovered an organism that caused Malta fever; he called it *Micrococcus melitensis*, but the genus was subsequently named *Brucella*. However, germ theory and medical microbiology were not immediately accepted by all or even most practitioners. Debate on **typhomalaria** remained lively, particularly in American medical literature. Leading physicians saw etiologic research and eventual etiologic definition of disease as the way to resolve clinical difficulties, but microbiological techniques remained largely in the realm of experimental pathology, not yet overly useful to practitioners. The possibility of specific diseases similar to typhoid and malaria yet etiologically unique remained viable, but the profession was divided on how prevalent such diseases might be. "Periodic typhoid" and "severe malaria" were clinically real and needed names. Debate continued, but the terms were changing.

In the 1890s, progress in medical microbiology and the development of serum diagnostic tests for typhoid and Malta fevers made etiologic definitions of disease more useful to practitioners, and doubts increased about the utility of typhomalarial fever as a diagnosis.

When America mobilized volunteers for the war with Spain in 1898, sanitation in the camps was very bad. Disease was widespread and Army Surgeon General George Sternberg appointed a commission of experts composed of Walter Reed, Victor Vaughan, and E. Shakespeare to investigate. Using modern techniques, the commission proved that most of the cases diagnosed as typhomalarial fever were typhoid. Because the conditions, particularly in camps in the Deep South, approximated those under which Woodward had originally postulated the existence of typhomalarial fever, these results were particularly significant. By the early twentieth century, the diagnosis of typhomalarial fever was widely regarded as an admission of diagnostic failure, and slowly it vanished from the medical literature.

Dale Smith

154. Typhus, Epidemic

Epidemic typhus is an acute **rickettsial disease** transmitted by lice. Characteristic symptoms include fever, prostration, aches, and a widespread rash covering trunk and limbs. Mortality in untreated cases varies widely. Broad-spectrum antibiotics provide effective therapy.

Associated with poor conditions, typhus has had many names. "Jail distemper," *morbus carcerum*, and "gaol fever" indicate its prevalence in prisons. "Ship fever," "camp fever," and "famine fever" reflect the poor hygiene characteristic of such circumstances. Typhus's characteristic rash has elicited other names, includ-

ing "spotted fever," *Fleckfieber* and *typhus exanthematicus* in German, *typhus exanthématique* in French, *tifo exantemático* and *tabardillo* in Spanish, and *typhus-esantematico* in Italian.

Hippocrates applied the word "typhus" (from Greek "smoky" or "hazy") to confused or stuporous states of mind associated with high fevers, but the word was not associated with the disease under discussion until the eighteenth century. After **murine typhus** was identified, the appellation *typhus historique* was sometimes applied to the classic epidemic disease.

Characteristics

Occurring naturally only in humans, epidemic typhus is caused by *Rickettsia prowazekii*. It is spread by the human body louse (*Pediculus humanus corporis*) and less often by the human head louse (*P. humanus capitis*). The body louse spends its entire existence in the clothes of humans. Eggs laid in the seams of the undergarments hatch after about 8 days, and the nymphs become adults in about 2 weeks, going through three molts. Each louse takes 4–6 blood meals a day from its host under natural conditions. Human blood constitutes its only food.

Typhus organisms in blood ingested by a louse multiply rapidly in the louse's intestines and are secreted in the feces of infected lice. Rickettsiae are transmitted to new hosts mechanically, usually by contact of infected louse feces with skin abrasions incurred when the human scratches the unpleasant itch caused by feeding lice. The disease spreads when lice leave feverish or dead victims for new hosts with normal temperatures. Unlike other rickettsiae, *R. prowazekii* is not passed from generation to generation in the eggs of its host arthropod.

Typhus is widely known as a disease of cold climates, with epidemics that peak in late winter and taper off in spring. This pattern clearly reflects favorable conditions for lice multiplication and transmission. Typhus flourishes when people crowd together in unsanitary surroundings and lack fuel, circumstances predisposing them to wear the same garments day and night for months. Persons of all ages are susceptible.

Mortality in untreated cases varies between 5 and 25 percent, occasionally reaching 40 percent. In children under 15, however, the disease is generally mild. As age increases, so does mortality.

After incubating from 5 to 15 days, onset of typhus is abrupt. Many patients can state the exact hour their illness began. Headache, loss of appetite, and malaise are followed by rapidly rising fever. Chills, nausea, and prostration characterize the first week. A widespread rash appears 4–6 days after onset. After recovery, the rash usually fades but in rare cases leaves a brownish stain that persists for several months.

During the first 2 or 3 days, the fever reaches its maximum, between 102° and 105°F, and persists another 5 days, after which it falls rapidly. In fatal cases, however, prostration becomes more progressive, with increasing neurological symptoms including deafness, stupor, delirium, and eventually coma preceding death. Since broad-spectrum antibiotics were introduced, however, no one need die of typhus with timely diagnosis.

An attack of typhus confers long immunity. Many children in endemic regions may contract mild cases that protect them somewhat from later infection. Because *R. prowazekii* persists in its victims even after recovery, symptoms may reappear years later, especially under conditions of stress, when a victim's immune system is depressed. This phenomenon was noted in 1898, when Nathan Brill described a disease frequently diagnosed as **typhoid** but having symptoms more closely related to typhus. In 1910, Brill published an exhaustive study, which led to the designation of **Brill's disease** as a catchall for unknown, typhus-like symptoms. Two years later, U.S. Public Health Service investigators John Anderson and Joseph Goldberger demonstrated reciprocal cross-immunity in monkeys between Brill's disease and epidemic typhus.

For the next two decades, because of ignorance surrounding rickettsial diseases, illnesses exhibiting typhus-like symptoms were often classified as Brill's disease. But in 1934, Hans Zinsser hypothesized that Brill's disease was a recrudescence of typhus in persons who had earlier suffered an attack. During the 1950s, investigations confirmed this, and the condition was renamed **Brill-Zinsser disease**.

History

Although some have speculated that certain ancient plagues were probably typhus, the first contemporary accounts of such a disease appeared during the late fifteenth century. In 1489–90 during the wars of Granada, physicians described a typhus-like disease that killed 17,000 Spanish soldiers – six times the number killed in combat with the Moors.

In the early sixteenth century, a similar malady appeared in Italy. During the French siege of Naples in 1528, an apparent typhus epidemic may have altered subsequent European history. The French were at the point of decisive victory when the disease struck down 30,000 French soldiers, forcing the remnants to withdraw. In 1546, Girolamo Fracastoro (Fracastorius), who had observed the epidemics in Italy, published the first clear description of what he termed a "lenticular or punctate or petechial" fever, also characterized by headache and general malaise.

In the Balkans, where European troops assembled to combat the Turks, many were struck by typhus even before they reached the battlefield. As it was disseminated across Europe by forces returning from Hungary, typhus became known as *morbus hungaricus*. Toward the end of the sixteenth century, typhus was also recorded in Mexico, where it killed over 2 million Amerindians. Whether the disease was brought to the New World by Spanish explorers or, as some evidence indicates, was known to pre-Columbian Mexicans is unclear.

Typhus increased dramatically in the early nineteenth century. In 1812, Napoleon's catastrophic Russian expedition was plagued by typhus. Between 1816 and 1819, a great epidemic struck 700,000 people in Ireland. For several decades, however, confusion characterized medical understanding. By the late eighteenth century, medical nosologist Boissier de Sauvages had begun using the word "typhus" to describe its neurological symptoms, but few attempted to distinguish between typhus and **typhoid fever**, which also produced a rash. Even into the twentieth century, confusion between typhoid and typhus was perpetuated in the nomenclature.

In 1837, William Gerhard, who had studied the intestinal lesions of typhoid, noted their absence in typhus victims. Gerhard's work, however, was not immediately accepted. Not until mid-century were most American physicians convinced that typhus and typhoid were distinct disease entities.

The European revolutions of 1848 spawned typhus epidemics, as did warfare in Ethiopia. During a particularly severe outbreak in Silesia, German physician Rudolph Virchow observed that the disease afflicted the poor, the uneducated, and the unclean, and he called for democracy, education, and public-health measures as proper "treatment" for the epidemic.

Although typhus subsided during the later nineteenth century, the advent of the germ theory of disease spurred bacteriologists to search for a microbial cause. In 1909, Charles Nicolle, director of the Institut Pasteur in Tunis, demonstrated that the body louse was the vector. The following year, Howard Ricketts described bacteria in the blood of typhus victims, in infected lice, and in lice feces. Before he could confirm his observations, however, Ricketts contracted and died of typhus. In 1916, Brazilian Henrique da Rocha Lima described similar organisms, which he named *Rickettsia prowazekii* after Ricketts and Stanislaus von Prowazek, who had also died from a laboratory-acquired typhus infection.

During World War I, the military on both sides acted on Nicolle's discovery, instituting delousing procedures including bathing and steam-treating clothing. Among poor Eastern European populations, with no such preventive measures, the disease exacted high mortality. In 1915, Serbia was particularly hard hit, and Russia and Poland after 1918. Research in Poland after World War I confirmed Rocha Lima's assertion that *R. prowazekii* caused typhus.

During the 1920s and 1930s, research on a typhus vaccine was hampered because rickettsiae could not be grown in necessary quantities outside of living cells. Then in 1937, U.S. Public Health Service investigator Herald Cox discovered that rickettsiae grew in fertile egg yolksacs. This method made vaccine production commercially feasible just as the onset of World War II again raised concern about large-scale epidemics.

The threat of typhus was a key factor in Allied military plans, and in 1942 President Roosevelt created the U.S. Typhus Commission to combat typhus wherever it might threaten military efforts. The so-called Cox vaccine was administered to all Allied personnel and, although failing to prevent the disease, clearly ameliorated its course. Intensive research demonstrated that lice could be controlled with dichlorodiphenyltrichloroethane (DDT), applied with a "blowing machine" to puff it under clothes without the wearer having to remove them. DDT proved highly effective in the 1943–44 epidemic in Naples, where a nascent outbreak collapsed with astonishing rapidity. Within two decades, however, adaptive resistance of lice to DDT was documented. Moreover, its ecological hazards were found unacceptable, and it is no longer widely used.

Prophylaxis and control during World War II reduced typhus from a major threat to a mere nuisance. Only 104 cases occurred among U.S. military personnel, with no deaths. In contrast, severe epidemics occurred in North Africa, Yugoslavia, German concentration camps, Japan, and Korea.

In 1948, the broad-spectrum antibiotics were discovered to be effective treatments for rickettsial diseases. Since then, efforts against typhus have depended on them almost exclusively. In 1980, concern about the limited efficacy and side effects of the Cox vaccine halted its production, and for now, at least, no typhus vaccine is commercially available.

Since 1950, typhus has been reported most frequently from the horn of Africa, from the high plains of the Andes, and from the Himalayan region – all areas characterized by rural poverty and cold weather. Since identification of the vector, the slogan of public-health efforts against typhus has been "no lice, no typhus." But as Zinsser has noted, typhus remains a threat, ready to break out whenever war, famine, and other catastrophes remove the barriers against it.

Victoria A. Harden

155. Typhus, Murine

Murine typhus is an acute illness characterized by symptoms similar to those of **epidemic typhus** but milder in character. Unlike its epidemic relative, it is a natural infection of rats and transmitted sporadically to humans by the rat flea, *Xenopsylla cheopis*. Its relation to the rat is reflected in the name "murine" typhus. The etiologic agent is *Rickettsia typhi*.

Characteristics

Symptoms and course of illness in murine typhus are similar to those in epidemic, louse-borne typhus; thus, distinguishing the two has been difficult. The flea-borne illness, however, is almost never fatal, with about 2 percent mortality in persons over 50.

Murine typhus is found worldwide. People living or working in areas where rats are abundant are most susceptible. Like epidemic typhus, murine typhus is transmitted mechanically, through rubbing infected flea feces into a skin abrasion, through the eye, or through mucous membranes of the respiratory tract. Following World War II, campaigns against rats and their fleas with DDT and rodenticides sharply reduced the incidence of murine typhus in the United States.

Some investigators prefer the name *Rickettsia mooseri* (over *R. typhi*) to honor Swiss pathologist Herman Mooser, who differentiated between this organism and *Rickettsia prowazekii*.

In guinea pigs, *R. typhi* causes a characteristic reaction in scrotal cells useful for distinguishing between murine and epidemic typhus. First noticed in 1917 by Mather Neill and confirmed nearly two decades later by Mooser, the reaction became known as the Neill-Mooser phenomenon.

History

Although murine typhus was identified only during the twentieth century, it may be even older than classic epidemic typhus. Neither the rat nor the rat flea suffers ill effects from the infection, whereas *R. prowazekii* inevitably kills its vector louse and causes serious illness in its human host.

Sporadic cases of typhus-like fevers in areas free from lice were reported early in the twentieth century in the United States, Malaya, and Australia. Often these infections were designated by local names, such as "urban" or "shop" typhus. Not until 1926, however, was the distinctiveness of this disease recognized. Investigating such cases in the southeastern United States, Kenneth Maxcy described an endemic form of typhus fever and postulated that some ectoparasite of the rat was its vector. By 1931, infected fleas had been found in nature, confirming Maxcy's hypothesis. Although the name **endemic typhus** was used for some time, it was observed that the disease could occur in epidemics as well as sporadically. In 1932, Mooser proposed the name "murine typhus" to indicate its relationship to rats.

Although broad-spectrum antibiotics provide effective treatment against the disease, its mild course and low fatality rate make these measures almost unnecessary. By the time it is diagnosed, the patient is usually in convalescence.

Victoria A. Harden

156. Typhus, Scrub (*Tsutsugamushi*)

In 1810, Hakuju Hashimoto described a *tsutsuga* (disease) along the Shinano River. A similar disease, thought to be carried by mites (*mushi*) had been known at least since the sixteenth century in China. Sometimes called "Japanese flood fever," *tsutsugamushi* is more commonly known in the United States as **scrub typhus** – a name widely used during World War II. The disease exhibits **typhus**-like symptoms of fever, headache, and rash.

Characteristics

The geography of *tsutsugamushi* is defined by the range of its vectors, which extend from India and Pakistan to Japan and northern Australia, including all of Southeast Asia, southern China, Korea, the Philippines, and Indonesia, as well as additional islands. During World War II, incidence of scrub typhus among troops was high, reaching 900 per 1,000 in some areas. It remains a problem in isolated rural areas.

The agent of scrub typhus, *Rickettsia tsutsugamushi*, is a natural infection of its several vector mites, most commonly *Leototrombidium deliensis*. Maintained in nature by generational transmission in mite eggs, the disease is communicated to humans only during the larval stage of the mite's life cycle. The six-legged larva, often called a "chigger," seeks to feed on tissue juices or lymph, usually from mice, rats, shrews, and other small mammals, but humans are satisfactory if they happen into the mite's environment. Ground-frequenting birds may also become infected and transport mites to a new location.

Scrub typhus incubates 10–12 days, after which it manifests itself suddenly, with chills and fever, headache, and other typhus-like symptoms. During the first week, fever increases to about 105°F. Between the fifth and eighth days, a macular rash appears on the trunk and may extend to arms and legs. During the second week, the pulse may increase, blood pressure falls, and neurological symptoms such as deafness, stupor, delirium, and twitching may appear in untreated patients. **Pneumonia** and signs of circulatory failure may also occur, but by the beginning of the third week, those who recover experience reduced symp-toms. Those who die usually do so by the end of the second week from circulatory failure, secondary pneumonia, or **encephalitis**. Even in recovered patients, neurological effects may continue, and convalescence is usually long. Fortunately, broad-spectrum antibiotics have reduced mortality in treated patients to nearly zero.

History

Bacteriologic investigations of *tsutsugamushi* began in Japan in the 1890s. Various researchers studied the disease through the first three decades of the twentieth century, identifying its causative microbe as a rickettsia.

Renewed investigation was stimulated by outbreaks in the Pacific and East Asia during World War II. With Allied countermoves to stem the Japanese advance, the occupation of islands often took place in haste, and troops would shortly become quite ill. From 1943 until war's end, scrub typhus disabled some 18,000 Allied troops, including 6,685 American servicemen. Mortality varied from a low of 0.6 percent in some regions to as high as 35 percent in others; 234 deaths occurred among U.S. troops.

Throughout the 1920s and 1930s, British researchers had observed that *tsutsugamushi* was distinguished from other typhus-like diseases by its reaction to a particular bacterial strain in the Weil-Felix test. When the U.S. Typhus Commission began to study scrub typhus, this test was virtually the only laboratory tool available. The army launched education efforts, including posters describing the mite, where it was likely to be found, and how soldiers should prepare their campsites to avoid it. In addition, chemicals were developed to impregnate clothing that would repel the *tsutsugamushi* mite. Benzyl benzoate proved to be effective and lasted 2 weeks before reapplication was necessary. Researchers also focused on developing a vaccine against *tsutsugamushi*. Then, in 1948, broad-spectrum antibiotics were found to be highly effective as treatment.

Victoria A. Harden

157. Urolithiasis

The major forms of **urolithiasis** consist of upper-tract stones within kidneys or ureters (renal stones) or lower-tract stones formed within the bladder. These two forms of urolithiasis have distinct differences and are considered separately.

Historical evidence exhibits a striking increase in **renal-stone disease** in developed countries over the past century. A simultaneous decrease in **bladder-stone disease** has occurred, demonstrating an inverse relationship between them. Changes in environment affect disease epidemiology, which is exemplified by the role of dietary change in the shifting pattern from bladder-stone to renal-stone disease.

Characteristics

Most bladder stones occur in young boys from rural or impoverished areas, where the disorder is termed **endemic bladder-stone disease**. A nutritional deficiency during infancy or possibly in utero appears to be the major factor. Other causes are **schistosomiasis** and, in elderly males, obstruction from **benign prostatic hypertrophy**.

Although deficiencies of vitamin A, vitamin B_6, or magnesium have been suggested in endemic bladder-stone disease, low intake of animal protein combined with high intake of grain carbohydrate is more important. Indeed, it seems that whereas low animal-protein intake in infancy may cause bladder stone, a high animal-protein diet provokes renal stones. This probably explains the enigma of disappearing endemic bladder stone as areas improved economically, with concomitant increasing incidence of renal stone.

Low intake of animal protein and high intake of grain carbohydrate produce more acidic urine and decreased urinary phosphate. These in turn decrease the solubility of calcium oxalate and uric acid, leading to bladder-stone formation. Conversely, greater animal-protein intake produces more urinary phosphate. Increased intake of refined sugar plus decreased intake of fiber increase intestinal absorption of calcium. Increased protein and sucrose intake cause increased urinary-calcium excretion. This sets the stage for calcium-phosphate- or calcium-oxalate-stone formation in the kidneys. Other less common renal stones have specific etiologies, and a multitude of other factors also operate in renal-stone formation or prevention.

Ancient physicians observed the frequent occurrence of bladder stone in young boys, and it still primarily affects boys under 10 years. Numerous studies confirm the early age of occurrence and the marked predominance of male patients. Anatomic differences between males and females probably account for the infrequency of bladder stone in females. The female urethra is short, wide, and straight, allowing stronger flow of urine and passage of gravel before large stones are formed.

Bladder-stone disease occurs in agricultural regions, particularly among lower economic classes. Historical accounts from the 1500s to the mid-1800s document the disease throughout Europe, Asia, and the Americas. Bladder stone remains common in Egypt, India, China, Thailand, Afghanistan, Iraq, Turkey, and Madagascar. Prior to 1940, it was also common in portions of Iceland, Russia, Hungary, Indonesia, Tunisia, and Sicily.

Renal-stone disease has mainly afflicted the industrialized, affluent countries of Europe, North America, and Japan and has been uncommon or unknown in impoverished regions and primitive societies. However, people in such areas have developed similar prevalence with improvement in living conditions and subsequent dietary changes.

Studies in North America and Europe show prevalence rates of renal stone up to 13 percent. Nearly 75 percent of people with so-called **idiopathic calcium-stone disease** have recurrences, implying a continuous exposure to risk factors such as diet. Incidence has risen continuously since the turn of the twentieth century except for brief declines during both world wars – again suggesting dietary changes as a factor. Unlike bladder-stone disease, renal stones occur predominantly in adults. Men are affected slightly more often than women.

History

Bladder stone is a disease of communities where diets are high in grain and low in animal protein. With dietary changes resulting from technology, migration, or cultural shift, bladder-stone disease is replaced by renal-stone disease. This is well demonstrated over the past two centuries in Europe, Russia, China, and Turkey. It is therefore not surprising that ancient references are almost entirely to bladder stone, with rare mention of upper-tract stones.

Bladder stone was common in ancient Persia, particularly in infants, and was considered a result of ingesting sour milk, fruits, or acidic drinks. The Babylonian *Talmud* refers to bladder-stone disease and includes the suggestion that patients urinate on the doorstep in order to see the stone.

In India, the *Rig Veda* and *Atharva Veda* (c. 1500 B.C.) consist of incantations against disease, including bladder stone. The *Ayur Veda*, composed about the first century A.D., described suprapubic incision for removing bladder stones. In the second century, Charaka described four types of stones almost certainly from the bladder.

In China, case histories of 25 patients treated by Shunyü I in the second century B.C. have been preserved, including one afflicted with **hematuria**, urinary retention, and bladder stones. This may represent a case of either schistosomiasis or endemic stone disease.

In Greece, Hippocrates recognized both renal and bladder stone and recommended diuretics and large quantities of water. He considered wounds of the bladder wall as invariably fatal and specifically forbade his followers to cut for the stone.

The Assyrian *Book of Medicine* (c. 300 B.C.) includes much of Hippocrates's teaching. Among numerous prescriptions are two for flushing out or dissolving renal stones; one contains 50 ingredients with particular emphasis on camphor and vinegar. Other Assyrian works include directions for infusing various preparations into the bladder through a bronze tube to dissolve bladder stones.

In Alexandria around 100 B.C., Ammonios developed an instrument for crushing stones within the bladder. In the first century A.D., Rufus gave detailed instructions for removing bladder stones through a transverse perineal incision.

In Rome during the same century, Celsus performed numerous operations for bladder stone in boys 9–14 years of age. His writings contain a description of transverse perineal lithotomy followed almost without modification until the sixteenth century. Galen described lateral perineal lithotomy and noted the frequent occurrence of bladder stone in young boys. He also administered stone solvents (lithotryptics).

In Arabic medicine, Rhazes at about the turn of the tenth century described both renal and bladder stones and implicated salt intake and hot weather as factors in renal stone formation. Around a century later, Avicenna thought that bladder stones formed when the urine contained excess matter.

By the eighteenth century, surgeons were increasingly attempting the dangerous lateral perineal lithotomy. Special hospitals for bladder-stone patients opened in England, France, Holland, and elsewhere. In 1753, Frère Come opened such a hospital in Paris, operating on more than 1,000 patients. The Norfolk and Norwich Hospital was founded in 1771, and one of every 55 admissions was for removal of bladder stone.

Through paleopathology and careful archaeological techniques, renal and bladder stones have been recovered from skeletal and mummified remains, testimony to the antiquity of these diseases.

R. Ted Steinbock

158. Varicella-Zoster Virus Disease (Chickenpox)

Varicella or **chickenpox** is an acute infection of short duration caused by varicella-zoster virus (VZV), spread in early stages by droplets from the nasopharynx. It is followed by lifetime latency – broken in occasional patients by reactivation of virus in sensory ganglia, which is manifested as **herpes zoster** or **shingles**.

Characteristics

Chickenpox is endemic worldwide, highly communicable, and commonly appears as epidemics among children, who are usually attacked between ages 2 and 8. Infants are protected by transplacental maternal antibodies. Few escape infection until adulthood, and these usually live in isolated communities. Probably most of those who have seemed to escape the disease had subclinical infections.

Sporadic reactivation of the virus as shingles is unrelated to exposure to exogenous infection and, in general, is uncommon even in populations in which practically all have had chickenpox. Its peak incidence is after age 50. Of those who develop shingles, only 1 percent have two attacks. Patients with impaired cellular immunity are at risk, and herpes zoster is not uncommon in those suffering from malignant disease. Although immunity is lifelong, it has been suggested that a waning of immunity in older age explains shingles.

After an incubation period of 10–20 days, and some 24 hours before the varicella rash appears, the prodromes of mild headache, malaise, and moderate fever appear. Because these are commonly unrecognized in children, the rash seemingly is the initial evidence of disease. It appears as a cutaneous blush, with the development of successive crops of macules, papules, and superficial vesicles surrounded by a red areola, which begin crusting within 24 hours. The acute phase lasts about a week.

Although the rash may be generalized, it usually involves the trunk and face, with fewer lesions on the extremities. Vesicles may appear in the mouth, and laryngeal involvement may cause **dyspnea**. Chickenpox is a benign disease in children unless they suffer from **leukemia** or are taking corticosteroids. Other than acute **encephalitis**, an occasional circumstance late in the disease, complications have rarely been reported. In adults, varicella tends to be less benign, and pulmonary infiltrates are commonly noted.

An attack of herpes zoster may begin with fever, chills, malaise, and gastrointestinal symptoms. With or without prodromal symptoms, the patient becomes aware of pain, at times with itching, in the area of the affected segmental nerves. After several days, crops of vesicles on an erythematous base appear in the distribution of nerves of one or several posterior root ganglia, usually accompanied by **hyperesthesia** and pain. The vesicles dry and become crusted in about a week, although the course may be slower in aged persons. Hyperesthesia or pain may last for weeks and months, especially in patients with malignant disease. In an occasional aged patient, these residua never disappear. **Herpes** of the ophthalmic branch of the trigeminal nerve is not uncommon and may be accompanied by **keratoconjunctivitis**, which may be followed by serious corneal scarring and **glaucoma**. **Zoster** of the geniculate ganglion produces **Ramsey Hunt's syndrome**. The characteristic pain syndrome of zoster may run its course without skin eruption.

History

Italian physician Giovanni Ingrassia is credited with differentiating chickenpox from **scarlet fever** in 1553, and English physician William Heberden gave the earliest clear description of varicella and distinguished it from **smallpox** in 1768. Jean Alibert in 1832 included varicella in his Group II category of **exanthematous dermatoses** – acute febrile contagious diseases. In the early twentieth century, American researchers described cellular inclusion bodies and isolated the virus.

P. Rayer in 1845 described the microscopic contents of zoster vesicles and the underlying skin. In the 1860s, F. von Bärensprung concluded that zoster was a disease of the posterior roots. In subsequent years, several reports described herpes zoster with postmortem findings of inflammation of posterior root ganglia. Bärensprung's suspicion that the Gasserian ganglion was affected in herpes zoster of the face was confirmed by O. Wyss in 1872. A. Campbell and Henry Head in 1900 established that herpes zoster results from hemorrhagic inflammation of the posterior nerve roots and homologous cranial ganglia. In 1925, Karl Kundratitz described inoculation of susceptible children with zoster vesicle fluid, resulting in varicella.

R. H. Kampmeier

159. Whooping Cough

Whooping cough, otherwise known as **pertussis**, after the causative bacillus *Bordetella pertussis*, is an infectious disease of childhood. Affecting the respiratory tract, it is characterized by paroxysms of coughing, culminating in the prolonged inspiration that provided its name. Before the twentieth century, the popular name was generally spelled without the initial "w"; indeed, it was not in general use until the end of the eighteenth century. Until the early nineteenth century, the commonest appellation was **chincough**. The term "pertussis" was first used by Thomas Sydenham in the latter seventeenth century.

Characteristics

The distribution of whooping cough is worldwide. It is generally an endemic disease that erupts in sporadic epidemics but in most developed countries has been controlled by immunization programs. Of clinical cases, 80 percent occur in the under-10 age group, and unlike most communicable diseases, whooping cough develops in females more often than males.

Although among the more important childhood diseases, whooping cough has been relatively neglected, and various aspects of its epidemiology are not fully understood. Transmission seems to be mainly airborne, apparently by droplet infection. Humans are the only reservoir of the disease; *B. pertussis* cannot survive long outside the host, and quickly succumbs to drying, ultraviolet light, and temperatures above 120°–130°F. It spreads primarily through household and schoolroom contact, although mild subclinical cases, perhaps in adolescents and adults, may play a further role in transmission. One attack confers immunity, and rare second attacks are probably explained by infection with the milder and rarer *Bordetella parapertussis*.

An incubation period of 7–10 days is followed by an initial catarrhal stage lasting 1–2 weeks. During this phase, the disease is highly communicable, but the symptoms are nonspecific and resemble many other infectious diseases and minor respiratory ailments. An increasingly persistent cough develops, which in the third stage becomes more severe and spasmodic, terminating in the characteristic whoop. In acute cases, paroxysms may occur 40–50 times in 24 hours. The whoop is frequently followed by vomiting. In young infants, who are unable to produce the whoop and resume effective breathing quickly, episodes of **cyanosis** follow paroxysms. The acute stage lasts up to 4 weeks, but paroxysms may continue for 3 months or longer. The patient is considered convalescent when vomiting ceases and severity of the paroxysms diminishes. Complications include collapsed lungs, **anoxic convulsions**, and exhaustion; secondary bacterial infections may cause **otitis media** or **pneumonia**. **Bronchiectasis** has become rare since the introduction of antimicrobial agents.

History

The history of whooping cough before the twentieth century is obscure. It cannot with certainty be traced back further than the mid-sixteenth century and was almost certainly unknown to the ancient world. Although the term "chincough" was current in the early sixteenth century, the first medical description of the disease dates from 1578, when Guillaume Baillou observed a severe epidemic in Paris. He wrote of it as a familiar affliction, for which there seemed to be several names already. Moreover, it was apparently the subject of medical discussion.

Nonetheless, the prevalence of the disease remains largely obscure until the mid-eighteenth century. August Hirsch in 1886 suggested that the native habitat of the disease was originally northern Europe. But widespread folklore regarding its treatment may indicate a more ancient existence in places such as southern India and Malabar.

Thomas Willis in 1675 described chincough as an epidemic disease of infants and children, usually occurring during summer and autumn. In his view, the cough, although difficult to cure, was rarely fatal or dangerous.

By contrast, his contemporary, Sydenham, thought it so formidable as to require the most rigorous treatment. The earliest statistics regarded as in any way reliable come from mid-eighteenth century Sweden, where Nils von Rosenstein described it as a familiar epidemic disease of variable fatality. The terms "whooping cough" and "chincough" first appear as causes of death in London in 1701, and an increasing number of deaths were attributed to them.

With the introduction of civil registration of deaths in 1838, English mortality figures became more reliable. Deaths from whooping cough peaked at some 1,500 per million population under age 15 annually around 1870, after which the rate began to decline. This was first manifest in agricultural regions, whereas in urban and industrial areas the death rates were slower to fall. During the 1880s, case fatality, so far as can be ascertained, stood at 10 percent, compared to 1.1 percent during World War II, and 0.1 percent in recent years. In underdeveloped countries today, hospital case-fatality rates are about 15 percent.

Although the infectious character of whooping cough was appreciated from at least the early eighteenth century, the nature of the clinical disease was a matter of debate. Both Willis and Sydenham, for example, thought the disease seated chiefly in the chest, whereas William Harvey and his followers held it to be in the stomach and the alimentary canal. Not until Robert Watt, stimulated by the deaths of two of his children from the disease, undertook a series of dissections in 1812–13 did the involvement of the respiratory tract become clear. Medical interest in the disease during the nineteenth century was minimal until discussion about prevention began in the 1880s.

In London during the nineteenth century, the highest whooping cough mortality was among children of the working classes; death generally resulted from complications involving the respiratory organs. The disease was made notifiable in the United States in 1922, but not until somewhat later in Britain.

Mortality and morbidity from whooping cough declined greatly in developed countries during the twentieth century. The causative organism was first isolated by Jules Bordet and Octave Gengou in 1900 but was not grown in vitro until 1906, when its morphology and cultural characteristics were established. Vaccines against the disease were first introduced in the 1930s and were in widespread use by the latter 1940s.

In the latter twentieth century, increasing public awareness of possible complications from whooping cough vaccine was stimulated by a relatively small number of cases in which the vaccine supposedly caused brain damage in children. Consequently, during the 1970s vaccination rates fell off in both Britain and Japan, where immunization was voluntary. In both countries, the disease began to increase in prevalence, and epidemic outbreaks in 1978 and 1982 were similar in scale to those of the 1950s, when the immunization program was new.

Afterward, intensive publicity concerning the benefits of vaccination caused immunization rates to rise again.

Anne Hardy

160. Yaws

This disease has suffered from confusing descriptions. It is now generally called **yaws**, although the term **framboesia** is still in use. Primary, secondary, and tertiary stages of the condition are recognized, and further subdivisions have been made that are associated with various alternative terminology.

Characteristics

Yaws is considered a highly contagious disease in tropical areas and in populations with limited hygiene. It is characterized in early stages by variable cutaneous changes and eventually affects joints and bones. The causal organism is considered to be *Treponema pertenue*, although the taxonomy of the pathogenic treponemes is in some doubt, and some reclassification may well take place in the near future. An incubation period of up to 28 days is followed by the appearance of the primary lesion, 2–5 centimeters in diameter, which develops into granular excrescences at times with lymph node enlargement. Further eruptions take place, which can be characterized by "waxing and waning" of successive lesions. Single or multiple lesions can eventually develop on the feet ("crab yaws" or **ulcerative plantar papules**) and are some of the most painful and disabling lesions of all. Eventually, in what some would see as a tertiary stage, there can be patchy depigmentation, deep destruction and remodeling of bones, and ***gangosa*** (damage of nasopharyngeal structures). Internal organs are not normally involved, and in this respect the disease contrasts markedly with its relative **venereal syphilis**.

As a result of the intensive campaign against yaws carried out in the 1950s by the World Health Organization, the disease is no longer present in many populations where previously it was a serious health threat. Before the mid-twentieth century, however, there were probably some 50 million yaws cases in the world.

In the 1940s and early 1950s, estimates of yaws prevalence were made in various areas of the world, partly for use by yaws-eradication programs. Although regional figures have dropped radically, it is pertinent to the history of the subject to note the extent of the previous evidence, and the variation found. In most of the New World, although yaws was probably introduced by slaves centuries ago, no significant incidence continued into this century. However, in the Caribbean area, which had been varyingly affected by the slave trade, yaws displayed some contrasts. Thus, Cuba was reported as having a low frequency of yaws, whereas in Haiti, 60–80 percent of the rural population were estimated to have had yaws. Similarly, Jamaica registered 70–80 percent frequency figures in some districts. In South America, Brazil was known to have many cases, especially in the northern regions, where 350,000 cases were at one time noted. In Colombia, there was also regional variation, with the Pacific coast regions reporting 80,000 cases (with a general rate of 43.5 per 100,000). In contrast to these two countries, yaws appears to have been only a modest health problem in Peru and Venezuela.

In the Old World, the disease was endemic in parts of Africa, Asia, and the Pacific. In Africa, high frequencies were found in some areas, although possibly the highest incidences occurred in Asia and the Pacific. For example, Congo, India, Indonesia, Samoa, and the Marianas appear to have suffered greatly from yaws; Tanganyika, Niger, Chad, and Laos were much less afflicted.

Yaws is one of four chronic infectious **treponemal diseases** that affect humans, and in contrast to **pinta**, **endemic syphilis**, and venereal syphilis, it appears to be especially adapted to hot and humid tropical and subtropical environments. Rural populations were probably more affected than urban groups. The causal organism has been given separate species status, *Treponema pertenue*, but the taxonomy of the **treponematoses** deserves reevaluation. The microorganism was discovered by Aldo Castellani in 1905, and since then its morphology has been to some extent revealed, especially by electron microscopy. Differences between the pathogenic treponemes have not, however, been resolved at this level, and it now seems unlikely that significant morphological differences will appear between *T. pertenue* and *Treponema pallidum* (which causes **syphilis**).

Humans appear to be the only natural hosts of all the pathogenic human treponemes. There is variable cross-protection once an individual has one variety of treponeme and comes into contact with another form.

The site of entry for yaws treponemes is often the legs, and large numbers of treponemes are probably unnecessary to instigate the disease. Transmission by flies is considered unimportant. Like endemic syphilis, yaws characteristically develops during childhood by nonvenereal contact. Eventually, after chronic progress of the disease, over 8 months or more, individuals commonly undergo spontaneous cure, although some cases continue to a tertiary stage.

There appears to be no significant natural resistance to infection by yaws or other pathogenic treponemes. However, there is clear evidence that some individuals can develop specific resistance or immunity following infection with these treponemes. The plasma cells and lymphocytes present in treponemal lesions indicate local antibody formation and some degree of immunologic response. Sera from yaws and the other pathogenic treponemes react to the same antigens.

The progress of yaws seems best described in two major stages: an early phase with initial and secondary lesions; then a late stage, which usually develops after some years. In the region of entry of the treponemes, primary lesions develop within the first 8 weeks, with the legs usually involved first. The lesion is a large, rounded, itching papule, usually less than 5–6 centime-

ters in size, which may ulcerate or become secondarily infected. The ulceration crusts, and eventually a raspberry-like granuloma develops beneath. Bleeding may occur, and there can be a yellowish discharge.

Within 3–6 weeks after the initial lesion, secondary eruptions occur, extending all over the body. These can continue up to 2 years. Annular lesions encircle an area of skin; macular eruptions may occur as well. These disappear within a few weeks or months. The "lichenous" rash can be regional or cover the whole body with small papules, usually for not more than a few weeks. Plantar and palmar lesions can be ulcerative or nonulcerative. In the case of painful ulcerating soles, the individual tends to walk on the outer border of the foot in a crablike fashion ("crab yaws").

In later stages of yaws, usually after 5 years, further lesions may occur in individuals whose condition has not become fully latent. In particular, there can be nodular "lupoid" involvement of the skin, with formation of granulation tissue, ulceration, and scars. One or a few large ulcers ("gummatous ulceration") may develop, lasting for years. Possibly the most significant of the late stages of yaws are significant changes in the bones. Parts of the skeleton, especially the long bones, may show a range of changes from **periostitis** to deep cavitation and shaft swelling. In children there can also be **dactylitis**, which can produce remodeling and expansion of one or more phalanges, especially of the fingers. Also, the vault of the skull may be affected, causing localized cratering or more widespread **osteitis** and eventual stellate scarring. Most destructive of all is *gangosa* (**rhinopharyngitis mutilans**), which is characterized by massive destruction of the nose, palate, turbinates, and vomer.

History

The history of yaws has been, to some extent, confused with that of syphilis. Early physicians and writers could easily mistake one condition for the other, or were vague about the actual nature of the disease under study. This does not mean that all earlier medical writers were wrong, and Robert Koch, in a 1900 report to the German government, perceptively wrote that in the Bismarck Archipelago he had seen places where practically all children were infected with yaws, and that framboesia was frequently mistaken for syphilis by both laypersons and medical practitioners. Koch went on to say that the alleged great epidemics of syphilis in the South Seas were in large part the result of this same misdiagnosis.

Although it has been suggested that the biblical condition **blains** could have been yaws, and similarly that a reference by Pliny (first century A.D.) to a yaws-like eruption of the face may indicate early treponemal disease, no ancient written records can be taken seriously as evidence. However, the archaeological record does appear to provide clear proof of the antiquity of treponemal diseases.

In 1367, Marco Pizziani explored along the African coast, and by 1470 others had sailed south as far as the Equator. Portuguese settlements were established, linked to the slave trade, and these intimate contacts between widely different peoples and environments provided opportunities for the movement of disease as well as people. Although the estimated figure of between 300,000 and 400,000 slaves arriving in Portugal by the end of the fifteenth century may well be too high, there is no doubt that this was a significant corridor for the potential shunting of disease, including yaws, to other areas, including Europe. Moreover, slaves did not simply move toward Europe and western Asia.

At the beginning of the sixteenth century, the first consignment of slaves from Africa arrived in Hispaniola and, following this, millions more reached the New World. It was thus that yaws became established to varying degrees in various parts of the Americas. In 1648, Willem Piso, a doctor with the Dutch West India Company in Brazil, wrote of treponematosis in that country, mentioning a condition called "bubas" which he distinguished from the "Spanish pocks." Earlier, in 1642, Jacobus Bontius, another Dutch doctor, had written of witnessing yaws during his travels in the East Indies. In the Moluccas, the frequency of yaws led Bontius to call it a "common plague."

From the mid-seventeenth century to the end of the eighteenth, a view of yaws as a distinct disease was consolidated. A 1720 "epidemic" in Scotland of "sibbens" offered symptoms suggestive of **intruded yaws**. John Brickell of North Carolina, writing in the 1730s, distinguished yaws from syphilis, noting that the former was of African origin. In the West Indies, physicians attending slaves came to know the condition well; they, too, believed it came from Africa. As in Africa, yaws was a disease mostly of children in the Caribbean, and many plantations erected yaws houses. Edward Bancroft, a physician who experienced yaws in South America, concluded that it could be transmitted by flies, a suggestion generally accepted in subsequent decades.

During the late eighteenth century and the first decades of the next, the stages of yaws development were slowly being understood. Vaccination was also attempted to prevent the disease, and positive results were claimed. Somewhat more alarming in humanitarian terms, experimental injection of slaves was practiced, at times with "success." Of special value were experiments on humans known to have already been infected, the negative results showing that immunity to secondary infection was possible.

Gangosa ("nasal voice") was first discussed by a Spanish medical committee in 1828, and by 1891 J. Numa Rat had discussed these lesions in rhinopharyngitis mutilans and viewed them as an indication of **tertiary yaws**. Similarly, "boomerang leg" (also called "sabre tibia"), a later-stage yaws feature in Australian aborigines, was first noted in 1894 by E. C. Stirling.

The question of the taxonomy of the pathogenic treponemes was opened up for debate in 1900 with the suggestion that, contrary to growing opinion, yaws and syphilis were simply different patterns of the same disease – an argument still strongly disputed 100 years later. But during the past century, researchers have tended to study the treponemal diseases singly. Thus, one might concentrate not only on yaws but specifically on **parangi**, a form that in the 1920s had some prevalence on Ceylon. Field work in the 1930s among Australian and African tribal communities and contributions dealing with bone changes in yaws and syphilis have been especially significant. Such findings in turn are helping physical anthropologists trace the history of these diseases in human skeletal remains. It is hoped that such efforts will soon produce major breakthroughs in our knowledge of the treponematoses.

Don R. Brothwell

161. Yellow Fever

Yellow fever is an acute viral disease transmitted to humans by various mosquitoes, especially *Aedes aegypti* (formerly *Stegomyia fasciata*). The disease remains endemic in tropical regions of Africa and the Americas in a sylvan or jungle form, but historically its greatest impact on humans has been in an epidemic or urban form. It presents symptoms ranging from mild to malignant, classically including fever, headache, **jaundice**, and gastrointestinal hemorrhage. High mortality rates were recorded during epidemics (20–70 percent), although today we know that yellow fever mortality is actually relatively low, suggesting that many cases were mild and undiagnosed.

The jaundice has prompted the appellation "yellow fever" and other designations such as *mal de Siam, fièvre jaune, gelbfieber,* and *virus amaril,* whereas the hemorrhaging of black blood underlies the name *vomito negro* ("black vomit"). Known early in the New World as "Barbados distemper," "bleeding fever," *maladie de Siam, el peste,* and "yellow jack" (from ships' quarantine flags), the disease has had some 150 names.

Characteristics

Yellow fever is normally a disease of nonhuman primates, particularly monkeys. Mosquitoes transmit the disease among them – but not mosquitoes that ordinarily bite humans. This form of the disease is **jungle yellow fever** or **sylvan yellow fever**; it is enzootic, meaning that transmission is from monkey to mosquito to monkey.

When the disease leaves the treetops, and mosquitoes (such as *Aedes africanus* and *Aedes simpsoni* in Africa, and species of *Haemogogus* in the Americas) begin transmission from nonhuman primate to mosquito to human, the disease is called **endemic yellow fever**. When the virus is carried by an infected human to populated areas, where transmission is from human to *A. aegypti* mosquito to human, the disease is termed **epidemic yellow fever** or **urban yellow fever**.

The habits of the female *A. aegypti* have much to do with shaping the characteristics of an epidemic. She is a domestic mosquito, living close to humans, depending on them for blood meals, and breeding in nearby loci of water. Her range is short, at most a few hundred yards, meaning that she requires a fairly dense human population. Because *A. aegypti* can survive only days without water (although her eggs can survive for years in dehydrated form) and requires water in which to breed, adequate rainfall is a prerequisite for epidemic yellow fever. Warm weather is another prerequisite: *A. aegypti* will not bite in temperatures under 62°F and hibernates in extended chilly weather.

The virus also has some distinctive requirements, especially for transmission – a process in which humans are best thought of as the site where the virus changes mosquitoes. This exchange can take place only during the first 3–6 days of infection of the yellow fever victim while the virus still remains in the blood (**viremia**); after the virus has entered the mosquito, it must incubate for another 9–18 days before the mosquito can infect another human. After this period of extrinsic incubation, however, the mosquito remains infective for the remainder of its life, which could be upward of 180 days, although generally the lifespan of the female *A. aegypti* is closer to a month or two.

In the Americas, epidemic yellow fever declined during the twentieth century, essentially because of efforts to eradicate *A. aegypti* in population centers. The last outbreak occurred in Trinidad in 1954. Nonetheless, the virus remains alive in the monkeys of Central and South America; consequently, some human cases are still reported among people who work or live close to the forests. Most cases occur in regions of Brazil, Ecuador, Venezuela, Colombia, and Peru that are drained by river networks contributing to the Orinoco, Magdalena, and Amazon systems. Earlier in the twentieth century, human cases were also reported fairly regularly in Central America, Bolivia, Argentina, and Paraguay.

In Africa, severe yellow fever epidemics still occur; a notable example, in Ethiopia in 1961, cost thousands of lives. Still more recently, a major outbreak in Nigeria claimed thousands more, and yet another was ongoing at the turn of the twenty-first century. A vast belt of endemic yellow fever stretches across Africa, but isolated cases are only irregulary reported.

One mystery surrounding yellow fever is its lack of incidence in Asia, despite the presence of *Aedes* mosquitoes. Some think that the mosquitoes themselves are resistant to infection. Others suspect that a population may support only so many arboviruses and that entrenched ones such as **dengue** and **Japanese encephalitis** may have forestalled the advance of yellow fever.

A yellow fever attack confers lifetime immunity on the host. Because the disease generally reserves severe symptoms for young adults and treats children more gently, whole populations in endemic or frequently visited areas can become more or less immune, with yellow fever just another childhood ailment. Under such circumstances, epidemics never occur unless groups of newcomers arrive, as was the case with immigrants, soldiers, and sailors reaching the Americas. It was this phenomenon that gave rise to yellow fever nicknames such as "strangers' fever," the "disease of acclimation," and "patriotic fever."

Many in the New World came to believe that blacks possessed a special ability to resist yellow fever. Most slaves reaching the Americas originated within the African endemic zone and would have acquired immunity before ever stepping aboard ship. Thus it is possible to explain blacks' refractoriness to yellow fever as acquired immunity.

On the other hand, genetic selection for yellow fever resistance as a result of prolonged exposure cannot be discounted, for many of the West African descendants of those first arrivals to the Americas lived for generations in areas untouched by yellow fever, yet, without any opportunity to acquire immunity in advance, suffered much less than whites when the disease finally did make an appearance. It has been suggested that related arboviruses or flaviviruses (dengue or Japanese encephalitis, for example) may confer some cross-protection against yellow fever, whereas others believe that certain strains of the illness may vary in mildness or severity, depending on the groups of individuals under attack. In this latter connection, it may be significant that Chinese in the New World were reputed to be almost as resistant to the illness as blacks, because although yellow fever has never invaded Asia, dengue and Japanese encephalitis are endemic to much of the region.

History

Much historical interest in yellow fever has focused on its place of origin: Africa or the Americas? Those favoring the latter emphasize that the disease was described in the Western Hemisphere over a century before it was recognized in Africa. The first recognizable epidemic struck Barbados in 1647 and spread during the next 2 years to Guadeloupe, St. Kitts, Cuba, and Yucatan. Moreover, Amerindian accounts and early Spanish records mention diseases that could have been yellow fever, such as a 1454 epidemic on the Mexican plateau, a 1477–97 outbreak in Yucatan, and a disease that assaulted Columbus's men in 1493.

By contrast, protagonists of an African origin dismiss these outbreaks as diseases other

than yellow fever, largely because of immunologic evidence. Whatever the illnesses were,
they argue, the Indians were quite susceptible;
however, any endemic yellow fever should have
engendered its own immunity. Moreover, American monkeys are susceptible to yellow fever,
whereas West African monkeys – and humans –
are resistant, suggesting long exposure.

Certainly the timing of yellow fever's recorded
appearance in the New World detracts nothing from the case for an African origin, for the
1640s saw an accelerated slave trade to Barbados as it converted to a slave-labor-based sugar-
plantation economy. The same slave ships that
could have delivered the virus in black bodies
doubtless carried the mosquito in water casks.
Many of the outbreaks to follow also seem to be
traceable directly to Africa via the slave trade.
It does seem, however, that Yucatan and the region around Vera Cruz became endemic foci at
an early date.

Having reached the Caribbean, yellow fever
moved northward, striking New York in 1668,
Philadelphia and Charleston in 1690, and
Boston in 1691. To the south, the disease regularly visited the port cities of Colombia, Ecuador,
and Peru. Interestingly, it disappeared from
Cuba after 1649–55 and, save for an oubreak
in 1695, did not return until 1761. A similar
phenomenon occurred in Brazil. There seems
no doubt that the epidemic that struck in 1685
was yellow fever, killing thousands before waning about 5 years later. As in the Caribbean, the
Brazilian outbreak has been attributed to ships
arriving from Africa. However, despite a thriving
slave trade that presumably could have brought
the disease, and a monkey population that some
believe already harbored the virus, Brazil reput-
edly was free of yellow fever for the next century and a half; the next outbreak was not until
1849.

Equally perplexing is the selectivity yellow
fever demonstrated in seeking out victims as it
spread from Bahia to other coastal cities, for, although the disease afflicted European newcomers with considerable fury, it treated local blacks
and whites far more gently, suggesting that it

may have been present all along – in jungle
form – quietly immunizing the population by
periodically producing mild cases in the young.
Significantly, in the years immediately prior to
the 1849 epidemic, Brazil had been the recipi-
ent of a sizable influx of European immigrants;
in addition, the population of Rio de Janeiro still
included a number of individuals on their way
to California. Thus in this epidemic, as in countless ones to follow, newcomers were the chief
sufferers.

Yellow fever sought out Europeans in their
homelands as well, apparently reaching there
from the Caribbean. The Iberian Peninsula
was the most common target, with epidemics
throughout the eighteenth and nineteenth centuries. Coastal cities such as Oporto, Lisbon, and
Barcelona bore the brunt of these attacks, although the disease did penetrate inland on occasion, even reaching Madrid in 1878. Small outbreaks also occurred in France, England, and
Italy.

Without doubt, however, yellow fever gained
its most fearsome reputation in the Caribbean
because Europeans, often military personnel,
provided the disease with a stream of nonim-
munes. In 1655, of 1,500 French soldiers occupying Saint Lucia, only 89 survived an onslaught of disease led by yellow fever. The 1690s
saw yellow fever sweep much of the region.
In 1693, the English attack on Martinique collapsed in face of yellow fever, whereas in 1741,
Admiral Edward Vernon's abortive attack on
Cartagena saw the loss of nearly half his force
of 19,000 to yellow fever.

Prisoners sent as workmen from Vera Cruz
to Havana in 1761 are credited with reintro-
ducing yellow fever in Cuba, where it proved
a formidable Spanish ally in an unsuccessful
effort to deny Havana to the English. But yellow fever deaths really peaked in the Caribbean
around the turn of the century. In 1793–96, the
British army lost 80,000 men, with over half the
deaths attributed to yellow fever. The disease
also decimated the French during their 1802 invasion of Hispaniola and accounted for many
of the 40,000 men lost. After their retreat to

Martinique and Guadeloupe, yellow fever raged among the survivors for another 3 years. The tremendous loss of life to yellow fever (and **malaria**) prompted the English to fill West Indies regiments with black troops thought to be immune to the diseases, who demonstrated over and over again that, indeed, many were.

Because of Philadelphia's brisk trade with the Caribbean, yellow fever appeared frequently in that port city during the eighteenth century, with epidemics in 1741, 1747, 1762, 1793, 1794, and 1797. The epidemic of 1793 was carried to the city by French refugees from revolution-torn San Domingue. With the turn of the nineteenth century, however, the U.S. South began to receive yellow fever's attention, with New Orleans, Savannah, Mobile, and Charleston the most frequent ports of call.

Chief among the victims of these epidemics were Northerners, foreigners (especially the Irish), and white Southerners from the interior. Permanent white residents, however, seldom died from yellow fever. Physicians reported that mulattoes were the most susceptible blacks (about the same as local whites). "Pure" blacks were believed to be totally immune, yet in the years just before the Civil War, physicians noted that blacks did contract mild yellow fever during epidemics – so mild that it had heretofore escaped notice.

In Brazil, the almost continual epidemic onslaught of yellow fever on coastal cities for the remainder of the century makes it reasonable to suppose that the disease was endemically established there. Cuba, like Brazil, was a nineteenth century destination of European laborers, and these, along with numerous refugees from Spanish America and Spanish soldiers, assured yellow fever a plenitude of hosts. Moreover, a contraband slave trade maintained contact with the yellow fever reservoir in Africa, and trade with Vera Cruz kept Cuba in touch with another endemic focus of the disease. Thus it is not surprising that Cuba became the yellow fever capital of the Caribbean. By contrast, the disease began to wane in most of the rest of the islands as the end of British and French slave

trading and the decline of the sugar industry turned them into economic backwaters seldom visited by outsiders.

The blockade of southern ports during the American Civil War, rather ironically, freed the South of yellow fever for the duration by curtailing West Indian shipping traffic. However, the disease returned to New Orleans in 1867, Montgomery in 1873, and Savannah in 1876, before ascending the Mississippi in 1878 to leave countless dead – 5,000 in Memphis alone.

This 1878 epidemic almost certainly reached the United States from Cuba, where the influx of Spanish soldiers sent since 1876 to end the Ten Years' War had provided the tinder for an epidemic that raged on that island from 1876 until 1879. Whether the Cuban epidemic also reached out to slaughter French workers arriving in Panama from 1878 onward to work on Ferdinand de Lesseps' abortive attempt to build a canal across the isthmus, or whether that outbreak came from an endemic jungle source, is a matter of speculation. But like their predecessors, who between 1851 and 1855 lost thousands of their numbers to yellow fever in building the Panamanian railroad for American financiers, the French canal workers died in droves, many even bringing their own caskets with them to the isthmus.

Just 3 years after the yellow fever disaster of 1878, Carlos Finlay y Barres of Cuba postulated that the *A. aegypti* mosquito transmitted the disease. The theory was confirmed in 1900 using human volunteers (three of whom died) by the U.S. Army Commission on Yellow Fever in Havana headed by Walter Reed. With this knowledge, William Gorgas rid Havana of the disease by eradicating *A. aegypti*. He later applied his methods in Panama, enabling workers on the American canal to avoid the fate of their French predecessors. These measures were applied elsewhere, so that the 1905 New Orleans outbreak and the 1908–9 Barbados epidemic represented, respectively, the last of yellow fever on North American soil, and its last appearance in the Caribbean for decades.

Gorgas suggested eradicating yellow fever from the entire globe, and in 1915 the Rockefeller Foundation launched this effort by creating its Yellow Fever Commission. Initially, the commission concentrated on Latin America but in 1920 turned its attention to Africa. In 1925, the Second Commission to West Africa established itself in Nigeria, soon discovering that the rhesus monkey was susceptible to yellow fever, which permitted use of monkeys rather than humans for experiments. Nonetheless, yellow fever research remained dangerous – Adrian Stokes, Hideyo Noguchi, William Young, and Theodore Hayne all perished from the disease in Africa during these "heroic days" of yellow fever research, which by 1929 had demonstrated beyond doubt that yellow fever was the result of infection by a virus.

In Brazil, Oswaldo Cruz began a mosquito-eradication campaign that freed coastal cities from yellow fever for the first time in more than 50 years. But the disease failed to disappear. Sporadic outbreaks continued in Brazil, Peru, Ecuador, Venezuela, and Colombia. In 1923, Brazil invited the International Health Division of the Rockefeller Foundation to administer the Brazilian Yellow Fever Service. Surveys conducted under Fred Soper showed that many Brazilians residing near forests had hosted yellow fever. In 1928, an epidemic triggered investigations revealing that yellow fever could spread without *A. aegypti* and that the disease was very much alive in the monkeys of the South American rain forest. Jungle yellow fever had been discovered, and thus most riddles of yellow fever transmission were resolved.

Meanwhile, by the late 1920s, the rhesus monkey was found to be susceptible to yellow fever; thus with an animal that could be used in laboratory experiments, efforts to isolate the yellow fever virus were begun. Shortly afterward, Max Theiler discovered that the virus could also be transmitted to mice, which were less expensive and easier to handle than monkeys. Soon, he showed that if the virus was transmitted among several mice, it weakened sufficiently to use in immunizing monkeys. By the late 1930s, a further attenuated strain called 17D Valline was developed. It is harmless to humans but immunizes them against yellow fever.

The development of a vaccine was crucial, for the discovery of jungle yellow fever meant that yellow fever could not be wiped out after all. The virus is always present in monkeys and perhaps other wild creatures of the forest as well.

For this reason, epidemiologists are particularly alarmed at the relaxation of mosquito-control measures in the Western Hemisphere, where few have been vaccinated. In the U.S. South, the Caribbean, and Central America, *A. aegypti* has reestablished itself, and Brazil, once apparently free of the mosquito, has reimported it from North America. With modern air travel, an infected individual – or even mosquito – could easily be whisked from the South American or African forests to any number of large cities where *A. aegypti* again resides in large numbers and stands ready to spread the disease throughout nonimmune populations. Moreover, *Aedes albopictus* has recently been introduced into the United States from its native Asian habitat. This close relative of *A. aegypti* is fully susceptible to the yellow fever virus and capable of transmitting it to vertebrates. The newcomer is more tolerant of cold weather and has spread widely in the United States. Its spread to the Caribbean and Central and South America is feared.

Donald B. Cooper and Kenneth F. Kiple

Name Index

Name Index

Bichat, Marie François, *69*
Bilharz, Theodor, 290–91
Bissell, A. D., 178
Black, Francis L., 171–74, 212
Blackall, John, 104–5, 146
Blacklock, D., 229
Blane, Sir Gilbert, 296–97
Blaud, P., 23
Blessed, Gary, 17
Blocq, Paul, 241
Boë, François de la, *69*
Boerhaave, Hermann, *69,* 103, 297
Boezo, M., 247
Bollet, Alfred Jay, 21–26
Bondy, Gustav, 211
Bontius, Jacobus, 75, 364
Bordet, Jules, 361
Borovsky, Peter, 192
Boswell, James, 152
Botallo, Leonardo, 315
Bouchardat, Apollinaire, 88
Bouchut, E., 83
Bouillaud, Jean Baptiste, 257
Boussingault, Jean Baptiste, 148
Bowman, William, 146
Boylston, Zabdiel, 302
Bozzolo, Camillo, 167
Bradford, William, 300
Brain, P., 25
Bramwell, Byron, 220
Brandt, Allan M., 1–5
Breschet, Gilbert, 273
Bretonneau, Pierre, 83, 95
Brickell, John, 364
Bright, Richard, 32, 104, 145–46, 170, 278,
    350
Brill, Nathan, 353
Bristowe, J. S., 178
Brooke, Bryan, 178
Brothwell, Don, 250–51, 332, 362–65
Brown, Audrey K., 21–26
Brown, J. Y., 177
Brown, Peter J., 123–25
Browne, John, 80
Bruce, David, 58, 60, 351
Bruch, Hilde, 28–29
Bruck, Carl, 317
Brumpt, E., 131
Buchwald, Alfred, 203
Budd, William, 78, 348, 351
Bumm, Ernst von, 152
Burgdorfer, Willy, 203, 283
Burnet, F., 269
Burns, Allan, 104
Butlin, Henry, 239
Bylon, David, 87

C

Cadawaler, Thomas, 187
Cailius Aurelianus, 257
Campbell, A., 360
Capivaccio, Girlamo, 102
Carini, A., *192*
Carlsson, A., 241
Carmichael, Ann G., 60–63, 94–96, 121–22,
    192–95, 251–54, 287–88, 311–12
Carpentier, A., 280
Carrión, Daniel, *69*
Carson, Paul E., 24
Carswell, Robert, 80
Carter, H. Vandyke, 131
Carter, K. Codell, 265–67
Casal, Gaspar, 243
Casserio, Giulio, 147
Castellani, Aldo, 363
Castle, William B., 22
Celsus, Aulus Cornelius, 102, 122, 129, 186, 232,
    246, 272, 358
Chagas, Carlos, 71
Chalmers, A. J., 131
Chapin, C., 344
Charaka, 358
Charcot, Jean, 32, 119, 241
Chatin, Adolphe, 148
Chauliac, Guy de, 233
Chaumette, Antoine, 315
Chen, Peter S. Y., 79–81
Chen, Thomas S. N., 79–81
Cherry, James D., 81–83
Chevreul, M. D. Eugène, 88
Cheyne, John, 32
Chien-i, 280
Chipley, William Stout, 27
Christie, A., 164
Clossey, Samuel, 104
Cobbold, T. Spencer, 127–28
Coburn, Alvin F., 278
Cockburn, T. A., 332
Coindet, J.-F., 148
Colles, Abraham, 328
Collier, Leslie, 312
Colombo, Realdo, 147
Colp, R., 178
Combe, C., 178
Come, Frère, 358
Cone, Thomas E., Jr., 218–20
Cooke, John, 32
Cooke, W. Trevor, 178
Cooper, Donald B., 14, 365–69
Correia, Gaspar, 75
Correns, Carl, 140–41
Corvisart, François, 330
Corvisart, Jean-Nicholas, 104, 257, 350

Name Index

Name Index

Name Index

Name Index

Withering, William, 104–5
Wolbach, Burt, 284
Wollaston, William H., 153
Wood, Corinne, 333
Woodward, Joseph, 349–50, 352
Wright, Almroth, 348
Wright, James, 192
Wucherer, Otto, 127–28
Wullstein, H., 211
Wunderlich, Karl, 340
Wyatt, H. V., 258–61
Wylie, John, 253, 312
Wyss, O., 360

Y
Yersin, Alexandre, 61, 95
Young, William, 369

Z
Zacharias, Pope, 171
Zammit, Themistocles, 60
Zenker, Friedrich, 336
Zilva, S. S., 298
Zimmerman, L. E., 132
Zinke, Georg Gottfried, 273
Zinsser, Hans, 252, 312, 353, 355
Zöllner, F., 211

Subject Index

Subject Index

Subject Index

Subject Index

AIDS and vaccines for, 6
characteristics, 300–1
chickenpox and, 359
eradication, 303–4
ergotism and, 120
eye diseases in, 234
hepatitis and vaccines for, 171
history, 301–4
introduction to North America, 206
measles and, 212, 301
as Plague of Athens, 252, 253
vaccine, 302–4
variolation, 302–4
Smallpox Eradication Programme, 303
smoking
arteriosclerosis and, 137
cancer and, 65–66
Crohn's disease and, 176
emphysema and, 113
heart disease and, 160
osteoporosis and, 237
"snail fever," 290
snakeroot poison, 218–20
sofersa, 213
soldier's heart, 158–59
"South African tick-bite fever," 285
South America
ainhum, 14
anemia, 26
anthrax, 30
arenaviruses, 38
ascariasis, 42
beriberi, 46–47
bleeding disorders, 56
Bolivian hemorrhagic fever, 39
brucellosis, 59
bubonic plague, 63
Carrión's disease, 68
Chagas' disease, 70–7
cholera, 77
dengue, 86
diabetes, 92
encephalitides, 37–38
fascioliasis, 123
filariasis, 127
fungus poisoning, 133–134
gallstones, 135
glomerulonephritis, 145
goiter, 148
heart-related diseases, 160
herpes simplex, 161
histoplasmosis, 163
hookworm infection, 166–167
hypertension, 170–171
influenza, 180
leishmaniasis, 191–192

leprosy, 193
leptospirosis, 196
malaria, 204, 206–207
mycoses, 130–132
onchocerciasis, 228
ophthalmia, 230
Paget's disease of bone, 238
paragonimiasis, 240
pica, 249
pinta, 250–251
poliomyelitis, 261
rabies, 274
ringworm, 129
Rocky Mountain spotted fever, 284–285
scarlet fever, 289
schistosomiasis, 290–291
syphilis, 313
tapeworm infection, 320
trichinosis, 334
tuberculosis, 338
tularemia, 343
yaws, 362, 364
yellow fever, 36, 366–369
South Asia
AIDS, 5
ainhum, 14
amebic dysentery, 20
anemia, 25–26
arthritis, 41
ascariasis, 42
beriberi, 46
Black Death, 49
brucellosis, 59
bubonic plague, 63
cholera, 74–77
diabetes, 89, 92
dracunculiasis, 98–100
encephalitides, 36
fasciolopsiasis, 123
favism, 124
filariasis, 125–127
fungus infections, 131–132
G6PD deficiency, 23
histoplasmosis, 163
hookworm infection, 165–167
infectious hepatitis, 172
lead poisoning, 186
leishmaniasis, 191–192
leprosy, 192–193, 195
malaria, 204
ophthalmia, 230
osteoporosis, 238
paragonimiasis, 240
pellagra, 244
pica, 249
poliomyelitis, 261

Subject Index

www.ingramcontent.com/pod-product-compliance
Ingram Content Group UK Ltd.
Pitfield, Milton Keynes, MK11 3LW, UK
UKHW050114180125
453697UK00008B/177